EUROPEAN PHARMACOPOEIA

Supplement 4.4 to the Fourth Edition

published 11ᵗʰ November 2002

The Fourth Edition of the European Pharmacopoeia consists of the main volume 4 dated 2002 and supplements 4.1, 4.2, 4.3 and 4.4. The **supplements are non-cumulative** and are to be kept for the duration of the Fourth Edition.

To use the Fourth Edition, make sure that you have all the published supplements and consult the index of the most recent volume to ensure that you use the latest versions of the monographs and general chapters.

EUROPEAN PHARMACOPOEIA CD-ROM

The Fourth Edition is also available as a CD-ROM with all the monographs and general chapters contained in the book. With the publication of each supplement the CD-ROM is replaced by a new fully updated cumulative version.

PHARMEUROPA
Quarterly Forum Publication

Pharmeuropa contains preliminary drafts of all new and revised monographs proposed for inclusion in the European Pharmacopoeia and gives an opportunity for all interested parties to comment on the specifications before they are finalised. Pharmeuropa also contains information on the work programme, the list of Certificates of Suitability of the Monographs of the European Pharmacopoeia issued by the EDQM, scientific articles on pharmacopoeial matters and other articles of general interest. Pharmeuropa is available on subscription from the EDQM (see opposite).

INTERNATIONAL HARMONISATION

Refer to information given in chapter *5.8. Pharmacopoeial Harmonisation.*

EUROPEAN PHARMACOPOEIA

FOURTH EDITION

SUPPLEMENT 4.4

EUROPEAN PHARMACOPOEIA

FOURTH EDITION

SUPPLEMENT 4.4

Published in accordance with the
Convention on the Elaboration of a European Pharmacopoeia
(European Treaty Series No. 50)

Council of Europe

Strasbourg

The European Pharmacopoeia is published by the Directorate for the Quality of Medicines of the Council of Europe (EDQM).

© Council of Europe, 67075 Strasbourg Cedex, France - 2002

ISBN: 92-871-4842-2

Printed in Germany by Druckerei C. H. Beck, Nördlingen
Bound in Germany by Sigloch Buchbinderei, Blaufelden

CONTENTS

Note: on the first page of each chapter/section there is a list of contents.

CONTENTS OF SUPPLEMENT 4.4

A vertical line in the margin indicates where part of a text has been revised or corrected. A horizontal line in the margin indicates where part of a text has been deleted. It is to be emphasized that these indications, which are not necessarily exhaustive, are given for information and do not form an official part of the texts. Editorial changes are not indicated.
Individual copies of texts will not be supplied.

NEW TEXTS

GENERAL CHAPTERS

2.5.36. Anisidine value

MONOGRAPHS

*The monographs below appear for the first time in the European Pharmacopoeia. They will be implemented on **1 April 2003** at the latest.*

Basic butylated methacrylate copolymer (1975)
Bitter-fennel fruit oil (1826)
Cefapirin sodium (1650)
Colophony (1862)

Levomethadone hydrochloride (1787)
Linseed oil, virgin (1908)
Magnesium acetate tetrahydrate (2035)
Meadowsweet (1868)
Nicotine resinate (1792)
Nifuroxazide (1999)
Oxaliplatin (2017)
Phenylmercuric acetate (2042)
Potassium clavulanate, diluted (1653)
Proguanil hydrochloride (2002)
Ribwort plantain (1884)
Rilmenidine dihydrogen phosphate (2020)
Sodium propionate (2041)
Squalane (1630)

REVISED TEXTS

GENERAL CHAPTERS

2.4.22. Composition of fatty acids by gas chromatography
2.4.27. Heavy metals in herbal drugs and fatty oils
2.5.29. Sulphur dioxide
2.9.5. Uniformity of mass of single-dose preparations
2.9.6. Uniformity of content of single-dose preparations
5.1.3. Efficacy of antimicrobial preservation

MONOGRAPHS

*The monographs below have been technically revised since their last publication. They will be implemented on **1 April 2003**.*

Dosage forms

Eye preparations (1163)
Granules (0499)
Liquid preparations for cutaneous application (0927)
Liquid preparations for oral use (0672)
Powders, oral (1165)
Preparations for inhalation (0671)

Monographs

Benzyl alcohol (0256)
Bromhexine hydrochloride (0706)

Carnauba wax (0597)
Chlortetracycline hydrochloride (0173)
Cholesterol (0993)
Cod-liver oil (type A) (1192)
Cod-liver oil (type B) (1193)
Colchicine (0758)
Crospovidone (0892)
Demeclocycline hydrochloride (0176)
Dextrin (1507)
Diphenhydramine hydrochloride (0023)
Disodium phosphate, anhydrous (1509)
Doxycycline hyclate (0272)
Doxycycline monohydrate (0820)
Estradiol benzoate (0139)
Estriol (1203)
Ethosuximide (0764)
Ethylcellulose (0822)
Isoconazole (1018)
Ketoconazole (0921)
Mannitol (0559)
Metformin hydrochloride (0931)
Nonoxinol 9 (1454)
Noscapine (0516)
Noscapine hydrochloride (0515)
Octoxinol 10 (1553)

CORRECTED TEXTS

The texts below have been corrected and are republished in their entirety. These corrections are to be taken into account from the publication date of Supplement 4.4.

TEXTS WHOSE TITLE HAS CHANGED

The title of the following texts has been changed in Supplement 4.4.

SUPPRESSION OF TEXTS

*The following texts are deleted on **1 January 2003**.*

*The following text was deleted on **1 April 2002**.*

2.3. IDENTIFICATION

2.3.2. IDENTIFICATION OF FATTY OILS BY THIN-LAYER CHROMATOGRAPHY

Examine by thin-layer chromatography (*2.2.27*), using as the coating substance a suitable octadecylsilyl silica gel for high performance thin-layer chromatography.

Test solution. Unless otherwise prescribed, dissolve about 20 mg (1 drop) of the fatty oil in 3 ml of *methylene chloride R*.

Reference solution. Dissolve about 20 mg (1 drop) of *maize oil R* in 3 ml of *methylene chloride R*.

Apply separately to the plate 1 μl of each solution. Develop twice over a path of 0.5 cm using *ether R*. Develop twice over a path of 8 cm using a mixture of 20 volumes of *methylene chloride R*, 40 volumes of *glacial acetic acid R* and 50 volumes of *acetone R*. Allow the plate to dry in air and spray with a 100 g/l solution of *phosphomolybdic acid R* in *alcohol R*. Heat the plate at 120 °C for about 3 min and examine in daylight.

The chromatogram obtained typically shows spots comparable to those in Figure 2.3.2.-1.

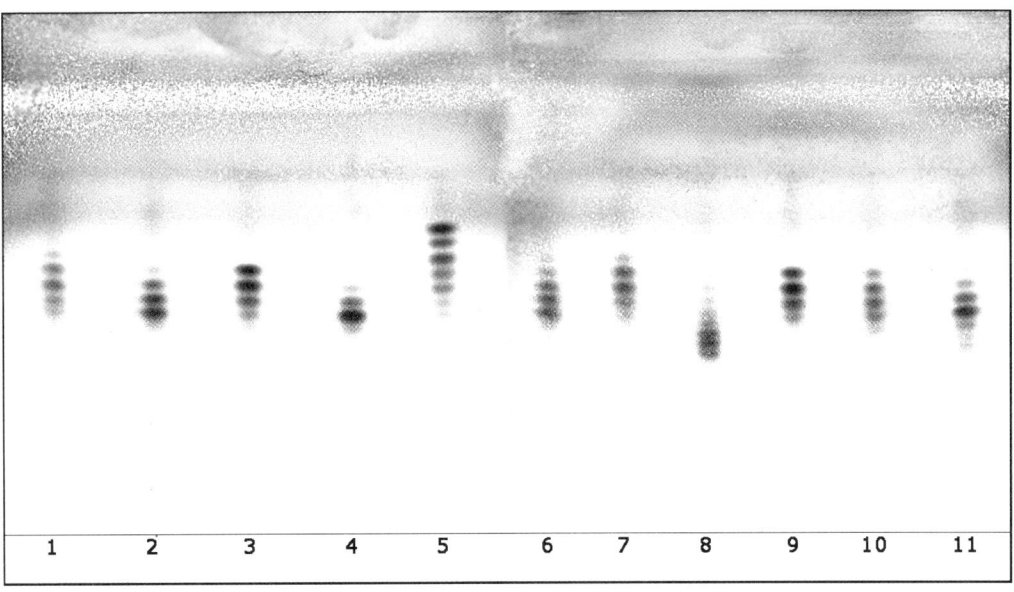

1. Arachis oil
2. Sesame oil
3. Maize oil
4. Rapeseed oil (erucic acid-free)
5. Soya-bean oil
6. Rapeseed oil

7. Linseed oil
8. Olive oil
9. Sunflower oil
10. Almond oil
11. Wheat-germ oil

Figure 2.3.2.-1. – *Chromatograms for the identification of fatty oils*

2.4. LIMIT TESTS

2. Methods of analysis

2.4.22. COMPOSITION OF FATTY ACIDS BY GAS CHROMATOGRAPHY

The test for foreign oils is carried out on the methyl esters of the fatty acids contained in the oil to be examined by gas chromatography (*2.2.28*).

METHOD A

This method is not applicable to oils that contain glycerides of fatty acids with an epoxy-, hydroepoxy-, cyclopropyl or cyclopropenyl group, or those that contain a large proportion of fatty acids of chain length less than 8 carbon atoms or to oils with an acid value greater than 2.0.

Test solution. When prescribed in the monograph, dry the oil to be examined before the methylation step. Weigh 1.0 g of the oil into a 25 ml round-bottomed flask with a ground-glass neck fitted with a reflux condenser and a gas port into the flask. Add 10 ml of *anhydrous methanol R* and 0.2 ml of a 60 g/l solution of *potassium hydroxide R* in *methanol R*. Attach the reflux condenser, pass *nitrogen R* through the mixture at a rate of about 50 ml/min, shake and heat to boiling. When the solution is clear (usually after about 10 min), continue heating for a further 5 min. Cool the flask under running water and transfer the contents to a separating funnel. Rinse the flask with 5 ml of *heptane R* and transfer the rinsings to the separating funnel and shake. Add 10 ml of a 200 g/l solution of *sodium chloride R* and shake vigorously. Allow to separate and transfer the organic layer to a vial containing *anhydrous sodium sulphate R*. Allow to stand, then filter.

Reference solution (a). Prepare 0.50 g of the mixture of calibrating substances with the composition described in one of the tables 2.4.22, as prescribed in the individual monograph (if the monograph does not mention a specific solution, use the composition described in Table 2.4.22.-1). Dissolve in *heptane R* and dilute to 50.0 ml with the same solvent.

Reference solution (b). Dilute 1.0 ml of reference solution (a) to 10.0 ml with *heptane R*.

Reference solution (c). Prepare 0.50 g of a mixture of fatty acid methyl esters[1], which corresponds in composition to the mixture of fatty acids indicated in the monograph of the substance to be examined. Dissolve in *heptane R* and dilute to 50.0 ml with the same solvent. Commercially available mixtures of fatty acid methyl esters may also be used.

Column:
- *material*: fused silica, glass or quartz,
- *size*: l = 10-30 m, Ø = 0.2-0.8 mm,
- *stationary phase*: *poly[(cyanopropyl)(methyl)][(phenyl)(methyl)]siloxane R* or *macrogol 20 000 R* (film thickness 0.1-0.5 μm) or some other suitable stationary phase.

Carrier gas: *helium for chromatography R* or *hydrogen for chromatography R*.

Flow rate: 1.3 ml/min (for a column Ø = 0.32 mm).

Split ratio: 1:100 or less, according to the internal diameter of the column used (1:50 when Ø = 0.32 mm).

Temperature:
- *column*: 160-200 °C, according to the length and type of column used (200 °C for a column 30 m long and coated with a layer of *macrogol 20 000 R*); if necessary, or where prescribed, raise the temperature of the column at a rate of 3 °C/min from 170 °C to 230 °C (for the *macrogol 20 000 R* column),

- *injection port*: 250 °C,
- *detector*: 250 °C.

Detection: flame ionisation.

Injection: 1 μl.

Sensitivity: the height of the principal peak in the chromatogram obtained with reference solution (a) is 50 per cent to 70 per cent of the full scale of the recorder.

System suitability when using the mixture of calibrating substances in Table 2.4.22.-1 or 2.4.22.-3:
- *resolution*: minimum 1.8 between the peaks due to methyl oleate and methyl stearate in the chromatogram obtained with reference solution (a),
- *signal-to-noise ratio*: minimum 5 for the peak due to methyl myristate in the chromatogram obtained with reference solution (b),
- *number of theoretical plates*: minimum 30 000 calculated for the peak due to methyl stearate in the chromatogram obtained with reference solution (a).

System suitability when using the mixture of calibrating substances in Table 2.4.22.-2:
- *resolution*: minimum 4.0 between the peaks due to methyl caprylate and methyl caprate in the chromatogram obtained with reference solution (a),
- *signal-to-noise ratio*: minimum 5 for the peak due to methyl caproate in the chromatogram obtained with reference solution (b),
- *number of theoretical plates*: minimum 15 000 calculated for the peak due to methyl caprate in the chromatogram obtained with reference solution (a).

ASSESSMENT OF CHROMATOGRAMS

Avoid working conditions tending to give masked peaks (presence of constituents with small differences between retention times, for example linolenic acid and arachidic acid).

Qualitative analysis. Identify the peaks in the chromatogram obtained with reference solution (c); the peaks may also be identified by drawing calibration curves using the chromatogram obtained with reference solution (a) and the information given in Tables 2.4.22.-1, 2.4.22.-2 and 2.4.22.-3:

a) using isothermal operating conditions giving the logarithms of reduced retention times as a function of the number of carbon atoms of the fatty acid; identify the peaks by means of the straight line thus obtained and the "equivalent chain lengths" of the different peaks. The calibration curve of the saturated acids is a straight line. The logarithms of reduced retention times of unsaturated acids are situated on this line at points corresponding to non-integer values of carbon atoms known as "equivalent chain lengths";

b) using linear temperature programming giving the retention time according to the number of carbon atoms of the fatty acid; identify by reference to the calibration curve.

Quantitative analysis. In general, the normalisation procedure is used in which the sum of the areas of the peaks in the chromatogram, except that of the solvent, is set at 100 per cent. The content of a constituent is calculated by determining the area of the corresponding peak as a percentage of the sum of the areas of all the peaks. Disregard any peak with an area less than 0.05 per cent of the total area.

In certain cases, for example in the presence of fatty acids with 12 or less carbon atoms, correction factors can be prescribed in the individual monograph to convert peak areas in per cent *m/m*.

---

(1) The fatty acid methyl esters used show a quality at least as good as that guaranteed by the BCR (Community Bureau of Reference) of the European Union.

METHOD B

This method is not applicable to oils that contain glycerides of fatty acids with an epoxy-, hydroepoxy-, cyclopropyl or cyclopropenyl group or to oils with an acid value greater than 2.0.

Test solution. Introduce 0.100 g of the substance to be examined in a 10 ml centrifuge tube with a screw cap. Dissolve with 1 ml of *heptane R* and 1 ml of *dimethyl carbonate R* and mix vigorously under gentle heating (50-60 °C). Add, while still warm, 1 ml of a 12 g/l solution of *sodium R* in *anhydrous methanol R*, prepared with the necessary precautions and mix vigorously for about 5 min. Add 3 ml of *distilled water R* and mix vigorously for about 30 s. Centrifuge for 15 min at 1500 *g*. Inject 1 µl of the organic phase.

Reference solutions and assessment of chromatograms. Without specific prescription in the individual monograph, proceed as described under Method A.

Column:
— *material*: fused silica,
— *size*: *l* = 30 m, Ø = 0.25 mm,
— *stationary phase*: *macrogol 20 000 R* (film thickness 0.25 µm),

Carrier gas: *helium for chromatography R*.

Flow rate: 0.9 ml/min.

Split ratio: 1:100.

Temperature:

	Time (min)	Temperature (°C)
	0 - 15	100
Column	15 - 36	100 → 225
	36 - 61	225
Injection port		250
Detector		250

Detection: flame ionisation.

Injection: 1 µl.

METHOD C

This method is not applicable to oils that contain glycerides of fatty acids with epoxy-, hydroperoxy-, aldehyde, ketone, cyclopropyl and cyclopropenyl groups, and conjugated polyunsaturated and acetylenic compounds because of partial or complete destruction of these groups.

Test solution. Dissolve 0.10 g of the substance to be examined in 2 ml of a 20 g/l solution of *sodium hydroxide R* in *methanol R* in a 25 ml conical flask and boil under a reflux condenser for 30 min. Add 2.0 ml of *boron trifluoride-methanol solution R* through the condenser and boil for 30 min. Add 4 ml of *heptane R* through the condenser and boil for 5 min. Cool and add 10.0 ml of *saturated sodium chloride solution R*, shake for about 15 s and add a quantity of *saturated sodium chloride solution R* such that the upper phase is brought into the neck of the flask. Collect 2 ml of the upper phase, wash with 3 quantities, each of 2 ml, of *water R* and dry over *anhydrous sodium sulphate R*.

Reference solutions, chromatographic procedure and assessment of chromatograms. Without specific prescription in the individual monograph, proceed as described under Method A.

Table 2.4.22.-1. - Mixture of calibrating substances[2]

Mixture of the following substances	Composition (per cent *m/m*)		
	Equivalent chain length[3]	Iso-thermal	Linear temperature programme
Methyl laurate R	12.0	5	10
Methyl myristate R	14.0	5	15
Methyl palmitate R	16.0	10	15
Methyl stearate R	18.0	20	20
Methyl arachidate R	20.0	40	20
Methyl oleate R	18.3	20	20

Table 2.4.22.-2. - Mixture of calibrating substances[2]

Mixture of the following substances	Composition (per cent *m/m*)		
	Equivalent chain length[3]	Iso-thermal	Linear temperature programme
Methyl caproate R	6.0	5	10
Methyl caprylate R	8.0	5	35
Methyl caprate R	10.0	10	35
Methyl laurate R	12.0	20	10
Methyl myristate R	14.0	40	10

Table 2.4.22.-3. - Mixture of calibrating substances[2]

Mixture of the following substances	Composition (per cent *m/m*)		
	Equivalent chain length[3]	Iso-thermal	Linear temperature programme
Methyl myristate R	14.0	5	15
Methyl palmitate R	16.0	10	15
Methyl stearate R	18.0	15	20
Methyl arachidate R	20.0	20	15
Methyl oleate R	18.3	20	15
Methyl eicosenoate R	20.2	10	10
Methyl behenate R	22.0	10	5
Methyl lignocerate R	24.0	10	5

2.4.27. HEAVY METALS IN HERBAL DRUGS AND FATTY OILS

Examine by atomic absorption spectrometry (*2.2.23*).

Caution: when using closed high-pressure digestion vessels and microwave laboratory equipment, be familiar with the safety and operating instructions given by the manufacturer.

APPARATUS

The apparatus typically consists of the following:

— as digestion flasks, polytetrafluoroethylene flasks with a volume of about 120 ml, fitted with an airtight closure, a valve to adjust the pressure inside the container and a polytetrafluoroethylene tube to allow release of gas,

— a system to make flasks airtight, using the same torsional force for each of them,

(2) For GC with capillary column and split inlet system, it is recommended that the component with the longest chain length of the mixture to be examined be added to the calibration mixture, when the qualitative analysis is done using calibration curves.
(3) This value, which is to be calculated using calibration curves, is given as an example for a column of *macrogol 20 000 R*.

— a microwave oven, with a magnetron frequency of 2450 MHz, with a selectable output from 0 to 630 ± 70 W in 1 per cent increments, a programmable digital computer, a polytetrafluoroethylene-coated microwave cavity with a variable speed exhaust fan, a rotating turntable drive system and exhaust tubing to vent fumes,

— an atomic absorption spectrometer, equipped with hollow-cathode lamps as source of radiation and a deuterium lamp as background corrector; the system is fitted with:

(a) a graphite furnace as atomisation device for cadmium, copper, iron, lead, nickel and zinc.

(b) an automated continuous-flow hydride vapour generation system for arsenic and mercury.

METHOD

In case alternative apparatus is used, an adjustment of the instrument parameters may be necessary.

Clean all the glassware and laboratory equipment with a 10 g/l solution of *nitric acid R* before use.

Test solution. In a digestion flask place the prescribed quantity of the substance to be examined (about 0.50 g of powdered drug (1400) or 0.50 g of fatty oil). Add 6 ml of *heavy metal-free nitric acid R* and 4 ml of *heavy metal-free hydrochloric acid R*. Make the flask airtight.

Place the digestion flasks in the microwave oven. Carry out the digestion in 3 steps according to the following programme, used for 7 flasks each containing the test solution: 80 per cent power for 15 min, 100 per cent power for 5 min, 80 per cent power for 20 min.

At the end of the cycle allow the flasks to cool in air and to each add 4 ml of *heavy metal-free sulphuric acid R*. Repeat the digestion programme. After cooling in air, open each digestion flask and introduce the clear, colourless solution obtained into a 50 ml volumetric flask. Rinse each digestion flask with 2 quantities, each of 15 ml, of *water R* and collect the rinsings in the volumetric flask. Add 1.0 ml of a 10 g/l solution of *magnesium nitrate R* and 1.0 ml of a 100 g/l solution of *ammonium dihydrogen phosphate R* and dilute to 50.0 ml with *water R*.

Blank solution. Mix 6 ml of *heavy metal-free nitric acid R* and 4 ml of *heavy metal-free hydrochloric acid R* in a digestion flask. Carry out the digestion in the same manner as for the test solution.

CADMIUM, COPPER, IRON, LEAD, NICKEL AND ZINC

Measure the content of cadmium, copper, iron, lead, nickel and zinc by the standard additions method (*2.2.23, Method II*), using reference solutions of each heavy metal and the instrumental parameters described in table 2.4.27.-1.

The absorbance value of the blank solution is automatically subtracted from the value obtained with the test solution.

Table 2.4.27.-1

		Cd	Cu	Fe	Ni	Pb	Zn
Wavelength	nm	228.8	324.8	248.3	232	283.5	213.9
Slit width	nm	0.5	0.5	0.2	0.2	0.5	0.5
Lamp current	mA	6	7	5	10	5	7
Ignition temperature	°C	800	800	800	800	800	800
Atomisation temperature	°C	1800	2300	2300	2500	2200	2000
Background corrector		on	off	off	off	off	off
Nitrogen flow	l/min	3	3	3	3	3	3

ARSENIC AND MERCURY

Measure the content of arsenic and mercury in comparison with the reference solutions of arsenic or mercury at a known concentration by direct calibration (*2.2.23, Method I*) using an automated continuous-flow hydride vapour generation system.

The absorbance value of the blank solution is automatically subtracted from the value obtained with the test solution.

Arsenic

Sample solution. To 19.0 ml of the test solution or of the blank solution as prescribed above, add 1 ml of a 200 g/l solution of *potassium iodide R*. Allow the test solution to stand at room temperature for about 50 min or at 70 °C for about 4 min.

Acid reagent. Heavy metal-free hydrochloric acid R.

Reducing reagent. A 6 g/l solution of *sodium tetrahydroborate R* in a 5 g/l solution of *sodium hydroxide R*.

The instrumental parameters in Table 2.4.27.-2 may be used.

Mercury

Sample solution. Test solution or blank solution, as prescribed above.

Acid reagent. A 515 g/l solution of *heavy metal-free hydrochloric acid R*.

Reducing reagent. A 10 g/l solution of *stannous chloride R* in *dilute heavy metal-free hydrochloric acid R*.

The instrumental parameters in Table 2.4.27.-2 may be used.

Table 2.4.27.-2

		As	Hg
Wavelength	nm	193.7	253.7
Slit width	nm	0.2	0.5
Lamp current	mA	10	4
Acid reagent flow rate	ml/min	1.0	1.0
Reducing reagent flow rate	ml/min	1.0	1.0
Sample solution flow rate	ml/min	7.0	7.0
Absorption cell		Quartz (heated)	Quartz (unheated)
Background corrector		off	off
Nitrogen flow rate	l/min	0.1	0.1

2. Methods of analysis

2.5. ASSAYS

2. Methods
of analysis

2.5.29. SULPHUR DIOXIDE

Introduce 150 ml of *water R* into the flask (*A*) (see Figure 2.5.29.-1) and pass *carbon dioxide R* through the whole system for 15 min at a rate of 100 ml/min. To 10 ml of *dilute hydrogen peroxide solution R* add 0.15 ml of a 1 g/l solution of *bromophenol blue R* in *alcohol (20 per cent V/V) R*. Add *0.1 M sodium hydroxide* until a violet-blue colour is obtained, without exceeding the end-point. Place the solution in the test-tube (*D*). Without interrupting the stream of carbon dioxide, remove the funnel (*B*) and introduce through the opening into the flask (*A*) 25.0 g of the substance to be examined (*m* g) with the aid of 100 ml of *water R*. Add through the funnel 80 ml of *dilute hydrochloric acid R* and boil for 1 h. Open the tap of the funnel and stop the flow of carbon dioxide and also the heating and the cooling water. Transfer the contents of the test-tube with the aid of a little *water R* to a 200 ml wide-necked, conical flask. Heat on a water-bath for 15 min and allow to cool. Add 0.1 ml of a 1 g/l solution of *bromophenol blue R* in *alcohol (20 per cent V/V) R* and titrate with *0.1 M sodium hydroxide* until the colour changes from yellow to violet-blue (V_1 ml). Carry out a blank titration (V_2 ml).

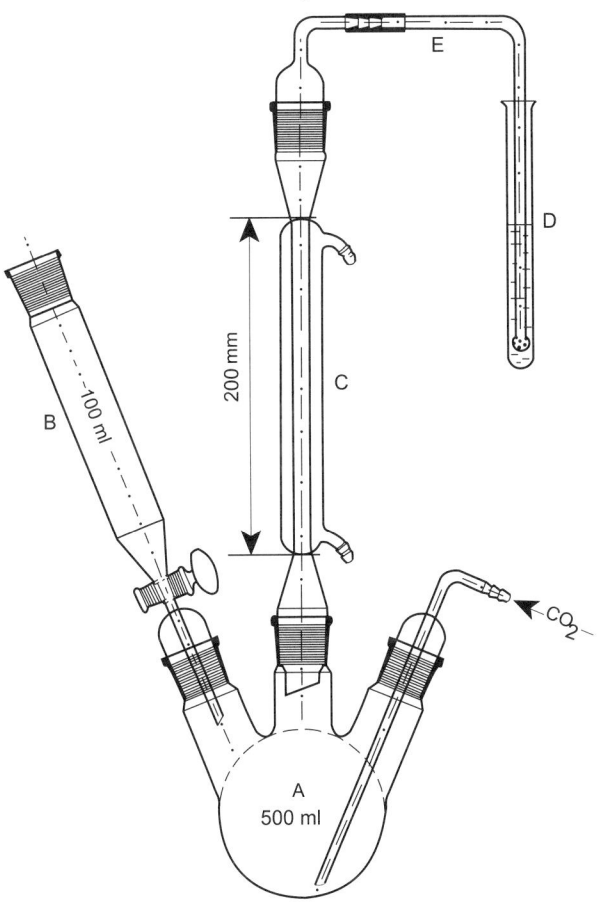

Figure 2.5.29.-1.– *Apparatus for the determination of sulphur dioxide*

Calculate the content of sulphur dioxide in parts per million from the expression:

$$32\,030 \times (V_1 - V_2) \times \frac{n}{m}$$

n = molarity of the sodium hydroxide solution used as titrant.

2.5.36. ANISIDINE VALUE

The anisidine value is defined as 100 times the optical density measured in a 1 cm cell of a solution containing 1 g of the substance to be examined in 100 ml of a mixture of solvents and reagents according to the following method.

Carry out the operations as rapidly as possible, avoiding exposure to actinic light.

Test solution (a). Dissolve 0.500 g of the substance to be examined in *trimethylpentane R* and dilute to 25.0 ml with the same solvent.

Test solution (b). To 5.0 ml of test solution (a) add 1.0 ml of a 2.5 g/l solution of *p-anisidine R* in *glacial acetic acid R*, shake and store protected from light.

Reference solution. To 5.0 ml of *trimethylpentane R* add 1.0 ml of a 2.5 g/l solution of *p-anisidine R* in *glacial acetic acid R*, shake and store protected from light.

Measure the absorbance (*2.2.25*) of test solution (a) at the maximum at 350 nm using *trimethylpentane R* as the compensation liquid. Measure the absorbance of test solution (b) at 350 nm exactly 10 min after its preparation, using the reference solution as the compensation liquid.

Calculate the anisidine value from the expression:

$$\frac{25 \times (1.2A_1 - A_2)}{m}$$

A_1 = absorbance of test solution (b) at 350 nm,

A_2 = absorbance of test solution (a) at 350 nm,

m = mass of the substance to be examined in test solution (a), in grams.

2.9. PHARMACEUTICAL TECHNICAL PROCEDURES

2.9.3. DISSOLUTION TEST FOR SOLID DOSAGE FORMS

The test is used to determine the dissolution rate of the active ingredients of solid dosage forms (for example, tablets, capsules and suppositories).

Unless otherwise justified and authorised, either the paddle apparatus or the basket apparatus or in special cases, the flow-through cell apparatus may be used.

The following are to be prescribed for each preparation to which the dissolution test is applied:

— the apparatus to be used, including in those cases where the flow-through cell apparatus is prescribed, which flow-through cell (Figures 2.9.3.-4/5/6) is to be used,

— the composition, the volume and the temperature of the dissolution medium,

— the rotation speed or the flow rate of the dissolution medium,

— the time, the method and the amount for sampling of the test solution or the conditions for continuous monitoring,

— the method of analysis,

— the quantity or quantities of active ingredients required to dissolve within a prescribed time.

APPARATUS

The choice of the apparatus to be used depends on the physico-chemical characteristics of the dosage form. All parts of the apparatus that may come into contact with the preparation or the dissolution medium are chemically inert and do not adsorb or react or interfere with the test sample. All metal parts of the apparatus that may come into contact with the preparation or the dissolution medium must be made from a suitable stainless steel or coated with a suitable material to ensure that such parts do not react or interfere with the preparation or the dissolution medium. No part of the assembly or its environment contributes significant motion, agitation or vibration beyond that resulting from the smoothly rotating element or from the flow-through system.

An apparatus that permits observation of the preparation to be examined and the stirrer during the test is preferable.

Paddle apparatus. The apparatus (see Figure 2.9.3.-1) consists of:

— a cylindrical vessel of borosilicate glass or other suitable transparent material with a hemispherical bottom and a nominal capacity of 1000 ml; a cover is fitted to retard evaporation; the cover has a central hole to accommodate the shaft of the stirrer and other holes for the thermometer and the devices used to withdraw liquid;

— a stirrer consisting of a vertical shaft to the lower end of which is attached a blade having the form of that part of a circle subtended by 2 parallel chords; the blade passes through the diameter of the shaft so that the bottom of the blade is flush with the bottom of the shaft; the shaft is placed so that its axis is within 2 mm of the axis of the vessel and the bottom of the blade is 25 ± 2 mm from the inner bottom of the vessel; the upper part of the shaft is connected to a motor provided with a speed regulator; the stirrer rotates smoothly without significant wobble;

— a water-bath that will maintain the dissolution medium at 37 ± 0.5 °C.

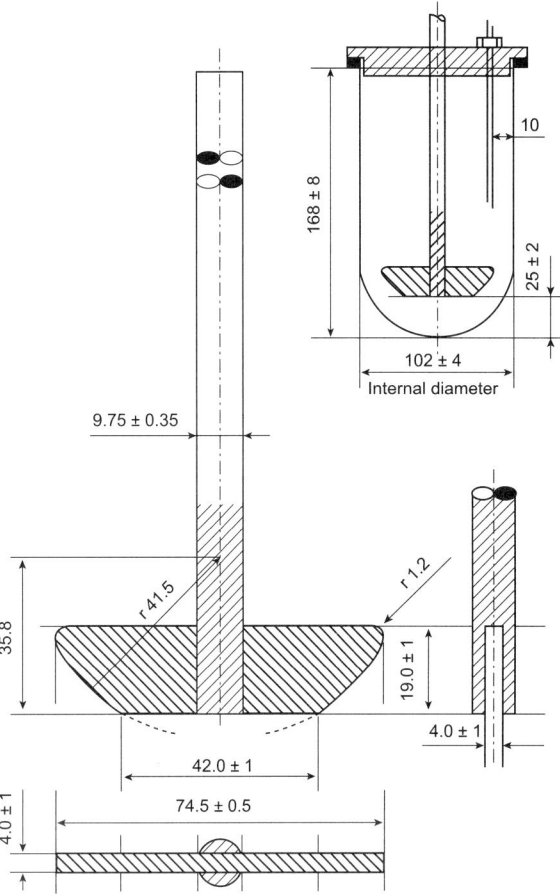

Figure 2.9.3.-1. — *Paddle apparatus*

Dimensions in millimetres

Basket apparatus. The apparatus (see Figure 2.9.3.-2) consists of:

— a vessel identical with that described for the paddle apparatus;

— a stirrer consisting of a vertical shaft to the lower part of which is attached a cylindrical basket; the basket has 2 parts: the upper part, with a 2 mm vent, is welded to the shaft and has 3 spring clips or other suitable device that allows removal of the lower part of the basket for introduction of the preparation to be examined and firmly holds the lower part concentric with the axis of the vessel during rotation; the lower part of the basket is made of welded-seam cloth formed into a cylinder with a narrow rim of sheet metal around the top and bottom; unless otherwise prescribed, the cloth has a wire thickness of 0.254 mm in diameter and 0.381 mm square openings; a basket with a gold coating 2.5 μm thick may be used for tests carried out in dilute acid medium; the bottom of the basket is 25 ± 2 mm from the inner bottom of the vessel during the test; the upper part of the shaft is connected to a motor provided with a speed regulator; the stirrer rotates smoothly without significant wobble;

— a water-bath that will maintain the dissolution medium at 37 ± 0.5 °C.

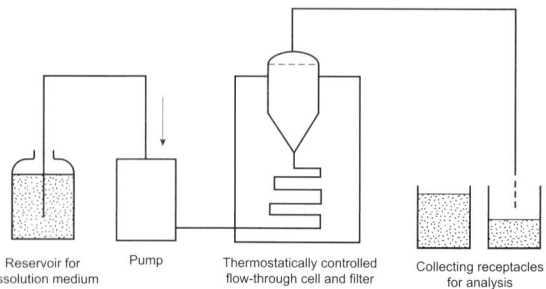

Figure 2.9.3.-3. — *Flow-through apparatus*

Dissolution medium. If the dissolution medium is buffered, adjust its pH to within ± 0.05 units of the prescribed value. Remove any dissolved gases from the dissolution medium before the test since they can cause the formation of bubbles that significantly affect the results.

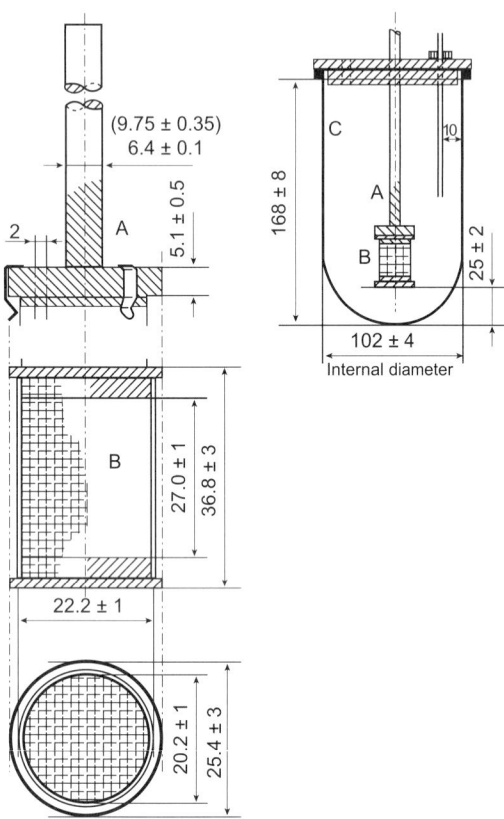

Figure 2.9.3.-2. — *Basket apparatus*

Dimensions in millimetres

Flow-through apparatus. The apparatus (see Figure 2.9.3.-3) consists of:

— a reservoir for the dissolution medium;

— a pump that forces the dissolution medium upwards through the flow-through cell;

— a flow-through cell (see Figures 2.9.3.-4/5/6) of transparent material mounted vertically with a filter system preventing escape of undissolved particles.

The flow-through cell shown in Figure 2.9.3.-6 is specifically intended for lipophilic solid dosage forms such as supposi-tories and soft capsules. It consists of 3 transparent parts which fit into each other. The lower part (1) is made up of 2 adjacent chambers connected to an overflow device.

The dissolution medium passes through chamber A and is subjected to an upwards flow. The flow in chamber B is downwards directed to a small-size bore exit which leads upwards to a filter assembly. The middle part (2) of the cell has a cavity designed to collect lipophilic excipients which float on the dissolution medium. A metal grill serves as a rough filter. The upper part (3) holds a filter unit for paper, glass fibre or cellulose filters.

— a water-bath that will maintain the dissolution medium at 37 ± 0.5 °C.

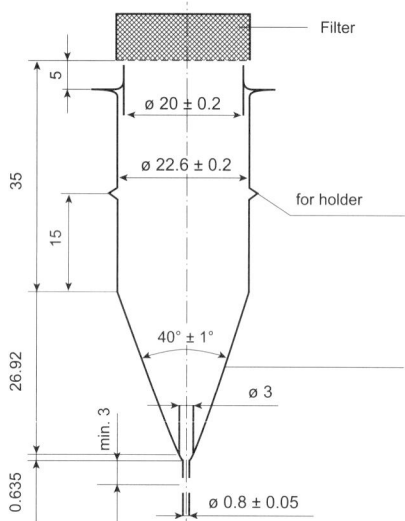

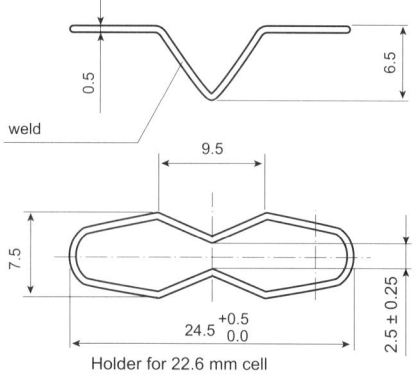

Holder for 22.6 mm cell

Figure 2.9.3.-4. — *Flow-through cell*
Dimensions in millimetres

METHOD

Paddle and basket apparatus

Place the prescribed volume of dissolution medium in the vessel, assemble the apparatus, warm the dissolution medium to 37 ± 0.5 °C and remove the thermometer.

Place one unit of the preparation to be examined in the apparatus. For the paddle apparatus, place the preparation at the bottom of the vessel before starting rotation of the blade; dosage forms that would otherwise float are kept horizontal at the bottom of the vessel using a suitable device, such as a wire or glass helix.

For the basket apparatus, place the preparation in a dry basket and lower into position before starting rotation.

Take care to avoid the presence of air bubbles on the surface of the preparation. Start the rotation of the apparatus immediately at the prescribed rate (± 4 per cent).

Flow-through apparatus

– Cells (see Figures 2.9.3.-4/5)

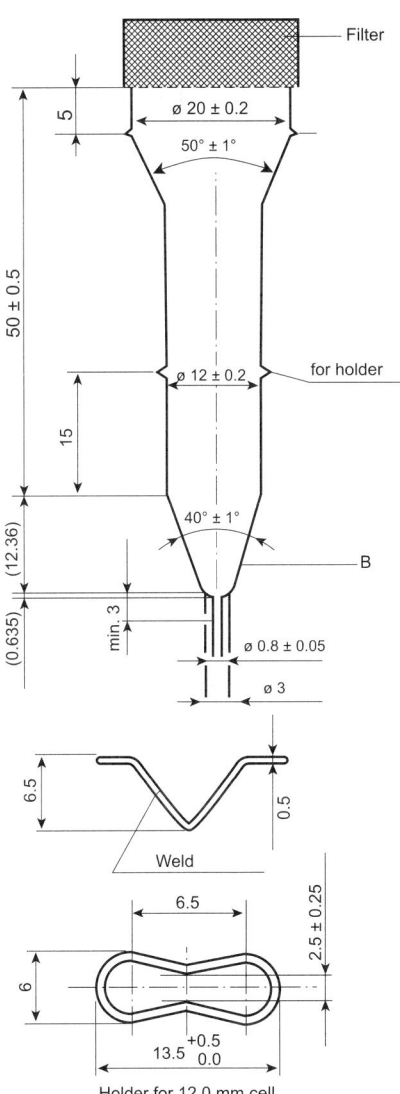

Figure 2.9.3.-5. — *Flow-through cell*

Dimensions in millimetres

Place 1 bead of 5 mm (± 0.5 mm) diameter at the bottom of the cone to protect the fluid entry of the tube and then glass beads of suitable size, preferably 1 mm (± 0.1 mm) diameter. Introduce 1 unit of the preparation in the cell on or within the layer of glass beads, by means of a holder. Assemble the filter head. Heat the dissolution medium to 37 ± 0.5 °C. Using a suitable pump, introduce the dissolution medium through the bottom of the cell to obtain a suitable continuous flow through an open or closed circuit at the prescribed rate (± 5 per cent).

– Cell (Figure 2.9.3.-6)

Place 1 unit of the preparation to be examined in chamber A. Close the cell with the prepared filter assembly. At the beginning of the test, chamber A requires air removal via a small orifice connected to the filter assembly. Heat the

dissolution medium to an appropriate temperature taking the melting point of the preparation into consideration. Using a suitable pump, introduce the warmed dissolution medium through the bottom of the cell to obtain a suitable continuous flow through an open or closed circuit at the prescribed rate (± 5 per cent). When the dissolution medium reaches the overflow, air starts to escape through the capillary and chamber B fills with the dissolution medium. The preparation spreads through the dissolution medium according to its physico-chemical properties.

In justified and authorised cases, representative fractions of large volume suppositories may be tested.

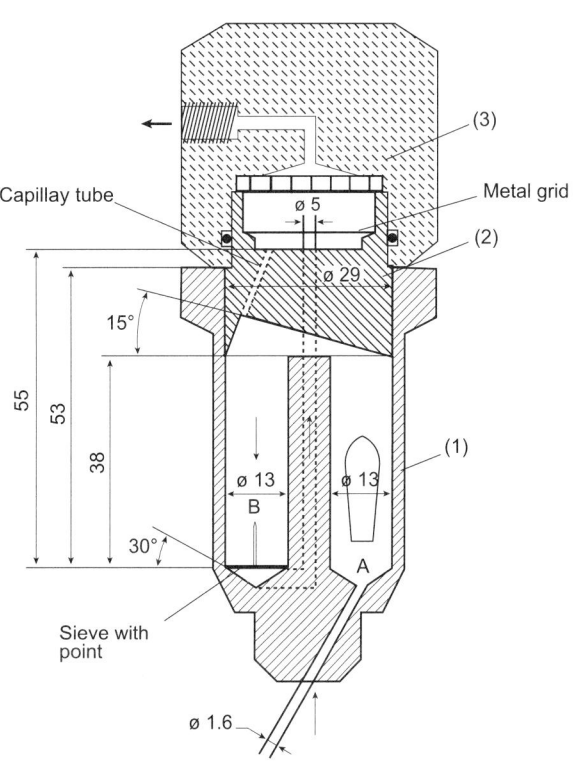

Figure 2.9.3.-6. — *Flow-through cell*

Dimensions in millimetres

SAMPLING AND EVALUATION

In the case of the paddle apparatus and the basket apparatus, withdraw at the prescribed time, or at the prescribed intervals or continuously, the prescribed volume or volumes from a position midway between the surface of the dissolution medium and the top of the basket or blade and not less than 10 mm from the vessel wall.

In the case of the flow-through apparatus, samples are always collected at the outlet of the cell, irrespective of whether the circuit is opened or closed.

Except where continuous measurement is used with the paddle or basket method (the liquid removed being returned to the vessel) or where a single portion of liquid is removed, add a volume of dissolution medium equal to the volume of liquid removed or compensate by calculation.

Filter the liquid removed using an inert filter of appropriate pore size that does not cause significant adsorption of the active ingredient from the solution and does not contain substances extractable by the dissolution medium that would interfere with the prescribed analytical method. Proceed with analysis of the filtrate as prescribed.

The quantity of the active ingredient dissolved in a specified time is expressed as a percentage of the content stated on the label.

2.9.5. UNIFORMITY OF MASS OF SINGLE-DOSE PREPARATIONS

Weigh individually 20 units taken at random or, for single-dose preparations presented in individual containers, the contents of 20 units, and determine the average mass. Not more than 2 of the individual masses deviate from the average mass by more than the percentage deviation shown in Table 2.9.5.-1 and none deviates by more than twice that percentage.

Table 2.9.5.-1

Pharmaceutical Form	Average Mass	Percentage deviation
Tablets (uncoated and film-coated)	80 mg or less	10
	More than 80 mg and less than 250 mg	7.5
	250 mg or more	5
Capsules, granules (uncoated, single-dose) and powders (single-dose)	Less than 300 mg	10
	300 mg or more	7.5
Powders for parenteral use* (single-dose)	More than 40 mg	10
Suppositories and pessaries	All masses	5
Powders for eye-drops and powders for eye lotions (single-dose)	Less than 300 mg	10
	300 mg or more	7.5

* When the average mass is equal to or below 40 mg, the preparation is not submitted to the test for uniformity of mass but to the test for uniformity of content of single-dose preparations (*2.9.6*).

For capsules and powders for parenteral use, proceed as described below.

CAPSULES

Weigh an intact capsule. Open the capsule without losing any part of the shell and remove the contents as completely as possible. For soft shell capsules, wash the shell with a suitable solvent and allow to stand until the odour of the solvent is no longer perceptible. Weigh the shell. The mass of the contents is the difference between the weighings. Repeat the procedure with another 19 capsules.

POWDERS FOR PARENTERAL USE

Remove any paper labels from a container and wash and dry the outside. Open the container and without delay weigh the container and its contents. Empty the container as completely as possible by gentle tapping, rinse it if necessary with *water R* and then with *alcohol R* and dry at 100-105 °C for 1 h, or, if the nature of the container precludes heating at this temperature, dry at a lower temperature to constant mass. Allow to cool in a desiccator and weigh. The mass of the contents is the difference between the weighings. Repeat the procedure with another 19 containers.

2.9.6. UNIFORMITY OF CONTENT OF SINGLE-DOSE PREPARATIONS

The test for uniformity of content of single-dose preparations is based on the assay of the individual contents of active substance(s) of a number of single-dose units to determine whether the individual contents are within limits set with reference to the average content of the sample.

The test is not required for multivitamin and trace-element preparations and in other justified and authorised circumstances.

Method. Using a suitable analytical method, determine the individual contents of active substance(s) of 10 dosage units taken at random.

Apply the criteria of test A, test B or test C as specified in the monograph for the dosage form in question.

TEST A

Tablets, powders for parenteral use, ophthalmic inserts, suspensions for injection. The preparation complies with the test if each individual content is between 85 per cent and 115 per cent of the average content. The preparation fails to comply with the test if more than one individual content is outside these limits or if one individual content is outside the limits of 75 per cent to 125 per cent of the average content.

If one individual content is outside the limits of 85 per cent to 115 per cent but within the limits of 75 per cent to 125 per cent, determine the individual contents of another 20 dosage units taken at random. The preparation complies with the test if not more than one of the individual contents of the 30 units is outside 85 per cent to 115 per cent of the average content and none is outside the limits of 75 per cent to 125 per cent of the average content.

TEST B

Capsules, powders other than for parenteral use, granules, suppositories, pessaries. The preparation complies with the test if not more than one individual content is outside the limits of 85 per cent to 115 per cent of the average content and none is outside the limits of 75 per cent to 125 per cent of the average content. The preparation fails to comply with the test if more than 3 individual contents are outside the limits of 85 per cent to 115 per cent of the average content or if one or more individual contents are outside the limits of 75 per cent to 125 per cent of the average content.

If 2 or 3 individual contents are outside the limits of 85 per cent to 115 per cent but within the limits of 75 per cent to 125 per cent, determine the individual contents of another 20 dosage units taken at random. The preparation complies with the test if not more than 3 individual contents of the 30 units are outside the limits of 85 per cent to 115 per cent of the average content and none is outside the limits of 75 per cent to 125 per cent of the average content.

TEST C

Transdermal patches. The preparation complies with the test if the average content of the 10 dosage units is between 90 per cent and 110 per cent of the content stated on the label and if the individual content of each dosage unit is between 75 per cent and 125 per cent of the average content.

4. REAGENTS

4. Reagents

4. REAGENTS

Exceptionally, a trademark or supplier may be indicated for certain reagents whose availability is limited. This information is given only to make it easier to obtain such reagents and this does not suggest in any way that the mentioned suppliers are especially recommended or certified by the European Pharmacopoeia Commission or the Council of Europe. It is therefore acceptable to use reagents from another source provided that they comply with the standards of the Pharmacopoeia.

4.1. REAGENTS, STANDARD SOLUTIONS, BUFFER SOLUTIONS

Where the name of substance or a solution is followed by the letter R (the whole in italics), this indicates a reagent included in the following list. The specifications given for reagents do not necessarily guarantee their quality for use in medicines.

Within the description of each reagent there is a seven-figure reference code in italics (for example, 1002501). This number, which will remain unchanged for a given reagent during subsequent revisions of the list, is used for identification purposes by the Secretariat, and users of the Pharmacopoeia may also find it useful, for example in the management of reagent stocks. The description may also include a CAS number (Chemical Abstract Service Registry Number) recognisable by its typical format, for example 9002-93-1.

Some of the reagents included in the list are toxic and should be handled in conformity with good quality control laboratory practice.

Reagents in aqueous solution are prepared using *water R*. Where a reagent solution is described using an expression such as "hydrochloric acid (10 g/l HCl)", the solution is prepared by an appropriate dilution with *water R* of a more concentrated reagent solution specified in this chapter. Reagent solutions used in the limit tests for barium, calcium and sulphates are prepared using *distilled water R*. Where the name of the solvent is not stated, an aqueous solution is intended.

The reagents and reagent solutions are to be stored in well-closed containers. The labelling should comply with the relevant national legislation and international agreements.

4.1.1. REAGENTS

Acacia. *1000100.*
See *Acacia (0307).*

> **Acacia solution.** *1000101.*
> Dissolve 100 g of *acacia R* in 1000 ml of *water R*. Stir with a mechanical stirrer for 2 h. Centrifuge at about 2000 *g* for 30 min to obtain a clear solution.
>
> Store in polyethylene containers of about 250 ml capacity at 0 °C to −20 °C.

Acetal. $C_6H_{14}O_2$. (M_r 118.2). *1112300.* [105-57-7].
Acetaldehyde diethyl acetal. 1,1-Diethoxyethane.
A clear, colourless, volatile liquid, miscible with water and with alcohol.
d_{20}^{20}: about 0.824.
n_D^{20}: about 1.382.
bp: about 103 °C.

Acetaldehyde. C_2H_4O. (M_r 44.1). *1000200.* [75-07-0].
Ethanal.
A clear, colourless flammable liquid, miscible with water and with alcohol.
d_{20}^{20}: about 0.788.
n_D^{20}: about 1.332.
bp: about 21 °C.

Acetaldehyde ammonia trimer trihydrate.
$C_6H_{15}N_3,3H_2O$. (M_r 183.3). *1133500.* [76231-37-3].
2,4,6-Trimethylhexahydro-1,3,5-triazine trihydrate.
mp: 95 °C to 97 °C.

Acetic acid, anhydrous. $C_2H_4O_2$. (M_r 60.1). *1000300.*
[64-19-7].
Contains not less than 99.6 per cent *m/m* of $C_2H_4O_2$.

A colourless liquid or white, shining, fern-like crystals, miscible with or very soluble in water, in alcohol, in ether, in glycerol (85 per cent), and in most fatty and essential oils.
d_{20}^{20}: 1.052 to 1.053.
bp: 117 °C to 119 °C.
A 100 g/l solution is strongly acid (*2.2.4*).

A 5 g/l solution neutralised with *dilute ammonia R2* gives reaction (b) of acetates (*2.3.1*).

Freezing point (*2.2.18*). Not below 15.8 °C.

Water (*2.5.12*). Not more than 0.4 per cent. If the water content is more than 0.4 per cent it may be adjusted by adding the calculated amount of *acetic anhydride R*.

Store protected from light.

Acetic acid, glacial. $C_2H_4O_2$. (M_r 60.1). *1000400.* [64-19-7].
See *Acetic acid, glacial (0590).*

> **Acetic acid.** *1000401.*
> Contains not less than 290 g/l and not more than 310 g/l of $C_2H_4O_2$ (M_r 60.1).
> Dilute 30 g of *glacial acetic acid R* to 100 ml with *water R*.

> **Acetic acid, dilute.** *1000402.*
> Contains not less than 115 g/l and not more than 125 g/l of $C_2H_4O_2$ (M_r 60.1).
> Dilute 12 g of *glacial acetic acid R* to 100 ml with *water R*.

Acetic anhydride. $C_4H_6O_3$. (M_r 102.1). *1000500.* [108-24-7].
Contains not less than 97.0 per cent *m/m* of $C_4H_6O_3$. A clear, colourless liquid.
bp: 136 °C to 142 °C.
Assay. Dissolve 2.00 g in 50.0 ml of *1 M sodium hydroxide* in a ground-glass-stoppered flask and boil under a reflux condenser for 1 h. Titrate with *1 M hydrochloric acid*, using 0.5 ml of *phenolphthalein solution R* as indicator. Calculate the number of millilitres of *1 M sodium hydroxide* required for 1 g (n_1). Dissolve 2.00 g in 20 ml of *cyclohexane R* in a ground-glass-stoppered flask, cool in ice and add a cold mixture of 10 ml of *aniline R* and 20 ml of *cyclohexane R*. Boil the mixture under a reflux condenser for 1 h, add 50.0 ml of *1 M sodium hydroxide* and shake vigorously. Titrate with *1 M hydrochloric acid*, using 0.5 ml of *phenolphthalein solution R* as indicator. Calculate the number of millilitres of *1 M sodium hydroxide* required for 1 g (n_2). Calculate the percentage of $C_4H_6O_3$ from the expression:

$$10.2\,(n_1 - n_2)$$

Acetic anhydride solution R1. *1000501.*
Dissolve 25.0 ml of *acetic anhydride R* in *anhydrous pyridine R* and dilute to 100.0 ml with the same solvent.

Store protected from light and air.

Acetic anhydride - sulphuric acid solution. *1000502.*
Carefully mix 5 ml of *acetic anhydride R* with 5 ml of *sulphuric acid R*. Add dropwise and with cooling to 50 ml of *ethanol R*.

Prepare immediately before use.

Acetone. *1000600.* [67-64-1].
See *Acetone (0872)*.

Acetonitrile. C_2H_3N. (M_r 41.05). *1000700.* [75-05-8]. Methyl cyanide. Ethanenitrile.
A clear, colourless liquid, miscible with water, with acetone, with ether and with methanol.
d_{20}^{20}: about 0.78.
n_D^{20}: about 1.344.
A 100 g/l solution is neutral to litmus paper.

Distillation range (2.2.11). Not less than 95 per cent distils between 80 °C and 82 °C.

Acetonitrile used in spectrophotometry complies with the following additional requirement:

Minimum transmittance (2.2.25). 98 per cent from 255 nm to 420 nm, using *water R* as compensation liquid.

> **Acetonitrile for chromatography.** *1000701.*
> See *Acetonitrile R.*
>
> *Acetonitrile used in chromatography complies with the following additional requirements:*
>
> *Minimum transmittance (2.2.25).* 98 per cent from 240 nm, using *water R* as compensation liquid.
>
> *Minimum purity (2.2.28).* 99.8 per cent.

> **Acetonitrile R1.** *1000702.*
>
> Complies with the requirements prescribed for *acetonitrile R* and with the following additional requirements:
>
> Contains not less than 99.9 per cent of C_2H_3N.
>
> *Absorbance (2.2.25).* The absorbance at 200 nm using *water R* as the compensation liquid is not more than 0.10.

Acetylacetamide. $C_4H_7NO_2$. (M_r 101.1). *1102600.* [5977-14-0]. 3-Oxobutanamide.
mp: 53 °C to 56 °C.

Acetylacetone. $C_5H_8O_2$. (M_r 100.1). *1000900.* [123-54-6]. 2,4-Pentanedione.
A colourless or slightly yellow, easily flammable liquid, freely soluble in water, miscible with acetone, with alcohol, with ether and with glacial acetic acid.
n_D^{20}: 1.452 to 1.453.
bp: 138 °C to 140 °C.

> **Acetylacetone reagent R1.** *1000901.*
> To 100 ml of *ammonium acetate solution R* add 0.2 ml of *acetylacetone R*.

N-Acetyl-ε-caprolactam. $C_8H_{13}NO_2$. (M_r 155.2). *1102700.* [1888-91-1]. *N*-Acetylhexane-6-lactam.
Colourless liquid, miscible with ethanol.
d_{20}^{20}: about 1.100.
n_D^{20}: about 1.489.
bp: about 135 °C.

Acetyl chloride. C_2H_3ClO. (M_r 78.5). *1000800.* [75-36-5].
A clear, colourless liquid, flammable, decomposes in contact with water and with alcohol, miscible with ethylene chloride.
d_{20}^{20}: about 1.10.
Distillation range (2.2.11). Not less than 95 per cent distils between 49 °C and 53 °C.

Acetylcholine chloride. $C_7H_{16}ClNO_2$. (M_r 181.7). *1001000.* [60-31-1].
A crystalline powder, very soluble in cold water and in alcohol, practically insoluble in ether; it decomposes in hot water and in alkalis.
Store at −20 °C.

Acetyleugenol. $C_{12}H_{14}O_3$. (M_r 206.2). *1100700.* [93-28-7]. 2-Methoxy-4-(2-propenyl)phenylacetate.
A yellow coloured, oily liquid, freely soluble in alcohol and ether, practically insoluble in water.
n_D^{20}: about 1.521.
bp: 281 °C to 282 °C.

Acetyleugenol used in gas chromatography complies with the following additional test:

Assay. Examine by gas chromatography (2.2.28) as prescribed in the monograph on *Clove oil (1091)* using the substance to be examined as the test solution.

The area of the principal peak is not less than 98.0 per cent of the total area of the peaks.

N-Acetylglucosamine. $C_8H_{15}NO_6$. (M_r 221.2). *1133600.* [7512-17-6]. 2-(Acetylamino)-2-deoxy-D-glucopyranose.
mp: about 202 °C.

N-Acetylneuraminic acid. $C_{11}H_{19}NO_9$. (M_r 309.3). *1001100.* [131-48-6]. *O*-Sialic acid.
White acicular crystals, soluble in water and in methanol, slightly soluble in ethanol, practically insoluble in acetone and in ether.
$[\alpha]_D^{20}$: about −36, determined on a 10 g/l solution.
mp: about 186 °C, with decomposition.

N-Acetyltryptophan. $C_{13}H_{14}N_2O_3$. (M_r 246.3). *1102800.* [1218-34-4]. 2-Acetylamino-3-(indol-3-yl)propanoic acid.
A white or almost white powder or colourless crystals, slightly soluble in water. It dissolves in dilute solutions of alkali hydroxides.
mp: about 205 °C.
Assay. Dissolve 10.0 mg in a mixture of 10 volumes of *acetonitrile R* and 90 volumes of *water R* and dilute to 100.0 ml with the same mixture of solvents. Examine as prescribed in the monograph on *Tryptophan (1272)* under "1,1′-Ethylidenebis(tryptophan) and other related substances". The area of the principal peak in the chromatogram obtained is not less than 99.0 per cent of the areas of all the peaks.

Acetyltyrosine ethyl ester. $C_{13}H_{17}NO_4, H_2O$. (M_r 269.3). *1001200.* [36546-50-6]. *N*-Acetyl-L-tyrosine ethyl ester monohydrate. Ethyl (*S*)-2-acetamido-3-(4-hydroxyphenyl)propionate monohydrate.
A white, crystalline powder suitable for the assay of chymo-trypsin.
$[\alpha]_D^{20}$: + 21 to + 25, determined on a 10 g/l solution in *alcohol R*.
$A_{1\ cm}^{1\%}$: 60 to 68, determined at 278 nm in *alcohol R*.

> **Acetyltyrosine ethyl ester 0.2 M.** *1001201.*
> Dissolve 0.54 g of *acetyltyrosine ethyl ester R* in *alcohol R* and dilute to 10.0 ml with the same solvent.

Acid blue 83. $C_{45}H_{44}N_3NaO_7S_2$. (M_r 826). *1012200.* [6104-59-2].
Colour Index No. 42660.
Brilliant blue R. Coomassie brilliant blue R 250.
Brown powder insoluble in cold water, slightly soluble in boiling water and in ethanol, soluble in sulphuric acid, glacial acetic acid and in dilute solutions of alkali hydroxides.

Acid blue 90. $C_{47}H_{48}N_3NaO_7S_2$. (M_r 854). *1001300*. [6104-58-1].
Colour Index No. 42655.
Sodium [4-[[4-[(4-ethoxyphenyl)amino]phenyl][[4-(ethyl)(3-sulphonatobenzyl)amino]phenyl]methylene]cyclo-hexa-2,5-dien-1-ylidene](ethyl)-(3-sulphonatobenzyl)ammonium.
A dark brown powder, with a violet sheen and some particles having a metallic lustre, soluble in water and in ethanol.
$A_{1\ cm}^{1\%}$: greater than 500, determined at 577 nm using a 0.01 g/l solution in buffer solution pH 7.0 and calculated with reference to the dried substance.
Loss on drying (2.2.32). Not more than 5.0 per cent, determined on 0.500 g by drying in an oven at 100 °C to 105 °C.

Acid blue 92. $C_{26}H_{16}N_3Na_3O_{10}S_3$. ($M_r$ 696). *1001400*. [3861-73-2].
Colour Index No. 13390.
Coomassie blue. Anazolene sodium. Trisodium 8-hydroxy-4′-(phenylamino)azonaphthalene-3,5′,6-trisulphonate.
Dark blue crystals slightly soluble in alcohol, soluble in water, in acetone and in ethylene glycol monoethylether.

> **Acid blue 92 solution.** *1001401*.
> Dissolve 0.5 g of *acid blue 92 R* in a mixture of 10 ml of *glacial acetic acid R*, 45 ml of *alcohol R* and 45 ml of *water R*.

Acid blue 93. $C_{37}H_{27}N_3Na_2O_9S_3$. ($M_r$ 800). *1134200*. [28983-56-4].
Colour Index No. 42780.
Methyl blue. Poirrier blue .
Mixture of triphenylrosaniline di- and trisulfonate and of triphenylpararosaniline.

Dark blue powder.

Colour change. pH 9.4 to pH 14.0.

> **Acid blue 93 solution.** *1134201*.
> Dissolve 0.2 g of *acid blue 93 R* in *water R* and dilute to 100 ml with the same solvent.

Acrylamide. C_3H_5NO. (M_r 71.1). *1001500*. [79-06-1].
Propenamide.
Colourless or white flakes or a white or almost white, crystalline powder, very soluble in water and in methanol, freely soluble in ethanol.
mp: about 84 °C.

> **30 per cent acrylamide/bisacrylamide (29:1) solution.** *1001501*.
> Prepare a solution containing 290 g of *acrylamide R* and 10 g of *methylenebisacrylamide R* per litre of *water R*. Filter.

> **30 per cent acrylamide/bisacrylamide (36.5:1) solution.** *1001502*.
> Prepare a solution containing 292 g of *acrylamide R* and 8 g of *methylenebisacrylamide R* per litre of *water R*. Filter.

Acrylic acid. $C_3H_4O_2$. (M_r 72.1). *1133700*. [79-10-7].
Prop-2-enoic acid. Vinylformic acid.

Contains not less than 99 per cent of $C_3H_4O_2$. It is stabilised with 0.02 per cent of hydroquinone monomethyl ether.

Corrosive liquid, miscible with water and alcohol. It polymerises readily in the presence of oxygen.
d_{20}^{20}: about 1.05.
n_D^{20}: about 1.421.
bp: about 141 °C.
mp: 12 °C to 15 °C.

Acteoside. $C_{29}H_{36}O_{15}$. (M_r 624.6). *1145100*. [61276-17-3]. 2-(3,4-Dihydroxyphenyl)ethyl 3-O-(6-deoxy-α-L-mannopyranosyl)-4-O-[(2E)-3-(3,4-dihydroxyphenyl)prop-2-enoyl]-β-D-glucopyranoside.
Light yellowish powder, freely soluble in water and in methanol.
mp: about 140 °C, with decomposition.

Adenosine. $C_{10}H_{13}N_5O_4$. (M_r 267.2). *1001600*. [58-61-7].
6-Amino-9-β-D-ribofuranosyl-9H-purine.
A white, crystalline powder, slightly soluble in water, practically insoluble in acetone, in alcohol and in ether. It dissolves in dilute solutions of acids.
mp: about 234 °C.

Adipic acid. $C_6H_{10}O_4$. (M_r 146.1). *1095600*. [124-04-9].
Prisms, freely soluble in methanol, soluble in acetone, practically insoluble in light petroleum.
mp: about 152 °C.

Aescin. *1001700*. [11072-93-8].
A mixture of related saponins obtained from the seeds of *Aesculus hippocastanum* L.

A fine, almost white or slightly reddish or yellowish, amorphous powder.
Chromatography. Examine as prescribed in the monograph on *Senega root (0202)* but apply 20 μl of the solution. After spraying with *anisaldehyde solution R* and heating, the chromatogram shows a principal band with an R_f of about 0.4.

Agarose/cross-linked polyacrylamide. *1002200*.
Agarose trapped within a cross-linked polyacrylamide network; it is used for the separation of globular proteins with relative molecular masses of 2×10^4 to 35×10^4.

Agarose-DEAE for ion-exchange chromatography. *1002100*. [57407-08-6].
Cross-linked agarose substituted with diethylaminoethyl groups, presented as beads.

Agarose for chromatography. *1001800*. [9012-36-6].
Swollen beads 60 μm to 140 μm in diameter presented as a 4 per cent suspension in *water R*. It is used in size-exclusion chromatography for the separation of proteins with relative molecular masses of 6×10^4 to 20×10^6 and of polysaccharides with relative molecular masses of 3×10^3 to 5×10^6.

Agarose for chromatography, cross-linked. *1001900*. [61970-08-9].
Prepared from agarose by reaction with 2,3-dibromopropanol in strongly alkaline conditions.
It occurs as swollen beads 60 μm to 140 μm in diameter and is presented as a 4 per cent suspension in *water R*. It is used in size-exclusion chromatography for the separation of proteins with relative molecular masses of 6×10^4 to 20×10^6 and of polysaccharides with relative molecular masses of 3×10^3 to 5×10^6.

> **Agarose for chromatography, cross-linked R1.** *1001901*. [65099-79-8].
> Prepared for agarose by reaction with 2,3-dibromo-propanol in strongly alkaline conditions.
> It occurs as swollen beads 60 μm to 140 μm in diameter and is presented as a 4 per cent suspension in *water R*. It is used in size-exclusion chromatography for the separation of proteins with relative molecular masses of 7×10^4 to 40×10^6 and of polysaccharides with relative molecular masses of 1×10^5 to 2×10^7.

4. Reagents

Agarose for electrophoresis. *1002000.* [9012-36-6].
A neutral, linear polysaccharide, the main component of which is derived from agar.

A white or almost white powder, practically insoluble in cold water, very slightly soluble in hot water.

Alanine. *1102900.* [56-41-7].
See *Alanine (0752)*.

β-Alanine. *1004500.* [107-95-9].
See *3-aminopropionic acid R*.

Albumin, bovine. *1002300.* [9048-46-8].
Bovine serum albumin containing about 96 per cent of protein.

A white to light-yellowish-brown powder.

Water (2.5.12). Not more than 3.0 per cent, determined on 0.800 g.

Bovine albumin used in the assay of tetracosactide should be pyrogen-free, free from proteolytic activity, when examined by a suitable means, for example using chromogenic substrate, and free from corticosteroid activity determined by measurement of fluorescence as described in the biological assay of Tetracosactide (0644).

Albumin, human. *1133800.*
Human serum albumin containing not less than 96 per cent of albumin.

Albumin solution, human. *1002400.* [9048-46-8].
See *Human albumin solution (0255)*.

Albumin solution, human R1. *1002401.*
Dilute *human albumin solution R* with a 9 g/l solution of *sodium chloride R* to a concentration of 1 g/l of protein. Adjust the pH to 3.5-4.5 with *glacial acetic acid R*.

Alcohol. C_2H_6O. (M_r 46.07). *1002500.* [64-17-5].
See *Ethanol (96 per cent) (1317)*.

Alcohol, aldehyde-free. *1002501.*
Mix 1200 ml of *alcohol R* with 5 ml of a 400 g/l solution of *silver nitrate R* and 10 ml of a cooled 500 g/l solution of *potassium hydroxide R*. Shake, allow to stand for a few days and filter. Distil the filtrate immediately before use.

Alcohol (*x* per cent *V/V*). *1002502.*
Mix appropriate volumes of *water R* and *alcohol R*, allowing for the effects of warming and volume contraction inherent to the preparation of such a mixture, to obtain a solution whose final content of alcohol corresponds to the value of *x*.

Aldehyde dehydrogenase. *1103000.*
Enzyme obtained from baker's yeast which oxidises acetaldehyde to acetic acid in the presence of nicotinamide-adenine dinucleotide, potassium salts and thiols, at pH 8.0.

Aldehyde dehydrogenase solution. *1103001.*
Dissolve in *water R* a quantity of *aldehyde dehydrogenase R*, equivalent to 70 units and dilute to 10 ml with the same solvent. This solution is stable for 8 h at 4 °C.

Aldrin. $C_{12}H_8Cl_6$. (M_r 364.9). *1123100.* [309-00-2].
bp: about 145 °C.
mp: about 104 °C.
A suitable certified reference solution (10 ng/μl in cyclohexane) may be used.

Aleuritic acid. $C_{16}H_{32}O_5$. (M_r 304.4). *1095700.* [533-87-9].
(9*RS*,10*SR*)-9,10,16-Trihydroxyhexadecanoic acid.
A white powder, greasy to the touch, soluble in methanol.
mp: about 101 °C.

Alizarin S. $C_{14}H_7NaO_7S,H_2O$. (M_r 360.3). *1002600.*
[130-22-3].
Schultz No. 1145.
Colour Index No. 58005.
Sodium 1,2-dihydroxyanthraquinone-3-sulphonate monohydrate. Sodium 3,4-dihydroxy-9,10-dioxo-9,10-dihydroanthracene-2-sulphonate monohydrate.
An orange-yellow powder, freely soluble in water and in alcohol.

Alizarin S solution. *1002601.*
A 1 g/l solution.

Test for sensitivity. If alizarin S solution is used for the standardisation of *0.05 M barium perchlorate*, it shows a colour change from yellow to orange-red when it is tested according to the standardisation of *0.05 M barium perchlorate (4.2.2)*.

Colour change. pH 3.7 (yellow) to pH 5.2 (violet).

Aluminium. Al. (A_r 26.98). *1118200.* [7429-90-5].
A white, malleable, flexible, bluish metal, available as bars, sheets, powder, strips or wire. In moist air an oxide film forms which protects the metal from corrosion.

Analytical grade.

Aluminium chloride. $AlCl_3,6H_2O$. (M_r 241.4). *1002700.*
[7784-13-6]. Aluminium chloride hexahydrate.
Contains not less than 98.0 per cent of $AlCl_3,6H_2O$.

A white to slightly yellowish, crystalline powder, hygroscopic, freely soluble in water and in alcohol, soluble in ether.
Store in an airtight container.

Aluminium chloride reagent. *1002702.*
Dissolve 2.0 g of *aluminium chloride R* in 100 ml of a 5 per cent *V/V* solution of *glacial acetic acid R* in *methanol R*.

Aluminium chloride solution. *1002701.*
Dissolve 65.0 g of *aluminium chloride R* in *water R* and dilute to 100 ml with the same solvent. Add 0.5 g of *activated charcoal R*, stir for 10 min, filter and add to the filtrate, with continuous stirring, sufficient of a 10 g/l solution of *sodium hydroxide R* (about 60 ml) to adjust the pH to about 1.5.

Aluminium nitrate. $Al(NO_3)_3,9H_2O$. (M_r 375.1). *1002800.*
[7784-27-2]. Aluminium nitrate nonahydrate.
Crystals, deliquescent, very soluble in water and alcohol, very slightly soluble in acetone.
Store in an airtight container.

Aluminium oxide, anhydrous. *1002900.* [1344-28-1].
An aluminium oxide, consisting of γ-Al_2O_3, dehydrated and activated by heat treatment. Particle size 75 μm to 150 μm.

Aluminium oxide, basic. *1118300.*
A basic grade of *anhydrous aluminium oxide R* suitable for column chromatography.

pH (2.2.3). Shake 1 g with 10 ml of *carbon dioxide-free water R* for 5 min. The pH of the suspension is 9 to 10.

Aluminium oxide, neutral. Al_2O_3. (M_r 102.0). *1118400.*
See *Aluminium oxide, hydrated (0311)*.

Aluminium potassium sulphate. *1003000.* [7784-24-9].
See *Alum (0006)*.

Amido black 10B. $C_{22}H_{14}N_6Na_2O_9S_2$. ($M_r$ 617). *1003100.*
[1064-48-8].
Schultz No. 299.
Colour Index No. 20470.
Disodium 5-amino-4-hydroxy-6-[(4-nitrophenyl)azo]-3-(phenylazo)naphthalene-2,7-disulphonate.
A dark-brown to black powder, sparingly soluble in water, soluble in alcohol.

Amido black 10B solution. *1003101.*
A 5 g/l solution of *amido black 10B R* in a mixture of 10 volumes of *acetic acid R* and 90 volumes of *methanol R*.

Aminoazobenzene. $C_{12}H_{11}N_3$. (M_r 197.2). *1003200.*
[60-09-3].
Colour Index No. 11000.
4-(Phenylazo)aniline.
Brownish-yellow needles with a bluish tinge, slightly soluble in water, freely soluble in alcohol and in ether.
mp: about 128 °C.

2-Aminobenzoic acid. $C_7H_7NO_2$. (M_r 137.1). *1003400.*
[118-92-3]. Anthranilic acid.
A white to pale-yellow, crystalline powder, sparingly soluble in cold water, freely soluble in hot water, in alcohol, in ether and in glycerol. Solutions in alcohol or in ether and, particularly, in glycerol show a violet fluorescence.
mp: about 145 °C.

4-Aminobenzoic acid. $C_7H_7NO_2$. (M_r 137.1). *1003300.*
[150-13-0].
A white, crystalline powder, slightly soluble in water, freely soluble in alcohol, practically insoluble in light petroleum.
mp: about 187 °C.
Chromatography. Examine as prescribed in the monograph on *Procaine hydrochloride (0050)*; the chromatogram shows only one principal spot.

Store protected from light.

4-Aminobenzoic acid solution. *1003301.*
Dissolve 1 g of *4-aminobenzoic acid R* in a mixture of 18 ml of *anhydrous acetic acid R*, 20 ml of *water R* and 1 ml of *phosphoric acid R*. Immediately before use, mix 2 volumes of the solution with 3 volumes of *acetone R*.

***N*-(4-Aminobenzoyl)-L-glutamic acid.** $C_{12}H_{14}N_2O_5$.
(M_r 266.3). *1141700.* [4271-30-1]. ABGA.
(2*S*)-2-[(4-Aminobenzoyl)amino]pentanedioic acid.
White or almost white, crystalline powder.
mp: about 175 °C, with decomposition.

4-Aminobutanoic acid. $C_4H_9NO_2$. (M_r 103.1). *1123200.*
[56-12-2]. γ-Aminobutyric acid. GABA.
Leaflets from methanol and ether, needles from water and alcohol. Freely soluble in water, practically insoluble or slightly soluble in other solvents.
mp: about 202 °C (decreases on rapid heating).

Aminobutanol. $C_4H_{11}NO$. (M_r 89.1). *1003500.* [5856-63-3].
2-Aminobutanol.
Oily liquid, miscible with water, soluble in alcohol.
d_{20}^{20}: about 0.94.
n_D^{20}: about 1.453.
bp: about 180 °C.

Aminochlorobenzophenone. $C_{13}H_{10}ClNO$. (M_r 231.7).
1003600. [719-59-5]. 2-Amino-5-chlorobenzophenone.
A yellow, crystalline powder, practically insoluble in water, freely soluble in acetone, soluble in alcohol.
mp: about 97 °C.
Chromatography. Examine as prescribed in the monograph on *Chlordiazepoxide hydrochloride (0474)* but apply 5 µl of a 0.5 g/l solution in *methanol R*; the chromatogram shows only one principal spot, at an R_f of about 0.9.

Store protected from light.

6-Aminohexanoic acid. $C_6H_{13}NO_2$. (M_r 131.2). *1103100.*
[60-32-2].
Colourless crystals, freely soluble in water, sparingly soluble in methanol, practically insoluble in ethanol.
mp: about 205 °C.

Aminohippuric acid. $C_9H_{10}N_2O_3$. (M_r 194.2). *1003700.*
[61-78-9]. (4-Aminobenzamido)acetic acid.
A white or almost white powder, sparingly soluble in water, soluble in alcohol, very slightly soluble in ether.
mp: about 200 °C.

Aminohippuric acid reagent. *1003701.*
Dissolve 3 g of *phthalic acid R* and 0.3 g of *aminohippuric acid R* in *alcohol R* and dilute to 100 ml with the same solvent.

Aminohydroxynaphthalenesulphonic acid.
$C_{10}H_9NO_4S$. (M_r 239.3). *1112400.* [116-63-2].
4-Amino-3-hydroxynaphthalene-1-sulphonic acid.
White or grey needles, turning pink on exposure to light, especially when moist, practically insoluble in water, in alcohol and in ether, soluble in solutions of alkali hydroxides and in hot solutions of sodium metabisulphite.
Store protected from light.

Aminohydroxynaphthalenesulphonic acid solution.
1112401.
Mix 5.0 g of *anhydrous sodium sulphite R* with 94.3 g of *sodium hydrogensulphite R* and 0.7 g of *aminohydroxynaphthalenesulphonic acid R*. Dissolve 1.5 g of the mixture in *water R* and dilute to 10.0 ml with the same solvent. Prepare the solution daily.

Aminomethylalizarindiacetic acid. $C_{19}H_{15}NO_8 , 2H_2O$.
(M_r 421.4). *1003900.* [3952-78-1]. 2,2′-[(3,4-dihydroxy-anthraquinon-3-yl)methylenenitrilo]diacetic acid dihydrate.
A fine, pale brownish-yellow to orange-brown powder, practically insoluble in water, soluble in solutions of alkali hydroxides.
mp: about 185 °C.
Loss on drying (2.2.32). Not more than 10.0 per cent, determined on 1.000 g.

Aminomethylalizarindiacetic acid reagent. *1003901.*

Solution I. Dissolve 0.36 g of *cerous nitrate R* in *water R* and dilute to 50 ml with the same solvent.

Solution II. Suspend 0.7 g of *aminomethylalizarindiacetic acid R* in 50 ml of *water R*. Dissolve with the aid of about 0.25 ml of *concentrated ammonia R*, add 0.25 ml of *glacial acetic acid R* and dilute to 100 ml with *water R*.

Solution III. Dissolve 6 g of *sodium acetate R* in 50 ml of *water R*, add 11.5 ml of *glacial acetic acid R* and dilute to 100 ml with *water R*.

To 33 ml of *acetone R* add 6.8 ml of solution III, 1.0 ml of solution II and 1.0 ml of solution I and dilute to 50 ml with *water R*.

Test for sensitivity. To 1.0 ml of *fluoride standard solution (10 ppm F) R* add 19.0 ml of *water R* and 5.0 ml of the aminomethylalizarindiacetic acid reagent. After 20 min, the solution assumes a blue colour.

Use the final solution within 5 days.

Aminomethylalizarindiacetic acid solution. *1003902.*
Dissolve 0.192 g of *aminomethylalizarindiacetic acid R* in 6 ml of freshly prepared *1 M sodium hydroxide*. Add 750 ml of *water R*, 25 ml of *succinate buffer solution pH 4.6 R* and, dropwise, *0.5 M hydrochloric acid* until the colour changes from violet-red to yellow (pH 4.5 to 5). Add 100 ml of *acetone R* and dilute to 1000 ml with *water R*.

Aminonitrobenzophenone. $C_{13}H_{10}N_2O_3$. (M_r 242.2). *1004000.* [1775-95-7]. 2-Amino-5-nitrobenzophenone.
A yellow, crystalline powder, practically insoluble in water, soluble in tetrahydrofuran, slightly soluble in methanol.
mp: about 160 °C.
$A_{1\,cm}^{1\%}$: 690 to 720, determined at 233 nm using a 0.01 g/l solution in *methanol R*.

Aminophenazone. $C_{13}H_{17}N_3O$. (231.3). *1133900.* [58-15-1]. 4-(Dimethylamino)-1,5-dimethyl-2-phenyl-1,2-dihydro-3*H*-pyrazol-3-one.
White, crystalline powder or colourless crystals, soluble in water, freely soluble in alcohol.
mp: about 108 °C.

4-Aminophenol. C_6H_7NO. (M_r 109.1). *1004300.* [123-30-8].
Contains not less than 95 per cent of C_6H_7NO.
A white or slightly coloured, crystalline powder, becoming coloured on exposure to air and light, sparingly soluble in water, soluble in ethanol.
mp: about 186 °C, with decomposition.
Store protected from light.

Aminopolyether. $C_{18}H_{36}N_2O_6$. (M_r 376.5). *1112500.* [23978-09-8]. 4,7,13,16,21,24-hexaoxa-1,10-diazabicyclo[8,8,8]hexacosane.
mp: 70 °C to 73 °C.

3-Aminopropanol. C_3H_9NO. (M_r 75.1). *1004400.* [156-87-6]. 3-Aminopropan-1-ol.
A clear, colourless, viscous liquid.
d_{20}^{20}: about 0.99.
n_D^{20}: about 1.461.
mp: about 11 °C.

3-Aminopropionic acid. $C_3H_7NO_2$. (M_r 89.1). *1004500.* [107-95-9]. β-Alanine.
Contains not less than 99 per cent of $C_3H_7NO_2$.
A white, crystalline powder, freely soluble in water, slightly soluble in alcohol, practically insoluble in acetone and in ether.
mp: about 200 °C, with decomposition.

Aminopyrazolone. $C_{11}H_{13}N_3O$. (M_r 203.2). *1004600.* [83-07-8]. 4-Amino-2,3-dimethyl-1-phenylpyrazolin-5-one.
Light-yellow needles or powder, sparingly soluble in water, freely soluble in alcohol, slightly soluble in ether.
mp: about 108 °C.

Aminopyrazolone solution. *1004601.*
A 1 g/l solution in *buffer solution pH 9.0 R*.

Ammonia, concentrated. *1004700.*
See *Concentrated ammonia solution (0877)*.

Ammonia. *1004701.*
Contains not less than 170 g/l and not more than 180 g/l of NH_3 (M_r 17.03).

Dilute 67 g of *concentrated ammonia R* to 100 ml with *water R*.
d_{20}^{20}: 0.931 to 0.934.
When used in the limit test for iron, *ammonia R* complies with the following additional requirement. Evaporate 5 ml of ammonia to dryness on a water-bath, add 10 ml of *water R*, 2 ml of a 200 g/l solution of *citric acid R* and 0.1 ml of *thioglycollic acid R*. Make alkaline by adding *ammonia R* and dilute to 20 ml with *water R*. No pink colour develops.
Store protected from atmospheric carbon dioxide, at a temperature below 20 °C.

Ammonia, dilute R1. *1004702.*
Contains not less than 100 g/l and not more than 104 g/l of NH_3 (M_r 17.03).
Dilute 41 g of *concentrated ammonia R* to 100 ml with *water R*.

Ammonia, dilute R2. *1004703.*
Contains not less than 33 g/l and not more than 35 g/l of NH_3 (M_r 17.03).
Dilute 14 g of *concentrated ammonia R* to 100 ml with *water R*.

Ammonia, dilute R3. *1004704.*
Contains not less than 1.6 g/l and not more than 1.8 g/l of NH_3 (M_r 17.03).
Dilute 0.7 g of *concentrated ammonia R* to 100 ml with *water R*.

Ammonia, lead-free. *1004705.*
Complies with the requirements prescribed for *dilute ammonia R1* and with the following additional test: to 20 ml of lead-free ammonia, add 1 ml of *lead-free potassium cyanide solution R*, dilute to 50 ml with *water R* and add 0.10 ml of *sodium sulphide solution R*. The solution is not more intensely coloured than a reference solution prepared without sodium sulphide.

Ammonia, concentrated R1. *1004800.*
Contains not less than 32.0 per cent *m/m* of NH_3 (M_r 17.03).
A clear, colourless liquid.
d_{20}^{20}: 0.883 to 0.889.
Assay. Weigh accurately a ground-glass-stoppered flask containing 50.0 ml of *1 M hydrochloric acid*. Introduce 2 ml of the concentrated ammonia and weigh again. Titrate the solution with *1 M sodium hydroxide*, using 0.5 ml of *methyl red mixed solution R* as indicator.
1 ml of *1 M hydrochloric acid* is equivalent to 17.03 mg of NH_3.
Store protected from atmospheric carbon dioxide, at a temperature below 20 °C.

Ammonium acetate. $C_2H_7NO_2$. (M_r 77.1). *1004900.* [631-61-8].
Colourless crystals, very deliquescent, very soluble in water and in alcohol.
Store in an airtight container.

Ammonium acetate solution. *1004901.*
Dissolve 150 g of *ammonium acetate R* in *water R*. Add 3 ml of *glacial acetic acid R* and dilute to 1000 ml with *water R*.
Use within one week.

Ammonium and cerium nitrate. $(NH_4)_2Ce(NO_3)_6$. (M_r 548.2). *1005000.* [16774-21-3].
An orange-yellow, crystalline powder, or orange transparent crystals, soluble in water.

Ammonium and cerium sulphate. $(NH_4)_4Ce(SO_4)_4,2H_2O$. (M_r 633). *1005100*. [10378-47-9].
Orange-yellow, crystalline powder or crystals, slowly soluble in water.

(1R)-(−)-Ammonium 10-camphorsulphonate. $C_{10}H_{19}NO_4S$. (M_r 249.3). *1103200*.
Contains not less than 97.0 per cent of (1R)-(−)-ammonium 10-camphorsulphonate.
$[\alpha]_D^{20}$: − 18 ± 2 (50 g/l solution in *water R*).

Ammonium carbonate. *1005200*. [506-87-6]. A mixture of varying proportions of ammonium hydrogen carbonate (NH_4HCO_3, M_r 79.1) and ammonium carbamate (NH_2COONH_4, M_r 78.1).
A white translucent mass, slowly soluble in about 4 parts of water. It is decomposed by boiling water. Ammonium carbonate liberates not less than 30 per cent *m/m* of NH_3 (M_r 17.03).
Assay. Dissolve 2.00 g in 25 ml of *water R*. Slowly add 50.0 ml of *1 M hydrochloric acid*, titrate with *1 M sodium hydroxide*, using 0.1 ml of *methyl orange solution R* as indicator.
1 ml of *1 M hydrochloric acid* is equivalent to 17.03 mg of NH_3. Store at a temperature below 20 °C.

> **Ammonium carbonate solution.** *1005201*.
> A 158 g/l solution.

Ammonium chloride. *1005300*. [12125-02-9].
See *Ammonium chloride (0007)*.

> **Ammonium chloride solution.** *1005301*.
> A 107 g/l solution.

Ammonium citrate. $C_6H_{14}N_2O_7$. (M_r 226.2). *1103300*. [3012-65-5]. Diammonium hydrogen citrate.
A white, crystalline powder or colourless crystals, freely soluble in water, slightly soluble in alcohol.
pH (2.2.3). The pH of a 22.6 g/l solution is about 4.3.

Ammonium dihydrogen phosphate. $(NH_4)H_2PO_4$. (M_r 115.0). *1005400*. [7722-76-1]. Monobasic ammonium phosphate.
A white, crystalline powder or colourless crystals, freely soluble in water.
pH (2.2.3). A 23 g/l solution has a pH of about 4.2.

Ammonium formate. CH_5NO_2. (M_r 63.1). *1112600*. [540-69-2].
Deliquescent crystals or granules, very soluble in water, soluble in alcohol.
mp: 119 °C to 121 °C.
Store in an airtight container.

Ammonium hexafluorogermanate (IV). $(NH_4)_2GeF_6$. (M_r 222.7). *1134000*. [16962-47-3].
White crystals, freely soluble in water.

Ammonium hydrogen carbonate. NH_4HCO_3. (M_r 79.1). *1005500*. [1066-33-7].
Contains not less than 99 per cent of NH_4HCO_3

Ammonium molybdate. $(NH_4)_6Mo_7O_{24},4H_2O$. (M_r 1236). *1005700*. [12054-85-2].
Colourless or slightly yellow or greenish crystals, soluble in water, practically insoluble in alcohol.

> **Ammonium molybdate reagent.** *1005701*.
> Mix, in the given order, 1 volume of a 25 g/l solution of *ammonium molybdate R*, 1 volume of a 100 g/l solution of *ascorbic acid R* and 1 volume of *sulphuric acid R* (294.5 g/l H_2SO_4). Add 2 volumes of *water R*.
> Use within one day.

Ammonium molybdate reagent R1. *1005706*.
Mix 10 ml of a 60 g/l solution of *disodium arsenate R*, 50 ml of *ammonium molybdate solution R*, 90 ml of *dilute sulphuric acid R* and dilute to 200 ml in *water R*.
The mixture is conditioned at 37 °C for 24 hours, and kept in amber flasks.

Ammonium molybdate solution. *1005702*.
A 100 g/l solution.

Ammonium molybdate solution R2. *1005703*.
Dissolve 5.0 g of *ammonium molybdate R* with heating in 30 ml of *water R*. Cool, adjust the pH to 7.0 with *dilute ammonia R2* and dilute to 50 ml with *water R*.

Ammonium molybdate solution R3. *1005704*.
Solution I. Dissolve 5 g of *ammonium molybdate R* in 20 ml of *water R* with heating.
Solution II. Mix 150 ml of *alcohol R* with 150 ml of *water R*. Add with cooling 100 ml of *sulphuric acid R*.
Immediately before use add 80 volumes of solution II to 20 volumes of solution I.

Ammonium molybdate solution R4. *1005705*.
Dissolve 1.0 g of *ammonium molybdate R* in *water R* and dilute to 40 ml with the same solvent. Add 3 ml of *hydrochloric acid R* and 5 ml of *perchloric acid R* and dilute to 100 ml with *acetone R*.
Store protected from light and use within 1 month.

Ammonium molybdate solution R5. *1005707*.
Dissolve 1.0 g of *ammonium molybdate R* in 40.0 ml of a 15 per cent *V/V* solution of *sulphuric acid R*. Prepare the solution daily.

Ammonium nitrate. NH_4NO_3. (M_r 80.0). *1005800*. [6484-52-2].
A white, crystalline powder or colourless crystals, hygroscopic, very soluble in water, freely soluble in methanol, soluble in alcohol.
Store in an airtight container.

> **Ammonium nitrate R1.** *1005801*. [6484-52-2].
> Complies with the requirements prescribed for *ammonium nitrate R* and with the following additional requirements.
> *Acidity.* The solution of the substance is faintly acid *(2.2.4)*.
> *Chlorides (2.4.4)*. 0.50 g complies with the limit test for chlorides (100 ppm).
> *Sulphates (2.4.13)*. 1.0 g complies with the limit test for sulphates (150 ppm).
> *Sulphated ash (2.4.14)*. Not more than 0.05 per cent, determined on 1.0 g.

Ammonium oxalate. $C_2H_8N_2O_4,H_2O$. (M_r 142.1). *1005900*. [6009-70-7].
Colourless crystals, soluble in water.

> **Ammonium oxalate solution.** *1005901*.
> A 40 g/l solution.

Ammonium persulphate. $(NH_4)_2S_2O_8$. (M_r 228.2). *1006000*. [7727-54-0].
White, crystalline powder or granular crystals, freely soluble in water.

Ammonium phosphate. $(NH_4)_2HPO_4$. (M_r 132.1). *1006100*. [7783-28-0]. Diammonium hydrogen phosphate.
White crystals or granules, hygroscopic, very soluble in water, practically insoluble in alcohol.
The pH of a 200 g/l solution is about 8.

Store in an airtight container.

Ammonium pyrrolidinedithiocarbamate. $C_5H_{12}N_2S_2$. (M_r 164.3). *1006200*. [5108-96-3]. Ammonium 1-pyrrolidinyl-dithioformate.
A white to pale yellow, crystalline powder, sparingly soluble in water, very slightly soluble in alcohol.
Store in a bottle containing a piece of ammonium carbonate in a muslin bag.

Ammonium reineckate. $NH_4[Cr(NCS)_4(NH_3)_2],H_2O$. ($M_r$ 354.4). *1006300*. [13573-16-5]. Ammonium diamine-tetrakis(isothiocyanato)chromate(III) monohydrate.
Red powder or crystals, sparingly soluble in cold water, soluble in hot water and in alcohol.

    Ammonium reineckate solution. *1006301*.
    A 10 g/l solution. Prepare immediately before use.

Ammonium sulphamate. $NH_2SO_3NH_4$. (M_r 114.1). *1006400*. [7773-06-0].
A white, crystalline powder or colourless crystals, hygroscopic, very soluble in water, slightly soluble in alcohol.
mp: about 130 °C.
Store in an airtight container.

Ammonium sulphate. $(NH_4)_2SO_4$. (M_r 132.1). *1006500*. [7783-20-2].
Colourless crystals or white granules, very soluble in water, practically insoluble in acetone and in alcohol.

pH (2.2.3). The pH of a 50 g/l solution in *carbon dioxide-free water R* is 4.5 to 6.0.
Sulphated ash (2.4.14). Not more than 0.1 per cent.

Ammonium sulphide solution. *1123300*.
Saturate 120 ml of *dilute ammonia R1* with *hydrogen sulphide R* and add 80 ml of *dilute ammonia R1*. Prepare immediately before use.

Ammonium thiocyanate. NH_4SCN. (M_r 76.1). *1006700*. [1762-95-4].
Colourless crystals, deliquescent, very soluble in water, soluble in alcohol.
Store in an airtight container.

    Ammonium thiocyanate solution. *1006701*.
    A 76 g/l solution.

Ammonium vanadate. NH_4VO_3. (M_r 117.0). *1006800*. [7803-55-6]. Ammonium trioxovanadate(V).
A white to slightly yellowish, crystalline powder, slightly soluble in water, soluble in *dilute ammonia R1*.

    Ammonium vanadate solution. *1006801*.
    Dissolve 1.2 g of *ammonium vanadate R* in 95 ml of *water R* and dilute to 100 ml with *sulphuric acid R*.

Amoxicillin trihydrate. *1103400*.
See *Amoxicillin trihydrate (0260)*.

α-Amylase. *1100800*. 1,4-α-D-glucane-glucanohydrolase (EC 3.2.1.1).
A white to light brown powder.

    α-Amylase solution. *1100801*.
    A solution of *α-amylase R* with an activity of 800 FAU/g.

β-Amyrin. $C_{30}H_{50}O$. (M_r 426.7). *1141800*. [559-70-6].
Olean-12-en-3β-ol.
White or almost white powder.
mp: 187 °C to 190 °C.

Anethole. $C_{10}H_{12}O$. (M_r 148.2). *1006900*. [4180-23-8].
1-Methoxy-4-(propen-1-yl)benzene.
A white, crystalline mass up to 20 °C to 21 °C, liquid above 23 °C, practically insoluble in water, freely soluble in ethanol, soluble in ethyl acetate and in light petroleum.
n_D^{25}: about 1.56.
bp: about 230 °C.
Anethole used in gas chromatography complies with the following test.

Assay. Examine by gas chromatography (*2.2.28*) under the conditions described in the monograph on *Anise oil (0804)* using the substance to be examined as the test solution.

The area of the principal peak, corresponding to *trans*-anethole, with a retention time of about 41 min, is not less than 99.0 per cent of the total area of the peaks.

***cis*-Anethole.** $C_{10}H_{12}O$. (M_r 148.2). *1007000*.
(Z)-1-Methoxy-4-(propen-1-yl)benzene.
A white, crystalline mass up to 20 °C to 21 °C, liquid above 23 °C, practically insoluble in water, freely soluble in ethanol, soluble in ethyl acetate and in light petroleum.
n_D^{25}: about 1.56.
bp: about 230 °C.
cis-Anethole used in gas chromatography complies with the following test.

Assay. Examine by gas chromatography (*2.2.28*) in the conditions described in the monograph on *Anise oil (0804)* using the substance to be examined as the test solution.

The area of the principal peak is not less than 92.0 per cent of the total area of the peaks.

Aniline. C_6H_7N. (M_r 93.1). *1007100*. [62-53-3].
Benzeneamine.
A colourless or slightly yellowish liquid, soluble in water, miscible with alcohol and with ether.
d_{20}^{20}: about 1.02.
bp: 183 °C to 186 °C.
Store protected from light.

Anion exchange resin. *1007200*.
A resin in chlorinated form containing quaternary ammonium groups [$CH_2N^+(CH_3)_3$] attached to a polymer lattice consisting of polystyrene cross-linked with 2 per cent of divinylbenzene. It is available as spherical beads and the particle size is specified in the monograph.

Wash the resin with *1 M sodium hydroxide* on a sintered-glass filter (40) until the washings are free from chloride, then wash with *water R* until the washings are neutral. Suspend in freshly prepared *ammonium-free water R* and protect from atmospheric carbon dioxide.

Anion exchange resin R1. *1123400*.
A resin containing quaternary ammonium groups [$CH_2N^+(CH_3)_3$] attached to a lattice consisting of methacrylate.

Anion exchange resin R2. *1141900*.
A conjugate of homogeneous 10 μm hydrophilic polyether particles, and a quaternary ammonium salt, providing a matrix suitable for strong anion-exchange chromatography of proteins.

Anion exchange resin for chromatography, strongly basic. *1112700*.
A resin with quaternary amine groups attached to a lattice of latex cross linked with divinylbenzene.

Anion exchange resin, strongly basic. *1026600.*

A gel-type resin in hydroxide form containing quaternary ammonium groups [$CH_2N^+(CH_3)_3$, type 1] attached to a polymer lattice consisting of polystyrene cross-linked with 8 per cent of divinylbenzene.

Brown transparent beads.

Particle size: 0.2 mm to 1.0 mm.

Moisture content: about 50 per cent.

Total exchange capacity: at least 1.2 meq/ml.

Anion exchange resin, weak. *1146700.*
A resin with diethylaminoethyl groups attached to a lattice consisting of poly(methyl methacrylate).

Anisaldehyde. $C_8H_8O_2$. (M_r 136.1). *1007300.* [123-11-5].
4-Methoxybenzaldehyde.
An oily liquid, very slightly soluble in water, miscible with alcohol and with ether.
bp: about 248 °C.

Anisaldehyde used in gas chromatography complies with the following test.

Assay. Examine by gas chromatography (*2.2.28*) in the conditions described in the monograph on *Anise oil (0804)* the substance to be examined as the test solution.

The area of the principal peak is not less than 99.0 per cent of the total area of the peaks.

> **Anisaldehyde solution.** *1007301.*
> Mix in the following order, 0.5 ml of *anisaldehyde R*, 10 ml of *glacial acetic acid R*, 85 ml of *methanol R* and 5 ml of *sulphuric acid R*.

> **Anisaldehyde solution R1.** *1007302.*
> To 10 ml of *anisaldehyde R* add 90 ml of *alcohol R*, mix, add 10 ml of *sulphuric acid R* and mix again.

***p*-Anisidine.** C_7H_9NO. (M_r 123.2). *1103500.* [104-94-9].
4-Methoxyaniline.
White crystals, sparingly soluble in water, soluble in ethanol.

Contains not less than 97.0 per cent of C_7H_9NO.

Caution: skin irritant, sensitiser.

Store protected from light at 0 °C to 4 °C.

On storage, *p*-anisidine tends to darken as a result of oxidation. A discoloured reagent can be reduced and decolorised in the following way: dissolve 20 g of *p-anisidine R* in 500 ml of *water R* at 75 °C. Add 1 g of *sodium sulphite R* and 10 g of *activated charcoal R* and stir for 5 min. Filter, cool the filtrate to about 0 °C and allow to stand at this temperature for at least 4 h. Filter, wash the crystals with a small quantity of *water R* at about 0 °C and dry the crystals in vacuum over *diphosphorus pentoxide R*.

Anolyte for isoelectric focusing pH 3 to 5. *1112800. 1 M Glutamic acid, 0.5 M phosphoric acid.*
Dissolve 14.71 g of *glutamic acid R* in *water R*. Add 33 ml of *phosphoric acid R* and dilute to 1000 ml with *water R*

Anthracene. $C_{14}H_{10}$. (M_r 178.2). *1007400.* [120-12-7].
A white, crystalline powder, practically insoluble in water, slightly soluble in chloroform.
mp: about 218 °C.

Anthrone. $C_{14}H_{10}O$. (M_r 194.2). *1007500.* [90-44-8].
9(10*H*)-Anthracenone.
A pale yellow, crystalline powder.
mp: about 155 °C.

Antimony potassium tartrate. $C_4H_4KO_7Sb,^1/_2H_2O$. (M_r 333.9). *1007600.* Potassium aqua[tartrato(4–)-O^1,O^2,O^3]-antimoniate(III) hemihydrate.
A white, granular powder or colourless, transparent crystals, soluble in water and in glycerol, freely soluble in boiling water, practically insoluble in alcohol. The aqueous solution is slightly acid.

Antimony trichloride. $SbCl_3$. (M_r 228.1). *1007700.*
[10025-91-9].
Colourless crystals or a transparent crystalline mass, hygroscopic, freely soluble in ethanol. Antimony trichloride is hydrolysed by water.
Store in an airtight container, protected from moisture.

> **Antimony trichloride solution.** *1007701.*
> Rapidly wash 30 g of *antimony trichloride R* with two quantities, each of 15 ml, of *ethanol-free chloroform R*, drain off the washings, and dissolve the washed crystals immediately in 100 ml of *ethanol-free chloroform R*, warming slightly.

> Store the solution over a few grams of *anhydrous sodium sulphate R*.

Antimony trichloride solution R1. *1007702.*

Solution I. Dissolve 110 g of *antimony trichloride R* in 400 ml of *ethylene chloride R*. Add 2 g of *anhydrous aluminium oxide R*, mix and filter through a sintered-glass filter (40). Dilute to 500.0 ml with *ethylene chloride R* and mix. The absorbance (*2.2.25*) of the solution, determined at 500 nm in a 2 cm cell, is not greater than 0.07.

Solution II. Under a hood, mix 100 ml of freshly distilled *acetyl chloride R* and 400 ml of *ethylene chloride R* and store in a cool place.

Mix 90 ml of solution I and 10 ml of solution II.

Store in brown ground-glass-stoppered bottles and use within 7 days. Discard any reagent in which colour develops.

Antithrombin III. *1007800.* [90170-80-2].
Antithrombin III is purified from human plasma by heparin agarose chromatography and should have a specific activity of at least 6 IU/mg.

Antithrombin III solution R1. *1007801.*
Reconstitute *antithrombin III R* as directed by the manufacturer and dilute with *tris(hydroxymethyl)aminomethane sodium chloride buffer solution pH 7.4 R* to 1 IU/ml.

Antithrombin III solution R2. *1007802.*
Reconstitute *antithrombin III R* as directed by the manufacturer and dilute with *tris(hydroxymethyl)aminomethane sodium chloride buffer solution pH 7.4 R* to 0.5 IU/ml.

Apigenin. $C_{15}H_{10}O_5$. (M_r 270.2). *1095800.* [520-36-5].
4′,5,7-Trihydroxyflavone.
Light yellowish powder; practically insoluble in water, sparingly soluble in alcohol.
mp: about 310 °C, with decomposition.
Chromatography. Examine as prescribed in the monograph on *Roman chamomile flower (0380)*, applying 10 μl of a 0.25 g/l solution in *methanol R*. The chromatogram shows in the upper third a principal zone of yellowish-green fluorescence.

Apigenin-7-glucoside. $C_{21}H_{20}O_{10}$. (M_r 432.6). *1095900*.
Light yellowish powder; practically insoluble in water,
sparingly soluble in alcohol.
mp: 198 °C to 201 °C.
Chromatography. Examine as prescribed in the monograph
on *Roman chamomile flower (0380)*, applying 10 µl of a
0.25 g/l solution in *methanol R*. The chromatogram shows
in the middle third a principal zone of yellowish fluorescence.

Aprotinin. *1007900*. [9087-70-1].
See *Aprotinin (0580)*.

Arabinose. $C_5H_{10}O_5$. (M_r 150.1). *1008000*. [87-72-9].
L-(+)-Arabinose.
A white, crystalline powder, freely soluble in water.
$[\alpha]_D^{20}$: + 103 to + 105, determined on a 50 g/l solution in
water R containing about 0.05 per cent of NH_3.

Arbutin. $C_{12}H_{16}O_7$. (M_r 272.3). *1008100*. [497-76-7].
Arbutoside. 4-Hydroxyphenyl-β-D-glucopyranoside.
Fine, white, shiny needles, freely soluble in water, very
soluble in hot water, soluble in alcohol.
$[\alpha]_D^{20}$: about − 64, determined on a 20 g/l solution.
mp: about 200 °C.
Chromatography. Examine by thin-layer chromatography
(2.2.27) as prescribed in the monograph *Bearberry leaf
(1054)*; the chromatogram shows only one principal spot.
*Arbutin used in the arbutin assay in the monograph
Bearberry leaf (1054) complies with the following
additional requirement.*
Assay. Examine by liquid chromatography *(2.2.29)* as
prescribed in the monograph *Bearberry leaf (1054)*.
The content of arbutin is not less than 95 per cent, calculated
by the normalisation procedure.

Arginine. *1103600*. [74-79-3].
See *Arginine (0806)*.

Argon. Ar. (A_r 39.95). *1008200*. [7440-37-1].
Contains not less than 99.995 per cent V/V of Ar.
Carbon monoxide. When used as described in the test for
carbon monoxide in medicinal gases (Method I, 2.5.25),
after passage of 10 litres of *argon R* at a flow rate of
4 litres per hour, not more than 0.05 ml of *0.002 M sodium
thiosulphate* is required for the titration (0.6 ppm V/V).

Aromadendrene. $C_{15}H_{24}$. (M_r 204.4). *1139100*. [489-39-4].
(1R,2S,4R,8R,11R)-3,3,11-Trimethyl-7-methylenetricyclo-
[6.3.0.0^{2,4}]undecane.
Clear, almost colourless liquid.
d_4^{20}: about 0.911.
n_D^{20}: about 1.497.
$[\alpha]_D^{20}$: about + 12.
bp: about 263 °C.
*Aromadendrene used in gas chromatography complies
with the following additional test:*
Assay. Examine by gas chromatography *(2.2.28)* as
prescribed in the monograph on *Tea tree oil (1837)*.
The content is not less than 92 per cent, calculated by the
normalisation procedure.

Arsenious trioxide. As_2O_3. (M_r 197.8). *1008300*. [1327-53-3].
Arsenious anhydride. Diarsenic trioxide.
A crystalline powder or a white mass, slightly soluble in
water, soluble in boiling water.

Arsenite solution. *1008301*.
Dissolve 0.50 g of *arsenious trioxide R* in 5 ml of *dilute
sodium hydroxide solution R*, add 2.0 g of *sodium
hydrogen carbonate R* and dilute to 100.0 ml with
water R.

Ascorbic acid. *1008400*. [50-81-7].
See *Ascorbic acid (0253)*.

Ascorbic acid solution. *1008401*.
Dissolve 50 mg in 0.5 ml of *water R* and dilute to 50 ml
with *dimethylformamide R*.

Asiaticoside. $C_{48}H_{78}O_{19}$. (M_r 959). *1123500*.
[16830-15-2]. *O*-6-Deoxy-α-L-mannopyranosyl-(1→4)-
O-β-D-glucopyranosyl-(1→6)-β-D-glucopyranosyl
2α,3β,23-trihydroxy-4α-urs-12-en-28-oate.
A white powder, hygroscopic, soluble in methanol, slightly
soluble in ethanol, insoluble in acetonitrile.
mp: about 232 °C, with decomposition.
Water (2.5.12): 6.0 per cent.
Store protected from humidity.
*Asiaticoside used in liquid chromatography complies with
the following additional test.*
Assay. Examine by liquid chromatography *(2.2.29)* as
prescribed in the monograph on *Centella (1498)*.
The content is not less than 97.0 per cent calculated by the
normalisation procedure.

Aspartic acid. *1134100*. [56-84-8].
See *Aspartic acid (0797)*.

L-Aspartyl-L-phenylalanine. $C_{13}H_{16}N_2O_5$. (M_r 280.3).
1008500. [13433-09-5]. (*S*)-3-Amino-*N*-[(*S*)-1-carboxy-2-
phenylethyl]-succinamic acid.
A white powder.
mp: about 210 °C, with decomposition.

Aucubin. $C_{15}H_{22}O_9$. (M_r 346.3). *1145200*. [479-98-1].
[1S,4aR,5S,7aS]-5-Hydroxy-7-(hydroxymethyl)-1,4a,5,7a-
tetrahydrocyclopenta[*c*]pyran-1-yl β-D-glucopyranoside.
Crystals, soluble in water, in alcohol and in methanol,
practically insoluble in light petroleum.
$[\alpha]_D^{20}$: about − 163.
mp: about 181 °C.

Azomethine H. $C_{17}H_{12}NNaO_8S_2$. (M_r 445.4). *1008700*.
[5941-07-1]. Sodium hydrogeno-4-hydroxy-5-(2-
hydroxybenzylideneamino)-2,7-naphthalenedisulphonate.

Azomethine H solution. *1008701*.
Dissolve 0.45 g of *azomethine H R* and 1 g of *ascorbic
acid R* with gentle heating in *water R* and dilute to 100 ml
with the same solvent.

Barbaloin. $C_{21}H_{22}O_9,H_2O$. (M_r 436.4). *1008800*. [1415-73-2].
Aloin. 1,8-Dihydroxy-3-hydroxymethyl-10-β-D-glucopyranosyl-
10*H*-anthracen-9-one.
A yellow to dark-yellow, crystalline powder, or yellow needles,
darkening on exposure to air and light, sparingly soluble in
water and in alcohol, soluble in acetone, in ammonia and in
solutions of alkali hydroxides, very slightly soluble in ether.
$A_{1\ cm}^{1\%}$: about 192 at 269 nm, about 226 at 296.5 nm, about
259 at 354 nm, determined on a solution in *methanol R* and
calculated with reference to the anhydrous substance.
Chromatography. Examine as prescribed in the monograph
on *Frangula bark (0025)*; the chromatogram shows only
one principal spot.

Barbital. *1008900*. [57-44-3].
See *Barbital (0170)*.

Barbital sodium. $C_8H_{11}N_2NaO_3$. (M_r 206.2). *1009000*.
[144-02-5].
Contains not less than 98.0 per cent of the sodium derivative
of 5,5-diethyl-1*H*,3*H*,5*H*-pyrimidine-2,4,6-trione.

A white, crystalline powder or colourless crystals, freely soluble in water, slightly soluble in alcohol, practically insoluble in ether.

Barbituric acid. $C_4H_4N_2O_3$. (M_r 128.1). *1009100*. [67-52-7]. $1H,3H,5H$-Pyrimidine-2,4,6-trione.
A white or almost white powder, slightly soluble in water, freely soluble in boiling water and in dilute acids.
mp: about 253 °C.

Barium carbonate. $BaCO_3$. (M_r 197.3). *1009200*. [513-77-9].
A white powder or friable masses, practically insoluble in water.

Barium chloride. $BaCl_2,2H_2O$. (M_r 244.3). *1009300*. [10326-27-9]. Barium dichloride.
Colourless crystals, freely soluble in water, slightly soluble in alcohol.

> **Barium chloride solution R1.** *1009301*.
> A 61 g/l solution.

> **Barium chloride solution R2.** *1009302*.
> A 36.5 g/l solution.

Barium hydroxide. $Ba(OH)_2,8H_2O$. (M_r 315.5). *1009400*. [12230-71-6]. Barium dihydroxide.
Colourless crystals, soluble in water.

> **Barium hydroxide solution.** *1009401*.
> A 47.3 g/l solution.

Barium sulphate. *1009500*. [7727-43-7].
See *Barium sulphate (0010)*.

Benzaldehyde. C_7H_6O. (M_r 106.1). *1009600*. [100-52-7].
A colourless or slightly yellow liquid, slightly soluble in water, miscible with alcohol and with ether.
d_{20}^{20}: about 1.05.
n_D^{20}: about 1.545.
Distillation range (2.2.11). Not less than 95 per cent distils between 177 °C and 180 °C.
Store protected from light.

Benzene. C_6H_6. (M_r 78.1). *1009800*. [71-43-2].
A clear, colourless, flammable liquid, practically insoluble in water, miscible with alcohol and with ether.
bp: about 80 °C.

Benzethonium chloride. $C_{27}H_{42}ClNO_2,H_2O$. (M_r 466.1). *1009900*. [121-54-0]. Benzyldimethyl[2-[2-[4-(1,1,3,3-tetramethylbutyl)phenoxy]ethoxy]ethyl]ammonium chloride monohydrate.
A fine, white powder or colourless crystals, soluble in water and in alcohol, slightly soluble in ether.
mp: about 163 °C.
Store protected from light.

Benzidine. $C_{12}H_{12}N_2$. (M_r 184.2). *1145300*. [92-87-5].
Biphenyl-4,4'-diamine.
Contains not less than 95 per cent of $C_{12}H_{12}N_2$.
White or slightly yellowish or reddish powder, darkening on exposure to air and light.
mp: about 120 °C.
Store protected from light.

Benzil. $C_{14}H_{10}O_2$. (M_r 210.2). *1117800*. [134-81-6].
Diphenylethanedione.
A yellow, crystalline powder, insoluble in water, soluble in alcohol, ethyl acetate and toluene.
mp: 95 °C.

Benzocaine. $C_9H_{11}NO_2$. (M_r 165.2). *1123600*. [94-09-7].
See *Benzocaine (0011)*.

Benzoic acid. *1010100*. [65-85-0].
See *Benzoic acid (0066)*.

Benzoin. $C_{14}H_{12}O_2$. (M_r 212.3). *1010200*. [579-44-2].
2-Hydroxy-1,2-diphenylethanone.
Slightly yellowish crystals, very slightly soluble in water, freely soluble in acetone, soluble in hot alcohol, sparingly soluble in ether.
mp: about 137 °C.

Benzophenone. $C_{13}H_{10}O$. (M_r 182.2). *1010300*. [119-61-9].
Diphenylmethanone.
Prismatic crystals, practically insoluble in water, freely soluble in alcohol and in ether.
mp: about 48 °C.

1,4-Benzoquinone. $C_6H_4O_2$. (M_r 108.1). *1118500*. [106-51-4].
Cyclohexa-2,5-diene-1,4-dione.
Contains not less than 98.0 per cent of $C_6H_4O_2$.

Benzoylarginine ethyl ester hydrochloride.
$C_{15}H_{23}ClN_4O_3$. (M_r 342.8). *1010500*. [2645-08-1].
N-Benzoyl-L-arginine ethyl ester hydrochloride. Ethyl (S)-2-benzamido-5-guanidinovalerate hydrochloride.
A white, crystalline powder, very soluble in water and in ethanol, practically insoluble in ether.
$[\alpha]_D^{20}$: − 15 to − 18, determined on a 10 g/l solution.
mp: about 129 °C.
$A_{1\,cm}^{1\%}$: 310 to 340, determined at 227 nm using a 0.01 g/l solution.

Benzoyl chloride. C_7H_5ClO. (M_r 140.6). *1010400*. [98-88-4].
A colourless, lachrymatory liquid, soluble in ether, decomposed by water and by alcohol.
d_{20}^{20}: about 1.21.
bp: about 197 °C.

***N*-Benzoyl-L-prolyl-L-phenylalanyl-L-arginine 4-nitroanilide acetate.** $C_{35}H_{42}N_8O_8$. (M_r 703). *1010600*.

2-Benzoylpyridine. $C_{12}H_9NO$. (M_r 183.2). *1134300*.
[91-02-1]. Phenyl(pyridin-2-yl)methanone.
Colourless crystals, soluble in alcohol.
mp: about 43 °C.

Benzyl alcohol. *1010700*. [100-51-6].
See *Benzyl alcohol (0256)*.

Benzyl benzoate. *1010800*. [120-51-4].
See *Benzyl benzoate (0705)*.

Chromatography. Examine as prescribed in the monograph on *Peru balsam (0754)* applying 20 µl of a 0.3 per cent V/V solution in *ethyl acetate R*. After spraying and heating, the chromatogram shows a principal band with an R_f of about 0.8.

Benzyl cinnamate. $C_{16}H_{14}O_2$. (M_r 238.3). *1010900*.
[103-41-3]. Benzyl 3-phenylprop-2-enoate.
Colourless or yellowish crystals, practically insoluble in water, soluble in alcohol and in ether.
mp: about 39 °C.
Chromatography. Examine as prescribed in the monograph on *Peru balsam (0754)* applying 20 µl of a 3 g/l solution in *ethyl acetate R*. After spraying and heating, the chromatogram shows a principal band with an R_f of about 0.6.

Benzyl ether. $C_{14}H_{14}O$. (M_r 198.3). *1140900*. [103-50-4].
Dibenzyl ether.
Clear, colourless liquid, practically insoluble in water, miscible with acetone and with ethanol.
d_{20}^{20}: about 1.043.

n_D^{20}: about 1.562.
bp: about 296 °C, with decomposition.

Benzylpenicillin sodium. *1011000.* [69-57-8].
See *Benzylpenicillin sodium (0114).*

2-Benzylpyridine. $C_{12}H_{11}N$. (M_r 169.2). *1112900.* [101-82-6].
Contains not less than 98.0 per cent of $C_{12}H_{11}N$.
A yellow liquid.
mp: 13 °C to 16 °C.

Bergapten. $C_{12}H_8O_4$. (M_r 216.2). *1103700.* [484-20-8].
5-Methoxypsoralen.
Colourless crystals, practically insoluble in water, sparingly soluble in alcohol and slightly soluble in glacial acetic acid.
mp: about 188 °C

Betulin. $C_{30}H_{50}O_2$. (M_r 442.7). *1011100.* [473-98-3].
Lup-20(39)-ene-3β,28-diol.
A white, crystalline powder.
mp: 248 °C to 251 °C.

Bibenzyl. $C_{14}H_{14}$. (M_r 182.3). *1011200.* [103-29-7].
1,2-Diphenylethane.
A white, crystalline powder, practically insoluble in water, very soluble in methylene chloride, freely soluble in acetone, soluble in alcohol.
mp: 50 °C to 53 °C.

Biphenyl-4-ol. $C_{12}H_{10}O$. (M_r 170.2). *1011300.* [90-43-7].
4-Phenylphenol.
A white, crystalline powder, practically insoluble in water.
mp: 164 °C to 167 °C.

Bisbenzimide. $C_{25}H_{27}Cl_3N_6O,5H_2O$. ($M_r$ 624). *1103800.*
[23491-44-3]. 4-[5-[5-(4-Methylpiperazin-1-yl)benzimidazol-2-yl]benzimidazol-2-yl]phenol trihydrochloride pentahydrate.

> **Bisbenzimide stock solution.** *1103801.*
> Dissolve 5 mg of *bisbenzimide R* in *water R* and dilute to 100 ml with the same solvent. Store in the dark.

> **Bisbenzimide working solution.** *1103802.*
> Immediately before use, dilute 100 µl of *bisbenzimide stock solution R* to 100 ml with *phosphate-buffered saline pH 7.4 R.*

Bismuth subnitrate. [$4BiNO_3(OH)_2,BiO(OH)$]. (M_r 1462).
1011500. [1304-85-4].
A white powder, practically insoluble in water.

> **Bismuth subnitrate R1.** *1011501.*
> Contains not less than 71.5 per cent and not more than 74.0 per cent of bismuth (Bi), and not less than 14.5 per cent and not more than 16.5 per cent of nitrate, calculated as nitrogen pentoxide (N_2O_5).

> **Bismuth subnitrate solution.** *1011502.*
> Dissolve 5 g of *bismuth subnitrate R1* in a mixture of 8.4 ml of *nitric acid R* and 50 ml of *water R* and dilute to 250 ml with *water R*. Filter if necessary.

> *Acidity.* To 10 ml add 0.05 ml of *methyl orange solution R.* 5.0 ml to 6.25 ml of *1 M sodium hydroxide* is required to change the colour of the indicator.

Biuret. $C_2H_5N_3O_2$. (M_r 103.1). *1011600.* [108-19-0].
White crystals, hygroscopic, soluble in water, sparingly soluble in alcohol, very slightly soluble in ether.
mp: 188 °C to 190 °C, with decomposition.
Store in an airtight container.

Biuret reagent. *1011601.*
Dissolve 1.5 g of *copper sulphate R* and 6.0 g of *sodium potassium tartrate R* in 500 ml of *water R*. Add 300 ml of a carbonate-free 100 g/l solution of *sodium hydroxide R*, dilute to 1000 ml with the same solution and mix.

Blocking solution. *1122400.*
A 10 per cent *V/V* solution of *acetic acid R*.

Blue dextran 2000. *1011700.* [9049-32-5].
Prepared from dextran having an average relative molecular mass of 2×10^6 by introduction of a polycyclic chromophore that colours the substance blue. The degree of substitution is 0.017. It is freeze-dried and dissolves rapidly and completely in water and aqueous saline solutions.
A 1 g/l solution in a *phosphate buffer solution pH 7.0 R* shows an absorption maximum (*2.2.25*) at 280 nm.

Boldine. $C_{19}H_{21}NO_4$. (M_r 327.3). *1118800.* [476-70-0].
1,10-Dimethoxy-6aα-aporphine-2,9-diol.
A white crystalline powder, very slightly soluble in water, soluble in alcohol and in dilute solutions of acids.
$[\alpha]_D^{25}$: about + 127, determined on a 1 g/l solution in *ethanol R*.
mp: about 163 °C.

Chromatography. Examined as prescribed in the monograph on *Boldo leaf (1396)* the chromatogram shows a single principal spot.

Assay. Examine by liquid chromatography (*2.2.29*) under the conditions described in the monograph on *Boldo leaf (1396)* using the substance to be examined as the test solution.

The area of the principal peak is not less than 99.0 per cent of the total area of the peaks.

Boric acid. *1011800.* [10043-35-3].
See *Boric acid (0001).*

Borneol. $C_{10}H_{18}O$. (M_r 154.3). *1011900.* [507-70-0].
endo-1,7,7-Trimethylbicyclo[2.2.1]heptan-2-ol.
Colourless crystals, readily sublimes, practically insoluble in water, freely soluble in alcohol, in ether and in light petroleum.
mp: about 208 °C.
Chromatography. Examine by thin-layer chromatography (*2.2.27*), using *silica gel G R* as the coating substance. Apply to the plate 10 µl of a 1 g/l solution in *toluene R*. Develop over a path of 10 cm using *chloroform R*. Allow the plate to dry in air, spray with *anisaldehyde solution R*, using 10 ml for a plate 200 mm square, and heat at 100 °C to 105 °C for 10 min. The chromatogram obtained shows only one principal spot.

Bornyl acetate. $C_{12}H_{20}O_2$. (M_r 196.3). *1012000.* [5655-61-8].
endo-1,7,7-Trimethylbicyclo[2.2.1]hept-2-yl acetate.
Colourless crystals or a colourless liquid, very slightly soluble in water, soluble in alcohol and in ether.
mp: about 28 °C.
Chromatography. Examine by thin-layer chromatography (*2.2.27*), using *silica gel G R* as the coating substance. Apply to the plate 10 µl of a 2 g/l solution in *toluene R*. Develop over a path of 10 cm using *chloroform R*. Allow the plate to dry in air, spray with *anisaldehyde solution R*, using 10 ml for a plate 200 mm square, and heat at 100 °C to 105 °C for 10 min. The chromatogram obtained shows only one principal spot.

Boron trichloride. BCl_3. (M_r 117.2). *1112000.* [10294-34-5].
Colourless gas. Reacts violently with water. Available as solutions in suitable solvents (2-chloroethanol, methylene chloride, hexane, heptane, methanol).

n_D^{20}: about 1.420.
bp: about 12.6 °C.
Caution: toxic, corrosive.

Boron trichloride-methanol solution. *1112001.*
A 120 g/l solution of BCl_3 in *methanol R.*

Store protected from light at -20 °C, preferably in sealed tubes.

Boron trifluoride. BF_3. (M_r 67.8). *1012100.* [7637-07-2].
Colourless gas.

Boron trifluoride-methanol solution. *1012101.*
A 140 g/l solution of *boron trifluoride R* in *methanol R.*

Brilliant blue. *1012200.* [6104-59-2].
See *acid blue 83 R.*

Bromelains. *1012300.* [37189-34-7].
A concentrate of proteolytic enzymes derived from *Ananas comosus* Merr.

A dull-yellow powder.
Activity. 1 g liberates about 1.2 g of amino-nitrogen from a solution of *gelatin R* in 20 min at 45 °C and pH 4.5.

Bromelains solution. *1012301.*
A 10 g/l solution of *bromelains R* in a mixture of 1 volume of *phosphate buffer solution pH 5.5 R* and 9 volumes of a 9 g/l solution of *sodium chloride R.*

Bromine. Br_2. (M_r 159.8). *1012400.* [7726-95-6].
A brownish-red fuming liquid, slightly soluble in water, soluble in alcohol and in ether.
d_{20}^{20}: about 3.1.

Bromine solution. *1012401.*
Dissolve 30 g of *bromine R* and 30 g of *potassium bromide R* in *water R* and dilute to 100 ml with the same solvent.

Bromine water. *1012402.*
Shake 3 ml of *bromine R* with 100 ml of *water R* to saturation.

Store over an excess of *bromine R*, protected from light.

Bromine water R1. *1012403.*
Shake 0.5 ml of *bromine R* with 100 ml of *water R.*

Store protected from light for not longer than 1 week.

Bromocresol green. $C_{21}H_{14}Br_4O_5S$. (M_r 698). *1012600.*
[76-60-8]. 3′,3″,5′,5″-Tetrabromo-*m*-cresol-sulfonphthalein.
4,4′-(3*H*-2,1-Benzoxathiol-3-ylidene)bis(2,6-dibromo-3-methylphenol)-*S,S*-dioxide.
A brownish-white powder, slightly soluble in water, soluble in alcohol and in dilute solutions of alkali hydroxides.

Bromocresol green-methyl red solution. *1012602.*
Dissolve 0.15 g of *bromocresol green R* and 0.1 g of *methyl red R* in 180 ml of *ethanol R* and dilute to 200 ml with *water R.*

Bromocresol green solution. *1012601.*
Dissolve 50 mg of *bromocresol green R* in 0.72 ml of *0.1 M sodium hydroxide* and 20 ml of *alcohol R* and dilute to 100 ml with *water R.*

Test for sensitivity. To 0.2 ml of the bromocresol green solution add 100 ml of *carbon dioxide-free water R.* The solution is blue. Not more than 0.2 ml of *0.02 M hydrochloric acid* is required to change the colour to yellow.

Colour change. pH 3.6 (yellow) to pH 5.2 (blue).

Bromocresol purple. $C_{21}H_{16}Br_2O_5S$. (M_r 540.2). *1012700.*
[115-40-2]. 3′,3″-Dibromo-*o*-cresolsulfonphthalein.
4,4′-(3*H*-2,1-Benzoxathiol-3-ylidene)bis(2-bromo-6-methylphenol)-*S,S*-dioxide.
A pinkish powder, practically insoluble in water, soluble in alcohol and in dilute solutions of alkali hydroxides.

Bromocresol purple solution. *1012701.*

Dissolve 50 mg of *bromocresol purple R* in 0.92 ml of *0.1 M sodium hydroxide* and 20 ml of *alcohol R* and dilute to 100 ml with *water R.*

Test for sensitivity. To 0.2 ml of the bromocresol purple solution add 100 ml of *carbon dioxide-free water R* and 0.05 ml of *0.02 M sodium hydroxide.* The solution is bluish-violet. Not more than 0.2 ml of *0.02 M hydrochloric acid* is required to change the colour to yellow.

Colour change. pH 5.2 (yellow) to pH 6.8 (bluish-violet).

5-Bromo-2′-deoxyuridine. $C_9H_{11}BrN_2O_5$. (M_r 307.1).
1012500. [59-14-3]. 5-Bromo-1-(2-deoxy-β-d-*erythro*-pentofuranosyl)-1*H*,3*H*-pyrimidine-2,4-dione.
mp: about 194 °C.
Chromatography. Examine as prescribed in the monograph on *Idoxuridine (0669)*, applying 5 µl of a 0.25 g/l solution. The chromatogram obtained shows only one principal spot.

Bromophenol blue. $C_{19}H_{10}Br_4O_5S$. (M_r 670). *1012800.*
[115-39-9]. 3′,3″,5′,5″-Tetrabromophenolsulfonphthalein.
4,4′-(3*H*-2,1-Benzoxathiol-3-ylidene)bis(2,6-dibromophenol) *S,S*-dioxide.
A light orange-yellow powder, very slightly soluble in water, slightly soluble in alcohol, freely soluble in solutions of alkali hydroxides.

Bromophenol blue solution. *1012801.*

Dissolve 0.1 g of *bromophenol blue R* in 1.5 ml of *0.1 M sodium hydroxide* and 20 ml of *alcohol R* and dilute to 100 ml with *water R.*

Test for sensitivity. To 0.05 ml of the bromophenol blue solution add 20 ml of *carbon dioxide-free water R* and 0.05 ml of *0.1 M hydrochloric acid.* The solution is yellow. Not more than 0.1 ml of *0.1 M sodium hydroxide* is required to change the colour to bluish-violet.

Colour change. pH 2.8 (yellow) to pH 4.4 (bluish-violet).

Bromophenol blue solution R1. *1012802.*
Dissolve 50 mg of *bromophenol blue R* with gentle heating in 3.73 ml of *0.02 M sodium hydroxide* and dilute to 100 ml with *water R.*

Bromophenol blue solution R2. *1012803.*
Dissolve with heating 0.2 g of *bromophenol blue R* in 3 ml of *0.1 M sodium hydroxide* and 10 ml of *alcohol R.* After solution is effected, allow to cool and dilute to 100 ml with *alcohol R.*

Bromophos. $C_8H_8BrCl_2O_3PS$. (M_r 366.0). *1123700.*
[2104-96-3].
A suitable certified reference solution (10 ng/µl in iso-octane) may be used.

Bromophos-ethyl. $C_{10}H_{12}BrCl_2O_3PS$. (M_r 394.0). *1123800.*
[4824-78-6].
A suitable certified reference solution (10 ng/µl in iso-octane) may be used.

Bromothymol blue. $C_{27}H_{28}Br_2O_5S$. (M_r 624). *1012900*.
[76-59-5]. 3′,3″-Dibromothymolsulfonphthalein.
4,4′-(3H-2,1-Benzoxathiol-3-ylidene)bis(2-bromo-6-isopropyl-3-methylphenol) S,S-dioxide.
A reddish-pink or brownish powder, practically insoluble in water, soluble in alcohol and in dilute solutions of alkali hydroxides.

Bromothymol blue solution R1. *1012901*.

Dissolve 50 mg of *bromothymol blue R* in a mixture of 4 ml of *0.02 M sodium hydroxide* and 20 ml of *alcohol R* and dilute to 100 ml with *water R*.

Test for sensitivity. To 0.3 ml of *bromothymol blue solution R1* add 100 ml of *carbon dioxide-free water R*. The solution is yellow. Not more than 0.1 ml of *0.02 M sodium hydroxide* is required to change the colour to blue.

Colour change. pH 5.8 (yellow) to pH 7.4 (blue).

Bromothymol blue solution R2. *1012902*.
A 10 g/l solution in *dimethylformamide R*.

Bromothymol blue solution R3. *1012903*.
Warm 0.1 g of *bromothymol blue R* with 3.2 ml of *0.05 M sodium hydroxide* and 5 ml of *alcohol (90 per cent V/V) R*. After solution is effected, dilute to 250 ml with *alcohol (90 per cent V/V) R*.

BRP indicator solution. *1013000*.
Dissolve 0.1 g of *bromothymol blue R*, 20 mg of *methyl red R* and 0.2 g of *phenolphthalein R* in *alcohol R* and dilute to 100 ml with the same solvent. Filter.

Brucine. $C_{23}H_{26}N_2O_4,2H_2O$. (M_r 430.5). *1013100*. [357-57-3].
10,11-Dimethoxystrychnine.
Colourless crystals, slightly soluble in water, freely soluble in alcohol and in ether.
mp: about 178 °C.

Butanal. C_4H_8O. (M_r 72.1). *1134400*. [123-72-8].
Butyraldehyde.
d_{20}^{20}: 0.806.
n_D^{20}: 1.380.
bp: 75 °C.

Butanol. $C_4H_{10}O$. (M_r 74.1). *1013200*. [71-36-3]. *n*-Butanol.
1-Butanol.
A clear, colourless liquid, miscible with alcohol.
d_{20}^{20}: about 0.81.
bp: 116 °C to 119 °C.

2-Butanol R1. $C_4H_{10}O$. (M_r 74.1). *1013301*. [78-92-2].
sec-Butyl alcohol.
Contains not less than 99.0 per cent of $C_4H_{10}O$. A clear, colourless liquid, soluble in water, miscible with alcohol and with ether.
d_{20}^{20}: about 0.81.

Distillation range (2.2.11). Not less than 95 per cent distils between 99 °C and 100 °C.

Assay. By gas chromatography as described in the monograph on *Isopropyl alcohol (0970)*.

Butyl acetate. $C_6H_{12}O_2$. (M_r 116.2). *1013400*. [123-86-4].
A clear, colourless liquid, flammable, slightly soluble in water, miscible with alcohol and with ether.
d_{20}^{20}: about 0.88.
n_D^{20}: about 1.395.
Distillation range (2.2.11). Not less than 95 per cent distils between 123 °C and 126 °C.

Butyl acetate R1. *1013401*.
A clear, colourless liquid, flammable, slightly soluble in water, miscible with alcohol and with ether.
d_{20}^{20}: about 0.883.
n_D^{20}: about 1.395.
Butanol. Not more than 0.2 per cent, determined by gas chromatography.

n-Butyl formate. Not more than 0.1 per cent, determined by gas chromatography.

n-Butyl propionate. Not more than 0.1 per cent, determined by gas chromatography.

Water. Not more than 0.1 per cent.

Assay. Not less than 99.5 per cent of $C_6H_{12}O_2$, determined by gas chromatography.

Butylamine. $C_4H_{11}N$. (M_r 73.1). *1013600*. [109-73-9].
1-Butanamine.
Distil and use within one month.
A colourless liquid, miscible with water, with alcohol and with ether.
n_D^{20}: about 1.401.
bp: about 78 °C.

***tert*-Butylamine.** *1100900*. [75-64-9].
See *1,1-dimethylethylamine R*.

Butylated hydroxytoluene. *1013800*. [128-37-0].
See *Butylhydroxytoluene R*.

Butylboronic acid. $C_4H_{11}BO_2$. (M_r 101.9). *1013700*.
[4426-47-5].
Contains not less than 98 per cent of $C_4H_{11}BO_2$.
mp: 90 °C to 92 °C.

***tert*-Butylhydroperoxide.** $C_4H_{10}O_2$. (M_r 90.1). *1118000*.
[75-91-2]. 1,1-Dimethylethylhydroperoxide.
Flammable liquid, soluble in organic solvents.
d_{20}^{20}: 0.898.
n_D^{20}: 1.401.
bp: 35 °C.

Butylhydroxytoluene. *1013800*. [128-37-0].
See *Butylhydroxytoluene (0581)*.

Butyl methacrylate. $C_8H_{14}O_2$. (M_r 142.2). *1145400*.
[97-88-1]. Butyl 2-methylpropenoate.
Clear, colourless solution.
d_4^{20}: about 0.894.
n_D^{20}: about 1.424.
bp: about 163 °C.

***tert*-Butyl methyl ether.** *1013900*. [1634-04-4].
See *1,1-dimethylethyl methyl ether R*.

Butyl parahydroxybenzoate. *1103900*. [94-26-8].
See *Butyl parahydroxybenzoate (0881)*.

Butyric acid. $C_4H_8O_2$. (M_r 88.1). *1014000*. [107-92-6].
Butanoic acid.
Contains not less than 99.0 per cent of $C_4H_8O_2$.

An oily liquid, miscible with water and with alcohol.
d_{20}^{20}: about 0.96.
n_D^{20}: about 1.398.
bp: about 163 °C.

Butyrolactone. $C_4H_6O_2$. (M_r 86.1). *1104000*. [96-48-0].
Dihydro-2(3H)-furanone. γ-Butyrolactone.
Oily liquid, miscible with water, soluble in methanol and in ether.
n_D^{25}: about 1.435.
bp: about 204 °C.

Cadmium. Cd. (A_r 112.4). *1014100.* [10108-64-2].
A silvery-white, lustrous metal, practically insoluble in water, freely soluble in nitric acid and in hot hydrochloric acid.

Caesium chloride. CsCl. (M_r 168.4). *1014200.* [7647-17-8].
A white powder, very soluble in water, freely soluble in methanol, practically insoluble in acetone.

Caffeic acid. $C_9H_8O_4$. (M_r 180.2). *1014300.* [331-39-5].
(*E*)-3-(3,4-Dihydroxyphenyl)propenoic acid.
White or almost white crystals or plates, freely soluble in hot water and in alcohol, sparingly soluble in cold water.
mp: about 225 °C, with decomposition.
A freshly prepared solution at pH 7.6 shows two absorption maxima (*2.2.25*), at 293 nm and 329 nm.

Caffeine. *1014400.* [58-08-2].
See *Caffeine (0267)*.

Calcium carbonate. *1014500.* [471-34-1].
See *Calcium carbonate (0014)*.

> **Calcium carbonate R1.** *1014501.*
> It complies with the requirements of *calcium carbonate R* and with the following additional requirement:
>
> *Chlorides (2.4.4).* Not more than 50 ppm.

Calcium chloride. *1014600.* [10035-04-8].
See *Calcium chloride (0015)*.

> **Calcium chloride solution.** *1014601.*
> A 73.5 g/l solution.

> **Calcium chloride solution 0.01 M.** *1014602.*
> Dissolve 0.147 g of *calcium chloride R* in *water R* and dilute to 100.0 ml with the same solvent.

> **Calcium chloride solution 0.02 M.** *1014603.*
> Dissolve 2.94 g of *calcium chloride R* in 900 ml of *water R*, adjust to pH 6.0 to 6.2 and dilute to 1000.0 ml with *water R*.
>
> Store at 2 °C to 8 °C.

Calcium chloride R1. $CaCl_2,4H_2O$. (M_r 183.1). *1014700.*
Calcium chloride tetrahydrate.
Contains not more than 0.05 ppm of Fe.

Calcium chloride, anhydrous. $CaCl_2$. (M_r 111.0). *1014800.*
[10043-52-4].
Contains not less than 98.0 per cent of $CaCl_2$, calculated with reference to the dried substance.
White granules, deliquescent, very soluble in water, freely soluble in alcohol and in methanol.
Loss on drying (2.2.32). Not more than 5.0 per cent, determined by drying in an oven at 200 °C.
Store in an airtight container, protected from moisture.

Calcium hydroxide. $Ca(OH)_2$. (M_r 74.1). *1015000.*
[1305-62-0]. Calcium dihydroxide.
A white powder, almost completely soluble in 600 parts of water.

> **Calcium hydroxide solution.** *1015001.*
> A freshly prepared saturated solution.

Calcium lactate. *1015100.* [41372-22-9].
See *Calcium lactate pentahydrate (0468)*.

Calcium sulphate. $CaSO_4,\frac{1}{2}H_2O$. (M_r 145.1). *1015200.*
[10034-76-1]. Calcium sulphate hemihydrate.
A white powder, soluble in about 1500 parts of water, practically insoluble in alcohol. When mixed with half its mass of water it rapidly solidifies to a hard and porous mass.

Calcium sulphate solution. *1015201.*
Shake 5 g of *calcium sulphate R* with 100 ml of *water R* for 1 h and filter.

Calconecarboxylic acid. $C_{21}H_{14}N_2O_7S,3H_2O$. ($M_r$ 492.5). *1015300.* [3737-95-9]. 2-Hydroxy-1-(2-hydroxy-4-sulpho-1-naphthylazo)naphthalene-3-carboxylic acid.
A brownish-black powder, slightly soluble in water, very slightly soluble in acetone and in alcohol, sparingly soluble in dilute solutions of sodium hydroxide.

> **Calconecarboxylic acid triturate.** *1015301.*
> Mix 1 part of *calconecarboxylic acid R* with 99 parts of *sodium chloride R*.
>
> *Test for sensitivity.* Dissolve 50 mg of calconecarboxylic acid triturate in a mixture of 2 ml of *strong sodium hydroxide solution R* and 100 ml of *water R*. The solution is blue but becomes violet on addition of 1 ml of a 10 g/l solution of *magnesium sulphate R* and 0.1 ml of a 1.5 g/l solution of *calcium chloride R* and turns pure blue on addition of 0.15 ml of *0.01 M sodium edetate*.

Camphene. $C_{10}H_{16}$. (M_r 136.2). *1139200.* [79-92-5].
2,2-Dimethyl-3-methylenebicyclo[2.2.1]heptane.
Camphene used in gas chromatography complies with the following additional test.
Assay. Examine by gas chromatography (*2.2.28*) as prescribed in the monograph on *Rosemary Oil (1846)*.
The content is not less than 90 per cent calculated by the normalisation procedure.

Camphor. *1113000.* [76-22-2]. See *Camphor, racemic (0655)*.
Camphor used in gas chromatography complies with the following additional test.
Assay. Examine by gas chromatography (*2.2.28*) as prescribed in the monograph on *Lavender oil (1338)*.
Test solution. A 10 g/l solution of the substance to be examined in *hexane R*.
The area of the principal peak is not less than 98.0 per cent of the area of all the peaks in the chromatogram obtained. Disregard the peak due to hexane.

(1*S*)-(+)-10-Camphorsulphonic acid. $C_{10}H_{16}O_4S$. (M_r 232.3). *1104100.* [3144-16-9]. (1*S*,4*R*)-(+)-2-Oxo-10-bornenesulphonic acid. [(1*S*)-7,7-Dimethyl-2-oxobicyclo[2.2.1]heptan-1-yl]methanesulphonic acid. Reychler's acid.
Prismatic crystals, hygroscopic, soluble in water.
Contains not less than 99.0 per cent of (1*S*)-(+)-10-camphorsulphonic acid.
$[\alpha]_D^{20}$: +20 ± 1 (43 g/l solution in *water R*).
mp: about 194 °C, with decomposition.
ΔA (*2.2.41*): 10.2×10^3 determined at 290.5 nm on a 1.0 g/l solution.

Capric acid. $C_{10}H_{20}O_2$. (M_r 172.3). *1142000.* [334-48-5].
Decanoic acid.
Crystalline solid, very slightly soluble in water, soluble in ethanol.
bp: about 270 °C.
mp: about 31.4 °C.
Capric acid used in the assay of total fatty acids in Saw palmetto fruit (1848) complies with the following additional requirement.
Assay. Examine by gas chromatography (*2.2.28*) as prescribed in the monograph on *Saw palmetto fruit (1848)*.
The content of capric acid is not less than 98 per cent, calculated by the normalisation procedure.

General Notices (1) apply to all monographs and other texts

4. Reagents

Capric alcohol. *1024700.*
See *Decanol R.*

Caproic acid. $C_6H_{12}O_2$. (M_r 116.2). *1142100.* [142-62-1].
Hexanoic acid.
Oily liquid, sparingly soluble in water.
d_4^{20}: about 0.926.
n_D^{20}: about 1.417.
bp: about 205 °C.
Caproic acid used in the assay of total fatty acids in Saw palmetto fruit (1848) complies with the following additional requirement.
Assay. Examine by gas chromatography (*2.2.28*) as prescribed in the monograph on *Saw palmetto fruit (1848)*.
The content of caproic acid is not less than 98 per cent, calculated by the normalisation procedure.

ε-Caprolactam. $C_6H_{11}NO$. (M_r 113.2). *1104200.* [105-60-2].
Hexane-6-lactam.
Hygroscopic flakes, freely soluble in water, in ethanol and in methanol.
mp: about 70 °C.

Caprylic acid. $C_8H_{16}O_2$. (M_r 144.2). *1142200.* [124-07-2].
Octanoic acid.
Slightly yellow, oily liquid.
d_4^{20}: about 0.910.
n_D^{20}: about 1.428.
bp: about 239.7 °C.
mp: about 16.7 °C.
Caprylic acid used in the assay of total fatty acids in Saw palmetto fruit (1848) complies with the following additional requirement.
Assay. Examine by gas chromatography (*2.2.28*) as prescribed in the monograph on *Saw palmetto fruit (1848)*.
The content of caprylic acid is not less than 98 per cent, calculated by the normalisation procedure.

Carbazole. $C_{12}H_9N$. (M_r 167.2). *1015400.* [86-74-8].
Dibenzopyrrole.
Crystals, practically insoluble in water, freely soluble in acetone, slightly soluble in ethanol.
mp: about 245 °C.

Carbomer. *1015500.* [9007-20-9].
A cross-linked polymer of acrylic acid; it contains a large proportion (56 per cent to 68 per cent) of carboxylic acid (CO_2H) groups after drying at 80 °C for 1 h. Average relative molecular mass about 3×10^6.
pH (*2.2.3*). The pH of a 10 g/l suspension is about 3.

Carbon dioxide. *1015600.* [124-38-9].
See *Carbon dioxide (0375)*.

Carbon dioxide R1. CO_2. (M_r 44.01). *1015700.*
Contains not less than 99.995 per cent V/V of CO_2.
Carbon monoxide: less than 5 ppm.
Oxygen: less than 25 ppm.
Nitric oxide: less than 1 ppm.

Carbon dioxide R2. CO_2. (M_r 44.01). *1134500.*
Contains not less than 99 per cent V/V of CO_2.

Carbon disulphide. CS_2. (M_r 76.1). *1015800.* [75-15-0].
A colourless or yellowish, flammable liquid, practically insoluble in water, miscible with ethanol and with ether.
d_{20}^{20}: about 1.26.
bp: 46 °C to 47 °C.

Carbon for chromatography, graphitised. *1015900.*
Carbon chains having a length greater than C_9 with a particle size of 400 µm to 850 µm.

Density: 0.72.
Surface area: 10 m²/g.
Do not use at a temperature higher than 400 °C.

Carbon monoxide. CO. (M_r 28.01). *1016000.* [630-08-0].
Contains not less than 99.97 per cent V/V of CO.

Carbon monoxide R1. CO. (M_r 28.01). *1134600.* [630-08-0].
Contains not less than 99 per cent V/V of CO.

Carbon tetrachloride. CCl_4. (M_r 153.8). *1016100.* [56-23-5].
Tetrachloromethane.
A clear, colourless liquid, practically insoluble in water, miscible with alcohol.
d_{20}^{20}: 1.595 to 1.598.
bp: 76 °C to 77 °C.

Carbophenothion. $C_{11}H_{16}ClO_2PS_3$. (M_r 342.9). *1016200.* [786-19-6]. *O,O*-Diethyl *S*-[[(4-chlorophenyl)thio]methyl]-phosphorodithioate.
Yellowish liquid, practically insoluble in water, miscible with organic solvents.
d_4^{25}: about 1.27.
For the monograph *Wool Fat (0134)*, a suitable certified reference solution (10 ng/µl in iso-octane) may be used.

Car-3-ene. $C_{10}H_{16}$. (M_r 136.2). *1124000.* [498-15-7]. 3,7,7-Trimethylbicyclo[4.1.0]hept-3-ene. 4,7,7-Trimethyl-3-norcarene.
A liquid with a pungent odour, slightly soluble in water, soluble in organic solvents.
d_{20}^{20}: about 0.864.
n_D^{20}: 1.473 to 1.474.
$[\alpha]_D^{20}$: + 15 to + 17.
bp: 170 °C to 172 °C.
Car-3-ene used in gas chromatography complies with the following additional test.
Assay. Examine by gas chromatography (*2.2.28*) as prescribed in the monograph on *Nutmeg oil (1552)*.
The content is not less than 95.0 per cent, calculated by the normalisation procedure.

Carob bean gum. *1104500.*
The ground endosperm of the fruit kernels of *Ceratonia siliqua* L. Taub.
A white powder containing 70 per cent to 80 per cent of a water-soluble gum consisting mainly of galactomannoglycone.

Carvacrol. $C_{10}H_{14}O$. (M_r 150.2). *1016400.* [499-75-2]. 5-Isopropyl-2-methylphenol.
Brownish liquid, practically insoluble in water, very soluble in alcohol and in ether.
d_{20}^{20}: about 0.975.
n_D^{20}: about 1.523.
bp: about 237 °C.
Carvacrol used in gas chromatography complies with the following additional test.
Assay. Examine by gas chromatography (*2.2.28*) as prescribed in the monograph on *Peppermint oil (0405)*.
Test solution. Dissolve 0.1 g in about 10 ml of *acetone R*.
The area of the principal peak is not less than 95.0 per cent of the area of all the peaks in the chromatogram obtained (disregard the peak due to acetone).

Carvone. $C_{10}H_{14}O$. (M_r 150.2). *1016500.* [2244-16-8]. (*S*)-*p*-Mentha-6,8-dien-2-one. (+)-2-Methyl-5-(1-methylethenyl)-cyclohex-2-enone.
A liquid, practically insoluble in water, miscible with alcohol.
d_{20}^{20}: about 0.965

n_D^{20}: about 1.500.

$[\alpha]_D^{20}$: about + 61.

bp: about 230 °C.

Carvone used in gas chromatography complies with the following additional test.

Assay. Examine by gas chromatography (*2.2.28*) as prescribed in the monograph on *Peppermint oil (0405)* using the substance to be examined as the test solution.

The area of the principal peak is not less than 98.0 per cent of the total area of the peaks.

β-Caryophyllene. $C_{15}H_{24}$. (M_r 204.4). *1101000*. [87-44-5]. (*E*)-(1*R*,9*S*)-4,11,11-Trimethyl-8-methylenebicyclo[7.2.0]undec-4-ene.

An oily liquid, practically insoluble in water, miscible with alcohol and with ether.

d_4^{17}: about 0.905.

n_D^{20}: about 1.492.

$[\alpha]_D^{15}$: about −5.2.

bp_{14}: 129 °C to 130 °C.

β-Caryophyllene used in gas chromatography complies with the following additional test.

Assay. Examine by gas chromatography (*2.2.28*) as prescribed in the monograph on *Clove oil (1091)* using the substance to be examined as the test solution.

The area of the principal peak is not less than 98.5 per cent of the total area of the peaks.

Casein. *1016600*. [9000-71-9].
A mixture of related phosphoproteins obtained from milk. White, amorphous powder or granules, very slightly soluble in water and in non-polar organic solvents. It dissolves in concentrated hydrochloric acid giving a pale-violet solution. It forms salts with acids and bases. Its isoelectric point is at about pH 4.7. Alkaline solutions are laevorotatory.

Catalpol. $C_{15}H_{22}O_{10}$. (M_r 362.3). *1142300*. [2415-24-9].
mp: 203 °C to 205 °C.

Catechin. $C_{15}H_{14}O_6 \cdot xH_2O$. ($M_r$ 290.3 for the anhydrous substance). *1119000*. [154-23-4]. (+)-(2*R*,3*S*)-2-(3,4-Dihydroxyphenyl)-3,4-dihydro-2*H*-chromene-3,5,7-triol. Catechol. Cianidanol. Cyanidol.

Catholyte for isoelectric focusing pH 3 to 5. *1113100*. 0.1 M β-Alanine.
Dissolve 8.9 g of *β-alanine R* in *water R* and dilute to 1000 ml with the same solvent.

Cation exchange resin. *1016700*.
A resin in protonated form with sulphonic acid groups attached to a polymer lattice consisting of polystyrene cross-linked with 8 per cent of divinylbenzene. It is available as beads and the particle size is specified after the name of the reagent in the tests where it is used.

Cation exchange resin R1. *1121900*.
A resin in protonated form with sulphonic acid groups attached to a polymer lattice consisting of polystyrene cross-linked with 4 per cent of divinylbenzene. It is available as beads and the particle size is specified after the name of the reagent in the tests where it is used.

Cation exchange resin (calcium form), strong. *1104600*.
A resin in calcium form with sulphonic acid groups attached to a polymer lattice consisting of polystyrene cross-linked with 8 per cent of divinylbenzene. The particle size is specified after the name of the reagent in the tests where it is used.

Cellulose for chromatography. *1016800*. [9004-34-6].
A fine, white, homogeneous powder with an average particle size less than 30 μm.
Preparation of a thin layer. Suspend 15 g in 100 ml of *water R* and homogenise in an electric mixer for 60 s. Coat carefully cleaned plates with a layer 0.1 mm thick using a spreading device. Allow to dry in air.

Cellulose for chromatography R1. *1016900*.
Microcrystalline cellulose. A fine, white homogeneous powder with an average particle size less than 30 μm.
Preparation of a thin layer. Suspend 25 g in 90 ml of *water R* and homogenise in an electric mixer for 60 s. Coat carefully cleaned plates with a layer 0.1 mm thick using a spreading device. Allow to dry in air.

Cellulose for chromatography F_{254}. *1017000*.
Microcrystalline cellulose F_{254}. A fine, white, homogeneous powder with an average particle size less than 30 μm, containing a fluorescent indicator having an optimal intensity at 254 nm.
Preparation of a thin layer. Suspend 25 g in 100 ml of *water R* and homogenise using an electric mixer for 60 s. Coat carefully cleaned plates with a layer 0.1 mm thick using a spreading device. Allow to dry in air.

Cephaëline dihydrochloride. $C_{28}H_{40}Cl_2N_2O_4, 7H_2O$. ($M_r$ 666). *1017100*. [5884-43-5]. (*R*)-1-[(2*S*,3*R*,11b*S*)-3-Ethyl-1,3,4,6,7,11b-hexahydro-9,10-dimethoxy-2*H*-benzo[*a*]quinolizin-2-ylmethyl]-1,2,3,4-tetrahydro-7-methoxyisoquinolin-6-ol dihydrochloride heptahydrate.
A white to yellowish, crystalline powder, freely soluble in water, soluble in acetone and in alcohol.
$[\alpha]_D^{20}$: about + 25, determined on a 20 g/l solution.

Cephalin. *1017200*.
To 0.5 g to 1 g of *acetone-dried ox brain R* add 20 ml of *acetone R* and allow to stand for 2 h. Centrifuge at 500 *g* for 2 min and decant the supernatant liquid. Dry the residue under reduced pressure and, to the dried material, add 20 ml of *chloroform R* and allow to stand for 2 h, shaking frequently. Remove the solid material by filtration or centrifugation and evaporate the chloroform under reduced pressure. Suspend the residue in 5 ml to 10 ml of a 9 g/l solution of *sodium chloride R*.

Solvents used to prepare the reagent should contain a suitable antioxidant, for example, 0.02 g/l of butylated hydroxyanisole.

Store frozen or freeze-dried and use within 3 months.

Cerium sulphate. $Ce(SO_4)_2, 4H_2O$. (M_r 404.3). *1017300*. [123333-60-8]. Cerium(IV) sulphate. Ceric sulphate.
Yellow or orange-yellow, crystalline powder or crystals, very slightly soluble in water, slowly soluble in dilute acids.

Cerous nitrate. $Ce(NO_3)_3, 6H_2O$. (M_r 434.3). *1017400*. [10294-41-4]. Cerium trinitrate hexahydrate.
A colourless or pale yellow, crystalline powder, freely soluble in water and in alcohol.

Cetostearyl alcohol. *1017500*. [67762-27-0].
See *Cetostearyl alcohol (0702)*.

Cetrimide. *1017600*. [8044-71-1].
See *Cetrimide (0378)*.

Cetyltrimethylammonium bromide. $C_{19}H_{42}BrN$. (M_r 364.5). *1017700*. [57-09-0]. Cetrimonium bromide.
N-Hexadecyl-*N*,*N*,*N*-trimethylammonium bromide.
A white, crystalline powder, soluble in water, freely soluble in alcohol.
mp: about 240 °C.

Charcoal, activated. *1017800.* [64365-11-3].
See *Activated charcoal (0313).*

Chloral hydrate. *1017900.* [302-17-0].
See *Choral hydrate (0265).*

   Chloral hydrate solution. *1017901.*
   A solution of 80 g in 20 ml of *water R.*

Chloramine. *1018000.* [7080-50-4].
See *Chloramine (0381).*

   Chloramine solution. *1018001.*
   A 20 g/l solution. Prepare immediately before use.

   Chloramine solution R1. *1018002.*
   A 0.1 g/l solution of *chloramine R.* Prepare immediately before use.

   Chloramine solution R2. *1018003.*
   A 0.2 g/l solution. Prepare immediately before use.

Chlordane. $C_{10}H_6Cl_8$. (M_r 409.8). *1124100.* [12789-03-6].
bp: about 175 °C.
mp: about 106 °C.
A suitable certified reference solution of technical grade (10 ng/µl in iso-octane) may be used.

Chlordiazepoxide. *1113200.* [58-25-3].
See *Chlordiazepoxide (0656).*

Chlorfenvinphos. $C_{12}H_{14}Cl_3O_4P$. (M_r 359.6). *1124200.* [470-90-6].
A suitable certified reference solution (10 ng/µl in cyclohexane) may be used.

Chloroacetanilide. C_8H_8ClNO. (M_r 169.6). *1018100.* [539-03-7]. 4'-Chloroacetanilide.
Contains not less than 95 per cent of C_8H_8ClNO.
A crystalline powder, practically insoluble in water, soluble in alcohol.
mp: about 178 °C.

Chloroacetic acid. $C_2H_3ClO_2$. (M_r 94.5). *1018200.* [79-11-8].
Colourless or white crystals, deliquescent, very soluble in water, soluble in alcohol and in ether.
Store in an airtight container.

Chloroaniline. C_6H_6ClN. (M_r 127.6). *1018300.* [106-47-8]. 4-Chloroaniline.
Crystals, soluble in hot water, freely soluble in alcohol and in ether.
mp: about 71 °C.

4-Chlorobenzenesulphonamide. $C_6H_6ClNO_2S$. (M_r 191.6). *1097400.* [98-64-6].
White powder.
mp: about 145 °C.

2-Chlorobenzoic acid. $C_7H_5ClO_2$. (M_r 156.7). *1139300.* [118-91-2].
Soluble in water, slightly soluble in ethanol.
bp: about 285 °C.
mp: about 140 °C.

Chlorobutanol. *1018400.* [57-15-8].
See *Anhydrous chlorobutanol (0382).*

2-Chloro-2-deoxy-D-glucose. $C_6H_{11}ClO_5$. (M_r 198.6). *1134700.* [14685-79-1].
A white crystalline, very hygroscopic powder, soluble in water and in dimethyl sulphoxide, insoluble in alcohol.

2-Chloroethanol. C_2H_5ClO. (M_r 80.5). *1097500.* [107-07-3].
Colourless liquid, soluble in alcohol.

d_{20}^{20}: about 1.197.
n_D^{20}: about 1.442.
bp: about 130 °C.
mp: about −89 °C.

   2-Chloroethanol solution. *1097501.*
   Dissolve 125 mg of *2-chloroethanol R* in *2-propanol R* and dilute to 50 ml with the same solvent. Dilute 5 ml of the solution to 50 ml with *2-propanol R.*

Chloroethylamine hydrochloride. $C_2H_7Cl_2N$. (M_r 116.0). *1124300.* [870-24-6]. 2-Chloroethanamine hydrochloride.
mp: about 145 °C.

(2-Chloroethyl)diethylamine hydrochloride. $C_6H_{15}Cl_2N$. (M_r 172.1). *1018500.* [869-24-9].
A white, crystalline powder, very soluble in water and in methanol, freely soluble in methylene chloride, practically insoluble in hexane.
mp: about 211 °C.

Chloroform. $CHCl_3$. (M_r 119.4). *1018600.* [67-66-3].
Trichloromethane.
A clear, colourless liquid, slightly soluble in water, miscible with alcohol.
d_{20}^{20}: 1.475 to 1.481.
bp: about 60 °C.
Chloroform contains 0.4 per cent *m/m* to 1.0 per cent *m/m* of ethanol.

Ethanol. Introduce 1.00 g (*m* g) into a ground-glass-stoppered flask. Add 15.0 ml of *nitrochromic reagent R*, close the flask, shake vigorously for 2 min and allow to stand for 15 min. Add 100 ml of *water R* and 5 ml of a 200 g/l solution of *potassium iodide R*. After 2 min titrate with *0.1 M sodium thiosulphate*, using 1 ml of *starch solution R* as indicator, until a light green colour is obtained (n_1 ml of *0.1 M sodium thiosulphate*). Carry out a blank assay (n_2 ml of *0.1 M sodium thiosulphate*). Calculate the percentage of ethanol using the expression:

$$\frac{(n_2 - n_1)\,0.115}{m}$$

   Chloroform, acidified. *1018601.*
   To 100 ml of *chloroform R* add 10 ml of *hydrochloric acid R.* Shake, allow to stand and separate the two layers.

   Chloroform, ethanol-free. *1018602.*
   Shake 200 ml of *chloroform R* with four quantities, each of 100 ml, of *water R.* Dry over 20 g of *anhydrous sodium sulphate R* for 24 h. Distil the filtrate over 10 g of *anhydrous sodium sulphate R.* Discard the first 20 ml of distillate. Prepare immediately before use.

Chloroform stabilised with amylene. $CHCl_3$. (M_r 119.4). *1018700.*

A clear, colourless liquid, slightly soluble in water, miscible with alcohol.

Water. Not more than 0.05 per cent.

Residue on evaporation. Not more than 0.001 per cent.

Minimum transmittance (2.2.25), determined using *water R* as compensation liquid:

not less than 50 per cent at 255 nm,

not less than 80 per cent at 260 nm,

not less than 98 per cent at 300 nm.

Assay. Not less than 99.8 per cent of $CHCl_3$, determined by gas chromatography.

Chlorogenic acid. $C_{16}H_{18}O_9$. (M_r 354.3). *1104700.*
[327-97-9]. (1S,3R,4R,5R)-3-[(3,4-Dihydroxycinnamoyl)oxy]-
1,4,5-trihydroxycyclohexanecarboxylic acid.
A white, crystalline powder or white needles, freely soluble
in boiling water, in acetone and in ethanol.
$[\alpha]_D^{26}$: about −35.2.
mp: about 208 °C.
Chromatography. Examined under the conditions described
on Identification A in the monograph on *Belladonna leaf
dry extract, standardised (1294)*, the chromatogram shows
only one principal zone.

3-Chloro-2-methylaniline. C_7H_8ClN. (M_r 141.6). *1139400.*
[87-60-5]. 6-Chloro-2-toluidine.
Not miscible with water, slightly soluble in ethanol.
d_{20}^{20}: : about 1.171.
n_D^{20}: : about 1.587.
bp: about 115 °C.
mp: about 2 °C.

2-Chloro-4-nitroaniline. $C_6H_5ClN_2O_2$. (M_r 172.6). *1018800.*
[121-87-9].
A yellow, crystalline powder, freely soluble in methanol.
mp: about 107 °C.
Store protected from light.

Chlorophenol. C_6H_5ClO. (M_r 128.6). *1018900.* [106-48-9].
4-Chlorophenol.
Colourless or almost colourless crystals, slightly soluble in
water, very soluble in alcohol, in ether and in solutions of
alkali hydroxides.
mp: about 42 °C.

Chloroplatinic acid. $H_2Cl_6Pt,6H_2O$. (M_r 517.9). *1019000.*
[18497-13-7]. Hydrogen hexachloroplatinate(IV)
hexahydrate.
Contains not less than 37.0 per cent m/m of platinum
(A_r 195.1).

Brownish-red crystals or a crystalline mass, very soluble in
water, soluble in alcohol.

Assay. Ignite 0.200 g to constant mass at 900 °C and weigh
the residue (platinum).

Store protected from light.

3-Chloropropane-1,2-diol. $C_3H_7ClO_2$. (M_r 110.5). *1097600.*
[96-24-2].
Colourless liquid, soluble in water, alcohol and ether.
d_{20}^{20}: about 1.322.
n_D^{20}: about 1.480
bp: about 213 °C.

5-Chlorosalicylic acid. $C_7H_5ClO_3$. (M_r 172.6). *1019100.*
[321-14-2].
A white or almost white, crystalline powder, soluble in
methanol.
mp: about 173 °C.

Chlorothiazide. *1112100.* [58-94-6].
See *Chlorothiazide (0385)*.

Chlorotrimethylsilane. C_3H_9ClSi. (M_r 108.6). *1019300.*
[75-77-4].
A clear, colourless liquid, fuming in air.
d_{20}^{20}: about 0.86.
n_D^{20}: about 1.388.
bp: about 57 °C.

Chlorpyriphos. $C_9H_{11}Cl_3NO_3PS$. (M_r 350.6). *1124400.*
[2921-88-2].
bp: about 200 °C.
mp: 42 °C to 44 °C.
A suitable certified reference solution (10 ng/µl in
cyclohexane) may be used.

Chlorpyriphos-methyl. $C_7H_7Cl_3NO_3PS$. (M_r 322.5). *1124500.*
[5598-13-0].
mp: 45 °C to 47 °C.
A suitable certified reference solution (10 ng/µl in
cyclohexane) may be used.

Chlortetracycline hydrochloride. *1145500.*
See *Chlortetracycline hydrochloride (0173)*.

Cholesterol. *1019400.* [57-88-5].
See *Cholesterol (0993)*.

Choline chloride. $C_5H_{14}ClNO$. (M_r 139.6). *1019500.*
[67-48-1]. (2-Hydroxyethyl)trimethylammonium chloride.
Deliquescent crystals, very soluble in water and in alcohol.
Chromatography. Examine as prescribed in the monograph
Suxamethonium chloride (0248), applying 5 µl of a 0.2 g/l
solution in *methanol R*. The chromatogram shows one
principal spot.

Store in an airtight container.

Chromazurol S. $C_{23}H_{13}Cl_2Na_3O_9S$. (M_r 605). *1019600.*
[1667-99-8].
Schultz No. 841.
Colour Index No. 43825.
Trisodium 5-[(3-carboxylato-5-methyl-4-oxocyclohexa-2,5-
dien-1-ylidene)(2,6-dichloro-3-sulphonatophenyl)methyl]-2-
hydroxy-3-methylbenzoate.
A brownish-black powder, soluble in water, slightly soluble
in alcohol.

Chromic acid cleansing mixture. *1019700.*
A saturated solution of *chromium trioxide R* in *sulphuric
acid R*.

Chromic potassium sulphate. $CrK(SO_4)_2,12H_2O$. (M_r 499.4).
1019800. [7788-99-0]. Chrome alum.
Large, violet-red to black crystals, freely soluble in water,
practically insoluble in alcohol.

Chromium(III) trichloride hexahydrate.
$[Cr(H_2O)_4Cl_2]Cl,2H_2O$. (M_r 266.5). *1104800.* [10060-12-5].
A dark green crystalline powder, hygroscopic.
Store protected from humidity and oxidising agents.

Chromium trioxide. CrO_3. (M_r 100.0). *1019900.* [1333-82-0].
Dark brownish-red needles or granules, deliquescent, very
soluble in water.
Store in an airtight glass container.

Chromophore substrate R1. *1020000.*
Dissolve N-α-benzyloxycarbonyl-D-arginyl-L-glycyl-
L-arginine-4-nitroanilide dihydrochloride in
water R to give a 0.003 M solution. Dilute in
*tris(hydroxymethyl)aminomethane-EDTA buffer solution
pH 8.4 R* to 0.0005 M before use.

Chromophore substrate R2. *1020100.*
Dissolve D-phenylalanyl-L-pipecolyl-L-arginine-4-nitroanilide
dihydrochloride in *water R* to give a 0.003 M
solution. Dilute before use in titrating in
*tris(hydroxymethyl)aminomethane-EDTA buffer
solution pH 8.4 R* to give a 0.0005 M solution.

Chromotrope II B. $C_{16}H_9N_3Na_2O_{10}S_2$. ($M_r$ 513.4). *1020200.*
[548-80-1].
Schultz No. 67.

Colour Index No. 16575.
Disodium 4,5-dihydroxy-3-(4-nitrophenylazo)naphthalene-2,7-disulphonate.
A reddish-brown powder, soluble in water giving a yellowish-red colour, practically insoluble in alcohol.

Chromotrope II B solution. *1020201.*
A 0.05 g/l solution in *sulphuric acid R*.

Chromotropic acid, sodium salt. $C_{10}H_6Na_2O_8S_2,2H_2O$. ($M_r$ 400.3). *1020300.* [5808-22-0].
Schultz No. 1136.
Disodium 4,5-dihydroxynaphthalene-2,7-disulphonate dihydrate. Disodium 1,8-dihydroxynaphthalene-3,6-disulphonate dihydrate.
A yellowish-white powder, soluble in water, practically insoluble in alcohol.

Chromotropic acid, sodium salt solution. *1020301.*
Dissolve 0.60 g of *chromotropic acid, sodium salt R* in about 80 ml of *water R* and dilute to 100 ml with the same solvent. Use this solution within 24 h.

Chrysanthemin. $C_{21}H_{21}ClO_{11}$. (M_r 485.5). *1134800.* [7084-24-4]. Kuromanin chloride. 2-(3,4-Dihydroxyphenyl)-3-(β-D-glucopyranosyl)oxy-5,7-dihydroxy-1-benzopyrylium chloride.

A reddish-brown crystalline powder, soluble in water and in alcohol.

Absorbance (*2.2.25*). A 0.01 g/l solution in a mixture of 1 volume of *hydrochloric acid R* and 999 volumes of *methanol R* shows a maximum at 528 nm.

α-Chymotrypsin for peptide mapping. *1142400.*
α-Chymotrypsin of high purity, treated to eliminate tryptic activity.

Cinchonidine. $C_{19}H_{22}N_2O$. (M_r 294.4). *1020400.* [485-71-2]. (*R*)-(Quinol-4-yl)[(2*S*,4*S*,5*R*)-5-vinylquinuclidin-2-yl]methanol.
A white, crystalline powder, very slightly soluble in water and in light petroleum, soluble in alcohol, slightly soluble in ether.
$[\alpha]_D^{20}$: − 105 to − 110, determined on a 50 g/l solution in *alcohol R*.
mp: about 208 °C, with decomposition.
Store protected from light.

Cinchonine. $C_{19}H_{22}N_2O$. (M_r 294.4). *1020500.* [118-10-5]. (*S*)-(Quinol-4-yl)[(2*R*,4*S*,5*R*)-5-vinylquinuclidin-2-yl]methanol.
A white, crystalline powder, very slightly soluble in water, sparingly soluble in alcohol and in methanol, slightly soluble in ether.
$[\alpha]_D^{20}$: + 225 to + 230, determined on a 50 g/l solution in *alcohol R*.
mp: about 263 °C.
Store protected from light.

Cineole. $C_{10}H_{18}O$. (M_r 154.3). *1020600.* [470-82-6].
1,8-Cineole. Eucalyptol. 1,8-Epoxy-*p*-menthane.
A colourless liquid, practically insoluble in water, miscible with ethanol and with ether.
d_{20}^{20}: 0.922 to 0.927.
n_D^{20}: 1.456 to 1.459.

Freezing point (*2.2.18*). 0 °C to 1 °C.

Distillation range (*2.2.11*). 174 °C to 177 °C.

Phenol. Shake 1 g with 20 ml of *water R*. Allow to separate and add to 10 ml of the aqueous layer 0.1 ml of *ferric chloride solution R1*. No violet colour develops.

Turpentine oil. Dissolve 1 g in 5 ml of *alcohol (90 per cent V/V) R*. Add dropwise freshly prepared *bromine water R*. Not more than 0.5 ml is required to give a yellow colour lasting for 30 min.

Residue on evaporation. Not more than 0.05 per cent. To 10.0 ml add 25 ml of *water R*, evaporate on a water-bath and dry the residue to constant mass at 100 °C to 105 °C.

Cineole used in gas chromatography complies with the following additional test.

Assay. Examine by gas chromatography (*2.2.28*) as prescribed in the monograph on *Peppermint oil (0405)* using the substance to be examined as the test solution.

The area of the principal peak is not less than 98.0 per cent of the total area of the peaks.

1,4-Cineole. $C_{10}H_{18}O$. (M_r 154.3). *1142500.* [470-67-7].
1-Methyl-4-(1-methylethyl)-7-oxabicyclo[2.2.1]heptane.
1-Isopropyl-4-methyl-7-oxabicyclo[2.2.1]heptane.
A colourless liquid.
d_4^{20}: about 0.900.
n_D^{20}: about 1.445.
bp: about 173 °C.

Cinnamic aldehyde. C_9H_8O. (M_r 132.1). *1020700.* [104-55-2].
3-Phenylpropenal.
A yellowish to greenish-yellow, oily liquid, slightly soluble in water, very soluble in alcohol and in ether.
d_{20}^{20}: 1.048 to 1.051.
n_D^{20}: about 1.620.
Store protected from light, in a cool place.

***trans*-Cinnamic aldehyde.** C_9H_8O. (M_r 132.2). *1124600.* [14371-10-9]. (*E*)-3-Phenylprop-2-enal.
trans-Cinnamic aldehyde used in gas chromatography complies with the following additional test.

Assay. Examine by gas chromatography (*2.2.28*) as prescribed in the monograph on *Cassia oil (1496)*.

The content is not less than 99.0 per cent, calculated by the normalisation procedure.

Cinnamyl acetate. $C_{11}H_{12}O_2$. (M_r 176.2). *1124700.* [103-54-8]. 3-Phenylprop-2-en-1-yl acetate.
n_D^{20}: about 1.542.
bp: about 262 °C.

Cinnamyl acetate used in gas chromatography complies with the following additional test.

Assay. Examine by gas chromatography (*2.2.28*) as prescribed in the monograph on *Cassia oil (1496)*.

The content is not less than 99.0 per cent, calculated by the normalisation procedure.

Citral. $C_{10}H_{16}O$. (M_r 152.2). *1020800.* [5392-40-5]. Mixture of (2*E*)- and (2*Z*)-3,7-Dimethylocta-2,6-dienal.
A light yellow liquid, practically insoluble in water, miscible with alcohol, with ether and with glycerol.
Chromatography. Examine by thin-layer chromatography (*2.2.27*), using *silica gel GF$_{254}$ R* as the coating substance. Apply to the plate 10 μl of a 1 g/l solution in *toluene R*. Develop over a path of 15 cm using a mixture of 15 volumes of *ethyl acetate R* and 85 volumes of *toluene R*. Allow the plate to dry in air and examine in ultraviolet light at 254 nm. The chromatogram obtained shows only one principal spot.

Citral used in gas chromatography complies with the following additional test.

Assay. Examine by gas chromatography (*2.2.28*) as prescribed in the monograph on *Citronella oil (1609)*.

The content of citral (neral + geranial) is not less than 95.0 per cent calculated by the normalisation procedure.

Citrated rabbit plasma. *1020900.*

Collect blood by intracardiac puncture from a rabbit kept fasting for 12 h, using a plastic syringe with a No. 1 needle containing a suitable volume of 38 g/l solution of *sodium citrate R* so that the final volume ratio of citrate solution to blood is 1 : 9. Separate the plasma by centrifugation at 1500 *g* to 1800 *g* at 15 °C to 20 °C for 30 min.

Store at 0 °C to 6 °C.

Use within 4 h of collection.

Citric acid. *1021000.* [5949-29-1]. See *Citric acid monohydrate (0456).*
When used in the limit test for iron, it complies with the following additional requirement:
Dissolve 0.5 g in 10 ml of *water R*, add 0.1 ml of *thioglycollic acid R*, mix and make alkaline with *ammonia R*. Dilute to 20 ml with *water R*. No pink colour appears in the solution.

Citric acid, anhydrous. *1021200.* [77-92-9]. See *Anhydrous citric acid (0455).*

Citronellal. $C_{10}H_{18}O$. (M_r 154.3). *1113300.* [106-23-0]. 3,7-Dimethyl-6-octenal.
Very slightly soluble in water, soluble in alcohols.
d_{20}^{20}: 0.848 to 0.856.
n_D^{20}: about 1.446.
$[\alpha]_D^{25}$: about + 11.50.

Citronellal used in gas chromatography complies with the following additional test.

Assay. Examine by gas chromatography (*2.2.28*) as prescribed in the monograph on *Citronella oil (1609).*

The content is not less than 95.0 per cent calculated by the normalisation procedure.

Citronellol. $C_{10}H_{20}O$. (M_r 156.3). *1134900.* [106-22-9]. 3,7-Dimethyloct-6-en-1-ol.
A clear, colourless liquid, practically insoluble in water, miscible with alcohol.
d_{20}^{20}: 0.857.
n_D^{20}: 1.456.
bp: 220 °C to 222 °C.

Citronellol used in gas chromatography complies with the following additional test.

Assay. Examine by gas chromatography (*2.2.28*) as prescribed in the monograph on *Citronella oil (1609).*

The content is not less than 95.0 per cent calculated by the normalisation procedure.

Store in an airtight container, protected from light.

Citronellyl acetate. $C_{12}H_{22}O_2$. (M_r 198.3). *1135000.* [150-84-5]. 3,7-Dimethyl-6-octen-1-yl acetate.
d_{20}^{20}: 0.890.
n_D^{20}: 1.443.
bp: 229 °C.

Citronellyl acetate used in gas chromatography complies with the following additional test.

Assay. Examine by gas chromatography (*2.2.28*) as prescribed in the monograph on *Citronella oil (1609).*

The content is not less than 97.0 per cent calculated by the normalisation procedure.

Store in an airtight container, protected from light.

Citropten. $C_{11}H_{10}O_4$. (M_r 206.2). *1021300.* [487-06-9]. Limettin. 5,7-Dimethoxy-2*H*-1-benzopyran-2-one.
Needle-shaped crystals, practically insoluble in water, in ether and in light petroleum, freely soluble in acetone and in alcohol.
mp: about 145 °C.
Chromatography. Examine by thin-layer chromatography (*2.2.27*), using *silica gel GF$_{254}$R* as the coating substance. Apply to the plate 10 µl of a 1 g/l solution in *toluene R*. Develop over a path of 15 cm using a mixture of 15 volumes of *ethyl acetate R* and 85 volumes of *toluene R*. Allow the plate to dry in air and examine in ultraviolet light at 254 nm. The chromatogram obtained shows only one principal spot.

Clobetasol propionate. $C_{25}H_{32}ClFO_5$. (M_r 467.0). *1097700.* [25122-46-7]. 21-Chloro-9-fluoro-11β,17-dihydroxy-16β-methylpregna-1,4-diene-3,20-dione 17-propionate.
A white crystalline powder, insoluble in water, soluble in alcohol and in acetone.
$[\alpha]_D^{20}$: about + 104 (in dioxan).
mp: about 196 °C.

Coagulation factor V solution. *1021400.*

Coagulation factor V solution may be prepared by the following method or by any other method which excludes factor VIII.

Prepare the factor V reagent from fresh oxalated bovine plasma, by fractionation at 4 °C with a saturated solution of *ammonium sulphate R* prepared at 4 °C. Separate the fraction which precipitates between 38 per cent and 50 per cent of saturation, which contains factor V without significant contamination with factor VIII. Remove the ammonium sulphate by dialysis and dilute the solution with a 9 g/l solution of *sodium chloride R* to give a solution containing between 10 per cent and 20 per cent of the quantity of factor V present in fresh human normal plasma.

Determination of factor V content. Prepare two dilutions of the preparation of factor V in *imidazole buffer solution pH 7.3 R* containing 1 volume of the preparation in 10 volumes and in 20 volumes of the buffer solution respectively. Test each dilution as follows: mix 0.1 ml of *plasma substrate deficient in factor V R*, 0.1 ml of the solution to be examined, 0.1 ml of *thromboplastin R* and 0.1 ml of a 3.5 g/l solution of *calcium chloride R* and measure the coagulation times, i.e. the interval between the moment at which the calcium chloride solution is added and the first indication of the formation of fibrin, which may be observed visually or by means of a suitable apparatus.

In the same manner, determine the coagulation time (in duplicate) of four dilutions of human normal plasma in *imidazole buffer solution pH 7.3 R*, containing respectively, 1 volume in 10 (equivalent to 100 per cent of factor V), 1 volume in 50 (20 per cent), 1 volume in 100 (10 per cent), and 1 volume in 1000 (1 per cent). Using two-way logarithmic paper plot the average coagulation times for each dilution of human plasma against the equivalent percentage of factor V and read the percentage of factor V for the two dilutions of the factor V solution by interpolation. The mean of the two results gives the percentage of factor V in the solution to be examined.

Store the solution in the frozen state at a temperature not higher than − 20 °C.

Cobalt chloride. $CoCl_2,6H_2O$. (M_r 237.9). *1021600.* [7791-13-1].
A red, crystalline powder or deep-red crystals, very soluble in water, soluble in alcohol.

Cobalt nitrate. Co(NO$_3$)$_2$,6H$_2$O. (M_r 291.0). *1021700*. [10026-22-9].
Small garnet-red crystals, very soluble in water.

Codeine. *1021800*. [6059-47-8].
See *Codeine (0076)*.

Codeine phosphate. *1021900*. [52-28-8].
See *Codeine phosphate hemihydrate (0074)*.

Congo red. C$_{32}$H$_{22}$N$_6$Na$_2$O$_6$S$_2$. (M_r 697). *1022000*. [573-58-0].
Schultz No. 360.
Colour Index No. 22120.
Disodium (biphenyl-4,4′-diyl-bis-2,2′-azo)bis(1-aminonaphthalene-4-sulphonate).
A brownish-red powder, soluble in water.

> **Congo red paper.** *1022002*.
> Immerse strips of filter paper for a few minutes in *congo red solution R*. Allow to dry.

> **Congo red solution.** *1022001*.
> Dissolve 0.1 g of *congo red R* in a mixture of 20 ml of *alcohol R* and *water R* and dilute to 100 ml with *water R*.
> *Test for sensitivity.* To 0.2 ml of the congo red solution add 100 ml of *carbon dioxide-free water R* and 0.3 ml of *0.1 M hydrochloric acid*. The solution is blue. Not more than 0.3 ml of *0.1 M sodium hydroxide* is required to change the colour to pink.
> Colour change: pH 3.0 (blue) to pH 5.0 (pink).

Coomassie blue. *1001400*. [3861-73-2].
See *acid blue 92 R*.

> **Coomassie blue solution.** *1001401*.
> See *acid blue 92 solution R*.

Coomassie staining solution. *1012201*.
A 1.25 g/l solution of *acid blue 83 R* in a mixture consisting of 1 volume of *glacial acetic acid R*, 4 volumes of *methanol R* and 5 volumes of *water R*. Filter.

Copper. Cu. (A_r 63.55). *1022100*. [7440-50-8].
Cleaned foil, turnings, wire or powder of the pure metal of electrolytic grade.

Copper acetate. C$_4$H$_6$CuO$_4$,H$_2$O. (M_r 199.7). *1022200*. [142-71-2].
Blue-green crystals or powder, freely soluble in boiling water, soluble in water and in alcohol, slightly soluble in ether and in glycerol (85 per cent).

Copper edetate solution. *1022300*.
To 2 ml of a 20 g/l solution of *copper acetate R* add 2 ml of *0.1 M sodium edetate* and dilute to 50 ml with *water R*.

Copper nitrate. Cu(NO$_3$)$_2$,3H$_2$O. (M_r 241.6). *1022400*. [10031-43-3]. Chloride dinitrate trihydrate.
Dark blue crystals, hygroscopic, very soluble in water giving a strongly acid reaction, freely soluble in alcohol and in dilute nitric acid.
Store in an airtight container.

Copper sulphate. CuSO$_4$,5H$_2$O. (M_r 249.7). *1022500*. [7758-99-8].
A blue powder or deep-blue crystals, slowly efflorescent, very soluble in water, slightly soluble in alcohol.

> **Copper sulphate solution.** *1022501*.
> A 125 g/l solution.

Copper tetrammine, ammoniacal solution of. *1022600*.
Dissolve 34.5 g of *copper sulphate R* in 100 ml of *water R* and, whilst stirring, add dropwise *concentrated ammonia R* until the precipitate which forms dissolves completely. Keeping the temperature below 20 °C, add dropwise with continuous shaking 30 ml of *strong sodium hydroxide solution R*. Filter through a sintered-glass filter (40), wash with *water R* until the filtrate is clear and take up the precipitate with 200 ml of *concentrated ammonia R*. Filter through a sintered-glass filter and repeat the filtration to reduce the residue to a minimum.

Cortisone acetate. *1097800*. [50-04-4].
See *Cortisone acetate (0321)*.

Coumaphos. C$_{14}$H$_{16}$ClO$_5$PS. (M_r 362.8). *1124800*. [56-72-4].
mp: 91 °C to 92 °C.
A suitable certified reference solution (10 ng/µl in iso-octane) may be used.

Coumarin. C$_9$H$_6$O$_2$. (M_r 146.1). *1124900*. [91-64-5].
2*H*-Chromen-2-one. 2*H*-1-Benzopyran-2-one.
A colourless, crystalline powder or orthorhombic or rectangular crystals, very soluble in boiling water, soluble in alcohol. It dissolves in solutions of alkali hydroxides.
mp: 68 °C to 70 °C.
Coumarin used in gas chromatography complies with the following additional test.
Assay. Examine by gas chromatography (*2.2.28*) as prescribed in the monograph on *Cassia oil (1496)*.
The content is not less than 98.0 per cent, calculated by the normalisation procedure.

Cresol. C$_7$H$_8$O. (M_r 108.1). *1022700*. [95-48-7]. *o*-Cresol.
2-Methylphenol.
Crystals or a super-cooled liquid becoming dark on exposure to light and air, miscible with ethanol and with ether, soluble in about 50 parts of water and soluble in solutions of alkali hydroxides.
d_{20}^{20}: about 1.05.
n_D^{20}: 1.540 to 1.550.
bp: about 190 °C.
Freezing point (2.2.18). Not below 30.5 °C.
Residue on evaporation. Not more than 0.1 per cent *m/m*, determined by evaporating on a water-bath and drying in an oven at 100 °C to 105 °C.
Distil before use.
Store protected from light, moisture and oxygen and distil before use.

***m*-Cresol purple.** C$_{21}$H$_{18}$O$_5$S. (M_r 382.44). *1121700*. [2303-01-7]. *m*-Cresolsulphonphthalein.
An olive-green, crystalline powder, slightly soluble in water, soluble in alcohol, in glacial acetic acid and in methanol.

> ***m*-Cresol purple solution.** *1121701*.
> Dissolve 0.1 g of *m-cresol purple R* in 13 ml of *0.01 M sodium hydroxide*, dilute to 100 ml with *water R* and mix.
> *Colour change.* pH 1.2 (red) to pH 2.8 (yellow); pH 7.4 (yellow) to pH 9.0 (purple).

Cresol red. C$_{21}$H$_{18}$O$_5$S. (M_r 382.4). *1022800*. [1733-12-6].
Cresolsulfonphthalein. 4,4′-(3*H*-2,1-Benzoxathiol-3-ylidene)bis-(2-methylphenol) *S,S*-dioxide.
A reddish-brown crystalline powder, slightly soluble in water, soluble in alcohol and in dilute solutions of alkali hydroxides.

> **Cresol red solution.** *1022801*.
> Dissolve 0.1 g of *cresol red R* in a mixture of 2.65 ml of *0.1 M sodium hydroxide* and 20 ml of *alcohol R* and dilute to 100 ml with *water R*.

Test for sensitivity. A mixture of 0.1 ml of the cresol red solution and 100 ml of *carbon dioxide-free water R* to which 0.15 ml of *0.02 M sodium hydroxide* has been added is purple-red. Not more than 0.15 ml of *0.02 M hydrochloric acid* is required to change the colour to yellow.

Colour change. pH 7.0 (yellow) to pH 8.6 (red).

Crystal violet. $C_{25}H_{30}ClN_3$. (M_r 408.0). *1022900.* [548-62-9].
Schultz No. 78.
Colour Index No. 42555.
Hexamethyl-pararosanilinium chloride.
Dark-green powder or crystals, soluble in water and in alcohol.

Crystal violet solution. *1022901.*

Dissolve 0.5 g of *crystal violet R* in *anhydrous acetic acid R* and dilute to 100 ml with the same solvent.

Test for sensitivity. To 50 ml of *anhydrous acetic acid R* add 0.1 ml of the crystal violet solution. On addition of 0.1 ml of *0.1 M perchloric acid* the bluish-purple solution turns bluish-green.

Cupric chloride. $CuCl_2,2H_2O$. (M_r 170.5). *1023000.*
[10125-13-0]. Cupric chloride dihydrate.
Greenish-blue powder or crystals, deliquescent in moist air, efflorescent in dry air, freely soluble in water, in alcohol and in methanol, sparingly soluble in acetone, slightly soluble in ether.
Store in an airtight container.

Cupri-citric solution. *1023100.*
Dissolve 25 g of *copper sulphate R*, 50 g of *citric acid R* and 144 g of *anhydrous sodium carbonate R* in *water R* and dilute to 1000 ml with the same solvent.

Cupri-citric solution R1. *1023200.*

Dissolve 25 g of *copper sulphate R*, 50 g of *citric acid R* and 144 g of *anhydrous sodium carbonate R* in *water R* and dilute to 1000 ml with the same solvent.

Adjust the solution so that it complies with the following requirements:

a) To 25.0 ml add 3 g of *potassium iodide R*. Add 25 ml of a 25 per cent *m/m* solution of *sulphuric acid R* with precaution and in small quantities. Titrate with *0.1 M sodium thiosulphate* using 0.5 ml of *starch solution R*, added towards the end of the titration, as indicator.

24.5 ml to 25.5 ml of *0.1 M sodium thiosulphate* is used in the titration.

b) Dilute 10.0 ml to 100.0 ml with *water R* and mix. To 10.0 ml of the solution, add 25.0 ml of *0.1 M hydrochloric acid* and heat for 1 h on a water-bath. Cool, adjust with *water R* to the initial volume and titrate with *0.1 M sodium hydroxide*, using 0.1 ml of *phenolphthalein solution R1* as indicator.

5.7 ml to 6.3 ml of *0.1 M sodium hydroxide* is used in the titration.

c) Dilute 10.0 ml to 100.0 ml with *water R* and mix. Titrate 10.0 ml of the solution with *0.1 M hydrochloric acid*, using 0.1 ml of *phenolphthalein solution R1* as indicator.

6.0 ml to 7.5 ml of *0.1 M hydrochloric acid* is used in the titration.

Cupri-tartaric solution. *1023300.*

Solution I. Dissolve 34.6 g of *copper sulphate R* in *water R* and dilute to 500 ml with the same solvent.

Solution II. Dissolve 173 g of *sodium potassium tartrate R* and 50 g of *sodium hydroxide R* in 400 ml of *water R*. Heat to boiling, allow to cool and dilute to 500 ml with *carbon dioxide-free water R*.

Mix equal volumes of the two solutions immediately before use.

Cupri-tartaric solution R2. *1023302.*
Add 1 ml of a solution containing 5 g/l of *copper sulphate R* and 10 g/l of *potassium tartrate R* to 50 ml of *sodium carbonate solution R1*. Prepare immediately before use.

Cupri-tartaric solution R3. *1023303.*
Prepare a solution containing 10 g/l of *copper sulphate R* and 20 g/l of *sodium tartrate R*. To 1.0 ml of the solution add 50 ml of *sodium carbonate solution R2*. Prepare immediately before use.

Cupri-tartaric solution R4. *1023304.*
Solution I. 150 g/l *copper sulphate R*.

Solution II. Dissolve 2.5 g of *anhydrous sodium carbonate R*, 2.5 g of *potassium sodium tartrate R*, 2.0 g of *sodium hydrogen carbonate R*, and 20.0 g of *anhydrous sodium sulphate R* in *water R* and dilute to 100 ml with the same solvent.

Mix 1 part of solution I with 25 parts of solution II immediately before use.

Curcumin. $C_{21}H_{20}O_6$. (M_r 368.4). *1023500.* [458-37-7]. 1,7-bis(4-Hydroxy-3-methoxyphenyl)hepta-1,6-diene-3,5-dione.
An orange-brown, crystalline powder, practically insoluble in water, soluble in glacial acetic acid, practically insoluble in ether.
mp: about 183 °C.

Cyanoacetic acid. $C_3H_3NO_2$. (M_r 85.1). *1097900.* [372-09-8].
White to yellowish-white, hygroscopic crystals, very soluble in water.
Store in an airtight container.

Cyanocobalamin. *1023600.* [68-19-9].
See *Cyanocobalamin (0547)*.

Cyanogen bromide solution. *1023700.* [506-68-3].
Add dropwise, with cooling *0.1 M ammonium thiocyanate* to *bromine water R* until the yellow colour disappears. Prepare immediately before use.

Cyanoguanidine. $C_2H_4N_4$. (M_r 84.1). *1023800.* [461-58-5].
Dicyandiamide. 1-Cyanoguanidine.
A white, crystalline powder, sparingly soluble in water and in alcohol, practically insoluble in ether and in methylene chloride.
mp: about 210 °C.

Cyclohexane. C_6H_{12}. (M_r 84.2). *1023900.* [110-82-7].
A clear, colourless, flammable liquid, practically insoluble in water, miscible with organic solvents.
d_{20}^{20}: about 0.78.
bp: about 80.5 °C.

Cyclohexane used in spectrophotometry complies with the following additional requirements.

Minimum transmittance (2.2.25), determined using *water R* as compensation liquid:

45 per cent at 220 nm,

70 per cent at 235 nm,

90 per cent at 240 nm,

98 per cent at 250 nm.

Cyclohexane R1. *1023901.*

Complies with the requirements prescribed for *cyclohexane R* and with the following additional requirement:

The fluorescence, measured at 460 nm, under illumination with an excitant light beam at 365 nm, is not more intense than that of a solution containing 0.002 ppm of *quinine R* in *0.05 M sulphuric acid.*

Cyclohexylamine. $C_6H_{13}N$. (M_r 99.2). *1024000.* [108-91-8]. A colourless liquid, soluble in water, miscible with usual organic solvents.
n_D^{20}: about 1.460.
bp: 134 °C to 135 °C.

Cyclohexylenedinitrilotetra-acetic acid. $C_{14}H_{22}N_2O_8,H_2O$. (M_r 364.4). *1024100.* *trans*-Cyclohexylene-1,2-dinitrilo-*N,N,N',N'*-tetra-acetic acid.
A white, crystalline powder.
mp: about 204 °C.

Cyclohexylmethanol. $C_7H_{14}O$. (M_r 114.2). *1135200.* [100-49-2]. Cyclohexylcarbinol.
A liquid with a slight odour of camphor, soluble in alcohol.
n_D^{25}: about 1.464.
bp: about 185 °C.

3-Cyclohexylpropionic acid. $C_9H_{16}O_2$. (M_r 156.2). *1119200.* [701-97-3].
A clear liquid.
d_{20}^{20}: about 0.998.
n_D^{20}: about 1.4648.
bp: about 130 °C.

Cyhalothrin. $C_{23}H_{19}ClF_3NO_3$. (M_r 449.9). *1125000.* [91465-08-6].
bp: 187 °C to 190 °C.
mp: about 49 °C.
A suitable certified reference solution (10 ng/µl in cyclohexane) may be used.

p-**Cymene.** $C_{10}H_{14}$. (M_r 134.2). *1113400.* [99-87-6]. 1-Isopropyl-4-methylbenzene.
A colourless liquid, practically insoluble in water, soluble in alcohol and in ether.
d_{20}^{20}: about 0.858.
n_D^{20}: about 1.4895.
bp: 175 °C to 178 °C.

p-*Cymene used in gas chromatography complies with the following additional test.*

Assay. Examine by gas chromatography (*2.2.28*) as prescribed in the monograph *Peppermint oil (0405).*

Test solution. The substance to be examined.

The area of the principal peak is not less than 96.0 per cent of the area of all the peaks in the chromatogram obtained.

Cypermethrin. $C_{22}H_{19}Cl_2NO_3$. (M_r 416.3). *1125100.* [52315-07-8].
bp: 170 °C to 195 °C.
mp: 60 °C to 80 °C.
A suitable certified reference solution (10 ng/µl in cyclohexane) may be used.

L-Cysteine. $C_3H_7NO_2S$. (M_r 121.1). *1024200.* [52-90-4]. A powder, freely soluble in water, in alcohol and in acetic acid, practically insoluble in acetone.

Cysteine hydrochloride. *1024300.* [7048-04-6]. See *Cysteine hydrochloride monohydrate (0895).*

L-Cystine. $C_6H_{12}N_2O_4S_2$. (M_r 240.3). *1024400.* [56-89-3]. A white, crystalline powder, practically insoluble in water and in alcohol. It dissolves in dilute solutions of alkali hydroxides. It decomposes at 250 °C.
$[\alpha]_D^{20}$: −218 to −224, determined in *1 M hydrochloric acid.*

Dantron. $C_{14}H_8O_4$. (M_r 240.2). *1024500.* [117-10-2]. 1,8-Dihydroxyanthraquinone. 1,8-Dihydroxyanthracene-9,10-dione.
A crystalline orange powder, practically insoluble in water, slightly soluble in alcohol, soluble in solutions of alkali hydroxides.
mp: about 195 °C.
Dantron used in the sesquiterpenic acids assay in Valerian root (0453) complies with the following additional requirements.
$A_{1\ cm}^{1\%}$: 355 to 375, determined at 500 nm in *1 M potassium hydroxide.*

Assay. Examine by liquid chromatography (*2.2.29*) as prescribed in the monograph on *Valerian Root (0453)* at the concentration of the reference solution. The content of dantron is not less than 95 per cent calculated by the normalisation procedure

o,p′-**DDD.** $C_{14}H_{10}Cl_4$. (M_r 320.0). *1125200.* [53-19-0]. 1-(2-Chlorophenyl)-1-(4-chlorophenyl)-2,2-dichloroethane.
A suitable certified reference solution (10 ng/µl in cyclohexane) may be used.

p,p′-**DDD.** $C_{14}H_{10}Cl_4$. (M_r 320.0). *1125300.* [72-54-8]. 1,1-bis(4-Chlorophenyl)-2,2-dichloroethane.
bp: about 193 °C.
mp: about 109 °C.
A suitable certified reference solution (10 ng/µl in cyclohexane) may be used.

o,p′-**DDE.** $C_{14}H_8Cl_4$. (M_r 318.0). *1125400.* [3424-82-6]. 1-(2-Chlorophenyl)-1-(4-chlorophenyl)-2,2-dichloroethylene.
A suitable certified reference solution (10 ng/µl in cyclohexane) may be used.

p,p′-**DDE.** $C_{14}H_8Cl_4$. (M_r 318.0). *1125500.* [72-55-9]. 1,1-bis(4-Chlorophenyl)-2,2-dichloroethylene.
bp: 316 °C to 317 °C.
mp: 88 °C to 89 °C.
A suitable certified reference solution (10 ng/µl in cyclohexane) may be used.

o,p′-**DDT.** $C_{14}H_9Cl_5$. (M_r 354.5). *1125600.* [789-02-6]. 1-(2-Chlorophenyl)-1-(4-chlorophenyl)-2,2,2-trichloroethane.
A suitable certified reference solution (10 ng/µl in cyclohexane) may be used.

p,p′-**DDT.** $C_{14}H_9Cl_5$. (M_r 354.5). *1125700.* [50-29-3]. 1,1-bis(4-Chlorophenyl)-2,2,2-trichloroethane.
bp: about 260 °C.
mp: 108 °C to 109 °C.
A suitable certified reference solution (10 ng/µl in cyclohexane) may be used.

Decane. $C_{10}H_{22}$. (M_r 142.3). *1024600.* [124-18-5]. A colourless liquid, practically insoluble in water.
n_D^{20}: about 1.411.
bp: about 174 °C.

Decanol. $C_{10}H_{22}O$. (M_r 158.3). *1024700.* [112-30-1]. *n*-Decyl alcohol.
A viscous liquid, solidifying at about 6 °C, practically insoluble in water, soluble in alcohol and in ether.
n_D^{20}: about 1.436.
bp: about 230 °C.

Deltamethrin. $C_{22}H_{19}Br_2NO_3$. (M_r 505.2). *1125800.* [52918-63-5].
bp: about 300 °C.
mp: about 98 °C.
A suitable certified reference solution (10 ng/µl in cyclohexane) may be used.

Demeclocycline hydrochloride. *1145600.*
See *Demeclocycline hydrochloride (0176)*.

2′-Deoxyuridine. $C_9H_{12}N_2O_5$. (M_r 228.2). *1024800.* [951-78-0]. 1-(2-Deoxy-β-d-*erythro*-pentofuranosyl)-1*H*,3*H*-pyrimidine-2,4-dione.
mp: about 165 °C.
Chromatography. Examine as prescribed in the monograph on *Idoxuridine (0669)*, applying 5 µl of a 0.25 g/l solution. The chromatogram obtained shows only one principal spot.

Destaining solution. *1012202.*
A mixture consisting of 1 volume of *glacial acetic acid R*, 4 volumes of *methanol R* and 5 volumes of *water R*.

Deuterated acetic acid. $C_2{}^2H_4O_2$. (M_r 64.1). *1101100.* [1186-52-3]. Tetradeuteroacetic acid. Acetic-d_3 acid-*d*.
The degree of deuteration is not less than 99.7 per cent.
d_{20}^{20}: about 1.12.
n_D^{20}: about 1.368.
bp: about 115 °C.
mp: about 16 °C.

Deuterated acetone. $C_3{}^2H_6O$. (M_r 64.1). *1024900.* [666-52-4]. Acetone-d_6. ($^2H_6$)-Acetone.
The degree of deuteration is not less than 99.5 per cent.
A clear, colourless liquid, miscible with water, with dimethylformamide, with ethanol, with ether and with methanol.
d_{20}^{20}: about 0.87.
n_D^{20}: about 1.357.
bp: about 55 °C.
Water and deuterium oxide: Not more than 0.1 per cent.

Deuterated chloroform. C^2HCl_3. (M_r 120.4). *1025000.* [865-49-6]. (^2H)-Chloroform. Chloroform-*d*.
The degree of deuteration is not less than 99.7 per cent.
A clear, colourless liquid, practically insoluble in water, miscible with acetone, with alcohol and with ether. It may be stabilised over silver foil.
d_{20}^{20}: about 1.51.
n_D^{20}: about 1.445.
bp: about 60 °C.
Water and deuterium oxide: Not more than 0.05 per cent.

Deuterated dimethyl sulphoxide. $C_2{}^2H_6OS$. (M_r 84.2). *1025100.* [2206-27-1]. ($^2H_6$)-Dimethyl sulphoxide. Dimethyl sulphoxide-d_6.
The degree of deuteration is not less than 99.8 per cent.
A very hygroscopic liquid, practically colourless, viscous, soluble in water, in acetone, in ethanol and in ether.
d_{20}^{20}: about 1.18.
mp: about 20 °C.
Water and deuterium oxide: Not more than 0.1 per cent.
Store in an airtight container.

Deuterated methanol. C^2H_4O. (M_r 36.1). *1025200.* [811-98-3]. (^2H)-Methanol. Methanol-*d*.
The degree of deuteration is not less than 99.8 per cent.
Clear, colourless liquid miscible with water, with alcohol and with methylene chloride.
d_{20}^{20}: about 0.888.
n_D^{20}: about 1.326.
bp: 65.4 °C.

Deuterium oxide. ^2H_2O. (M_r 20.03). *1025300.* [7789-20-0]. Deuterated water.
The degree of deuteration is not less than 99.7 per cent.
d_{20}^{20}: about 1.11.
n_D^{20}: about 1.328.
bp: about 101 °C.

Developer solution. *1122500.*
Dilute 2.5 ml of a 20 g/l solution of *citric acid R* and 0.27 ml of *formaldehyde R* to 500.0 ml with *water R*.

Dextran for chromatography, cross-linked R2. *1025500.*
A bead-form dextran with a fraction range suitable for the separation of peptides and proteins with relative molecular masses of 15×10^2 to 30×10^3. When dry, the beads have a diameter of 20 µm to 80 µm.

Dextran for chromatography, cross-linked R3. *1025600.*
A bead-form dextran with a fraction range suitable for the separation of peptides and proteins with relative molecular masses of 4×10^3 to 15×10^4. When dry, the beads have a diameter of 40 µm to 120 µm.

Dextrose. *1025700.* [50-99-7].
See *glucose R*.

3,3′-Diaminobenzidine tetrahydrochloride.
$C_{12}H_{18}Cl_4N_4$, $2H_2O$. (M_r 396.1). *1098000.* [7411-49-6]. 3,3′,4,4′-Biphenyl-tetramine.
An almost white or slightly pink powder, soluble in water.
mp: about 280 °C, with decomposition.

Diatomaceous earth. *1025900.* [91053-39-3].
A white or almost white, fine granular powder, made up of siliceous frustules of fossil diatoms or of debris of fossil diatoms, practically insoluble in water, in alcohol and in ether.
The substance may be identified by microscopic examination with a magnification of × 500.

Diatomaceous earth for gas chromatography. *1026000.*
A white or almost white, fine granular powder, made up of siliceous frustules of fossil diatoms or of debris of fossil diatoms, practically insoluble in water, in alcohol and in ether. The substance may be identified by microscopic examination with a magnification of × 500. The substance is purified by treating with *hydrochloric acid R* and washing with *water R*.
Particle size. Not more than 5 per cent is retained on a sieve No. 180. Not more than 10 per cent passes a sieve No. 125.

Diatomaceous earth for gas chromatography R1. *1026100.*
A white or almost white, fine granular powder, made up of siliceous frustules of fossil diatoms or of debris of fossil diatoms, practically insoluble in water, in alcohol and in ether. The substance may be identified by microscopic examination with a magnification of × 500. The substance is purified by treating with *hydrochloric acid R* and washing with *water R*.
Particle size. Not more than 5 per cent is retained on a sieve No. 250. Not more than 10 per cent passes a sieve No. 180.

Diatomaceous earth for gas chromatography R2. *1026200.*
A white or almost white, fine granular powder with a specific surface area of about 0.5 m²/g, made up of siliceous frustules of fossil diatoms or of debris of fossil diatoms, practically insoluble in water, in alcohol and in ether. The substance may be identified by microscopic examination with a magnification of × 500. The substance is purified by treating with *hydrochloric acid R* and washing with *water R*.
Particle size. Not more than 5 per cent is retained on a sieve No. 180. Not more than 10 per cent passes a sieve No. 125.

Diatomaceous earth for gas chromatography, silanised. *1026300.*

Diatomaceous earth for gas chromatography R silanised with dimethyldichlorosilane or other suitable silanising agents.

Diatomaceous earth for gas chromatography, silanised R1. *1026400.*

Prepared from crushed pink firebrick and silanised with dimethyldichlorosilane or other suitable silanising agents. The substance is purified by treating with *hydrochloric acid R* and washing with *water R*.

Diazinon. $C_{12}H_{21}N_2O_3PS$. (M_r 304.3). *1125900.* [333-41-5]. bp: about 306 °C.

A suitable certified reference solution (10 ng/µl in iso-octane) may be used.

Diazobenzenesulphonic acid solution R1. *1026500.*

Dissolve 0.9 g of *sulphanilic acid R* in a mixture of 30 ml of *dilute hydrochloric acid R* and 70 ml of *water R*. To 3 ml of the solution add 3 ml of a 50 g/l solution of *sodium nitrite R*. Cool in an ice-bath for 5 min, add 12 ml of the sodium nitrite solution and cool again. Dilute to 100 ml with *water R* and keep the reagent in an ice-bath. Prepare extemporaneously but allow to stand for 15 min before use.

Dibutylamine. $C_8H_{19}N$. (M_r 129.3). *1126000.* [111-92-2]. *N*-Butylbutan-1-amine.

Colourless liquid.

n_D^{20}: about 1.417.

bp: about 159 °C.

Dibutyl ether. $C_8H_{18}O$. (M_r 130.2). *1026700.* [142-96-1].

A colourless, flammable liquid, practically insoluble in water, miscible with ethanol and with ether.

d_{20}^{20}: about 0.77.

n_D^{20}: about 1.399.

Do not distil if the dibutyl ether does not comply with the test for peroxides.

Peroxides. Place 8 ml of *potassium iodide and starch solution R* in a 12 ml ground-glass-stoppered cylinder about 1.5 cm in diameter. Fill completely with the substance to be examined, shake vigorously and allow to stand protected from light for 30 min. No colour is produced.

The name and concentration of any added stabiliser are stated on the label.

Dibutyl phthalate. $C_{16}H_{22}O_4$. (M_r 278.3). *1026800.* [84-74-2]. Dibutyl benzene-1,2-dicarboxylate.

A clear, colourless or faintly coloured, oily liquid, very slightly soluble in water, miscible with acetone, with alcohol and with ether.

d_{20}^{20}: 1.043 to 1.048.

n_D^{20}: 1.490 to 1.495.

Dicarboxidine hydrochloride. $C_{20}H_{26}Cl_2N_2O_6$. (M_r 461.3). *1026900.* [56455-90-4]. 4,4′-[(4,4′-Diaminobiphenyl-3,3′-diyl)dioxy]dibutanoic acid dihydrochloride.

Dichlofenthion. $C_{10}H_{13}Cl_2O_3PS$. (M_r 315.2). *1126100.* [97-17-6].

A suitable certified reference solution (10 ng/µl in cyclohexane) may be used.

Dichloroacetic acid. $C_2H_2Cl_2O_2$. (M_r 128.9). *1027000.* [79-43-6].

Colourless liquid, miscible with water, alcohol and ether.

d_{20}^{20}: about 1.566.

n_D^{20}: about 1.466.

bp: about 193 °C.

Dichloroacetic acid solution. *1027001.*

Dilute 67 ml of *dichloroacetic acid R* to 300 ml with *water R* and neutralise to *blue litmus paper R* using *ammonia R*. Cool, add 33 ml of *dichloroacetic acid R* and dilute to 600 ml with *water R*.

Dichlorobenzene. $C_6H_4Cl_2$. (M_r 147.0). *1027100.* [95-50-1]. 1,2-Dichlorobenzene.

A colourless, oily liquid, practically insoluble in water, soluble in ethanol and in ether.

d_{20}^{20}: about 1.31.

bp: about 180 °C.

(S)-3,5-Dichloro-2,6-dihydroxy-*N*-[(1-ethylpyrrolidin-2-yl)methyl]benzamide hydrobromide. $C_{14}H_{19}BrCl_2O_3$. (M_r 441.1). *1142600.* [113310-88-6].

White, crystalline powder.

$[\alpha]_D^{22}$: + 11.4, determined on a 15.0 g/l solution in *ethanol R*.

mp: about 212 °C.

Dichlorofluorescein. $C_{20}H_{10}Cl_2O_5$. (M_r 401.2). *1027200.* [76-54-0]. 2,7-Dichlorofluorescein.

2-(2,7-Dichloro-6-hydroxy-3-oxo-3*H*-xanthen-9-yl)benzoic acid.

A yellowish-brown to yellow-orange powder, slightly soluble in water, freely soluble in alcohol and in dilute solutions of alkali hydroxides giving a solution showing a yellowish-green fluorescence; practically insoluble in ether.

Dichlorophenolindophenol, sodium salt.

$C_{12}H_6Cl_2NNaO_2,2H_2O$. ($M_r$ 326.1). *1027300.* [620-45-1]. The sodium derivative of 2,6-dichloro-*N*-(4-hydroxyphenyl)-1,4-benzoquinone monoimine dihydrate.

A dark-green powder, freely soluble in water and in ethanol. The aqueous solution is dark blue; when acidified it becomes pink.

Dichlorophenolindophenol standard solution. *1027301.*

Dissolve 50.0 mg of *dichlorophenolindophenol, sodium salt R* in 100.0 ml of *water R* and filter.

Standardisation. Dissolve 20.0 mg of *ascorbic acid R* in 10 ml of a freshly prepared 200 g/l solution of *metaphosphoric acid R* and dilute to 250.0 ml with *water R*. Titrate 5.0 ml rapidly with the dichloro-phenolindophenol standard solution, added from a microburette graduated in 0.01 ml, until the pink colour persists for 10 s, the titration occupying not more than 2 min. Dilute the dichlorophenolindophenol solution with *water R* to make 1 ml of the solution equivalent to 0.1 mg of ascorbic acid ($C_6H_8O_6$).

Use within three days of preparation. Standardise immediately before use.

Dichloroquinonechlorimide. $C_6H_2Cl_3NO$. (M_r 210.4). *1027400.* [101-38-2]. 2,6-Dichloro-*N*-chloro-1,4-benzoquinone mono-imine.

A pale yellow or greenish-yellow crystalline powder, practically insoluble in water, soluble in alcohol and in dilute alkaline solutions.

mp: about 66 °C.

Dichlorvos. $C_4H_7Cl_2O_4P$. (M_r 221). *1101200.* [62-73-7]. 2,2-Dichlorovinyl dimethyl phosphate.

Colourless or brownish-yellow liquid, soluble in water, miscible with most organic solvents.

n_D^{25}: about 1.452.

Dicyclohexyl. $C_{12}H_{22}$. (M_r 166.3). *1135300.* [92-51-3]. Bicyclohexyl.

d_{20}^{20}: about 0.864.

bp: about 227 °C.

mp: about 4 °C.

Dicyclohexylamine. $C_{12}H_{23}N$. (M_r 181.3). *1027500*.
[101-83-7]. *N,N*-Dicyclohexylamine.
Colourless liquid, sparingly soluble in water, miscible with
the usual organic solvents.
n_D^{20}: about 1.484.
bp: about 256 °C.
Freezing point (2.2.18). 0 °C to 1 °C.

Dicyclohexylurea. $C_{13}H_{24}N_2O$. (M_r 224.4). *1027600*.
[2387-23-7]. 1,3-Dicyclohexylurea.
A white, crystalline powder.
mp: about 232 °C.

Didocosahexaenoin. $C_{47}H_{68}O_5$. (M_r 713.0). *1142700*.
[88315-12-2]. Diglyceride of docosahexaenoic acid (C22:6).
Glycerol didocosahexaenoate. (*all-Z*)-Docosahexaenoic acid,
diester with propane-1,2,3-triol.
The reagent from Nu-Chek Prep, Inc. has been found
suitable.

Didodecyl 3,3′-thiodipropionate. $C_{30}H_{58}O_4S$. (M_r 514.8).
1027700. [123-28-4].
A white, crystalline powder, practically insoluble in water,
freely soluble in acetone and in light petroleum, slightly
soluble in alcohol.
mp: about 39 °C.

Dieldrin. $C_{12}H_8Cl_6O$. (M_r 380.9). *1126200*. [60-57-1].
bp: about 385 °C.
mp: about 176 °C.
A suitable certified reference solution (10 ng/µl in
cyclohexane) may be used.

Diethanolamine. $C_4H_{11}NO_2$. (M_r 105.1). *1027800*.
[111-42-2]. 2,2′-Iminobisethanol.
A viscous, clear, slightly yellow liquid or deliquescent crystals
melting at about 28 °C, very soluble in water, in acetone and
in methanol.
d_{20}^{20}: about 1.09.

pH (2.2.3). 10.0 to 11.5, determined on a 50 g/l solution.

*Diethanolamine used in the test for alkaline phosphatase
complies with the following additional test.*

Ethanolamine. Not more than 1.0 per cent. Examine by gas
chromatography (2.2.28), using *propanolamine R* as the
internal standard.

Internal standard solution. Dissolve 1.00 g of
propanolamine R in *acetone R* and dilute to 10.0 ml with
the same solvent.

Test solution (a). Dissolve 5.00 g of the substance to be
examined in *acetone R* and dilute to 10.0 ml with the same
solvent.

Test solution (b). Dissolve 5.00 g of the substance to be
examined in *acetone R*, add 1.0 ml of the internal standard
solution and dilute to 10.0 ml with the same solvent.

Reference solutions. Dissolve 0.50 g of *ethanolamine R*
in *acetone R* and dilute to 10.0 ml with the same solvent.
To 0.5 ml, 1.0 ml and 2.0 ml of this solution, add 1.0 ml of
the internal standard solution and dilute to 10.0 ml with
acetone R.

The chromatographic procedure may be carried out using:

- a column 1 m long and 4 mm in internal diameter packed
  with *diphenylphenylene oxide polymer R* (180 µm to
  250 µm),

- *nitrogen for chromatography R* as the carrier gas at a
  flow rate of 40 ml/min,

- a flame-ionisation detector.

Maintain the temperature of the column at 125 °C for 3 min
and then raise to 300 °C at a rate of 12 °C/min. Maintain
the temperature of the injection port at 250 °C and that of
the detector at 280 °C. Inject 1.0 µl of each test solution and
1.0 µl of each reference solution.

Store in an airtight container.

Diethoxytetrahydrofuran. $C_8H_{16}O_3$. (M_r 160.2). *1027900*.
[3320-90-9]. 2,5-Diethoxytetrahydrofuran. A mixture of the
cis and *trans* isomers.
A clear, colourless or slightly yellowish liquid, practically
insoluble in water, soluble in alcohol, in ether and in most
other organic solvents.
d_{20}^{20}: about 0.98.
n_D^{20}: about 1.418.

Diethylamine. $C_4H_{11}N$. (M_r 73.1). *1028000*. [109-89-7].
A clear, colourless, flammable liquid, strongly alkaline,
miscible with water and with alcohol.
d_{20}^{20}: about 0.71.
bp: about 55 °C.

Diethylaminoethyldextran. *1028200*.
Anion exchange resin presented as the hydrochloride.
A powder forming gels with water.

N,N-Diethylaniline. $C_{10}H_{15}N$. (M_r 149.2). *1028400*. [91-66-7].
d_{20}^{20}: about 0.938.
bp: about 217 °C.
mp: about −38 °C.

Diethylene glycol. $C_4H_{10}O_3$. (M_r 106.1). *1028300*. [111-46-6].
2,2′-Oxydiethanol.
Contains not less than 99.5 per cent *m/m* of $C_4H_{10}O_3$.

A clear, colourless liquid, hygroscopic, miscible with water,
with acetone and with alcohol.
d_{20}^{20}: about 1.118.
n_D^{20}: about 1.447.
bp: 244 °C to 246 °C.
Store in an airtight container.

N,N-Diethylethane-1,2-diamine. *1028500*. [100-36-7].
See *N,N-diethylethylenediamine R*.

N,N-Diethylethylenediamine. $C_6H_{16}N_2$. (M_r 116.2).
1028500. [100-36-7].

Contains not less than 98.0 per cent of $C_6H_{16}N_2$.

A slightly oily liquid, colourless or slightly yellow, strong
odour of ammonia, irritant to the skin, eyes and mucous
membranes.
d_{20}^{20}: 0.827.
bp: 145 °C to 147 °C.
Water (2.5.12). Not more than 1.0 per cent, determined on
0.500 g.

Di(2-ethylhexyl) phthalate. $C_{24}H_{38}O_4$. (M_r 390.5). *1028100*.
Di(2-ethylhexyl) benzene-1,2-dicarboxylate.
A colourless, oily liquid, practically insoluble in water,
soluble in organic solvents.
d_{20}^{20}: about 0.98.
n_D^{20}: about 1.486.
Viscosity (2.2.9). About 80 mPa·s.

Diethylphenylenediamine sulphate. $C_{10}H_{18}N_2O_4S$.
(M_r 262.3). *1028600*. [6283-63-2]. *N,N′*-Diethyl-*p*-
phenylenediamine sulphate. *N,N′*-Diethylbenzene-1,4-
diamine sulphate.
A white or slightly yellow powder, soluble in water.
mp: about 185 °C, with decomposition.
Store protected from light.

Diethylphenylenediamine sulphate solution. *1028601.*
To 250 ml of *water R* add 2 ml of *sulphuric acid R* and 25 ml of *0.02 M sodium edetate.* Dissolve in this solution 1.1 g of *diethylphenylenediamine sulphate R* and dilute to 1000 ml with *water R*.

Do not use if the solution is not colourless.

Store protected from light and heat and use within 1 month.

Digitonin. $C_{56}H_{92}O_{29}$. (M_r 1229). *1028700.* [11024-24-1].
3β-[*O*-β-D-Glucopyranosyl-(1→3)-*O*-β-D-galactopyranosyl-(1→2)-*O*-[β-D-xylopyranosyl-(1→3)]-*O*-β-D-galactopyranosyl-(1→4)-*O*-β-D-galactopyranosyloxy]-(25*R*)-5α-spirostan-2α,15β-diol.
Crystals, practically insoluble in water, sparingly soluble in ethanol, slightly soluble in alcohol, practically insoluble in ether.

Digitoxin. *1028800.* [71-63-6].
See *Digitoxin (0078).*

10,11-Dihydrocarbamazepine. $C_{15}H_{14}N_2O$. (M_r 238.3). *1028900.* [3564-73-6]. 10,11-Dihydro-5*H*-dibenzo[*b,f*]azepine-5-carboxamide.
mp: 205 °C to 210 °C.

Dihydroxynaphthalene. *1029000.* [132-86-5].
See *1,3-dihydroxynaphthalene R.*

1,3-Dihydroxynaphthalene. $C_{10}H_8O_2$. (M_r 160.2). *1029000.* [132-86-5]. Naphthalene-1,3-diol.
A crystalline, generally brownish-violet powder, freely soluble in water and in alcohol.
mp: about 125 °C.

2,7-Dihydroxynaphthalene. $C_{10}H_8O_2$. (M_r 160.2). *1029100.* [582-17-2]. Naphthalene-2,7-diol.
Needles, soluble in water, in alcohol and in ether.
mp: about 190 °C.

2,7-Dihydroxynaphthalene solution. *1029101.*
Dissolve 10 mg of *2,7-dihydroxynaphthalene R* in 100 ml of *sulphuric acid R* and allow to stand until decolorised.
Use within 2 days.

Di-isobutyl ketone. $C_9H_{18}O$. (M_r 142.2). *1029200.* [108-83-8].
A clear, colourless liquid, slightly soluble in water, miscible with most organic solvents.
n_D^{20}: about 1.414
bp: about 168 °C.

Di-isopropyl ether. $C_6H_{14}O$. (M_r 102.2). *1029300.* [108-20-3].
A clear, colourless liquid, very slightly soluble in water, miscible with alcohol and with ether.
d_{20}^{20}: 0.723 to 0.728.
bp: 67 °C to 69 °C.

Do not distil if the di-isopropyl ether does not comply with the test for peroxides.

Peroxides. Place 8 ml of *potassium iodide and starch solution R* in a 12 ml ground-glass-stoppered cylinder about 1.5 cm in diameter. Fill completely with the substance to be examined, shake vigorously and allow to stand protected from light for 30 min. No colour is produced.

The name and concentration of any added stabiliser are stated on the label.

Store protected from light.

***N,N*-Diisopropylethylenediamine.** $C_8H_{20}N_2$. (M_r 144.3). *1140600.* [4013-94-9]. *N,N*-bis(1-Methylethyl)-1,2-ethanediamine.
Colourless to yellowish, corrosive, flammable, hygroscopic liquid.

d_{20}^{20}: about 0.798.
n_D^{20}: about 1.429.
bp: about 170 °C.

4,4′-Dimethoxybenzophenone. $C_{15}H_{14}O_3$. (M_r 242.3). *1126300.* [90-96-0]. bis(4-Methoxyphenyl)methanone.
A white powder, practically insoluble in water and slightly soluble in alcohol.
mp: about 142 °C.

Dimethoxypropane. $C_5H_{12}O_2$. (M_r 104.1). *1105200.* [77-76-9]. 2,2-Dimethoxypropane.
A colourless liquid, decomposing on exposure to moist air or water.
d_{20}^{20}: about 0.847.
n_D^{20}: about 1.378.
bp: about 83 °C.

Dimethylacetamide. C_4H_9NO. (M_r 87.1). *1029700.* [127-19-5]. *N,N*-Dimethylacetamide.
Contains not less than 99.5 per cent of C_4H_9NO.
A colourless liquid, miscible with water and with many organic solvents.
d_{20}^{20}: about 0.94.
n_D^{20}: about 1.437.
bp: about 165 °C.

Dimethylaminobenzaldehyde. $C_9H_{11}NO$. (M_r 149.2). *1029800.* [100-10-7]. 4-Dimethylaminobenzaldehyde.
White or yellowish-white crystals, soluble in alcohol and in dilute acids.
mp: about 74 °C.

Dimethylaminobenzaldehyde solution R1. *1029801.*
Dissolve 0.2 g of *dimethylaminobenzaldehyde R* in 20 ml of *alcohol R* and add 0.5 ml of *hydrochloric acid R*.
Shake the solution with *activated charcoal R* and filter. The colour of the reagent is less intense than that of *iodine solution R3*. Prepare immediately before use.

Dimethylaminobenzaldehyde solution R2. *1029802.*
Dissolve 0.2 g of *dimethylaminobenzaldehyde R*, without heating, in a mixture of 4.5 ml of *water R* and 5.5 ml of *hydrochloric acid R*. Prepare immediately before use.

Dimethylaminobenzaldehyde solution R6. *1029803.*
Dissolve 0.125 g of *dimethylaminobenzaldehyde R* in a cooled mixture of 35 ml of *water R* and 65 ml of *sulphuric acid R*. Add 0.1 ml of a 50 g/l solution of *ferric chloride R*. Before use allow to stand for 24 h, protected from light.

When stored at room temperature it must be used within one week; when kept in a refrigerator, it may be stored for several months.

Dimethylaminobenzaldehyde solution R7. *1029804.*
Dissolve 1.0 g of *dimethylaminobenzaldehyde R* in 50 ml of *hydrochloric acid R* and add 50 ml of *alcohol R*.

Store protected from light and use within 4 weeks.

Dimethylaminobenzaldehyde solution R8. *1029805.*
Dissolve 0.25 g of *dimethylaminobenzaldehyde R* in a mixture of 5 g of *phosphoric acid R*, 45 g of *water R* and 50 g of *anhydrous acetic acid R*. Prepare immediately before use.

4-Dimethylaminocinnamaldehyde. $C_{11}H_{13}NO$. (M_r 175.2). *1029900.* [6203-18-5]. 3-(4-Dimethylaminophenyl)prop-2-enal.
Orange to orange-brown crystals or powder. Sensitive to light.
mp: about 138 °C.

4-Dimethylaminocinnamaldehyde solution. *1029901.* Dissolve 2 g of *4-dimethylaminocinnamaldehyde R* in a mixture of 100 ml of *hydrochloric acid R1* and 100 ml of *ethanol R*. Store in a cool place. Dilute the solution to four times its volume with *ethanol R* immediately before use.

Store in a cool place.

2-(Dimethylamino)ethyl methacrylate. $C_8H_{15}NO_2$. (M_r 157.2). *1147200.* [2867-47-2]. 2-(Dimethylamino)ethyl 2-methylpropenoate.
d_4^{20}: about 0.930.
bp: about 187 °C.

Dimethylaminonaphthalenesulphonyl chloride. $C_{12}H_{12}ClNO_2S$. (M_r 269.8). *1030000.* [605-65-2]. 5-Dimethyl-amino-1-naphthalenesulphonyl chloride.
A yellow, crystalline powder, slightly soluble in water, soluble in methanol.
mp: about 70 °C.
Store in a cool place.

Dimethylaniline. $C_8H_{11}N$. (M_r 121.2). *1030100.* [121-69-7]. *N,N*-Dimethylaniline.
A clear, oily liquid, almost colourless when freshly distilled, darkening on storage to reddish-brown, practically insoluble in water, freely soluble in alcohol and in ether.
n_D^{20}: about 1.558.
Distillation range (2.2.11). Not less than 95 per cent distils between 192 °C and 194 °C.

***N,N*-Dimethylaniline.** *1030100.* [121-69-7].
See *Dimethylaniline R*.

2,3-Dimethylaniline. $C_8H_{11}N$. (M_r 121.2). *1105300.* [87-59-2]. 2,3-Xylidine.
A yellowish liquid, sparingly soluble in water, soluble in alcohol.
d_{20}^{20}: 0.993 to 0.995.
n_D^{20}: about 1.569.
bp: about 224 °C.

2,6-Dimethylaniline. $C_8H_{11}N$. (M_r 121.2). *1030200.* [87-62-7]. 2,6-Xylidine.
A colourless liquid, sparingly soluble in water, soluble in alcohol.
d_{20}^{20}: about 0.98.

2,4-Dimethyl-6-*tert*-butylphenol. $C_{12}H_{18}O$. (M_r 178.3). *1126500.* [1879-09-0].

Dimethyl carbonate. $C_3H_6O_3$. (M_r 90.1). *1119300.* [616-38-6]. Carbonic acid dimethyl ester.
Liquid, insoluble in water, miscible with alcohol.
d_4^{17}: 1.065.
n_D^{20}: 1.368.
bp: about 90 °C.

Dimethyldecylamine. $C_{12}H_{27}N$. (M_r 185.4). *1113500.* [1120-24-7]. *N,N*-dimethyldecylamine.
Contains not less than 98.0 per cent *m/m* of $C_{12}H_{27}N$.
bp: about 234 °C.

1,1-Dimethylethylamine. $C_4H_{11}N$. (M_r 73.1). *1100900.* [75-64-9]. 2-Amino-2-methylpropane. *tert*-Butylamine.
Liquid, miscible with alcohol.
d_{20}^{20}: about 0.694.
n_D^{20}: about 1.378.
bp: about 46 °C.

1,1-Dimethylethyl methyl ether. $C_5H_{12}O$. (M_r 88.1). *1013900.* [1634-04-4]. 2-Methoxy-2-methylpropane. *tert*-Butyl methyl ether.
A colourless, clear, flammable liquid.
n_D^{20}: about 1.376.
Minimum transmittance (2.2.25), determined using *water R* as compensation liquid:
not less than 50 per cent at 240 nm,
not less than 80 per cent at 255 nm,
not less than 98 per cent at 280 nm.

1,1-Dimethylethyl methyl ether R1. *1126400.*
It contains not less than 99.5 per cent of $C_5H_{12}O$.
d_{20}^{20}: about 0.741.
n_D^{20}: about 1.369.
bp: about 55 °C.

Dimethylformamide. C_3H_7NO. (M_r 73.1). *1030300.* [68-12-2].
A clear, colourless neutral liquid, miscible with water and with alcohol.
d_{20}^{20}: 0.949 to 0.952.
bp: about 153 °C.
Water (2.5.12). Not more than 0.1 per cent.

Dimethylformamide diethylacetal. $C_7H_{17}NO_2$. (M_r 147.2). *1113600.* [1188-33-6]. *N,N*-Dimethylformamide diethylacetal.
n_D^{20}: about 1.40.
bp: 128 °C to 130 °C.

***N,N*-Dimethylformamide dimethylacetal.** $C_5H_{13}NO_2$. (M_r 119.2). *1140700.* [4637-24-5]. 1,1-Dimethoxytrimethylamine.
Clear, colourless liquid.
d_{20}^{20}: about 0.896.
n_D^{20}: about 1.396.
bp: about 103 °C.

Dimethylglyoxime. $C_4H_8N_2O_2$. (M_r 116.1). *1030400.* [95-45-4]. 2,3-Butanedione dioxime.
A white, crystalline powder or colourless crystals, practically insoluble in cold water, very slightly soluble in boiling water, soluble in alcohol and in ether.
mp: about 240 °C, with decomposition.
Sulphated ash (2.4.14). Not more than 0.05 per cent.

1,3-Dimethyl-2-imidazolidinone. $C_5H_{10}N_2O$. (M_r 114.2). *1135400.* [80-73-9]. *N,N'*-Dimethylethylene urea.
1,3-Dimethyl-2-imidazolidone.
n_D^{20}: 1.4720
bp: about 224 °C.

***N,N*-Dimethyloctylamine.** $C_{10}H_{23}N$. (M_r 157.3). *1030500.* [7378-99-6]. Octyldimethylamine.
Colourless liquid.
d_{20}^{20}: about 0.765.
n_D^{20}: about 1.424.
bp: about 195 °C.

2,6-Dimethylphenol. $C_8H_{10}O$. (M_r 122.2). *1030600.* [576-26-1].
Colourless needles, slightly soluble in water, very soluble in alcohol and in ether.
bp: about 203 °C.
mp: 46 °C to 48 °C.

3,4-Dimethylphenol. $C_8H_{10}O$. (M_r 122.2). *1098100.* [95-65-8].
White or almost white crystals, slightly soluble in water, freely soluble in alcohol.
bp: about 226 °C.
mp: 25 °C to 27 °C.

Dimethylpiperazine. $C_6H_{14}N_2$. (M_r 114.2). *1030700*. [106-58-1]. 1,4-Dimethylpiperazine.
A colourless liquid, miscible with water and with alcohol.
d_{20}^{20}: about 0.85.
n_D^{20}: about 1.446.
bp: about 131 °C.

Dimethylstearamide. $C_{20}H_{41}NO$. (M_r 311.6). *1030800*.
N,N-Dimethylstearamide.
A white or almost white solid mass, soluble in many organic solvents, including acetone.
mp: about 51 °C.

Dimethylstearylamide. *1030800*.
See *dimethylstearamide R*.

Dimethyl sulphone. $C_2H_6O_2S$. (M_r 94.1). *1030900*. [67-71-0].
A white, crystalline powder, freely soluble in water, soluble in acetone and alcohol.
mp: 108 °C to 110 °C.

Dimethyl sulphoxide. C_2H_6OS. (M_r 78.1). *1029500*.
[67-68-5].
A clear, colourless, oily liquid, hygroscopic, miscible with water and with alcohol.
d_{20}^{20}: about 1.10.
bp: about 189 °C.

Water (2.5.12). Not more than 10 g/l.

Dimethyl sulphoxide used in spectrophotometry complies with the requirements prescribed for dimethyl sulphoxide R with the modified water content shown below and with the following additional test.

Minimum transmittance (2.2.25), determined using *water R* as compensation liquid:

10 per cent at 262 nm,

35 per cent at 270 nm,

70 per cent at 290 nm,

98 per cent at 340 nm and at higher wavelengths.

Water (2.5.12). Not more than 0.2 per cent *m/m*.

Store in an airtight container.

Dimethyl sulphoxide R1. *1029501*.
Contains not less than 99.7 per cent of C_2H_6OS, determined by gas chromatography.

Dimeticone. *1105400*. [9006-65-9].
See *Dimeticone (0138)*.

Dimidium bromide. $C_{20}H_{18}BrN_3$. (M_r 380.3). *1031100*.
[518-67-2]. 3,8-Diamino-5-methyl-6-phenylphenanthridinium bromide.
Dark-red crystals, slightly soluble in water at 20 °C, sparingly soluble in water at 60 °C and in alcohol, practically insoluble in ether.

Dimidium bromide-sulphan blue mixed solution.
1031101.
Dissolve separately 0.5 g of *dimidium bromide R* and 0.25 g of *sulphan blue R* in 30 ml of a hot mixture of 1 volume of *ethanol R* and 9 volumes of *water R*, stir, mix the two solutions, and dilute to 250 ml with the same mixture of solvents. Mix 20 ml of this solution with 20 ml of a 14.0 per cent *V/V* solution of *sulphuric acid R* previously diluted with about 250 ml of *water R* and dilute to 500 ml with *water R*.

Store protected from light.

Dinitrobenzene. $C_6H_4N_2O_4$. (M_r 168.1). *1031200*. [528-29-0].
1,3-Dinitrobenzene.
Yellowish crystalline powder or crystals, practically insoluble in water, slightly soluble in alcohol.
mp: about 90 °C.

Dinitrobenzene solution. *1031201*.
A 10 g/l solution in *alcohol R*.

Dinitrobenzoic acid. $C_7H_4N_2O_6$. (M_r 212.1). *1031300*.
[99-34-3]. 3,5-Dinitrobenzoic acid.
Almost colourless crystals, slightly soluble in water, very soluble in alcohol.
mp: about 206 °C.

Dinitrobenzoic acid solution. *1031301*.
A 20 g/l solution in *alcohol R*.

Dinitrobenzoyl chloride. $C_7H_3ClN_2O_5$. (M_r 230.6). *1031400*.
[99-33-2]. 3,5-Dinitrobenzoyl chloride.
A pale-yellow, crystalline powder or colourless crystals.
mp: about 68 °C.

Dinitrophenylhydrazine. $C_6H_6N_4O_4$. (M_r 198.1). *1031500*.
[119-26-6]. 2,4-Dinitrophenylhydrazine.
Reddish-orange crystals, very slightly soluble in water, slightly soluble in alcohol.
mp: about 203 °C (instantaneous method).

Dinitrophenylhydrazine-aceto-hydrochloric solution.
1031501.
Dissolve 0.2 g of *dinitrophenylhydrazine R* in 20 ml of *methanol R* and add 80 ml of a mixture of equal volumes of *acetic acid R* and *hydrochloric acid R1*. Prepare immediately before use.

Dinitrophenylhydrazine-hydrochloric solution.
1031502.
Dissolve by heating 0.50 g of *dinitrophenylhydrazine R* in *dilute hydrochloric acid R* and complete to 100 ml with the same solvent. Allow to cool and filter. Prepare immediately before use.

Dinitrophenylhydrazine-sulphuric acid solution.
1031503.
Dissolve 1.5 g of *dinitrophenylhydrazine R* in 50 ml of a 20 per cent *V/V* solution of *sulphuric acid R*. Prepare immediately before use.

Dinonyl phthalate. $C_{26}H_{42}O_4$. (M_r 418.6). *1031600*.
[28553-12-0].
A colourless to pale yellow, viscous liquid.
d_{20}^{20}: 0.97 to 0.98.
n_D^{20}: 1.482 to 1.489.
Acidity. Shake 5.0 g with 25 ml of *water R* for 1 min. Allow to stand, filter the separated aqueous layer and add 0.1 ml of *phenolphthalein solution R*. Not more than 0.3 ml of *0.1 M sodium hydroxide* is required to change the colour of the solution (0.05 per cent, calculated as phthalic acid).

Water (2.5.12). Not more than 0.1 per cent.

Dioctadecyl disulphide. $C_{36}H_{74}S_2$. (M_r 571.1). *1031700*.
[1844-09-3].
A white powder, practically insoluble in water.
mp: 53 °C to 58 °C.

2,2′-Di(octadecyloxy)-5,5′-spirobi(1,3,2-dioxaphosphorin-ane). $C_{41}H_{82}O_6P_2$. (M_r 733). *1031800*.
White, waxy solid, practically insoluble in water, soluble in hydrocarbons.
mp: 40 °C to 70 °C.

Dioctadecyl 3,3′-thiodipropionate. $C_{42}H_{82}O_4S$. (M_r 683). *1031900*. [693-36-7].
A white, crystalline powder, practically insoluble in water, freely soluble in methylene chloride, sparingly soluble in acetone, in alcohol and in light petroleum.
mp: 58 °C to 67 °C.

Dioxan. $C_4H_8O_2$. (M_r 88.1). *1032000*. [123-91-1]. 1,4-Dioxan.
A clear, colourless liquid, miscible with water and with most organic solvents.
d_{20}^{20}: about 1.03.
Freezing-point (2.2.18). 9 °C to 11 °C.
Water (2.5.12). Not more than 0.5 per cent.
Do not distil if the dioxan does not comply with the test for peroxides.
Peroxides. Place 8 ml of *potassium iodide and starch solution R* in a 12 ml ground-glass-stoppered cylinder about 1.5 cm in diameter. Fill completely with the substance to be examined, shake vigorously and allow to stand in the dark for 30 min. No colour is produced.
Dioxan used for liquid scintillation is of a suitable analytical grade.

Dioxan solution. *1032002*.
Dilute 50.0 ml of *dioxan stock solution R* to 100.0 ml with *water R*. (0.5 mg/ml of dioxan).

Dioxan solution R1. *1032003*.
Dilute 10.0 ml of *dioxan solution R* to 50.0 ml with *water R*. (0.1 mg/ml of dioxan).

Dioxan stock solution. *1032001*.
Dissolve 1.00 g of *dioxan R* in *water R* and dilute to 100.0 ml with the same solvent. Dilute 5.0 ml of this solution to 50.0 ml with *water R* (1.0 mg/ml).

Diphenylamine. $C_{12}H_{11}N$. (M_r 169.2). *1032100*. [122-39-4].
White crystals, slightly soluble in water, soluble in alcohol.
mp: about 55 °C.
Store protected from light.

Diphenylamine solution. *1032101*.
A 1 g/l solution in *sulphuric acid R*.
Store protected from light.

Diphenylamine solution R1. *1032102*.
A 10 g/l solution in *sulphuric acid R*. The solution is colourless.

Diphenylamine solution R2. *1032103*.
Dissolve 1 g of *diphenylamine R* in 100 ml of *glacial acetic acid R* and add 2.75 ml of *sulphuric acid R*. Use immediately.

Diphenylanthracene. $C_{26}H_{18}$. (M_r 330.4). *1032200*.
[1499-10-1]. 9,10-Diphenylanthracene.
Yellowish to yellow, crystalline powder, practically insoluble in water, freely soluble in ether.
mp: about 248 °C.

Diphenylbenzidine. $C_{24}H_{20}N_2$. (M_r 336.4).
1032300. [531-91-9]. *N,N′*-Diphenylbenzidine.
N,N′-Diphenylbiphenyl-4,4′-diamine.
A white or faintly grey, crystalline powder, practically insoluble in water, slightly soluble in acetone and in alcohol.
mp: about 248 °C.
Nitrates. Dissolve 8 mg in a cooled mixture of 5 ml of *water R* and 45 ml of *nitrogen-free sulphuric acid R*. The solution is colourless or very pale blue.
Sulphated ash (2.4.14). Not more than 0.1 per cent.

Store protected from light.

Diphenylboric acid aminoethyl ester. $C_{14}H_{16}BNO$. (M_r 225.1). *1032400*. [524-95-8].
A white or slightly yellow, crystalline powder, practically insoluble in water, soluble in alcohol.
mp: about 193 °C.

Diphenylcarbazide. $C_{13}H_{14}N_4O$. (M_r 242.3). *1032500*.
[140-22-7]. 1,5-Diphenylcarbonodihydrazide.
A white, crystalline powder which gradually becomes pink on exposure to air, very slightly soluble in water, soluble in acetone, in alcohol and in glacial acetic acid.
mp: about 170 °C.
Sulphated ash (2.4.14). Not more than 0.1 per cent.
Store protected from light.

Diphenylcarbazide solution. *1032501*.
Dissolve 0.2 g of *diphenylcarbazide R* in 10 ml of *glacial acetic acid R* and dilute to 100 ml with *ethanol R*. Prepare immediately before use.

Diphenylcarbazone. $C_{13}H_{12}N_4O$. (M_r 240.3). *1032600*.
[538-62-5]. 1,5-Diphenylcarbazone.
An orange-yellow, crystalline powder, practically insoluble in water, freely soluble in alcohol.
mp: about 157 °C, with decomposition.

Diphenylcarbazone mercuric reagent. *1032601*.
Solution I. Dissolve 0.1 g of *diphenylcarbazone R* in *ethanol R* and dilute to 50 ml with the same solvent.
Solution II. Dissolve 1 g of *mercuric chloride R* in *ethanol R* and dilute to 50 ml with the same solvent.
Mix equal volumes of the two solutions.

1,2-Diphenylhydrazine. $C_{12}H_{12}N_2$. (M_r 184.3). *1140800*.
[122-66-7]. Hydrazobenzene. 1,2-Diphenyldiazane.
Orange powder.
mp: about 125 °C.

Diphenylmethanol. $C_{13}H_{12}O$. (M_r 184.2). *1145700*. [91-01-0].
Benzhydrol.
A white, crystalline powder.
mp: about 66 °C.

Diphenyloxazole. $C_{15}H_{11}NO$. (M_r 221.3). *1032700*. [92-71-7].
2,5-Diphenyloxazole.
A white powder, practically insoluble in water, soluble in methanol, sparingly soluble in dioxan and in glacial acetic acid.
mp: about 70 °C.
$A_{1\,cm}^{1\%}$: about 1260 determined at 305 nm in *methanol R*.
Diphenyloxazole used for liquid scintillation is of a suitable analytical grade.

Diphenylphenylene oxide polymer. *1032800*.
2,6-Diphenyl-*p*-phenylene oxide polymer.
White or almost white, porous beads. The size range of the beads is specified after the name of the reagent in the tests where it is used.

Diphosphorus pentoxide. P_2O_5. (M_r 141.9). *1032900*.
[1314-56-3]. Phosphorus pentoxide. Phosphoric anhydride.
A white powder, amorphous, deliquescent. It is hydrated by water with the evolution of heat.
Store in an airtight container.

Dipotassium hydrogen phosphate. K_2HPO_4. (M_r 174.2).
1033000. [7758-11-4].
A white, crystalline powder, hygroscopic, very soluble in water, slightly soluble in alcohol.
Store in an airtight container.

Dipotassium sulphate. K_2SO_4. (M_r 174.3). *1033100.* [7778-80-5].
Colourless crystals, soluble in water.

Disodium arsenate. $Na_2HAsO_4,7H_2O$. (M_r 312.0). *1102500.*
[10048-95-0]. Disodium hydrogen arsenate heptahydrate.
Dibasic sodium arsenate.
Crystals, efflorescent in warm air, freely soluble in water,
soluble in glycerol, slightly soluble in alcohol. The aqueous
solution is alcaline to litmus.
d_{20}^{20}: about 1.87.
mp: about 57 °C when rapidly heated.

Disodium bicinchoninate. $C_{20}H_{10}N_2Na_2O_4$.
(M_r 388.3). *1126600.* [979-88-4]. Disodium
2,2'-biquinoline-4-4'-dicarboxylate.

Disodium hydrogen citrate. $C_6H_6Na_2O_7,1^1/_2H_2O$. (M_r
263.1). *1033200.* [144-33-2]. Sodium acid citrate.
Disodium hydrogen 2-hydroxypropane-1,2,3-tricarboxylate
sesquihydrate.
A white powder, soluble in less than 2 parts of water,
practically insoluble in alcohol.

Disodium hydrogen phosphate. *1033300.* [10039-32-4].
See *Disodium phosphate dodecahydrate (0118).*

> **Disodium hydrogen phosphate solution.** *1033301.*
> A 90 g/l solution.

Disodium hydrogen phosphate, anhydrous. Na_2HPO_4. (M_r
142.0). *1033400.* [7558-79-4].

Disodium hydrogen phosphate dihydrate. *1033500.*
[10028-24-7].
See *Disodium phosphate dihydrate (0602).*

Disodium tetraborate. *1033600.* [1303-96-4].
See *Borax (0013).*

> **Borate solution.** *1033601.*
> Dissolve 9.55 g of *disodium tetraborate R* in *sulphuric
> acid R*, heating on a water-bath, and dilute to 1 litre with
> the same acid.

Ditalimphos. $C_{12}H_{14}NO_4PS$. (M_r 299.3). *1126700.*
[5131-24-8]. *O,O*-Diethyl (1,3-dihydro-1,3-dioxo-2*H*-isoindol-2-
yl)phosphonothioate.
Very slightly soluble in water, in ethyl acetate and in ethanol.
A suitable certified reference solution may be used.

5,5'-Dithiobis(2-nitrobenzoic acid). $C_{14}H_8N_2O_8S_2$.
(M_r 396.4). *1097300.* [69-78-3]. 3-Carboxy-4-
nitrophenyldisulphide. Ellman's reagent. DTNB.
Yellow powder sparingly soluble in alcohol.
mp: about 242 °C.

Dithiol. $C_7H_8S_2$. (M_r 156.3). *1033800.* [496-74-2].
Toluene-3,4-dithiol. 4-Methylbenzene-1,2-dithiol.
White crystals, hygroscopic, soluble in methanol and in
solutions of alkali hydroxides.
mp: about 30 °C.
Store in an airtight container.

> **Dithiol reagent.** *1033801.*
> To 1 g of *dithiol R* add 2 ml of *thioglycollic acid R*
> and dilute to 250 ml with a 20 g/l solution of *sodium
> hydroxide R*. Prepare immediately before use.

Dithiothreitol. $C_4H_{10}O_2S_2$. (M_r 154.2). *1098200.*
[27565-41-9]. *threo*-1,4-Dimercaptobutane-2,3-diol.
Slightly hygroscopic needles, freely soluble in water, in
acetone and in ethanol.
Store in an airtight container.

Dithizone. $C_{13}H_{12}N_4S$. (M_r 256.3). *1033900.* [60-10-6].
1,5-Diphenylthiocarbazone.
A bluish-black, brownish-black or black powder, practically
insoluble in water, soluble in alcohol.
Store protected from light.

> **Dithizone solution.** *1033901.*
> A 0.5 g/l solution in *chloroform R*. Prepare immediately
> before use.

> **Dithizone solution R2.** *1033903.*
> Dissolve 40.0 mg of *dithizone R* in *chloroform R* and
> dilute to 1000.0 ml with the same solvent. Dilute 30.0 ml
> of the solution to 100.0 ml with *chloroform R*.
>
> *Standardisation.* Dissolve a quantity of *mercuric
> chloride R* equivalent to 0.1354 g of $HgCl_2$ in a mixture
> of equal volumes of *dilute sulphuric acid R* and *water R*
> and dilute to 100.0 ml with the same mixture of solvents.
> Dilute 2.0 ml of this solution to 100.0 ml with a mixture
> of equal volumes of *dilute sulphuric acid R* and *water R*.
> (This solution contains 20 ppm of Hg). Transfer 1.0 ml
> of the solution to a separating funnel and add 50 ml of
> *dilute sulphuric acid R*, 140 ml of *water R* and 10 ml of
> a 200 g/l solution of *hydroxylamine hydrochloride R*.
> Titrate with the dithizone solution; after each addition,
> shake the mixture twenty times and towards the end of
> the titration allow to separate and discard the chloroform
> layer. Titrate until a bluish-green colour is obtained.
> Calculate the equivalent in micrograms of mercury per
> millilitre of the dithizone solution from the expression
> $20/V$, where V is the volume in millilitres of the dithizone
> solution used in the titration.

Dithizone R1. $C_{13}H_{12}N_4S$. (M_r 256.3). *1105500.* [60-10-6].
1,5-Diphenylthiocarbazone.
Contains not less than 98.0 per cent of $C_{13}H_{12}N_4S$.
A bluish-black, brownish-black or black powder, practically
insoluble in water, soluble in alcohol.
Store protected from light.

Divanadium pentoxide. V_2O_5. (M_r 181.9). *1034000.*
[1314-62-1]. Vanadic anhydride.
Contains not less than 98.5 per cent of V_2O_5.
A yellow-brown to rust-brown powder, slightly soluble in
water, soluble in strong mineral acids and in solutions of
alkali hydroxides with formation of salts.

Appearance of solution. Heat 1 g for 30 min with 10 ml of
sulphuric acid R. Allow to cool and dilute to 10 ml with the
same acid. The solution is clear (*2.2.1*).

Sensitivity to hydrogen peroxide. Dilute 1.0 ml of the
solution prepared for the test for appearance of solution
cautiously to 50.0 ml with *water R*. To 0.5 ml of the solution
add 0.1 ml of a solution of *hydrogen peroxide R* (0.1 g/l of
H_2O_2). The solution has a distinct orange colour compared
with a blank prepared from 0.5 ml of the solution to be
examined and 0.1 ml of *water R*. After the addition of 0.4 ml
of hydrogen peroxide solution (0.1 g/l H_2O_2), the orange
solution becomes orange-yellow.

Loss on ignition. Not more than 1.0 per cent, determined
on 1.00 g at 700 °C.

Assay. Dissolve 0.200 g with heating in 20 ml of a 70 per
cent *m/m* solution of *sulphuric acid R*. Add 100 ml of
water R and *0.02 M potassium permanganate* until a reddish
colour is obtained. Decolorise the excess of potassium
permanganate by the addition of a 30 g/l solution of *sodium
nitrite R*. Add 5 g of *urea R* and 80 ml of a 70 per cent *m/m*
solution of *sulphuric acid R*. Cool. Using 0.1 ml of *ferroin R*
as indicator, titrate the solution immediately with *0.1 M
ferrous sulphate* until a greenish-red colour is obtained.

1 ml of *0.1 M ferrous sulphate* is equivalent to 9.095 mg of V_2O_5.

Divanadium pentoxide solution in sulphuric acid.
1034001.
Dissolve 0.2 g of *divanadium pentoxide R* in 4 ml of *sulphuric acid R* and dilute to 100 ml with *water R*.

Docosahexaenoic acid methyl ester. $C_{23}H_{34}O_2$. (M_r 342.5). *1142800.* [301-01-9]. DHA methyl ester. Cervonic acid methyl ester. (all-*Z*)-Docosa-4,7,10,13,16,19-hexaenoic acid methyl ester.
Contains not less than 90.0 per cent of $C_{23}H_{34}O_2$, determined by gas chromatography.

Docusate sodium. *1034100.* [577-11-7].
See *Docusate sodium (1418)*.

Dodecyltrimethylammonium bromide. $C_{15}H_{34}BrN$. (M_r 308.4). *1135500.* [1119-94-4]. *N,N,N*-Trimethyldodecan-1-aminium bromide.
White crystals.
mp: about 246 °C.

Dotriacontane. $C_{32}H_{66}$. (M_r 450.9). *1034200.* [544-85-4].
n-Dotriacontane.
White plates, practically insoluble in water, sparingly soluble in hexane, slightly soluble in ether.
mp: about 69 °C.
Impurities. Not more than 0.1 per cent of impurities with the same t_R value as α-tocopherol acetate, determined by the gas chromatographic method prescribed in the monograph on *α-Tocopherol acetate (0439)*.

Doxycycline. *1145800.*
See *Doxycycline monohydrate (0820)*.

Electrolyte reagent for the micro determination of water.
1113700.
Commercially available anhydrous reagent or a combination of anhydrous reagents for the coulometric titration of water, containing suitable organic bases, sulphur dioxide and iodide dissolved in a suitable solvent.

Elementary standard solution for atomic spectrometry (1.000 g/l). *5004000.*
This solution is prepared, generally in acid conditions, from the element or a salt of the element whose minimum content is not less than 99.0 per cent. The quantity per litre of solution is greater than 0.995 g throughout the guaranteed period, as long as the vial has not been opened. The starting material (element or salt) and the characteristics of the final solvent (nature and acidity, etc.) are mentioned on the label.

Emetine dihydrochloride. *1034300.* [316-42-7].
See *Emetine hydrochloride pentahydrate (0081)*.

Emodin. $C_{15}H_{10}O_5$. (M_r 270.2). *1034400.* [518-82-1].
1,3,8-Trihydroxy-6-methylanthraquinone.
Orange-red needles, practically insoluble in water, slightly soluble in ether, soluble in alcohol and in solutions of alkali hydroxides.
Chromatography. Examine as prescribed in the monograph on *Rhubarb (0291)*; the chromatogram shows only one principal spot.

α-Endosulphan. $C_9H_6Cl_6O_3S$. (M_r 406.9). *1126800.*
[959-98-8].
bp: about 200 °C.
mp: about 108 °C.
A suitable certified reference solution (10 ng/μl in cyclohexane) may be used.

β-Endosulphan. $C_9H_6Cl_6O_3S$. (M_r 406.9). *1126900.*
[33213-65-9].
bp: about 390 °C.
mp: about 207 °C.
A suitable certified reference solution (10 ng/μl in cyclohexane) may be used.

Endrin. $C_{12}H_8Cl_6O$. (M_r 380.9). *1127000.* [72-20-8].
A suitable certified reference solution (10 ng/μl in cyclohexane) may be used.

Erucamide. $C_{22}H_{43}NO$. (M_r 337.6). *1034500.* [112-84-5].
(*Z*)-Docos-13-enoamide.
Yellowish or white powder or granules, practically insoluble in water, very soluble in methylene chloride, soluble in ethanol.
mp: about 70 °C.

Erythritol. *1113800.* [149-32-6].
See *Erythritol (1803)*.

Esculin. $C_{15}H_{16}O_9,1^1/_2H_2O$. ($M_r$ 367.3). *1119400.* [531-75-9].
6-(β-D-Glucopyranosyloxy)-7-hydroxy-2*H*-chromen-2-one.
A white to almost white powder or colourless crystals, sparingly soluble in water and in alcohol, freely soluble in hot water and in hot alcohol.
Chromatography (*2.2.27*). Examine as prescribed in the monograph on *Eleutherococcus (1419)*. The chromatogram shows only one principal spot.

Estradiol. $C_{18}H_{24}O_2$. (M_r 272.4). *1135600.* [50-28-2].
Estra-1,3,5(10)-triène-3,17β-diol. β-Estradiol.
Prisms stable in air, practically insoluble in water, freely soluble in alcohol, soluble in acetone and in dioxane, sparingly soluble in vegetable oils.
mp: 173 °C to 179 °C.

17α-Estradiol. $C_{18}H_{24}O_2$. (M_r 272.4). *1034600.* [57-91-0].
A white or almost white, crystalline powder or colourless crystals.
mp: 220 °C to 223 °C.

Estragole. $C_{10}H_{12}O$. (M_r 148.2). *1034700.* [140-67-0].
1-Methoxy-4-prop-2-enylbenzene.
Liquid, miscible with alcohol.
n_D^{20}: about 1.52.
bp: about 216 °C.
Estragole used in gas chromatography complies with the following test.
Assay. Examine by gas chromatography (*2.2.28*) under the conditions described in the monograph on *Anise oil (0804)* using the substance to be examined as the test solution.
The area of the principal peak is not less than 98.0 per cent of the total area of the peaks.

Ethanol. C_2H_6O. (M_r 46.07). *1034800.* [64-17-5].
See *Ethanol anhydrous (1318)*.

Ethanol R1. *1034801.*
Complies with the requirements prescribed for the monograph *Ethanol, anhydrous (1318)* and with the following requirement.
Methanol. Not more than 0.005 per cent *V/V*, determined by gas chromatography (*2.2.28*).
Test solution. Use the substance to be examined.
Reference solution. Dilute 0.50 ml of *anhydrous methanol R* to 100.0 ml with the substance to be examined. Dilute 1.0 ml of this solution to 100.0 ml with the substance to be examined.
The chromatographic procedure may be carried out using:

— a glass column 2 m long and 2 mm in internal diameter packed with *ethylvinylbenzene-divinyl-benzene copolymer R* (75 μm to 100 μm),

— *nitrogen for chromatography R* as the carrier gas at a flow rate of 30 ml/min,

— a flame-ionisation detector.

Maintain the temperature of the column at 130 °C, that of the injection port at 150 °C and that of the detector at 200 °C.

Inject 1 μl of the test solution and 1 μl of the reference solution, alternately, three times. After each chromatography, heat the column to 230 °C for 8 min. Integrate the methanol peak. Calculate the percentage methanol content from the expression:

$$\frac{a \times b}{c - b}$$

a = percentage V/V content of methanol in the reference solution,

b = area of the methanol peak in the chromatogram obtained with the test solution,

c = area of the methanol peak in the chromatogram obtained with the reference solution.

Ethanol (96 per cent). *1002500.* [64-17-5].
See *Alcohol R.*

Ethanol, anhydrous. *1034800.* [64-17-5].
See *Ethanol R.*

Ethanolamine. C_2H_7NO. (M_r 61.1). *1034900.* [141-43-5].
2-Aminoethanol.
A clear, colourless, viscous, hygroscopic liquid, miscible with water and with methanol, sparingly soluble in ether.
d_{20}^{20}: about 1.04.
n_D^{20}: about 1.454.
mp: about 11 °C.
Store in an airtight container.

Ether. $C_4H_{10}O$. (M_r 74.1). *1035000.* [60-29-7].
A clear, colourless, volatile and very mobile liquid, very flammable, hygroscopic, soluble in water, miscible with alcohol.
d_{20}^{20}: 0.713 to 0.715.
bp: 34 °C to 35 °C.

Do not distil if the ether does not comply with the test for peroxides.

Peroxides. Place 8 ml of *potassium iodide and starch solution R* in a 12 ml ground-glass-stoppered cylinder about 1.5 cm in diameter. Fill completely with the substance to be examined, shake vigorously and allow to stand in the dark for 30 min. No colour is produced.

The name and concentration of any added stabilisers are stated on the label.

Store in an airtight container, protected from light, at a temperature not exceeding 15 °C.

Ether, peroxide-free. *1035100.*
See *Anaesthetic ether (0367).*

Ethion. $C_9H_{22}O_4P_2S_4$. (M_r 384.5). *1127100.* [563-12-2].
mp: −24 °C to −25 °C.
A suitable certified reference solution (10 ng/μl in cyclohexane) may be used.

Ethoxychrysoidine hydrochloride. $C_{14}H_{17}ClN_4O$. (M_r 292.8). *1035200.* [2313-87-3]. 4-[(4-Ethoxyphenyl)diazenyl]phenylene-1,3-diamine hydrochloride.
A reddish powder, soluble in alcohol.

Ethoxychrysoidine solution. *1035201.*
A 1 g/l solution in *alcohol R.*
Test for sensitivity. To a mixture of 5 ml of *dilute hydrochloric acid R* and 0.05 ml of the ethoxy-chrysoidine solution add 0.05 ml of *0.0167 M bromide-bromate.* The colour changes from red to light yellow within 2 min.

Ethyl acetate. $C_4H_8O_2$. (M_r 88.1). *1035300.* [141-78-6].
A clear, colourless liquid, soluble in water, miscible with alcohol.
d_{20}^{20}: 0.901 to 0.904.
bp: 76 °C to 78 °C.

Ethyl acetate, treated. *1035301.*
Disperse 200 g of *sulphamic acid R* in *ethyl acetate R* and make up to 1000 ml with the same solvent. Stir the suspension obtained for three days and filter through a filter paper.

The solution should be used within one month of its preparation.

Ethyl acrylate. $C_5H_8O_2$. (M_r 100.1). *1035400.* [140-88-5].
Ethyl prop-2-enoate.
A colourless liquid.
d_{20}^{20}: about 0.924.
n_D^{20}: about 1.406.
bp: about 99 °C.
mp: about −71 °C.

4-[(Ethylamino)methyl]pyridine. $C_8H_{12}N_2$. (M_r 136.2). *1101300.* [33403-97-3].
A pale yellow liquid.
d_{20}^{20}: about 0.98.
n_D^{20}: about 1.516.
bp: about 98 °C.

Ethylbenzene. C_8H_{10}. (M_r 106.2). *1035800.* [100-41-4].
Contains not less than 99.5 per cent *m/m* of C_8H_{10}, determined by gas chromatography. A clear, colourless liquid, practically insoluble in water, soluble in acetone, and in alcohol.
d_{20}^{20}: about 0.87.
n_D^{20}: about 1.496.
bp: about 135 °C.

Ethyl benzoate. $C_9H_{10}O_2$. (M_r 150.2). *1135700.* [93-89-0].
A clear, colourless, refractive liquid, practically insoluble in water, miscible with alcohol and with light petroleum.
d_4^{25}: about 1.050.
n_D^{20}: about 1.506.
bp: 211 °C to 213 °C.

Ethyl 5-bromovalerate. $C_7H_{13}BrO_2$. (M_r 209.1). *1142900.* [14660-52-7]. Ethyl 5-bromopentanoate.
Clear, colourless liquid.
d_{20}^{20}: about 1.321.
bp: 104 °C to 109 °C.

Ethyl cyanoacetate. $C_5H_7NO_2$. (M_r 113.1). *1035500.* [105-56-6].
A colourless to pale yellow liquid, slightly soluble in water, miscible with alcohol and with ether.
bp: 205 °C to 209 °C, with decomposition.

Ethylene chloride. $C_2H_4Cl_2$. (M_r 99.0). *1036000.* [107-06-2].
1,2-Dichloroethane.
A clear, colourless liquid, soluble in about 120 parts of water and in 2 parts of alcohol, miscible with ether.

d_{20}^{20}: about 1.25.

Distillation range (2.2.11). Not less than 95 per cent distils between 82 °C and 84 °C.

Ethylenediamine. $C_2H_8N_2$. (M_r 60.1). *1036500.* [107-15-3]. Ethane-1,2-diamine.

A clear, colourless, fuming liquid, strongly alkaline, miscible with water and with alcohol, slightly soluble in ether.

bp: about 116 °C.

Ethylene bis[3,3-di(3-*tert*-butyl-4-hydroxyphenyl)butyrate]. *1035900.* [32509-66-3].

See *ethylene bis[3,3-di-(3-(1,1-dimethylethyl)-4-hydroxyphenyl)butyrate] R.*

Ethylene bis[3,3-di(3-(1,1-dimethylethyl)-4-hydroxyphenyl)butyrate]. $C_{50}H_{66}O_8$. (M_r 795). *1035900.* [32509-66-3]. Ethylene bis[3,3-di(3-*tert*-butyl-4-hydroxyphenyl)butyrate].

A crystalline powder, practically insoluble in water and in light petroleum, very soluble in acetone, in ether and in methanol.

mp: about 165 °C.

(Ethylenedinitrilo)tetra-acetic acid. $C_{10}H_{16}N_2O_8$. (M_r 292.2). *1105800.* [60-00-4]. *N,N'*-1,2-Ethanediylbis[*N*-(carboxymethyl)glycine]. Edetic acid.

A white crystalline powder, very slightly soluble in water.

mp: about 250 °C, with decomposition.

Ethylene glycol. $C_2H_6O_2$. (M_r 62.1). *1036100.* [107-21-1]. Ethane-1,2-diol.

A colourless, slightly viscous liquid, hygroscopic, miscible with water and with alcohol, slightly soluble in ether.

d_{20}^{20}: 1.113 to 1.115.

n_D^{20}: about 1.432.

bp: about 198 °C.

mp: about − 12 °C.

Acidity. To 10 ml add 20 ml of *water R* and 1 ml of *phenolphthalein solution R.* Not more than 0.15 ml of *0.02 M sodium hydroxide* is required to change the colour of the indicator to pink.

Water (2.5.12). Not more than 0.2 per cent

Ethylene glycol monoethyl ether. $C_4H_{10}O_2$. (M_r 90.1). *1036200.* [110-80-5]. 2-Ethoxyethanol.

A clear, colourless liquid, miscible with water, with acetone, with alcohol and with ether.

d_{20}^{20}: about 0.93.

n_D^{25}: about 1.406

bp: about 135 °C.

Ethylene glycol monomethyl ether. $C_3H_8O_2$. (M_r 76.1). *1036300.* [109-86-4]. 2-Methoxyethanol.

A clear, colourless liquid, miscible with water, with acetone, with alcohol and with ether.

d_{20}^{20}: about 0.97.

n_D^{20}: about 1.403.

bp: about 125 °C.

Ethylene oxide. C_2H_4O. (M_r 44.05). *1036400.* [75-21-8]. Oxirane.

Colourless, flammable gas, very soluble in water and in ethanol.

Liquefaction point: about 12 °C.

Ethylene oxide solution. *1036402.*

Weigh a quantity of cool *ethylene oxide stock solution R* equivalent to 2.5 mg of ethylene oxide into a cool flask and dilute to 50.0 g with *macrogol 200 R1.* Mix well and dilute 2.5 g of this solution to 25.0 ml with *macrogol 200 R1* (5 µg of ethylene oxide per gram of solution). Prepare immediately before use.

Ethylene oxide solution R1. *1036403.*

Dilute 1.0 ml of cooled *ethylene oxide stock solution R* (check the exact volume by weighing) to 50.0 ml with *macrogol 200 R1.* Mix well and dilute 2.5 g of this solution to 25.0 ml with *macrogol 200 R1.* Calculate the exact amount of ethylene oxide in ppm from the volume determined by weighing and taking the density of *macrogol 200 R1* as 1.127. Prepare immediately before use.

Ethylene oxide solution R2. *1036404.*

Weigh 1.00 g of cold *ethylene oxide stock solution R* (equivalent to 2.5 mg of ethylene oxide) into a cold flask containing 40.0 g of cold *macrogol 200 R1.* Mix and determine the exact mass and dilute to a calculated mass to obtain a solution containing 50 µg of ethylene oxide per gram of solution. Weigh 10.00 g into a flask containing about 30 ml of *water R*, mix and dilute to 50.0 ml with *water R* (10 µg/ml of ethylene oxide). Prepare immediately before use.

Ethylene oxide solution R3. *1036405.*

Dilute 10.0 ml of *ethylene oxide solution R2* to 50.0 ml with *water R* (2 µg/ml of ethylene oxide). Prepare immediately before use.

Ethylene oxide solution R4. *1036407.*

Dilute 1.0 ml of *ethylene oxide stock solution R1* to 100.0 ml with *water R.* Dilute 1.0 ml of this solution to 25.0 ml with *water R.*

Ethylene oxide solution R5. *1036408.*

A 50 g/l solution of *ethylene oxide R* in *methylene chloride R.*

Either use a commercially available reagent or prepare the solution corresponding to the above-mentioned composition.

Ethylene oxide stock solution. *1036401.*

All operations carried out in the preparation of these solutions must be conducted in a fume-hood. The operator must protect both hands and face by wearing polyethylene protective gloves and an appropriate face mask.

Store all solutions in an airtight container in a refrigerator at 4 °C to 8 °C. Carry out all determinations three times.

Into a dry, clean test-tube, cooled in a mixture of 1 part of *sodium chloride R* and 3 parts of crushed ice, introduce a slow current of *ethylene oxide R* gas, allowing condensation onto the inner wall of the test-tube. Using a glass syringe, previously cooled to − 10 °C, inject about 300 µl (corresponding to about 0.25 g) of liquid *ethylene oxide R* into 50 ml of *macrogol 200 R1.* Determine the absorbed quantity of ethylene oxide by weighing before and after absorption (M_{eo}). Dilute to 100.0 ml with *macrogol 200 R1.* Mix well before use.

Assay. To 10 ml of a 500 g/l suspension of *magnesium chloride R* in *ethanol R* add 20.0 ml of *0.1 M alcoholic hydrochloric acid* in a flask. Stopper and shake to obtain a saturated solution and allow to stand overnight to equilibrate. Weigh 5.00 g of *ethylene oxide stock solution (2.5 g/l) R* into the flask and allow to stand for 30 min. Titrate with *0.1 M alcoholic potassium hydroxide* determining the end-point potentiometrically (2.2.20). Carry out a blank titration, replacing the substance to be examined with the same quantity of *macrogol 200 R1.*

Ethylene oxide content in milligrams per gram is given by:

$$\frac{(V_0 - V_1) \times f \times 4.404}{m}$$

Where V_0 and V_1 are the volumes of alcoholic potassium hydroxide used respectively for the blank titration and the assay,

f = factor of the alcoholic potassium hydroxide solution,

m = mass of the sample taken (g).

Ethylene oxide stock solution R1. *1036406.*
A 50 mg/ml solution of *ethylene oxide R* in *methanol R*.

Ethyl formate. $C_3H_6O_2$. (M_r 74.1). *1035600.* [109-94-4].
Ethyl methanoate.
A clear, colourless, flammable liquid, freely soluble in water, miscible with alcohol and with ether.
d_{20}^{20}: about 0.919.
n_D^{20}: about 1.36.
bp: about 54 °C.

2-Ethylhexane-1,3-diol. $C_8H_{18}O_2$. (M_r 146.2). *1105900.*
[94-96-2].
A slightly oily liquid, soluble in ethanol, 2-propanol, propylene glycol and castor oil.
d_{20}^{20}: about 0.942.
n_D^{20}: about 1.451.
bp: about 244 °C.

2-Ethylhexanoic acid. $C_8H_{16}O_2$. (M_r 144.2). *1036600.*
[149-57-5].
A colourless liquid.
d_{20}^{20}: about 0.91.
n_D^{20}: about 1.425.
Related substances. Examine by gas chromatography (*2.2.28*). Inject 1 µl of a solution prepared as follows: suspend 0.2 g of the 2-ethylhexanoic acid in 5 ml of *water R*, add 3 ml of *dilute hydrochloric acid R* and 5 ml of *hexane R*, shake for 1 min, allow the layers to separate and use the upper layer. Carry out the chromatographic procedure as prescribed in the test for 2-ethylhexanoic acid in the monograph on *Amoxicillin sodium (0577)*. The sum of the area of any peaks, apart from the principal peak and the peak due to the solvent, is not greater than 2.5 per cent of the area of the principal peak.

1,1'-Ethylidenebis(tryptophan). $C_{24}H_{26}N_4O_4$. (M_r 434.5).
1106000. [132685-02-0]. 3,3'-[Ethylidenebis(1*H*-indole-1,3-diyl)]bis[(2*S*)-2-aminopropanoic acid].
Contains not less than 98.0 per cent of $C_{24}H_{26}N_4O_4$.
A white or almost white, crystalline powder, slightly soluble in water, very slightly soluble in alcohol, practically insoluble in ether.
mp: about 223 °C, with decomposition.
Assay. Proceed as prescribed in the monograph on *Tryptophan (1272)* under "1,1'-Ethylidenebis(tryptophan) and other related substances". The area of the principal peak in the chromatogram obtained with reference solution (a) is not less than 98.0 per cent of the areas of all the peaks.

N-Ethylmaleimide. $C_6H_7NO_2$. (M_r 125.1). *1036700.*
[128-53-0]. 1-Ethyl-1*H*-pyrrole-2,5-dione.
Colourless crystals, sparingly soluble in water, freely soluble in alcohol.
mp: 41 °C to 45 °C.
Store at a temperature of 2 °C to 8 °C.

Ethyl methyl ketone. *1054100.* [78-93-3].
See *methyl ethyl ketone R*.

2-Ethyl-2-methylsuccinic acid. $C_7H_{12}O_4$. (M_r 160.2).
1036800. [631-31-2]. 2-Ethyl-2-methylbutanedioic acid.
mp: 104 °C to 107 °C.

Ethyl parahydroxybenzoate. *1035700.* [120-47-8].
See *Ethyl parahydroxybenzoate (0900)*.

2-Ethylpyridine. C_7H_9N. (M_r 107.2). *1133400.* [100-71-0].
Colourless or brownish liquid.
d_{20}^{20}: about 0.939.
n_D^{20}: about 1.496.
bp: about 149 °C.

Ethylvinylbenzene-divinylbenzene copolymer. *1036900.*
Porous, rigid, cross-linked polymer beads. Several grades are available with different sizes of bead. The size range of the beads is specified after the name of the reagent in the tests where it is used.

Ethylvinylbenzene-divinylbenzene copolymer R1.
1036901.
Porous, rigid, cross-linked polymer beads, with a nominal specific surface area of 500 m²/g to 600 m²/g and having pores with a mean diameter of 7.5 nm. Several grades are available with different sizes of beads. The size range of the beads is specified after the name of the reagent in the tests where it is used.

Eugenol. $C_{10}H_{12}O_2$. (M_r 164.2). *1037000.* [97-53-0].
4-Allyl-2-methoxyphenol.
A colourless or pale yellow, oily liquid, darkening on exposure to air and light and becoming more viscous, practically insoluble in water, miscible with alcohol, with ether and with fatty and essential oils.
d_{20}^{20}: about 1.07.
bp: about 250 °C.

Eugenol used in gas chromatography complies with the following additional test.

Assay. Examine by gas chromatography (*2.2.28*) as prescribed in the monograph on *Clove oil (1091)* using the substance to be examined as the test solution.

The area of the principal peak is not less than 98.0 per cent of the total area of the peaks.

Store protected from light.

Euglobulins, bovine. *1037100.*

Use fresh bovine blood collected into an anticoagulant solution (for example, sodium citrate solution). Discard any haemolysed blood. Centrifuge at 1500 *g* to 1800 *g* at 15 °C to 20 °C to obtain a supernatant plasma poor in platelets.

To 1 litre of bovine plasma add 75 g of *barium sulphate R* and shake for 30 min. Centrifuge at not less than 1500 *g* to 1800 *g* at 15 °C to 20 °C and draw off the clear supernatant liquid. Add 10 ml of a 0.2 mg/ml solution of *aprotinin R* and shake to ensure mixing. In a container with a minimum capacity of 30 litres in a chamber at 4 °C introduce 25 litres of *distilled water R* at 4 °C and add about 500 g of solid carbon dioxide. Immediately add, while stirring, the supernatant liquid obtained from the plasma. A white precipitate is formed. Allow to settle at 4 °C for 10 h to 15 h. Remove the clear supernatant solution by siphoning. Collect the precipitate by centrifuging at 4 °C. Suspend the precipitate by dispersing mechanically in 500 ml of *distilled water R* at 4 °C, shake for 5 min and collect the precipitate by centrifuging at 4 °C. Disperse the precipitate mechanically in 60 ml of a solution containing 9 g/l of *sodium chloride R* and 0.9 g/l *sodium citrate R* and adjust to pH 7.2 to 7.4 by adding a 10 g/l solution of *sodium hydroxide R*. Filter through a sintered glass filter; to facilitate the dissolution of the precipitate crush the particles of the precipitate with a suitable instrument. Wash the filter and the instrument with 40 ml of the chloride-citrate solution described above and dilute to 100 ml with the same solution. Freeze-dry the solution. The yields are generally 6 g to 8 g of euglobulins per litre of bovine plasma.

Test for suitability. For this test, prepare the solutions using *phosphate buffer solution pH 7.4 R* containing 30 g/l of *bovine albumin R*.

Into a test-tube 8 mm in diameter placed in a water-bath at 37 °C introduce 0.2 ml of a solution of a reference preparation of urokinase containing 100 IU/ml and 0.1 ml of a solution of *human thrombin R* containing 20 IU/ml. Add rapidly 0.5 ml of a solution containing 10 mg of bovine euglobulins per millilitre. A firm clot forms in less than 10 s. Note the time that elapses between the addition of the solution of bovine euglobulins and the lysis of the clot. The lysis time does not exceed 15 min.

Store protected from moisture at 4 °C and use within 1 year.

Euglobulins, human. *1037200.*

For the preparation, use fresh human blood collected into an anticoagulant solution (for example sodium citrate solution) or human blood for transfusion that has been collected in plastic blood bags and which has just reached its expiry date. Discard any haemolysed blood. Centrifuge at 1500 *g* to 1800 *g* at 15 °C to obtain a supernatant plasma poor in platelets. Iso-group plasmas may be mixed.

To 1 litre of the plasma add 75 g of *barium sulphate R* and shake for 30 min. Centrifuge at not less than 15 000 *g* at 15 °C and draw off the clear supernatant liquid. Add 10 ml of a solution of *aprotinin R* containing 0.2 mg/ml and shake to ensure mixing. In a container with a minimum capacity of 30 litres in a chamber at 4 °C introduce 25 litres of *distilled water R* at 4 °C and add about 500 g of solid carbon dioxide. Immediately add while stirring the supernatant liquid obtained from the plasma. A white precipitate is formed. Allow to settle at 4 °C for 10 h to 15 h. Remove the clear supernatant solution by siphoning. Collect the precipitate by centrifuging at 4 °C. Suspend the precipitate by dispersing mechanically in 500 ml of *distilled water R* at 4 °C, shake for 5 min and collect the precipitate by centrifuging at 4 °C. Disperse the precipitate mechanically in 60 ml of a solution containing 9 g/l of *sodium chloride R* and 0.9 g/l of *sodium citrate R*, and adjust the pH to 7.2 to 7.4 by adding a 10 g/l solution of *sodium hydroxide R*. Filter through a sintered-glass filter; to facilitate the dissolution of the precipitate crush the particles of the precipitate with a suitable instrument. Wash the filter and the instrument with 40 ml of the chloride-citrate solution described above and dilute to 100 ml with the same solution. Freeze-dry the solution. The yields are generally 6 g to 8 g of euglobulins per litre of human plasma.

Test for suitability. For this test, prepare the solutions using *phosphate buffer solution pH 7.2 R* containing 30 g/l of *bovine albumin R*. Into a test-tube 8 mm in diameter placed in a water-bath at 37 °C introduce 0.1 ml of a solution of a reference preparation of streptokinase containing 10 IU of streptokinase activity per millilitre and 0.1 ml of a solution of *human thrombin R* containing 20 IU/ml. Add rapidly 1 ml of a solution containing 10 mg of human euglobulins per millilitre. A firm clot forms in less than 10 s. Note the time that elapses between the addition of the solution of human euglobulins and the lysis of the clot. The lysis time does not exceed 15 min.

Store in an airtight container at 4 °C and use within 1 year.

Factor Xa, bovine, coagulation. *1037300.* [9002-05-5]. An enzyme which converts prothrombin to thrombin. The semi-purified preparation is obtained from liquid bovine plasma and it may be prepared by activation of the zymogen factor X with a suitable activator such as Russell's viper venom.

Store freeze-dried preparation at −20 °C and frozen solution at a temperature lower than −20 °C.

Factor Xa solution, bovine. *1037301.* Reconstitute as directed by the manufacturer and dilute with *tris(hydroxymethyl)aminomethane sodium chloride buffer solution pH 7.4 R*.

Any change in the absorbance of the solution, measured at 405 nm (*2.2.25*) against *tris(hydroxymethyl)aminomethane sodium chloride buffer solution pH 7.4 R* as the blank is not more than 0.15 to 0.20 per minute.

Fast blue B salt. $C_{14}H_{12}Cl_2N_4O_2$. (M_r 339.2). *1037400.* [84633-94-3].
Schultz No. 490.
Colour Index No. 37235.
3,3′-Dimethoxy(biphenyl)-4,4′-bisdiazonium dichloride.
A dark green powder, soluble in water. It is stabilised by addition of zinc chloride.
Store in an airtight container, at a temperature between 2 °C and 8 °C.

Fast red B salt. $C_{17}H_{13}N_3O_9S_2$. (M_r 467.4). *1037500.* [56315-29-8].
Schultz No. 155.
Colour Index No. 37125.
2-Methoxy-4-nitrobenzenediazonium hydrogen naphthalene-1,5-disulphonate.
An orange-yellow powder, soluble in water, slightly soluble in alcohol.
Store in an airtight container, protected from light, at 2 °C to 8 °C.

Fenchlorphos. $C_8H_8Cl_3O_3PS$. (M_r 321.5). *1127200.* [299-84-3].
mp: about 35 °C.
A suitable certified reference solution (10 ng/µl in cyclohexane) may be used.

Fenchone. $C_{10}H_{16}O$. (M_r 152.2). *1037600.* [7787-20-4].
1,3,3-Trimethylbicyclo[2.2.1]heptan-2-one.
An oily liquid, miscible with alcohol and with ether, practically insoluble in water.
n_D^{20}: about 1.46.
bp_{15mm}: about 66 °C.
Fenchone used in gas chromatography complies with the following test.

Assay. Examine by gas chromatography (*2.2.28*) under the conditions described in the monograph on *Bitter fennel (0824)* using the substance to be examined as the test solution.

The area of the principal peak is not less than 98.0 per cent of the total area of the peaks.

Fenvalerate. $C_{25}H_{22}ClNO_3$. (M_r 419.9). *1127300.* [51630-58-1].
bp: about 300 °C.
A suitable certified reference solution (10 ng/µl in cyclohexane) may be used.

Ferric ammonium sulphate. $FeNH_4(SO_4)_2,12H_2O$. (M_r 482.2). *1037700.* [7783-83-7]. Ammonium iron disulphate dodecahydrate.
Pale-violet crystals, efflorescent, very soluble in water, practically insoluble in alcohol.

Ferric ammonium sulphate solution R2. *1037702.*
A 100 g/l solution. If necessary filter before use.

Ferric ammonium sulphate solution R5. *1037704.*
Shake 30.0 g of *ferric ammonium sulphate R* with 40 ml of *nitric acid R* and dilute to 100 ml with *water R*. If the solution is turbid, centrifuge or filter it.

Store protected from light.

Ferric ammonium sulphate solution R6. *1037705.*
Dissolve 20 g of *ferric ammonium sulphate R* in 75 ml of *water R*, add 10 ml of a 2.8 per cent *V/V* solution of *sulphuric acid R* and dilute to 100 ml with *water R*.

Ferric chloride. $FeCl_3,6H_2O$. (M_r 270.3). *1037800.*
[10025-77-1]. Iron trichloride hexahydrate.
Yellowish-orange or brownish crystalline masses, deliquescent, very soluble in water, soluble in alcohol and in ether. On exposure to light, ferric chloride and its solutions are partly reduced.
Store in an airtight container.

Ferric chloride solution R1. *1037801.*
A 105 g/l solution.

Ferric chloride solution R2. *1037802.*
A 13 g/l solution.

Ferric chloride solution R3. *1037803.*
Dissolve 2.0 g of *ferric chloride R* in *ethanol R* and dilute to 100.0 ml with the same solvent.

Ferric chloride-sulphamic acid reagent. *1037804.*
A solution containing 10 g/l of *ferric chloride R* and 16 g/l of *sulphamic acid R*.

Ferric nitrate. $Fe(NO_3)_3,9H_2O$. (M_r 404). *1106100.*
[7782-61-8].
Contains not less than 99.0 per cent *m/m* of $Fe(NO_3)_3,9H_2O$.

Light-purple crystals or crystalline mass, very soluble in water.
Free acid: not more than 0.3 per cent (as HNO_3).

Ferric sulphate. $Fe_2(SO_4)_3,xH_2O$. *1037900.* [10028-22-5].
Iron(III) trisulphate hydrated.
A yellowish-white powder, very hygroscopic, decomposes in air, slightly soluble in water and in alcohol.
Store in an airtight container, protected from light.

Ferrocyphene. $C_{26}H_{16}FeN_6$. (M_r 468.3). *1038000.*
[14768-11-7]. Dicyanobis(1,10-phenanthroline)iron(II).
A violet-bronze, crystalline powder, practically insoluble in water and in alcohol.
Store protected from light and moisture.

Ferroin. *1038100.* [14634-91-4].
Dissolve 0.7 g of *ferrous sulphate R* and 1.76 g of *phenanthroline hydrochloride R* in 70 ml of *water R* and dilute to 100 ml with the same solvent.
Test for sensitivity. To 50 ml of *dilute sulphuric acid R* add 0.15 ml of *osmium tetroxide solution R* and 0.1 ml of the ferroin. After the addition of 0.1 ml of *0.1 M ammonium and cerium nitrate* the colour changes from red to light blue.

Ferrous ammonium sulphate. $Fe(NH_4)_2(SO_4)_2,6H_2O$. (M_r 392.2). *1038200.* [7783-85-9]. Diammonium iron disulphate hexahydrate.
Pale bluish-green crystals or granules, freely soluble in water, practically insoluble in alcohol.
Store protected from light.

Ferrous sulphate. *1038300.* [7782-63-0].
See *Ferrous sulphate (0083)*.

Ferrous sulphate solution R2. *1038301.*
Dissolve 0.45 g of *ferrous sulphate R* in 50 ml of *0.1 M hydrochloric acid* and dilute to 100 ml with *carbon dioxide-free water R*. Prepare immediately before use.

Fibrin blue. *1101400.*
Mix 1.5 g of fibrin with 30 ml of a 5 g/l solution of *indigo carmine R* in 1 per cent *V/V* dilute hydrochloric acid R. Heat the mixture to 80 °C and maintain at this temperature whilst stirring for about 30 min. Allow to cool. Filter. Wash extensively by resuspension in 1 per cent *V/V* dilute hydrochloric acid R and mixing for about 30 min; filter. Repeat the washing operation three times. Dry at 50 °C. Grind.

Fibrin congo red. *1038400.*
Take 1.5 g of fibrin and leave overnight in 50 ml of a 20 g/l solution of *congo red R* in *alcohol (90 per cent V/V) R*. Filter, rinse the fibrin with *water R* and store under *ether R*.

Fibrinogen. *1038500.* [9001-32-5].
See *Human fibrinogen, freeze-dried (0024)*.

Fixing solution. *1122600.*
To 250 ml of *methanol R*, add 0.27 ml of *formaldehyde R* and dilute to 500.0 ml with *water R*.

Fixing solution for isoelectric focusing in polyacrylamide gel. *1138700.*
A solution containing 35 g of *sulphosalicylic acid R* and 100 g of *trichloroacetic acid R* per litre of *water R*.

Flufenamic acid. $C_{14}H_{10}F_3NO_2$. (M_r 281.2). *1106200.*
[530-78-9]. 2-[[3-(Trifluoromethyl)phenyl]amino]benzoic acid.
Pale yellow, crystalline powder or needles, practically insoluble in water, freely soluble in alcohol.
mp: 132 °C to 135 °C.

Fluoranthene. $C_{16}H_{10}$. (M_r 202.3). *1038600.* [206-44-0].
1,2-(1,8-Naphtylene)benzene. 1,2-Benzacenaphtene.
Yellow or yellowish-brown crystals.
bp: about 384 °C.
mp: 109 °C to 110 °C.

Fluorene. $C_{13}H_{10}$. (M_r 166.2). *1127400.* [86-73-7].
Diphenylenemethane.
White crystals, freely soluble in anhydrous acetic acid, soluble in hot alcohol.
mp: 113 °C to 115 °C.

Fluorescamine. $C_{17}H_{10}O_4$. (M_r 278.3). *1135800.*
[38183-12-9]. 4-Phenylspiro[furan-2(3*H*),1'(3'*H*)-isobenzofuran]-3,3'-dione.
mp: 154 °C to 155 °C.

Fluorescein. $C_{20}H_{12}O_5$. (M_r 332.3). *1106300.* [2321-07-5].
3',6'-Dihydroxyspiro[isobenzofurane-1(3*H*),9'-[9*H*]xanthen]-3-one.
An orange-red powder, practically insoluble in water, soluble in warm alcohol, practically insoluble in ether, soluble in alkaline solutions. In solution, fluorescein displays a green fluorescence.
mp: about 315 °C.

Fluorescein-conjugated rabies antiserum. *1038700.*
Immunoglobulin fraction with a high rabies antibody titre, prepared from the sera of suitable animals that have been immunised with inactivated rabies virus; the immunoglobulin is conjugated with fluorescein isothiocyanate.

2-Fluoro-2-deoxy-D-glucose. $C_6H_{11}FO_5$. (M_r 182.2). *1113900*. [86783-82-6].
A white crystalline powder.
mp: 174 °C to 176 °C.

Fluorodinitrobenzene. $C_6H_3FN_2O_4$. (M_r 186.1). *1038800*. [70-34-8]. 1-Fluoro-2,4-dinitrobenzene.
Pale yellow crystals, soluble in ether and in propylene glycol.
mp: about 29 °C.

1-Fluoro-2-nitro-4-(trifluoromethyl)benzene. $C_7H_3F_4NO_2$. (M_r 209.1). *1038900*. [367-86-2].
mp: about 197 °C.

Folic acid. *1039000*. [75708-92-8].
See *Folic acid (0067)*.

Formaldehyde. *1039100*. [50-00-0].
See *Formaldehyde solution R*.

> **Formaldehyde solution.** *1039101*.
> See *Formaldehyde solution (35 per cent) (0826)*.

Formamide. CH_3NO. (M_r 45.0). *1039200*. [75-12-7].
A clear, colourless, oily liquid, hygroscopic, miscible with water and with alcohol. It is hydrolysed by water.
bp: about 103 °C, determined at a pressure of 2 kPa.
Store in an airtight container.

> **Formamide R1.** *1039202*.
> Complies with the requirements prescribed for *formamide R* and with the following additional test.
> *Water (2.5.12)*. Not more than 0.1 per cent determined with an equal volume of *anhydrous methanol R*.

> **Formamide, treated.** *1039201*.
> Disperse 1.0 g of *sulphamic acid R* in 20.0 ml of *formamide R* containing 5 per cent *V/V* of *water R*.

Formic acid, anhydrous. CH_2O_2. (M_r 46.03). *1039300*. [64-18-6].
Contains not less than 98.0 per cent *m/m* of CH_2O_2.
A colourless liquid, corrosive, miscible with water and with alcohol.
d_{20}^{20}: about 1.22.
Assay. Weigh accurately a conical flask containing 10 ml of *water R*, quickly add about 1 ml of the acid and weigh again. Add 50 ml of *water R* and titrate with *1 M sodium hydroxide*, using 0.5 ml of *phenolphthalein solution R* as indicator.
1 ml of *1 M sodium hydroxide* is equivalent to 46.03 mg of CH_2O_2.

Fructose. *1106400*. [57-48-7].
See *Fructose (0188)*.

Fuchsin, basic. *1039400*. [632-99-5].
A mixture of rosaniline hydrochloride ($C_{20}H_{20}ClN_3$; M_r 337.9; Colour Index No. 42510; Schultz No. 780) and *para*-rosaniline hydrochloride ($C_{19}H_{18}ClN_3$; M_r 323.8; Colour Index No. 42500; Schultz No. 779).
If necessary, purify in the following manner. Dissolve 1 g in 250 ml of *dilute hydrochloric acid R*. Allow to stand for 2 h at room temperature, filter and neutralise with *dilute sodium hydroxide solution R* and add 1 ml to 2 ml in excess. Filter the precipitate through a sintered-glass filter (40) and wash with *water R*. Dissolve the precipitate in 70 ml of *methanol R*, previously heated to boiling, and add 300 ml of *water R* at 80 °C. Allow to cool to room temperature, filter and dry the crystals *in vacuo*.
Crystals with a greenish-bronze sheen, soluble in water and in alcohol.

Store protected from light.

Fuchsin solution, decolorised. *1039401*.
Dissolve 0.1 g of *basic fuchsin R* in 60 ml of *water R*. Add a solution containing 1 g of *anhydrous sodium sulphite R* or 2 g of *sodium sulphite R* in 10 ml of *water R*. Slowly and with continuous shaking add 2 ml of *hydrochloric acid R*. Dilute to 100 ml with *water R*. Allow to stand protected from light for at least 12 h, decolorise with *activated charcoal R* and filter. If the solution becomes cloudy, filter before use. If on standing the solution becomes violet, decolorise again by adding *activated charcoal R*.
Test for sensitivity. To 1.0 ml add 1.0 ml of *water R* and 0.1 ml of *aldehyde-free alcohol R*. Add 0.2 ml of a solution containing 0.1 g/l of formaldehyde (CH_2O, M_r 30.0). A pale-pink colour develops within 5 min.
Store protected from light.

Fuchsin solution, decolorised R1. *1039402*.
To 1 g of *basic fuchsin R* add 100 ml of *water R*. Heat to 50 °C and allow to cool with occasional shaking. Allow to stand for 48 h, shake and filter. To 4 ml of the filtrate add 6 ml of *hydrochloric acid R*, mix and dilute to 100 ml with *water R*. Allow to stand for at least 1 h before use.

Fucose. $C_6H_{12}O_5$. (M_r 164.2). *1039500*. [6696-41-9].
6-Deoxy-L-galactose.
A white powder, soluble in water and in alcohol.
$[\alpha]_D^{20}$: about −76, determined on a 90 g/l solution 24 h after dissolution.
mp: about 140 °C.

Furfural. $C_5H_4O_2$. (M_r 96.1). *1039600*. [98-01-1].
2-Furaldehyde. 2-Furanecarbaldehyde.
A clear, colourless to brownish-yellow, oily liquid, miscible in 11 parts of water, miscible with alcohol and with ether.
d_{20}^{20}: 1.155 to 1.161.
Distillation range (2.2.11). Not less than 95 per cent distils between 159 °C and 163 °C.
Store in a dark place.

Galactose. $C_6H_{12}O_6$. (M_r 180.2). *1039700*. [59-23-4].
D-(+)-Galactose.
A white, crystalline powder, freely soluble in water.
$[\alpha]_D^{20}$: + 79 to + 81, determined on a 100 g/l solution in *water R* containing about 0.05 per cent of NH_3.

Gallic acid. $C_7H_6O_5,H_2O$. (M_r 188.1). *1039800*. [5995-86-8].
3,4,5-Trihydroxybenzoic acid monohydrate.
A crystalline powder or long needles, colourless or slightly yellow, soluble in water, freely soluble in hot water, in alcohol and in glycerol, slightly soluble in ether.
It loses its water of crystallisation at 120 °C and it melts at about 260 °C, with decomposition.
Chromatography. Examine as prescribed in the monograph on *Bearberry leaf (1054)*; the chromatogram shows only one principal spot.

Gastric juice, artificial. *1039900*.
Dissolve 2.0 g of *sodium chloride R* and 3.2 g of *pepsin powder R* in *water R*. Add 80 ml of *1 M hydrochloric acid* and dilute to 1000 ml with *water R*.

GC concentrical column. *1135100*.
A commercially available system consisting of 2 concentrically arranged tubes. The outer tube is packed with molecular sieves and the inner tube is packed with a porous polymer mixture. The main application is the separation of gases.

Gelatin. *1040000*. [9000-70-8].
See *Gelatin (0330)*.

Gelatin, hydrolysed. *1040100.*
Dissolve 50 g of *gelatin R* in 1000 ml of *water R*. Autoclave in saturated steam at 121 °C for 90 min and freeze dry.

Geraniol. $C_{10}H_{18}O$. (M_r 154.2). *1135900.* [106-24-1].
(*E*)-3,7-Dimethylocta-2,6-dien-1-ol.
An oily liquid, slight odour of rose, practically insoluble in water, miscible with alcohol.
d_{20}^{20}: 0.890.
n_D^{20}: 1.477.
bp: 229 °C to 230 °C.

Geraniol used in gas chromatography complies with the following additional test.

Assay. Examine by gas chromatography (*2.2.28*) as prescribed in the monograph on *Citronella oil (1609)*.

The content is not less than 98.5 per cent calculated by the normalisation procedure.

Store in an airtight container, protected from light

Geranyl acetate. $C_{12}H_{20}O_2$. (M_r 196.3). *1106500.* [105-87-3].
(*E*)-3,7-Dimethylocta-2,6-dien-1-yl acetate.
A colourless or slightly yellow liquid, slight odour of rose and lavender.
d_{25}^{25}: 0.896 to 0.913.
n_D^{15}: about 1.463.
bp_{25}: about 138 °C.

Geranyl acetate used in gas chromatography complies with the following additional test.

Assay. Examine by gas chromatography (*2.2.28*) as prescribed in the monograph on *Bitter-orange-flower oil (1175)*, using the substance to be examined as the test solution. The area of the principal peak is not less than 99.0 per cent of the total area of the peaks.

Ginsenoside Rb1. $C_{54}H_{92}O_{23},3H_2O$. (M_r 1163). *1127500.*
[41753-43-9]. (20*S*)-3β-di-D-Glucopyranosyl-20-di-D-glucopyranosylprotopanaxadiol. (20*S*)-3β-[(2-*O*-β-D-Glucopyranosyl-β-D-glucopyranosyl)oxy]-20-[(6-*O*-β-D-glucopyranosyl-β-D-glucopyranosyl)oxy]-5α-dammar-24-en-12β-ol. (20*S*)-3β-[(2-*O*-β-D-Glucopyranosyl-β-D-glucopyranosyl)oxy]-20-[(6-*O*-β-D-glucopyranosyl-β-D-glucopyranosyl)oxy]-4,4,8,14-tetramethyl-18-nor-5α-cholest-24-en-12β-ol.
A colourless solid, soluble in water, in ethanol and in methanol.
$[\alpha]_D^{20}$: + 11.3 determined on a 10 g/l solution in *methanol R*.
mp: about 199 °C.

Water (2.5.12). Not more than 6.8 per cent.

Assay. Examined by liquid chromatography (*2.2.29*) as prescribed in the monograph on *Ginseng (1523)*.

Test solution. Dissolve 3.0 mg, accurately weighted, of ginsenoside Rb1 in 10 ml of *methanol R*.

The content is not less than 95.0 per cent calculated by the normalisation procedure.

Ginsenoside Rf. $C_{42}H_{72}O_{14},2H_2O$. (M_r 837). *1127700.*
[52286-58-5]. (20*S*)-6-*O*-[β-D-Glucopyranosyl-(1→2)-β-D-glycopyranoside]-dammar-24-ene-3β,6α,12β,20-tetrol.
A colourless solid, soluble in water, in ethanol and in methanol.
$[\alpha]_D^{20}$: + 12.8 determined on a 10 g/l solution in *methanol R*.
mp: about 198 °C.

Ginsenoside Rg1. $C_{42}H_{72}O_{14},2H_2O$. (M_r 837).
1127600. [22427-39-0]. (20*S*)-6β-D-Glucopyranosyl-D-glucopyranosylprotopanaxatriol. (20*S*)-6α,20-bis(β-

D-Glucopyranosyloxy)-5α-dammar-24-ene-3β,12β-diol.
(20*S*)-6α,20-bis(β-D-Glucopyranosyloxy)-4,4,8,14-tetramethyl-18-nor-5α-cholest-24-ene-3β,12β-diol.
A colourless solid, soluble in water, in ethanol and in methanol.
$[\alpha]_D^{20}$: + 31.2 determined on a 10 g/l solution in *methanol R*.
mp: 188 °C to 191 °C.

Water (2.5.12). Not more than 4.8 per cent.

Assay. Examined by liquid chromatography (*2.2.29*) as prescribed in the monograph on *Ginseng (1523)*.

Test solution. Dissolve 3.0 mg, accurately weighted, of ginsenoside Rg1 in 10 ml of *methanol R*.

The content is not less than 95.0 per cent calculated by the normalisation procedure.

Gitoxin. $C_{41}H_{64}O_{14}$. (M_r 781). *1040200.* [4562-36-1].
Glycoside of *Digitalis purpurea* L. 3β-(*O*-2,6-Dideoxy-β-d-*ribo*-hexopyranosyl-(1→4)-*O*-2,6-dideoxy-β-d-*ribo*-hexopyranosyl-(1→4)-2,6-dideoxy-β-d-*ribo*-hexopyranosyloxy)-14,16β-dihydroxy-5β,14β-card-20(22)-enolide.
A white, crystalline powder, practically insoluble in water and in most common organic solvents, soluble in pyridine.
$[\alpha]_D^{20}$: + 20 to + 24, determined on a 5 g/l solution in a mixture of equal volumes of *chloroform R* and *methanol R*.
Chromatography. Examine as prescribed in the monograph on *Digitalis leaf (0117)*; the chromatogram shows only one principal spot.

Glucosamine hydrochloride. $C_6H_{14}ClNO_5$. (M_r 215.6). *1040300.* [66-84-2]. D-Glucosamine hydrochloride.
Crystals, soluble in water, practically insoluble in ether.
$[\alpha]_D^{20}$: + 100, decreasing to + 47.5 after 30 min, determined on a 100 g/l solution in *water R*.

Glucose. *1025700.* [50-99-7].
See *Anhydrous glucose (0177)*.

D-Glucuronic acid. $C_6H_{10}O_7$. (M_r 194.1). *1119700.*
[6556-12-3].
It contains not less than 96.0 per cent of $C_6H_{10}O_7$, calculated with reference to the substance dried *in vacuo* (*2.2.32*).

Soluble in water and in alcohol.
Shows mutarotation: $[\alpha]_D^{24}$: + 11.7 → + 36.3

Assay. Dissolve 0.150 g in 50 ml of *anhydrous methanol R* while stirring under nitrogen. Titrate with *0.1 M tetrabutylammonium hydroxide*, protecting the solution from atmospheric carbon dioxide throughout solubilisation and titration. Determine the end-point potentiometrically (*2.2.20*).

1 ml of *0.1 M tetrabutylammonium hydroxide* is equivalent to 19.41 mg of $C_6H_{10}O_7$.

Glutamic acid. *1040400.* [56-86-0].
See *Glutamic acid (0750)*.

Glutaraldehyde. $C_5H_8O_2$. (M_r 100.1). *1098300.* [111-30-8].
An oily liquid, soluble in water.
n_D^{25}: about 1.434.
bp: about 188 °C.

Glycerol. *1040500.* [56-81-5].
See *Glycerol (0496)*.

Glycerol (85 per cent). *1040600.*
See *Glycerol (85 per cent) (0497)*.

Glycidol. $C_3H_6O_2$. (M_r 74.1). *1127800.* [556-52-5].
A slightly viscous liquid, miscible with water.
d_4^{20}: about 1.115.
n_D^{20}: about 1.432.

Glycine. *1040700.* [56-40-6].
See *Glycine (0614)*.

Glycollic acid. $C_2H_4O_3$. (M_r 76.0). *1040800.* [79-14-1].
2-Hydroxyacetic acid.
Crystals, soluble in water, in acetone, in alcohol, in ether and in methanol.
mp: about 80 °C.

Glycyrrhetic acid. $C_{30}H_{46}O_4$. (M_r 470.7). *1040900.*
[471-53-4]. Glycyrrhetinic acid. 12,13-Didehydro-3β-hydroxy-11-oxo-olean-30-oic acid.
A mixture of α- and β-glycyrrhetic acids in which the β-isomer is predominant.

A white or yellowish-brown powder, practically insoluble in water, soluble in ethanol and in glacial acetic acid.
$[\alpha]_D^{20}$: + 145 to + 155, determined on a 10.0 g/l solution in *ethanol R*.
Chromatography. Examine by thin-layer chromatography (*2.2.27*) using *silica gel GF$_{254}$R* as the coating substance; prepare the slurry using a 0.25 per cent V/V solution of *phosphoric acid R*. Apply to the plate 5 µl of a 5 g/l solution of the glycyrrhetic acid in a mixture of equal volumes of *chloroform R* and *methanol R*. Develop over a path of 10 cm using a mixture of 5 volumes of *methanol R* and 95 volumes of *chloroform R*. Examine the chromatogram in ultraviolet light at 254 nm. The chromatogram shows a dark spot (R_f about 0.3) corresponding to β-glycyrrhetic acid and a smaller spot (R_f about 0.5) corresponding to α-glycyrrhetic acid. Spray with *anisaldehyde solution R* and heat at 100 °C to 105 °C for 10 min. Both spots are coloured bluish-violet. Between them a smaller bluish-violet spot may be present.

18α-Glycyrrhetinic acid. $C_{30}H_{46}O_4$. (M_r 470.7). *1127900.*
[1449-05-4]. (20β)-3β-Hydroxy-11-oxo-18α-olean-12-en-29-oic acid.
A white or almost white powder, practically insoluble in water, soluble in ethanol, sparingly soluble in methylene chloride.

Glyoxalhydroxyanil. $C_{14}H_{12}N_2O_2$. (M_r 240.3). *1041000.*
[1149-16-2]. Glyoxal bis(2-hydroxyanil).
White crystals, soluble in hot alcohol.
mp: about 200 °C.

Glyoxal solution. *1098400.* [107-22-2].
Contains about 40 per cent (m/m) glyoxal.

Assay. In a ground-glass stoppered flask place 1.000 g of glyoxal solution, 20 ml of a 70 g/l solution of *hydroxylamine hydrochloride R* and 50 ml of *water R*. Allow to stand for 30 min and add 1 ml of *methyl red mixed solution R* and titrate with *1 M sodium hydroxide* until the colour changes from red to green. Carry out a blank titration.

1 ml of *1 M sodium hydroxide* is equivalent to 29.02 mg of glyoxal ($C_2H_2O_2$).

Gonadotrophin, chorionic. *1041100.* [9002-61-3].
See *Chorionic gonadotrophin (0498)*.

Gonadotrophin, serum. *1041200.*
See *Equine serum gonadotrophin for veterinary use (0719)*.

Guaiacum resin. *1041400.*
Resin obtained from the heartwood of *Guaiacum officinale* L. and *Guaiacum sanctum* L.

Reddish-brown or greenish-brown, hard, glassy fragments; fracture shiny.

Guaiazulene. $C_{15}H_{18}$. (M_r 198.3). *1041500.* [489-84-9].
1,4-Dimethyl-7-isopropylazulene.
Dark-blue crystals or blue liquid, very slightly soluble in water, miscible with fatty and essential oils and with liquid paraffin, sparingly soluble in alcohol, soluble in 500 g/l sulphuric acid and 80 per cent m/m phosphoric acid, giving a colourless solution.
mp: about 30 °C.
Store protected from light and air.

Guanidine hydrochloride. CH_5N_3HCl. (M_r 95.5). *1098500.*
[50-01-1].
Crystalline powder, freely soluble in water and in alcohol.

Guanine. $C_5H_5N_5O$. (M_r 151.1). *1041600.* [73-40-5].
2-Amino-1,7-dihydro-6*H*-purin-6-one.
An amorphous white powder, practically insoluble in water, slightly soluble in alcohol. It dissolves in ammonia and in dilute solutions of alkali hydroxides.

Haemoglobin. *1041700.* [9008-02-0].
Nitrogen. 15 per cent to 16 per cent.
Iron. 0.2 per cent to 0.3 per cent.
Loss on drying (2.2.32). Not more than 2 per cent.
Sulphated ash (2.4.14). Not more than 1.5 per cent.

Haemoglobin solution. *1041701.*
Transfer 2 g of *haemoglobin R* to a 250 ml beaker and add 75 ml of *dilute hydrochloric acid R2*. Stir until solution is complete. Adjust the pH to 1.6 ± 0.1 (*2.2.3*) using *1 M hydrochloric acid*. Transfer to a 100 ml flask with the aid of *dilute hydrochloric acid R2*. Add 25 mg of *thiomersal R*. Prepare daily, store at 5 ± 3 °C and readjust to pH 1.6 before use.
Store at 2 °C to 8 °C.

Harpagoside. $C_{24}H_{30}O_{11}$. (M_r 494.5). *1098600.*
A white, crystalline powder, very hygroscopic, soluble in water and in alcohol.
mp: 117 °C to 121 °C.
Store in an airtight container.

Helium for chromatography. He. (A_r 4.003). *1041800.*
[7440-59-7].
Contains not less than 99.995 per cent V/V of He.

Heparin. *1041900.* [9041-08-1].
See *Heparin sodium (0333)*.

Heptachlor. $C_{10}H_5Cl_7$. (M_r 373.3). *1128000.* [76-44-8].
bp: about 135 °C.
mp: about 95 °C.
A suitable certified reference solution (10 ng/µl in cyclohexane) may be used.

Heptachlor epoxide. $C_{10}H_5Cl_7O$. (M_r 389.3). *1128100.*
[1024-57-3].
bp: about 200 °C.
mp: about 160 °C.
A suitable certified reference solution (10 ng/µl in cyclohexane) may be used.

Heptafluoro-*N*-methyl-*N*-(trimethylsilyl)butanamide.
$C_8H_{12}F_7NOSi$. (M_r 299.3). *1139500.* [53296-64-3]. 2,2,3,3,4,4,4-Heptafluoro-*N*-methyl-*N*-(trimethylsilyl)butyramide.
Clear, colourless liquid, flammable.
n_D^{20}: about 1.351.
bp: about 148 °C.

Heptane. C_7H_{16}. (M_r 100.2). *1042000.* [142-82-5].
A colourless, flammable liquid, practically insoluble in water, miscible with ethanol and with ether.

d_{20}^{20}: 0.683 to 0.686.
n_D^{20}: 1.387 to 1.388.
Distillation range (2.2.11). Not less than 95 per cent distils between 97 °C and 98 °C.

Hesperidin. $C_{28}H_{34}O_{15}$. (M_r 611). *1139000.* [520-26-3].
(S)-7-[[6-O-(6-Deoxy–α-L-mannopyranosyl)-β-D-glucopyranosyl]oxy]-5-hydroxy-2-(3-hydroxy-4-methoxyphenyl)-2,3-dihydro-4H-1-benzopyran-4-one.
Hygroscopic powder, slightly soluble in water and in methanol.
mp: 258 °C to 262 °C.

Hexachlorobenzene. C_6Cl_6. (M_r 284.8). *1128200.* [118-74-1].
bp: about 332 °C.
mp: about 230 °C.
A suitable certified reference solution (10 ng/µl in cyclohexane) may be used.

α-Hexachlorocyclohexane. $C_6H_6Cl_6$. (M_r 290.8). *1128300.* [319-84-6].
bp: about 288 °C.
mp: about 158 °C.
A suitable certified reference solution (10 ng/µl in cyclohexane) may be used.

β-Hexachlorocyclohexane. $C_6H_6Cl_6$. (M_r 290.8). *1128400.* [319-85-7].
A suitable certified reference solution (10 ng/µl in cyclohexane) may be used.

δ-Hexachlorocyclohexane. $C_6H_6Cl_6$. (M_r 290.8). *1128500.* [319-86-8].
A suitable certified reference solution (10 ng/µl in cyclohexane) may be used.

Hexacosane. $C_{26}H_{54}$. (M_r 366.7). *1042200.* [630-01-3].
Colourless or white flakes.
mp: about 57 °C.

Hexadimethrine bromide. $(C_{13}H_{30}Br_2N_2)_n$. *1042300.* [28728-55-4]. 1,5-Dimethyl-1,5-diazaundecamethylene polymethobromide. Poly(1,1,5,5-tetramethyl-1,5-azonia-undecamethylene dibromide).
A white, amorphous powder, hygroscopic, soluble in water. Store in an airtight container.

2,2′,2″,6,6′,6″-Hexa(1,1-dimethylethyl)-4,4′,4″-[(2,4,6-trimethyl-1,3,5-benzenetriyl)trismethylene]triphenol.
$C_{54}H_{78}O_3$. (M_r 775). *1042100.* 2,2′,2″,6,6′,6″-Hexa-*tert*-butyl-4,4′,4″-[(2,4,6-trimethyl-1,3,5-benzenetriyl)trismethylene]triphenol.
A crystalline powder, practically insoluble in water, soluble in acetone, slightly soluble in alcohol.
mp: about 244 °C.

1,1,1,3,3,3-Hexafluoropropan-2-ol. $C_3H_2F_6O$. (M_r 168.0). *1136000.* [920-66-1].
Contains not less than 99.0 per cent of $C_3H_2F_6O$, determined by gas chromatography.
A clear, colourless liquid, miscible with water and with ethanol.
d^{20}_{20}: about 1.596.
bp: about 59 °C.

Hexamethyldisilazane. $C_6H_{19}NSi_2$. (M_r 161.4). *1042400.* [999-97-3].
A clear, colourless liquid.
d_{20}^{20}: about 0.78.
n_D^{20}: about 1.408.
bp: about 125 °C.
Store in an airtight container.

Hexamethylenetetramine. $C_6H_{12}N_4$. (M_r 140.2). *1042500.* [100-97-0]. Hexamine. 1,3,5,7-Tetra-azatricyclo [3.3.1.1^{3,7}]decane.
A colourless, crystalline powder, very soluble in water.

Hexane. C_6H_{14}. (M_r 86.2). *1042600.* [110-54-3].
A colourless, flammable liquid, practically insoluble in water, miscible with ethanol and with ether.
d_{20}^{20}: 0.659 to 0.663.
n_D^{20}: 1.375 to 1.376.
Distillation range (2.2.11). Not less than 95 per cent distils between 67 °C and 69 °C.

Hexane used in spectrophotometry complies with the following additional test.

Minimum transmittance (2.2.25), determined using *water R* as compensation liquid: 97 per cent from 260 nm to 420 nm.

Hexylamine. $C_6H_{15}N$. (M_r 101.2). *1042700.* [111-26-2].
Hexanamine.
A colourless liquid, slightly soluble in water, soluble in alcohol and in ether.
d_{20}^{20}: about 0.766.
n_D^{20}: about 1.418.
bp: 127 °C to 131 °C.

Histamine dihydrochloride. *1042800.* [56-92-8].
See *Histamine dihydrochloride (0143)*.

Histamine phosphate. *1042900.* [23297-93-0].
See *Histamine phosphate (0144)*.

Histamine solution. *1042901.*
A 9 g/l solution of *sodium chloride R* containing 0.1 µg per millilitre of histamine base (as the phosphate or dihydrochloride).

Histidine monohydrochloride. $C_6H_{10}ClN_3O_2,H_2O$. (M_r 209.6). *1043000.* [123333-71-1]. (RS)-2-Amino-3-(imidazol-4-yl)propionic acid hydrochloride monohydrate.
A crystalline powder or colourless crystals, soluble in water.
mp: about 250 °C, with decomposition.
Chromatography. Examine as prescribed in the monograph on *Histamine dihydrochloride (0143)*; the chromatogram shows only one principal spot.

Holmium oxide. Ho_2O_3. (M_r 377.9). *1043100.* [12055-62-8].
Diholmium trioxide.
A yellowish powder, practically insoluble in water.

Holmium perchlorate solution. *1043101.*
A 40 g/l solution of *holmium oxide R* in a solution of *perchloric acid R* containing 141 g/l of $HClO_4$.

DL-Homocysteine. $C_5H_{11}NO_2S$. (M_r 135.2). *1136100.* [454-29-5]. (2RS)-2-Amino-4-sulphanylbutanoic acid.
A white, crystalline powder.
mp: about 232 °C.

L-Homocysteine thiolactone hydrochloride.
C_4H_8ClNOS. (M_r 153,6). *1136200.* [6038-19-3]. (3S)-3-Aminodihydrothiophen-2(3H)-one hydrochloride.
A white, crystalline powder.
mp: about 202 °C.

Hyaluronidase diluent. *1043300.*
Mix 100 ml of *phosphate buffer solution pH 6.4 R* with 100 ml of *water R*. Dissolve 0.140 g of *hydrolysed gelatin R* in the solution at 37 °C.
Use the solution within 2 h.

Hydrazine. H_4N_2. (M_r 32.05). *1136300*. [302-01-2]. Diazane. A slightly oily liquid, colourless, with a strong odour of ammonia, miscible with water. Dilute solutions in water are commercially available.

Caution: toxic and corrosive.
n_D^{20}: about 1.470.
bp: about 113 °C.
mp: about 1.5 °C.

Hydrazine sulphate. $H_6N_2O_4S$. (M_r 130.1). *1043400*. [10034-93-2].
Colourless crystals, sparingly soluble in cold water, soluble in hot water (50 °C) and freely soluble in boiling water, practically insoluble in alcohol.

Arsenic (2.4.2). 1.0 g complies with limit test A (1 ppm).

Sulphated ash (2.4.14). Not more than 0.1 per cent.

Hydriodic acid. HI. (M_r 127.9). *1098900*. [10034-85-2]. Prepare by distilling hydriodic acid over red phosphorus, passing *carbon dioxide R* or *nitrogen R* through the apparatus during the distillation. Use the colourless or almost colourless, constant-boiling mixture (55 per cent to 58 per cent of HI) distilling between 126 °C and 127 °C. Place the acid in small, amber, glass-stoppered bottles previously flushed with *carbon dioxide R* or *nitrogen R*, seal with paraffin.

Store in a dark place.

Hydrobromic acid, 30 per cent. *1098700*. [10035-10-6]. 30 per cent hydrobromic acid in *glacial acetic acid R*. Degas with caution the contents before opening.

Hydrobromic acid, dilute. *1098701*.
Place 5.0 ml of *30 per cent hydrobromic acid R* in amber vials equipped with polyethylene stoppers. Seal under *argon R* and store in the dark. Add 5.0 ml of *glacial acetic acid R* immediately before use. Shake.

Store in the dark.

Hydrobromic acid, 47 per cent. *1118900*.
A 47 per cent *m/m* solution of hydrobromic acid in *water R*.

Hydrobromic acid, dilute R1. *1118901*.
Contains 7,9 g/l of HBr.

Dissolve 16.81 g of *47 per cent hydrobromic acid R* in *water R* and dilute to 1000 ml with the same solvent.

Hydrochloric acid. *1043500*. [7647-01-0].
See *Concentrated hydrochloric acid (0002)*.

Hydrochloric acid R1. *1043501*.
Contains 250 g/l of HCl.

Dilute 70 g of *hydrochloric acid R* to 100 ml with *water R*.

Hydrochloric acid, brominated. *1043507*.
To 1 ml of *bromine solution R* add 100 ml of *hydrochloric acid R*.

Hydrochloric acid, dilute. *1043503*.
Contains 73 g/l of HCl.

Dilute 20 g of *hydrochloric acid R* to 100 ml with *water R*.

Hydrochloric acid, dilute, heavy metal-free. *1043509*.
Complies with the requirements prescribed for *dilute hydrochloric acid R* and with the following maximum contents of heavy metals:

As: 0.005 ppm;
Cd: 0.003 ppm;
Cu: 0.003 ppm;
Fe: 0.05 ppm;
Hg: 0.005 ppm;
Ni: 0.004 ppm;
Pb: 0.001 ppm;
Zn: 0.005 ppm.

Hydrochloric acid, dilute R1. *1043504*.
Contains 0.37 g/l of HCl.
Dilute 1.0 ml of *dilute hydrochloric acid R* to 200.0 ml with *water R*.

Hydrochloric acid, dilute R2. *1043505*.
Dilute 30 ml of *1 M hydrochloric acid* to 1000 ml with *water R*; adjust to pH 1.6 ± 0.1.

Hydrochloric acid, ethanolic. *1043506*.
Dilute 5.0 ml of *1 M hydrochloric acid* to 500.0 ml with *alcohol R*.

Hydrochloric acid, heavy metal-free. *1043510*.
Complies with the requirements prescribed for *hydrochloric acid R* and with the following maximum contents of heavy metals:

As: 0.005 ppm;
Cd: 0.003 ppm;
Cu: 0.003 ppm;
Fe: 0.05 ppm;
Hg: 0.005 ppm;
Ni: 0.004 ppm;
Pb: 0.001 ppm;
Zn: 0.005 ppm.

Hydrochloric acid, lead-free. *1043508*.
Complies with the requirements prescribed for *hydrochloric acid R* and with the following additional test.

Lead. Not more than 20 ppm of Pb determined by atomic emission spectrometry (*Method I, 2.2.22*).

Test solution. In a quartz crucible evaporate 200 g of the acid to be examined almost to dryness. Take up the residue in 5 ml of nitric acid prepared by sub-boiling distillation of *nitric acid R* and evaporate to dryness. Take up the residue in 5 ml of nitric acid prepared by sub-boiling distillation of *nitric acid R*.

Reference solutions. Prepare the reference solutions using *lead standard solution (0.1 ppm Pb) R* diluted with nitric acid prepared by sub-boiling distillation of *nitric acid R*. Measure the emission intensity at 220.35 nm.

Hydrocortisone acetate. *1098800*. [50-03-3].
See *Hydrocortisone acetate (0334)*.

Hydrofluoric acid. HF. (M_r 20.01). *1043600*. [7664-39-3]. Contains not less than 40.0 per cent *m/m* of HF.

A clear, colourless liquid.

Residue on ignition. Not more than 0.05 per cent *m/m*. Evaporate the hydrofluoric acid in a platinum crucible and gently ignite the residue to constant mass.

Assay. Weigh accurately a glass-stoppered flask containing 50.0 ml of *1 M sodium hydroxide*. Introduce 2 g of the hydrofluoric acid and weigh again. Titrate the solution with *0.5 M sulphuric acid*, using 0.5 ml of *phenolphthalein solution R* as indicator.

1 ml of *1 M sodium hydroxide* is equivalent to 20.01 mg of HF.

Store in a polyethylene container.

Hydrogen for chromatography. H_2. (M_r 2.016). *1043700*. [1333-74-0].
Contains not less than 99.95 per cent *V/V* of H_2.

Hydrogen peroxide solution, dilute. *1043800.* [7722-84-1]. See *Hydrogen peroxide solution (3 per cent) (0395)*.

Hydrogen peroxide solution, strong. *1043900.* [7722-84-1]. See *Hydrogen peroxide solution (30 per cent) (0396)*.

Hydrogen sulphide. H_2S. (M_r 34.08). *1044000.* [7783-06-4]. A gas, slightly soluble in water.

> **Hydrogen sulphide solution.** *1136400.*
> A recently prepared solution of *hydrogen sulphide R* in *water R*. The saturated solution contains about 0.4 per cent to 0.5 per cent of H_2S at 20 °C.

Hydrogen sulphide R1. H_2S. (M_r 34.08). *1106600.* Contains not less than 99.7 per cent *V/V* of H_2S.

Hydroquinone. $C_6H_6O_2$. (M_r 110.1). *1044100.* [123-31-9]. Benzene-1,4-diol.
Fine, colourless or white needles, darkening on exposure to air and light, soluble in water, in alcohol and in ether.
mp: about 173 °C.
Store protected from light and air.

4-Hydroxybenzohydrazide. $C_7H_8N_2O_2$. (M_r 152.2). *1145900.* [5351-23-5]. *p*-Hydroxybenzohydrazide.

4-Hydroxybenzoic acid. $C_7H_6O_3$. (M_r 138.1). *1106700.* [99-96-7].
Crystals, slightly soluble in water, very soluble in alcohol, soluble in acetone and in ether.
mp: 214 °C to 215 °C.

2-[4-(2-Hydroxyethyl)piperazin-1-yl]ethanesulphonic acid. $C_8H_{18}N_2O_4S$. (M_r 238.3). *1106800.* [7365-45-9]. HEPES.
A white powder.
mp: about 236 °C, with decomposition

4-Hydroxyisophthalic acid. $C_8H_6O_5$. (M_r 182.1). *1106900.* [636-46-4]. 4-Hydroxybenzene-1,3-dicarboxylic acid.
Needles or platelets, very slightly soluble in water, freely soluble in alcohol and in ether.
mp: about 314 °C, with decomposition.

Hydroxylamine hydrochloride. NH_4ClO. (M_r 69.5). *1044300.* [5470-11-1].
A white, crystalline powder, very soluble in water, soluble in alcohol.

> **Hydroxylamine hydrochloride solution R2.** *1044304.*
> Dissolve 2.5 g of *hydroxylamine hydrochloride R* in 4.5 ml of hot *water R* and add 40 ml of *alcohol R* and 0.4 ml of *bromophenol blue solution R2*. Add *0.5 M alcoholic potassium hydroxide* until a greenish-yellow colour is obtained. Dilute to 50.0 ml with *alcohol R*.

> **Hydroxylamine solution, alcoholic.** *1044301.*
> Dissolve 3.5 g of *hydroxylamine hydrochloride R* in 95 ml of *alcohol (60 per cent V/V) R*, add 0.5 ml of a 2 g/l solution of *methyl orange R* in *alcohol (60 per cent V/V) R* and sufficient *0.5 M potassium hydroxide in alcohol (60 per cent V/V)* to give a pure yellow colour. Dilute to 100 ml with *alcohol (60 per cent V/V) R*.

> **Hydroxylamine solution, alkaline.** *1044302.*
> Immediately before use, mix equal volumes of a 139 g/l solution of *hydroxylamine hydrochloride R* and a 150 g/l solution of *sodium hydroxide R*.

> **Hydroxylamine solution, alkaline R1.** *1044303.*
> *Solution A*. Dissolve 12.5 g of *hydroxylamine hydrochloride R* in *methanol R* and dilute to 100 ml with the same solvent.

Solution B. Dissolve 12.5 g of *sodium hydroxide R* in *methanol R* and dilute to 100 ml with the same solvent.

Mix equal volumes of solution A and solution B immediately before use.

Hydroxymethylfurfural. $C_6H_6O_3$. (M_r 126.1). *1044400.* [67-47-0]. 5-Hydroxymethylfurfural.
Acicular crystals, freely soluble in water, in acetone and in alcohol, soluble in ether.
mp: about 32 °C.

Hydroxynaphthol blue, sodium salt. $C_{20}H_{11}N_2Na_3O_{11}S_3$. ($M_r$ 620). *1044500.* [63451-35-4]. Trisodium 2,2′-dihydroxy-1,1′-azonaphthalene-3′,4,6′-trisulphonate.

2-Hydroxypropylbetadex for chromatography R. *1146000.* Betacyclodextrin modified by the bonding of (*R*) or (*RS*) propylene oxide groups on the hydroxyl groups.

Hydroxypropyl-β-cyclodextrin. $[C_6H_{10-x}O_5,(C_3H_7O)_x]_7$ where x = molecular substitution degree (M_r 1371-1432, depending on the degree of molar substitution). *1128600.* [94035-02-6]. Hydroxypropylbetadex.
A white to almost white powder.
pH (*2.2.3*): 5.0-7.5 (20 g/l solution).

Hydroxyquinoline. C_9H_7NO. (M_r 145.2). *1044600.* [148-24-3]. 8-Hydroxyquinoline. Quinolin-8-ol.
A white or slightly yellowish, crystalline powder, slightly soluble in water, freely soluble in acetone, in alcohol and in dilute mineral acids.
mp: about 75 °C.
Sulphated ash (2.4.14). Not more than 0.05 per cent.

12-Hydroxystearic acid. $C_{18}H_{36}O_3$. (M_r 300.5). *1099000.* [106-14-9]. 12-Hydroxyoctadecanoic acid.
White powder.
mp: 71 °C to 74 °C.

5-Hydroxyuracil. $C_4H_4N_2O_3$. (M_r 128.1). *1044700.* [496-76-4]. Isobarbituric acid. Pyrimidine-2,4,5-triol.
A white, crystalline powder.
mp: about 310 °C, with decomposition.
Chromatography. Examined as prescribed in the monograph on *Fluorouracil (0611)*, the chromatogram shows a principal spot with an R_f of about 0.3.

Store in an airtight container.

Hyoscine hydrobromide. *1044800.* [6533-68-2]. See *Hyoscine hydrobromide (0106)*.

Hyoscyamine sulphate. *1044900.* [620-61-1]. See *Hyoscyamine sulphate (0501)*.

Hyperoside. $C_{21}H_{20}O_{12}$. (M_r 464.4). *1045000.* 2-(3,4-Dihydroxyphenyl)-3-β-D-galactopyranosyloxy-5,7-dihydroxy-chromen-4-one.
Faint yellow needles, soluble in methanol.
$[\alpha]_D^{20}$: −8.3, determined on a 2 g/l solution in *pyridine R*.
mp: about 240 °C, with decomposition.
A solution in *methanol R* shows two absorption maxima (*2.2.25*), at 259 nm and at 364 nm.

Hypophosphorous reagent. *1045200.*
Dissolve with the aid of gentle heat, 10 g of *sodium hypophosphite R* in 20 ml of *water R* and dilute to 100 ml with *hydrochloric acid R*. Allow to settle and decant or filter through glass wool.

Hypoxanthine. $C_5H_4N_4O$. (M_r 136.1). *1045300*. [68-94-0].
1*H*-Purin-6-one.
A white, crystalline powder, very slightly soluble in water, sparingly soluble in boiling water, soluble in dilute acids and in dilute alkali hydroxide solutions, decomposes without melting at about 150 °C.
Chromatography. Examine as prescribed in the monograph on *Mercaptopurine (0096)*; the chromatogram shows only one principal spot.

Imidazole. $C_3H_4N_2$. (M_r 68.1). *1045400*. [288-32-4].
A white, crystalline powder, soluble in water and in alcohol.
mp: about 90 °C.

Iminodibenzyl. $C_{14}H_{13}N$. (M_r 195.3). *1045500*. [494-19-9].
10,11-Dihydrodibenz[*b,f*]azepine.
A pale yellow, crystalline powder, practically insoluble in water, freely soluble in acetone.
mp: about 106 °C.

Indigo carmine. $C_{16}H_8N_2Na_2O_8S_2$. (M_r 466.3). *1045600*.
[860-22-0].
Schultz No. 1309.
Colour Index No. 73015.
3,3′-Dioxo-2,2′-bisindolylidene-5,5′-disulphonate disodium.
E 132.
It usually contains sodium chloride.

A blue or violet-blue powder or blue granules with a coppery lustre, sparingly soluble in water, practically insoluble in alcohol. It is precipitated from an aqueous solution by sodium chloride.

Indigo carmine solution. *1045601*.

To a mixture of 10 ml of *hydrochloric acid R* and 990 ml of 200 g/l *nitrogen-free sulphuric acid R* add 0.2 g of *indigo carmine R*.

The solution complies with the following test.

Add 10 ml to a solution of 1.0 mg of *potassium nitrate R* in 10 ml of *water R*, rapidly add 20 ml of *nitrogen-free sulphuric acid R* and heat to boiling. The blue colour is discharged within 1 min.

Indigo carmine solution R1. *1045602*.

Dissolve 4 g of *indigo carmine R* in about 900 ml of *water R* added in several portions. Add 2 ml of *sulphuric acid R* and dilute to 1000 ml with *water R*.

Standardisation. Place in a 100 ml conical flask with a wide neck 10.0 ml of *nitrate standard solution (100 ppm NO$_3$) R*, 10 ml of *water R*, 0.05 ml of the *indigo carmine solution R1*, and then in a single addition, but with caution, 30 ml of *sulphuric acid R*. Titrate the solution immediately, using the *indigo carmine solution R1*, until a stable blue colour is obtained.

The number of millilitres used, *n*, is equivalent to 1 mg of NO$_3$.

Indometacin. *1101500*. [53-86-1].
See *Indometacin (0092)*.

Iodine. *1045800*. [7553-56-2].
See *Iodine (0031)*.

Iodine solution R1. *1045801*.
To 10.0 ml of *0.05 M iodine* add 0.6 g of *potassium iodide R* and dilute to 100.0 ml with *water R*. Prepare immediately before use.

Iodine solution R2. *1045802*.
To 10.0 ml of *0.05 M iodine* add 0.6 g of *potassium iodide R* and dilute to 1000.0 ml with *water R*. Prepare immediately before use.

Iodine solution R3. *1045803*.
Dilute 2.0 ml of *iodine solution R1* to 100.0 ml with *water R*. Prepare immediately before use.

Iodine solution R4. *1045806*.
Dissolve 14 g of *iodine R* in 100 ml of a 400 g/l solution of *potassium iodide R*, add 1 ml of *dilute hydrochloric acid R* and dilute to 1000 ml with *water R*.

Store protected from light.

Iodine solution, alcoholic. *1045804*.
A 10 g/l solution in *alcohol R*.

Store protected from light.

Iodine solution, chloroformic. *1045805*.
A 5 g/l solution in *chloroform R*.

Store protected from light.

Iodine bromide. IBr. (M_r 206.8). *1045900*. [7789-33-5].
Bluish-black or brownish-black crystals, freely soluble in water, in alcohol, in ether and in glacial acetic acid.
bp: about 116 °C.
mp: about 40 °C.
Store protected from light, in a cool place.

Iodine bromide solution. *1045901*.
Dissolve 20 g of *iodine bromide R* in *glacial acetic acid R* and dilute to 1000 ml with the same solvent. Store protected from light.

Iodine chloride. ICl. (M_r 162.4). *1143000*. [7790-99-0].
Black crystals, soluble in water, in acetic acid and in alcohol.
bp: about 97.4 °C.

Iodine chloride solution. *1143001*.
Dissolve 1.4 g of *iodine chloride R* in *glacial acetic acid R* and dilute to 100 ml with the same acid.

Store protected from light.

Iodine pentoxide, recrystallised. I_2O_5. (M_r 333.8). *1046000*.
[12029-98-0]. Di-iodine pentoxide. Iodic anhydride.
Contains not less than 99.5 per cent of I_2O_5.

A white, crystalline powder, or white or greyish-white granules, hygroscopic, very soluble in water forming HIO_3.

Stability on heating. Dissolve 2 g, previously heated for 1 h at 200 °C, in 50 ml of *water R*. A colourless solution is obtained.

Assay. Dissolve 0.100 g in 50 ml of *water R*, add 3 g of *potassium iodide R* and 10 ml of *dilute hydrochloric acid R*. Titrate the liberated iodine with *0.1 M sodium thiosulphate*, using 1 ml of *starch solution R* as indicator.

1 ml of *0.1 M sodium thiosulphate* is equivalent to 2.782 mg of I_2O_5.

Store in an airtight container, protected from light.

Iodoacetic acid. $C_2H_3IO_2$. (M_r 185.9). *1107000*. [64-69-7].
Colourless or white crystals, soluble in water and in alcohol.
mp: 82 °C to 83 °C.

2-Iodobenzoic acid. $C_7H_5IO_2$. (M_r 248.0). *1046100*. [88-67-5].
A white or slightly yellow, crystalline powder, slightly soluble in water, soluble in alcohol.
mp: about 160 °C.
Chromatography. Examine by thin-layer chromatography (*2.2.27*), using cellulose for chromatography f_{254} R as the coating substance. Apply to the plate 20 µl of a solution of the 2-iodobenzoic acid, prepared by dissolving 40 mg in 4 ml of *0.1 M sodium hydroxide* and diluting to 10 ml with *water R*. Develop over a path of about 12 cm using as the mobile phase the upper layer obtained by shaking together 20 volumes of *water R*, 40 volumes of *glacial acetic acid R* and 40 volumes of *toluene R*. Allow the plate to dry in air and examine in ultraviolet light at 254 nm. The chromatogram shows only one principal spot.

Iodoethane. C_2H_5I. (M_r 155.9). *1099100*. [75-03-6].
Colourless to slightly yellowish liquid, darkening on exposure to air and light, miscible with alcohol and most organic solvents.
d_{20}^{20}: about 1.95.
n_D^{20}: about 1.513.
bp: about 72 °C.
Store in an airtight container.

2-Iodohippuric acid. $C_9H_8INO_3,2H_2O$. (M_r 341.1). *1046200*. [147-58-0]. 2-(2-Iodobenzamido)acetic acid.
A white or almost white, crystalline powder, sparingly soluble in water.
mp: about 170 °C.
Water (2.5.12). 9 per cent to 13 per cent, determined on 1.000 g.
Chromatography. Examine by thin-layer chromatography (*2.2.27*), using *cellulose for chromatography F_{254} R* as the coating substance. Apply to the plate 20 µl of a solution of the 2-iodohippuric acid, prepared by dissolving 40 mg in 4 ml of *0.1 M sodium hydroxide* and diluting to 10 ml with *water R*. Develop over a path of about 12 cm using as the mobile phase the upper layer obtained by shaking together 20 volumes of *water R*, 40 volumes of *glacial acetic acid R* and 40 volumes of *toluene R*. Allow the plate to dry in air and examine in ultraviolet light at 254 nm. The chromatogram shows only one principal spot.

Iodoplatinate reagent. *1046300*.
To 3 ml of a 100 g/l solution of *chloroplatinic acid R* add 97 ml of *water R* and 100 ml of a 60 g/l solution of *potassium iodide R*.
Store protected from light.

Iodosulphurous reagent. *1046400*.
The apparatus, which must be kept closed and dry during the preparation, consists of a 3000 ml to 4000 ml round-bottomed flask with three inlets for a stirrer and a thermometer and fitted with a drying tube. To 700 ml of *anhydrous pyridine R* and 700 ml of *ethyleneglycol monomethyl ether R* add, with constant stirring, 220 g of finely powdered *iodine R*, previously dried over *diphosphorus pentoxide R*. Continue stirring until the iodine has completely dissolved (about 30 min). Cool to − 10 °C, and add quickly, still stirring, 190 g of *sulphur dioxide R*. Do not allow the temperature to exceed 30 °C. Cool.
Standardisation. Add about 20 ml of *anhydrous methanol R* to a titration vessel and titrate to the end-point with the iodosulphurous reagent (*2.5.12*). Introduce in an appropriate form a suitable amount of *water R*, accurately weighed, and repeat the determination of water. Calculate the water equivalent in milligrams per millilitre of iodosulphurous reagent.

The minimum water equivalent is 3.5 mg of water per millilitre of reagent.
Work protected from humidity. Standardise immediately before use.
Store in a dry container.

5-Iodouracil. $C_4H_3IN_2O_2$. (M_r 238.0). *1046500*. [696-07-1].
5-Iodo-1*H*,3*H*-pyrimidine-2,4-dione.
mp: about 276 °C, with decomposition.
Chromatography. Examine as prescribed in the monograph on *Idoxuridine (0669)*, applying 5 µl of a 0.25 g/l solution. The chromatogram obtained shows only one principal spot.

Ion-exclusion resin for chromatography. *1131000*.
A resin with sulphonic acid groups attached to a polymer lattice consisting of polystyrene cross-linked with divinylbenzene.

Ion-exchange resin, strongly acidic. *1085400*.
A resin in protonated form with sulphonic acid groups attached to a lattice consisting of polystyrene cross-linked with 8 per cent of divinylbenzene. It is available as spherical beads; unless otherwise prescribed, the particle size is 0.3 mm to 1.2 mm.
Capacity. 4.5 mmol to 5 mmol per gram, with a water content of 50 per cent to 60 per cent.
Preparation of a column. Unless otherwise prescribed, use a tube with a fused-in sintered glass disc having a length of 400 mm, an internal diameter of 20 mm and a filling height of about 200 mm. Introduce the resin, mixing it with *water R* and pouring the slurry into the tube, ensuring that no air bubbles are trapped between the particles. When in use, the liquid must not be allowed to fall below the surface of the resin. If the resin is in its protonated form, wash with *water R* until 50 ml requires not more than 0.05 ml of *0.1 M sodium hydroxide* for neutralisation, using 0.1 ml of *methyl orange solution R* as indicator.
If the resin is in its sodium form or if it requires regeneration, pass about 100 ml of a mixture of equal volumes of *hydrochloric acid R1* and *water R* slowly through the column and then wash with *water R* as described above.

Iron. Fe. (A_r 55.85). *1046600*. [7439-89-6].
Grey powder or wire, soluble in dilute mineral acids.

Iron salicylate solution. *1046700*.
Dissolve 0.1 g of *ferric ammonium sulphate R* in a mixture of 2 ml of *dilute sulphuric acid R* and 48 ml of *water R* and dilute to 100 ml with *water R*. Add 50 ml of a 11.5 g/l solution of *sodium salicylate R*, 10 ml of *dilute acetic acid R*, 80 ml of a 136 g/l solution of *sodium acetate R* and dilute to 500 ml with *water R*. The solution should be recently prepared.
Store in an airtight container, protected from light.

Isatin. $C_8H_5NO_2$. (M_r 147.1). *1046800*. [91-56-5].
Indoline-2,3-dione.
Small, yellowish-red crystals, slightly soluble in water, soluble in hot water, in alcohol and in ether, soluble in solutions of alkali hydroxides giving a violet colour becoming yellow on standing.
mp: about 200 °C, with partial sublimation.
Sulphated ash (2.4.14). Not more than 0.2 per cent.

Isatin reagent. *1046801*.
Dissolve 6 mg of *ferric sulphate R* in 8 ml of *water R* and add cautiously 50 ml of *sulphuric acid R*. Add 6 mg of *isatin R* and stir until dissolved.
The reagent should be pale yellow, but not orange or red.

Isoamyl alcohol. $C_5H_{12}O$. (M_r 88.1). *1046900*. [123-51-3]. 3-Methylbutan-1-ol.
A colourless liquid, slightly soluble in water, miscible with alcohol and with ether.
bp: about 130 °C.

Isoandrosterone. $C_{19}H_{30}O_2$. (M_r 290.4). *1107100*. [481-29-8]. Epiandrosterone. 3β-Hydroxy-5α-androstan-17-one.
A white powder, practically insoluble in water, soluble in organic solvents.
$[\alpha]_D^{20}$: + 88, determined on 20 g/l solution in *methanol R*.
mp: 172 °C to 174 °C.
ΔA (*2.2.41*): 14.24×10^3, determined at 304 nm on a 1.25 g/l solution.

Isodrin. $C_{12}H_8Cl_6$. (M_r 364.9). *1128700*. [465-73-6].
1,2,3,4,10,10-Hexachloro-1,4,4a,5,8,8a-hexahydro-*endo,endo*-1,4:5,8-dimethanonaphthalene.
Practically insoluble in water, soluble in common organic solvents such as acetone.
A suitable certified reference solution may be used.

Isomenthol. $C_{10}H_{20}O$. (M_r 156.3). *1047000*. [23283-97-8]. (+)-*Isomenthol*: (1*S*,2*R*,5*R*)-2-isopropyl-5-methylcyclohexanol.
(±)-*Isomenthol*: a mixture of equal parts of (1*S*,2*R*,5*R*)- and (1*R*,2*S*,5*S*)-2-isopropyl-5-methylcyclohexanol.
Colourless crystals, practically insoluble in water, very soluble in alcohol and in ether.
$[\alpha]_D^{20}$: (+)-*Isomenthol*: about + 24, determined on a 100 g/l solution in *alcohol R*.
bp: (+)-*Isomenthol*: about 218 °C. (±)-*Isomenthol*: about 218 °C.
mp: (+)-*Isomenthol*: about 80 °C. (±)-*Isomenthol*: about 53 °C.

(+)-Isomenthone. $C_{10}H_{18}O$. (M_r 154.2). *1047100*. (1R)-*cis-p*-Menthan-3-one. (1R)-*cis*-2-Isopropyl-5-methylcyclohexanone.
Contains variable amounts of menthone. A colourless liquid, very slightly soluble in water, soluble in alcohol and in ether.
d_{20}^{20}: about 0.904.
n_D^{20}: about 1.453.
$[\alpha]_D^{20}$: about + 93.2.
Isomenthone used in gas chromatography complies with the following additional test.

Assay. Examine by gas chromatography (*2.2.28*) as prescribed in the monograph on *Peppermint oil (0405)* using the substance to be examined as the test solution.

The area of the principal peak is not less than 80.0 per cent of the total area of the peaks.

Isopropylamine. C_3H_9N. (M_r 59.1). *1119800*. [75-31-0]. Propan-2-amine.
A colourless, highly volatile, flammable liquid.
n_D^{20}: about 1.374.
bp: 32 °C to 34 °C.

Isopropyl myristate. *1047200*. [110-27-0].
See *Isopropyl myristate (0725)*.

4-Isopropylphenol. $C_9H_{12}O$. (M_r 136.2). *1047300*. [99-89-8].
Contains not less than 98 per cent of $C_9H_{12}O$.
bp: about 212 °C.
mp: 59 °C to 61 °C.

Isopulegol. $C_{10}H_{18}O$. (M_r 154.2). *1139600*. [89-79-2]. (−)-Isopulegol. (1*R*,2*S*,5*R*)-2-Isopropenyl-5-methylcyclohexanol.
d_4^{20}: about 0.911.
n_D^{20}: about 1.472.
bp: about 91 °C.
Isopulegol used in gas chromatography complies with the following additional test.

Assay. Examine by gas chromatography (*2.2.28*) as prescribed in the monograph on *Mint oil, partly dementholised (1838)*.

The content is not less than 99 per cent, calculated by the normalisation procedure.

Isoquercitroside. $C_{21}H_{20}O_{12}$. (M_r 464.4). *1136500*. [21637-25-2]. Isoquercitrin. 2-(3,4-Dihydroxyphenyl)-3-(β-D-glucofuranosyloxy)-5,7-dihydroxy-4*H*-1-benzopyran-4-one. 3,3′,4′,5,7-Pentahydroxyflavone-3-glucoside.

Kaolin, light. *1047400*. [1332-58-7].
A purified native hydrated aluminium silicate. It contains a suitable dispersing agent.

A light, white powder free from gritty particles, unctuous to the touch, practically insoluble in water and in mineral acids.

Coarse particles. Place 5.0 g in a ground-glass-stoppered cylinder about 160 mm long and 35 mm in diameter and add 60 ml of a 10 g/l solution of *sodium pyrophosphate R*. Shake vigorously and allow to stand for 5 min. Using a pipette, remove 50 ml of the liquid from a point about 5 cm below the surface. To the remaining liquid add 50 ml of *water R*, shake, allow to stand for 5 min and remove 50 ml as before. Repeat the operations until a total of 400 ml has been removed. Transfer the remaining suspension to an evaporating dish. Evaporate to dryness on a water-bath and dry the residue to constant mass at 100 °C to 105 °C. The residue weighs not more than 25 mg (0.5 per cent).

Fine particles. Disperse 5.0 g in 250 ml of *water R* by shaking vigorously for 2 min. Immediately pour into a glass cylinder 50 mm in diameter and, using a pipette, transfer 20 ml to a glass dish, evaporate to dryness on a water-bath and dry to constant mass at 100 °C to 105 °C. Allow the remainder of the suspension to stand at 20 °C for 4 h and, using a pipette with its tip exactly 5 cm below the surface, withdraw a further 20 ml without disturbing the sediment, place in a glass dish, evaporate to dryness on a water-bath and dry to constant mass at 100 °C to 105 °C. The mass of the second residue is not less than 70 per cent of that of the first residue.

Kieselguhr for chromatography. *1047500*.

A white or yellowish-white, light powder, practically insoluble in water, in dilute acids and in organic solvents.

Filtration rate. Use a chromatography column 0.25 m long and 10 mm in internal diameter with a sintered-glass (100) plate and two marks at 0.10 m and 0.20 m above the plate. Place sufficient of the substance to be examined in the column to reach the first mark and fill to the second mark with *water R*. When the first drops begin to flow from the column, fill to the second mark again with *water R* and measure the time required for the first 5 ml to flow from the column. The flow rate is not less than 1 ml/min.

Appearance of the eluate. The eluate obtained in the test for filtration rate is colourless (*Method I, 2.2.2*).

Acidity or alkalinity. To 1.00 g add 10 ml of *water R*, shake vigorously and allow to stand for 5 min. Filter the suspension on a filter previously washed with hot *water R* until the washings are neutral. To 2.0 ml of the filtrate add 0.05 ml of *methyl red solution R*; the solution is yellow. To 2.0 ml of the filtrate add 0.05 ml of *phenolphthalein solution R1*; the solution is at most slightly pink.

Water-soluble substances. Place 10.0 g in a chromatography column 0.25 m long and 10 mm in internal diameter and elute with *water R*. Collect the first 20 ml of eluate, evaporate to dryness and dry the residue at 100 °C to 105 °C. The residue weighs not more than 10 mg.

Iron (2.4.9). To 0.50 g add 10 ml of a mixture of equal volumes of *hydrochloric acid R1* and *water R*, shake vigorously, allow to stand for 5 min and filter. 1.0 ml of the filtrate complies with the limit test for iron (200 ppm).

Loss on ignition. Not more than 0.5 per cent. During heating to red heat (600 °C) the substance does not become brown or black.

Kieselguhr G. *1047600.*

Consists of kieselguhr treated with hydrochloric acid and calcined, to which is added about 15 per cent of calcium sulphate hemihydrate.

A fine greyish-white powder; the grey colour becomes more pronounced on triturating with water. The average particle size is 10 μm to 40 μm.

Calcium sulphate content. Determine by the method prescribed for *silica gel G R.*

pH (2.2.3). Shake 1 g with 10 ml of *carbon dioxide-free water R* for 5 min. The pH of the suspension is 7 to 8.

Chromatographic separation. Examine by thin-layer chromatography (2.2.27). Prepare plates using a slurry of the kieselguhr G with a 2.7 g/l solution of *sodium acetate R.* Apply 5 μl of a solution containing 0.1 g/l of lactose, sucrose, glucose and fructose in *pyridine R.* Develop over a path of 14 cm using a mixture of 12 volumes of *water R*, 23 volumes of *2-propanol R* and 65 volumes of *ethyl acetate R.* The migration time of the solvent is about 40 min. Dry, spray onto the plate about 10 ml of *anisaldehyde solution R* and heat for 5 min to 10 min at 100 °C to 105 °C. The chromatogram shows four well-defined spots without tailing and well separated from each other.

Lactic acid. *1047800.* [50-21-5].
See *Lactic acid (0458).*

> **Lactic reagent.** *1047801.*
> *Solution A.* To 60 ml of *lactic acid R* add 45 ml of previously filtered *lactic acid R* saturated without heating with *Sudan red G R;* as lactic acid saturates slowly without heating, an excess of colorant is always necessary.
>
> *Solution B.* Prepare 10 ml of a saturated solution of *aniline R.* Filter.
>
> *Solution C.* Dissolve 75 mg of *potassium iodide R* in water and dilute to 70 ml with the same solvent. Add 10 ml of *alcohol R* and 0.1 g of *iodine R.* Shake.
>
> Mix solutions A and B. Add solution C.

Lactobionic acid. $C_{12}H_{22}O_{12}$. (M_r 358.3). *1101600.* [96-82-2]. A white, crystalline powder, freely soluble in water, practically insoluble in alcohol.
mp: about 115 °C.

Lactose. *1047900.* [5989-81-1].
See *Lactose (0187).*

Lanthanum nitrate. $La(NO_3)_3, 6H_2O$. (M_r 433.0). *1048000.* [10277-43-7]. Lanthanum trinitrate hexahydrate. Colourless crystals, deliquescent, freely soluble in water. Store in an airtight container.

> **Lanthanum nitrate solution.** *1048001.*
> A 50 g/l solution.

Lanthanum trioxide. La_2O_3. (M_r 325.8). *1114000.* [1312-81-8].
An almost white, amorphous powder, practically insoluble in *water R.* It dissolves in dilute solutions of mineral acids and absorbs atmospheric carbon dioxide.
Calcium. Not more than 5 ppm.

Lanthanum chloride solution. *1114001.*
To 58.65 g of *lanthanum trioxide R* slowly add 100 ml of *hydrochloric acid R.* Heat to boiling. Allow to cool and dilute to 1000.0 ml with *water R.*

Lauric acid. $C_{12}H_{24}O_2$. (M_r 200.3). *1143100.* [143-07-7]. Dodecanoic acid.
White, crystalline powder, practically insoluble in water, freely soluble in alcohol.
mp: about 44 °C.
Lauric acid used in the assay of total fatty acids in Saw palmetto fruit (1848) complies with the following additional requirement.
Assay. Examine by gas chromatography (2.2.28) as prescribed in the monograph on *Saw palmetto fruit (1848).*
The content of lauric acid is not less than 98 per cent, calculated by the normalisation procedure.

Lauryl alcohol. $C_{12}H_{26}O$. (M_r 186.3). *1119900.* [112-53-8]. 1-Dodecanol.
d_{20}^{20}: about 0.820.
mp: 24 °C to 27 °C.

Lavandulol. $C_{10}H_{18}O$. (M_r 154.2). *1114100.* [498-16-8]. (R)-5-Methyl-2-(1-methylethenyl)-4-hexen-1-ol.
An oily liquid with a characteristic odour.
d_{20}^{20}: about 0.875.
n_D^{20}: about 1.407.
$[\alpha]_D^{20}$: about − 10.2.
bp_{13}: about 94 °C.
Lavandulol used in gas chromatography complies with the following additional test.
Assay. Examine by gas chromatography (2.2.28) as prescribed in the monograph on *Lavender oil (1338).*
Test solution. The substance to be examined.
The area of the principal peak is not less than 98.0 per cent of the area of all the peaks in the chromatogram obtained.

Lavandulyl acetate. $C_{12}H_{20}O_2$. (M_r 196.3). *1114200.* [50373-59-6]. 2-Isopropenyl-5-methylhex-4-en-1-yl acetate.
A colourless liquid with a characteristic odour.
d_{20}^{20}: about 0.911.
n_D^{20}: about 1.454.
bp_{13}: 106 °C to 107 °C.
Lavandulyl acetate used in gas chromatography complies with the following additional test.
Assay. Examine by gas chromatography (2.2.28) as prescribed in the monograph on *Lavender oil (1338).*
Test solution. The substance to be examined.
The area of the principal peak is not less than 93.0 per cent of the area of all the peaks in the chromatogram obtained.

Lead acetate. $C_4H_6O_4Pb, 3H_2O$. (M_r 379.3). *1048100.* [6080-56-4]. Lead di-acetate.
Colourless crystals, efflorescent, freely soluble in water, soluble in alcohol.

> **Lead acetate cotton.** *1048101.*
> Immerse absorbent cotton in a mixture of 1 volume of *dilute acetic acid R* and 10 volumes of *lead acetate solution R.* Drain off the excess of liquid, without squeezing the cotton, by placing it on several layers of filter paper. Allow to dry in air.
> Store in an airtight container.

> **Lead acetate paper.** *1048102.*
> Immerse filter paper weighing about 80 g/m² in a mixture of 1 volume of *dilute acetic acid R* and 10 volumes of *lead acetate solution R.* After drying, cut the paper into strips 15 mm by 40 mm.

Lead acetate solution. *1048103.*
A 95 g/l solution in *carbon dioxide-free water R.*

Lead dioxide. PbO_2. (M_r 239.2). *1048200.* [1309-60-0].
A dark brown powder, evolving oxygen when heated, practically insoluble in water, soluble in hydrochloric acid with evolution of chlorine, soluble in dilute nitric acid in the presence of hydrogen peroxide, oxalic acid or other reducing agents, soluble in hot, concentrated alkali hydroxide solutions.

Lead nitrate. $Pb(NO_3)_2$. (M_r 331.2). *1048300.* [10099-74-8].
Lead dinitrate.
A white, crystalline powder or colourless crystals, freely soluble in water.

Lead nitrate solution. *1048301.*
A 33 g/l solution.

Lead subacetate solution. *1048400.* [1335-32-6]. Basic lead acetate solution.
Contains not less than 16.7 per cent *m/m* and not more than 17.4 per cent *m/m* of Pb (A_r 207.2) in a form corresponding approximately to the formula $C_8H_{14}O_{10}Pb_3$.
Dissolve 40.0 g of *lead acetate R* in 90 ml of *carbon dioxide-free water R.* Adjust the pH to 7.5 with *strong sodium hydroxide solution R.* Centrifuge and use the clear colourless supernatant solution.

The solution remains clear when stored in a well-closed container.

Lemon oil. *1101700.*
See *Lemon oil (0620).*

Leucine. *1048500.* [61-90-5].
See *Leucine (0771).*

Levomenol. $C_{15}H_{26}O$. (M_r 222.4). *1128800.* [23089-26-1].
(−)-(2S)-6-Methyl-2-[(1S)-4-methylcyclohex-3-enyl]hept-5-en-2-ol. (−)-α-Bisabolol.
A colourless viscous liquid with a slight characteristic odour; practically insoluble in water freely soluble in alcohol, in methanol, in toluene, in fatty oils and in essential oils.
d_{20}^{20}: 0.925 to 0.935.
n_D^{20}: 1.493 to 1.500.
$[\alpha]_D^{20}$: −54.5 to 58.0, determined on a 50 mg/ml solution in *alcohol R.*

Limonene. $C_{10}H_{16}$. (M_r 136.2). *1048600.*
[5989-27-5]. D-Limonene. (+)-*p*-Mentha-1,8-diene.
(R)-4-Isopropenyl-1-methylcyclohex-1-ene.
A colourless liquid, practically insoluble in water, soluble in alcohol.
d_{20}^{20}: about 0.84.
n_D^{20}: 1.471 to 1.474.
$[\alpha]_D^{20}$: + 96 to + 106.
bp: 175 °C to 177 °C.
Limonene used in gas chromatography complies with the following additional test.

Assay. Examine by gas chromatography (*2.2.28*) as prescribed in the monograph on *Peppermint oil (0405)* using the substance to be examined as the test solution.

The area of the principal peak is not less than 99.0 per cent of the total area of the peaks.

Linalol. $C_{10}H_{18}O$. (M_r 154.2). *1048700.* [78-70-6].
(RS)-3,7-Dimethylocta-1,6-dien-3-ol.
Mixture of two stereoisomers (licareol and coriandrol).

Liquid, practically insoluble in water, soluble in ether.

d_{20}^{20}: about 0.860.
n_D^{20}: about 1.462.
bp: about 200 °C.
Linalol used in gas chromatography complies with the following test.

Assay. Examine by gas chromatography (*2.2.28*) under the conditions described in the monograph on *Anise oil (0804)* using the substance to be examined as the test solution.

The area of the principal peak is not less than 98.0 per cent of the total area of the peaks.

Linalyl acetate. $C_{12}H_{20}O_2$. (M_r 196.3). *1107200.* [115-95-7].
(RS)-1,5-Dimethyl-1-vinylhex-4-enyl acetate.
A colourless or slightly yellow liquid with a strong odour of bergamot and lavender.
d_{25}^{25}: : 0.895 to 0.912.
n_D^{20}: 1.448 to 1.451.
bp: about 215 °C.
Linalyl acetate used in gas chromatography complies with the following additional test.

Assay. Examine by gas chromatography (*2.2.28*) as prescribed in the monograph on *Bitter-orange-flower oil (1175)*, using the substance to be examined as the test solution.

The area of the principal peak is not less than 95.0 per cent of the total area of the peaks.

Lindane. $C_6H_6Cl_6$. (M_r 290.8). *1128900.* [58-89-9].
γ-Hexachlorocyclohexane.
See *Lindane (0772).*
For the monograph *Wool fat (0134)*, a suitable certified reference solution (10 ng/μl in cyclohexane) may be used.

Linoleic acid. $C_{18}H_{32}O_2$. (M_r 280.5). *1143200.* [60-33-3].
(9Z,12Z)-Octadeca-9,12-dienoic acid.
Colourless, oily liquid.
d_4^{20}: about 0.903.
n_D^{20}: about 1.470.
Linoleic acid used in the assay of total fatty acids in Saw palmetto fruit (1848) complies with the following additional requirement.

Assay. Examine by gas chromatography (*2.2.28*) as prescribed in the monograph on *Saw palmetto fruit (1848).*

The content of linoleic acid is not less than 98 per cent, calculated by the normalisation procedure.

Linolenic acid. $C_{18}H_{30}O_2$. (M_r 278.4). *1143300.* [463-40-1].
(9Z,12Z,15Z)-Octadeca-9,12,15-trienoic acid.
Colourless liquid, practically insoluble in water, soluble in organic solvents.
d_4^{20}: about 0.915.
n_D^{20}: about 1.480.
Linolenic acid used in the assay of total fatty acids in Saw palmetto fruit (1848) complies with the following additional requirement.

Assay. Examine by gas chromatography (*2.2.28*) as prescribed in the monograph on *Saw palmetto fruit (1848).*

The content of linolenic acid is not less than 98 per cent, calculated by the normalisation procedure.

Lithium. Li. (A_r 6.94). *1048800.* [7439-93-2].
A soft metal whose freshly cut surface is silvery-grey. It rapidly tarnishes in contact with air. It reacts violently with water, yielding hydrogen and giving a solution of lithium hydroxide; soluble in methanol, yielding hydrogen and a solution of lithium methoxide; practically insoluble in ether and in light petroleum.
Store under light petroleum or liquid paraffin.

General Notices (1) apply to all monographs and other texts

Lithium carbonate. Li_2CO. (M_r 73.9). *1048900.* [554-13-2].
Dilithium carbonate.
A white, light powder, sparingly soluble in water, very slightly soluble in alcohol. A saturated solution at 20 °C contains about 13 g/l of Li_2CO_3.

Lithium chloride. LiCl. (M_r 42.39). *1049000.* [7447-41-8].
Crystalline powder or granules or cubic crystals, deliquescent, freely soluble in water, soluble in acetone and in alcohol. Aqueous solutions are neutral or slightly alkaline. Store in an airtight container.

Lithium hydroxide. $LiOH,H_2O$. (M_r 41.96). *1049100.* [1310-66-3]. Lithium hydroxide monohydrate.
A white, granular powder, strongly alkaline, it rapidly absorbs water and carbon dioxide, soluble in water, sparingly soluble in alcohol.
Store in an airtight container.

Lithium metaborate, anhydrous. $LiBO_2$. (M_r 49.75). *1120000.* [13453-69-5].

Lithium sulphate. Li_2SO_4,H_2O. (M_r 128.0). *1049200.* [10102-25-7]. Dilithium sulphate monohydrate.
Colourless crystals, freely soluble in water, practically insoluble in alcohol.

Litmus. *1049300.* [1393-92-6].
Schultz No. 1386.
Indigo-blue fragments prepared from various species of Rocella, Lecanora or other lichens, soluble in water, practically insoluble in alcohol.
Colour change. pH 5 (red) to pH 8 (blue).

Litmus paper, blue. *1049301.*
Boil 10 parts of coarsely powdered *litmus R* for 1 h with 100 parts of *alcohol R*. Decant the alcohol and add to the residue a mixture of 45 parts of *alcohol R* and 55 parts of *water R*. After 2 days decant the clear liquid. Impregnate strips of filter paper with the solution and allow to dry.
Test for sensitivity. Immerse a strip measuring 10 mm by 60 mm in a mixture of 10 ml of *0.02 M hydrochloric acid* and 90 ml of *water R*. On shaking the paper turns red within 45 s.

Litmus paper, red. *1049302.*
To the blue litmus extract, add *dilute hydrochloric acid R* dropwise until the blue colour becomes red. Impregnate strips of filter paper with the solution and allow to dry.
Test for sensitivity. Immerse a strip measuring 10 mm by 60 mm in a mixture of 10 ml of *0.02 M sodium hydroxide* and 90 ml of *water R*. On shaking the paper turns blue within 45 s.

Loganin. $C_{17}H_{26}O_{10}$. (M_r 390.4). *1136700.* [18524-94-2].
Methyl (1S,4aS,6S,7R,7aS)-1-(β-D-glucopyranosyloxy)-6-hydroxy-7-methyl-1,4a,5,6,7,7a-hexahydrocyclopenta[c]pyran-4-carboxylate.
mp: 220 °C to 221 °C.

Low-vapour-pressure hydrocarbons (type L). *1049400.*
Unctuous mass, soluble in benzene and in toluene.

Lumiflavine. $C_{13}H_{12}N_4O_2$. (M_r 256.3). *1141000.* [1088-56-8].
7,8,10-Trimethylbenzo[g]pteridine-2,4(3H,10H)-dione.
Yellow powder or orange crystals, very slightly soluble in water, freely soluble in methylene chloride.

Macrogol 23 lauryl ether. *1129000.*
Complies with the monograph *Macrogol lauryl ether (1124)*, the nominal value for the amount of ethylene oxide reacted with lauryl alcohol being 23.

Macrogol 200. *1099200.* [25322-68-3]. Polyethyleneglycol 200.
A clear, colourless or almost colourless viscous liquid, very soluble in acetone and in ethanol, practically insoluble in ether and in fatty oils.
d_{20}^{20}: about 1.127.
n_D^{20}: about 1.450.

Macrogol 200 R1. *1099201.*
Introduce 500 ml of *macrogol 200 R* into a 1000 ml round bottom flask. Using a rotation evaporator remove any volatile components applying for 6 h a temperature of 60 °C and a vacuum with a pressure of 1.5 kPa to 2.5 kPa.

Macrogol 300. *1067100.* [25322-68-3]. Polyethyleneglycol 300.
See *Macrogols (1444)*.

Macrogol 400. *1067200.* [25322-68-3]. Polyethyleneglycol 400.
See *Macrogols (1444)*.

Macrogol 1000. *1067300.* [25322-68-3]. Polyethyleneglycol 1000.
See *Macrogols (1444)*.

Macrogol 1500. *1067400.* [25322-68-3]. Polyethyleneglycol 1500.
See *Macrogols (1444)*.

Macrogol 20 000. *1067600.* Polyethyleneglycol 20 000.
See *Macrogols (1444)*.

Macrogol 20 000 2-nitroterephthalate. *1067601.*
Polyethyleneglycol 20 000 2-nitroterephthalate.
Macrogol 20 000 R modified by treating with 2-nitroterephthalate acid.
A hard, white or almost white, waxy solid, soluble in acetone.

Magnesium. Mg. (A_r 24.30). *1049500.* [7439-95-4].
Silver-white ribbon, turnings or wire, or a grey powder.

Magnesium acetate. $C_4H_6MgO_4,4H_2O$. (M_r 214.5). *1049600.* [16674-78-5]. Magnesium diacetate tetrahydrate.
Colourless crystals, deliquescent, freely soluble in water and in alcohol.
Store in an airtight container.

Magnesium chloride. *1049700.* [7791-18-6].
See *Magnesium chloride hexahydrate (0402)*.

Magnesium nitrate. $Mg(NO_3)_2,6H_2O$. (M_r 256.4). *1049800.* [13446-18-9]. Magnesium nitrate hexahydrate.
Colourless, clear crystals, deliquescent, very soluble in water, freely soluble in alcohol.
Store in an airtight container.

Magnesium nitrate solution. *1049801.*
Dissolve 17.3 g of *magnesium nitrate R* in 5 ml of *water R* warming gently and add 80 ml of *alcohol R*. Cool and dilute to 100.0 ml with the same solvent.

Magnesium oxide. *1049900.* [1309-48-4].
See *Light magnesium oxide (0040)*.

Magnesium oxide R1. *1049901.*
Complies with the requirements prescribed for *magnesium oxide R* with the following modifications.
Arsenic (2.4.2). Dissolve 0.5 g in a mixture of 5 ml of *water R* and 5 ml of *hydrochloric acid R1*. The solution complies with limit test A for arsenic (2 ppm).

Heavy metals (*2.4.8*). Dissolve 1.0 g in a mixture of 3 ml of *water R* and 7 ml of *hydrochloric acid R1*. Add 0.05 ml of *phenolphthalein solution R* and *concentrated ammonia R* until a pink colour is obtained. Neutralise the excess of ammonia by the addition of *glacial acetic acid R*. Add 0.5 ml in excess and dilute to 20 ml with *water R*. Filter, if necessary. 12 ml of the solution complies with limit test A for heavy metals (10 ppm). Prepare the standard using a mixture of 5 ml of *lead standard solution (1 ppm Pb) R* and 5 ml of *water R*.

Iron (*2.4.9*). Dissolve 0.2 g in 6 ml of *dilute hydrochloric acid R* and dilute to 10 ml with *water R*. The solution complies with the limit test for iron (50 ppm).

Magnesium oxide, heavy. *1050000*. [1309-48-4]. See *Heavy magnesium oxide (0041)*.

Magnesium silicate for pesticide residue analysis. *1129100*. [1343-88-0]. Magnesium silicate for chromatography (60-100 mesh).

Magnesium sulphate. *1050200*. [10034-99-8]. See *Magnesium sulphate (0044)*.

Maize oil. *1050400*. See *Maize oil, refined (1342)*.

Malachite green. $C_{23}H_{25}ClN_2$. (M_r 364.9). *1050500*. [123333-61-9]. Schultz No. 754. Colour Index No. 42000. [4-[[4-(Dimethylamino)phenyl]phenylmethylene]cyclohexa-2,5-dien-1-ylidene]dimethylammonium chloride. Green crystals with a metallic lustre, very soluble in water giving a bluish-green solution, soluble in alcohol and in methanol. A 0.01 g/l solution in *alcohol R* shows an absorption maximum (*2.2.25*) at 617 nm.

> **Malachite green solution.** *1050501*.
> A 5 g/l solution in *anhydrous acetic acid R*.

Malathion. $C_{10}H_{19}O_6PS_2$. (M_r 330.3). *1129200*. [121-75-5]. bp: about 156 °C. A suitable certified reference solution (10 ng/µl in iso-octane) may be used.

Maleic acid. *1050600*. [110-16-7]. See *Maleic acid (0365)*.

Maleic anhydride. $C_4H_2O_3$. (M_r 98.1). *1050700*. [108-31-6]. Butenedioic anhydride. 2,5-Furandione. White crystals, soluble in water forming maleic acid, very soluble in acetone and in ethyl acetate, freely soluble in toluene, soluble in alcohol with ester formation, very slightly soluble in light petroleum. mp: about 52 °C. Any residue insoluble in toluene does not exceed 5 per cent (maleic acid).

> **Maleic anhydride solution.** *1050701*.
> Dissolve 5 g of *maleic anhydride R* in *toluene R* and dilute to 100 ml with the same solvent. Use within one month. If the solution becomes turbid, filter.

Maltitol. *1136800*. [585-88-6]. See *Maltitol (1235)*.

Manganese sulphate. $MnSO_4,H_2O$. (M_r 169.0). *1050900*. [10034-96-5]. Manganese sulphate monohydrate. Pale-pink, crystalline powder or crystals, freely soluble in water, practically insoluble in alcohol. *Loss on ignition*. 10.0 per cent to 12.0 per cent, determined on 1.000 g at 500 °C.

Mannitol. *1051000*. [69-65-8]. See *Mannitol (0559)*.

Mannose. $C_6H_{12}O_6$. (M_r 180.2). *1051100*. [3458-28-4]. D-(+)-Mannose. A white, crystalline powder or small, white crystals, very soluble in water, slightly soluble in ethanol. $[\alpha]_D^{20}$: + 13.7 + 14.7, determined on a 200 g/l solution in *water R* containing about 0.05 per cent of NH_3. mp: about 132 °C, with decomposition.

Meclozine hydrochloride. *1051200*. [1104-22-9]. See *Meclozine hydrochloride (0622)*.

Melamine. $C_3H_6N_6$. (M_r 126.1). *1051300*. [108-78-1]. 1,3,5-Triazine-2,4,6-triamine. A white, amorphous powder, very slightly soluble in water and in alcohol.

Menadione. *1051400*. [58-27-5]. See *Menadione (0507)*.

Menthofuran. $C_{10}H_{14}O$. (M_r 150.2). *1051500*. [17957-94-7]. 3,9-Epoxy-*p*-mentha-3,8-diene. 3,6-Dimethyl-4,5,6,7-tetrahydro-benzofuran. A slightly bluish liquid, very slightly soluble in water, soluble in alcohol. d_{15}^{20}: about 0.965. n_D^{20}: about 1.480. $[\alpha]_D^{20}$: about + 93. bp: 196 °C. *Menthofuran used in gas chromatography complies with the following additional test.*

Assay. Examine by gas chromatography (*2.2.28*) as prescribed in the monograph on *Peppermint oil (0405)* using the substance to be examined as the test solution.

The area of the principal peak is not less than 97.0 per cent of the total area of the peaks.

Menthol. *1051600*. [2216-51-5]. See *Levomenthol (0619)* and *Racemic menthol (0623)*. *Menthol used in gas chromatography complies with the following additional test.*

Assay. Examine by gas chromatography (*2.2.28*) as prescribed in the Related substances test included in the monograph on *Racemic menthol (0623)*.

The area of the principal peak is not less than 98.0 per cent of the total area of the peaks, disregarding any peak due to the solvent.

Menthone. $C_{10}H_{18}O$. (M_r 154.2). *1051700*. [14073-97-3]. (2*S*,5*R*)-2-Isopropyl-5-methylcyclohexanone. (−)-*trans*-*p*-Menthan-3-one. Contains variable amounts of isomenthone. A colourless liquid, very slightly soluble in water, very soluble in alcohol and in ether. d_{20}^{20}: about 0.897. n_D^{20}: about 1.450. *Menthone used in gas chromatography complies with the following additional test.*

Assay. Examine by gas chromatography (*2.2.28*) as prescribed in the monograph on *Peppermint oil (0405)* using the substance to be examined as the test solution.

The area of the principal peak is not less than 90.0 per cent of the total area of the peaks.

Menthyl acetate. $C_{12}H_{22}O_2$. (M_r 198.3). *1051800*. [16409-45-3]. 2-Isopropyl-5-methylcyclohexyl acetate. A colourless liquid, slightly soluble in water, miscible with alcohol and with ether. d_{20}^{20}: about 0.92.

n_D^{20}: about 1.447.
bp: about 225 °C.
Menthyl acetate used in gas chromatography complies with the following additional test.

Assay. Examine by gas chromatography (*2.2.28*) as prescribed in the monograph on *Peppermint oil (0405)* using the substance to be examined as the test solution.

The area of the principal peak is not less than 98.0 per cent of the total area of the peaks.

2-Mercaptoethanol. C_2H_6OS. (M_r 78.1). *1099300*. [60-24-2].
A liquid, miscible with water.
d_{20}^{20}: about 1.116.
bp: about 157 °C.

Mercaptopurine. *1051900*. [6112-76-1].
See *Mercaptopurine (0096)*.

Mercuric acetate. $C_4H_6HgO_4$. (M_r 318.7). *1052000*.
[1600-27-7]. Mercury diacetate.
White crystals, freely soluble in water, soluble in alcohol.

Mercuric acetate solution. *1052001*.
Dissolve 3.19 g of *mercuric acetate R* in *anhydrous acetic acid R* and dilute to 100 ml with the same acid. If necessary, neutralise the solution with *0.1 M perchloric acid* using 0.05 ml of *crystal violet solution R* as indicator.

Mercuric bromide. $HgBr_2$. (M_r 360.4). *1052100*. [7789-47-1].
Mercury dibromide.
White or faintly yellow crystals or a crystalline powder, slightly soluble in water, soluble in alcohol.

Mercuric bromide paper. *1052101*.
In a rectangular dish place a 50 g/l solution of *mercuric bromide R* in *ethanol R* and immerse in it pieces of white filter paper weighing 80 g per square metre (speed of filtration = filtration time expressed in seconds for 100 ml of water at 20 °C with a filter surface of 10 cm² and constant pressure of 6.7 kPa: 40 s to 60 s), each measuring 1.5 cm by 20 cm and folded in two. Allow the excess liquid to drain and allow the paper to dry, protected from light, suspended over a non-metallic thread. Discard 1 cm from each end of each strip and cut the remainder into 1.5 cm squares or discs of 1.5 cm diameter.

Store in a glass-stoppered container wrapped with black paper.

Mercuric chloride. *1052200*. [7487-94-7].
See *Mercuric chloride (0120)*.

Mercuric chloride solution. *1052201*.
A 54 g/l solution.

Mercuric iodide. HgI_2. (M_r 454.4). *1052300*. [7774-29-0].
Mercury di-iodide.
A dense, scarlet, crystalline powder, slightly soluble in water, sparingly soluble in acetone, in alcohol and in ether, soluble in an excess of *potassium iodide solution R*.
Store protected from light.

Mercuric nitrate. $Hg(NO_3)_2,H_2O$. (M_r 342.6). *1052400*.
[7782-86-7]. Mercury dinitrate monohydrate.
Colourless or slightly coloured crystals, hygroscopic, soluble in water in the presence of a small quantity of nitric acid.
Store in an airtight container, protected from light.

Mercuric oxide. HgO. (M_r 216.6). *1052500*. [21908-53-2].
Yellow mercuric oxide. Mercury oxide.
A yellow to orange-yellow powder, practically insoluble in water and in alcohol.
Store protected from light.

Mercuric sulphate solution. *1052600*. [7783-35-9].
Dissolve 1 g of *mercuric oxide R* in a mixture of 20 ml of *water R* and 4 ml of *sulphuric acid R*.

Mercuric thiocyanate. $Hg(SCN)_2$. (M_r 316.7). *1052700*.
[592-85-8]. Mercury di(thiocyanate).
A white, crystalline powder, very slightly soluble in water, slightly soluble in alcohol and in ether, soluble in solutions of sodium chloride.

Mercuric thiocyanate solution. *1052701*.
Dissolve 0.3 g of *mercuric thiocyanate R* in *ethanol R* and dilute to 100 ml with the same solvent.
Use within 1 week.

Mercury. Hg. (A_r 200.6). *1052800*. [7439-97-6].
A silver-white liquid, breaking into spherical globules which do not leave a metallic trace when rubbed on paper.
d_{20}^{20}: about 13.5.
bp: about 357 °C.

Mercury, nitric acid solution of. *1052801*.
Carefully dissolve 3 ml of *mercury R* in 27 ml of *fuming nitric acid R*. Dilute the solution with an equal volume of *water R*.
Store protected from light and use within 2 months.

Mesityl oxide. C_6H_{10}. (M_r 98.). *1120100*. [141-79-7].
4-Methylpent-3-en-2-one.
Colourless, oily liquid, soluble in 30 parts of water, miscible with most organic solvents.
d_{20}^{20}: about 0.858.
bp: 129 °C to 130 °C.

Metanil yellow. $C_{18}H_{14}N_3NaO_3S$. (M_r 375.4). *1052900*.
[587-98-4].
Schultz No. 169.
Colour Index No. 13065.
Sodium 3-[4-(phenylamino)phenylazo]benzenesulphonate.
A brownish-yellow powder, soluble in water and in alcohol, very slightly soluble in ether.

Metanil yellow solution. *1052901*.
A 1 g/l solution in *methanol R*.
Test for sensitivity. To 50 ml of *anhydrous acetic acid R* add 0.1 ml of the metanil yellow solution. Add 0.05 ml of *0.1 M perchloric acid*; the colour changes from pinkish-red to violet.
Colour change. pH 1.2 (red) to pH 2.3 (orange-yellow).

Metaphosphoric acid. $(HPO_3)_x$. *1053000*. [37267-86-0].
Glassy lumps or sticks containing a proportion of sodium metaphosphate, hygroscopic, very soluble in water.
Nitrates. Boil 1.0 g with 10 ml of *water R*, cool, add 1 ml of *indigo carmine solution R*, 10 ml of *nitrogen-free sulphuric acid R* and heat to boiling. The blue colour is not entirely discharged.

Reducing substances. Not more than 0.01 per cent, calculated as H_3PO_3. Dissolve 35.0 g in 50 ml of *water R*. Add 5 ml of a 200 g/l solution of *sulphuric acid R*, 50 mg of *potassium bromide R* and 5.0 ml of *0.02 M potassium bromate* and heat on a water-bath for 30 min. Allow to cool and add 0.5 g of *potassium iodide R*. Titrate the liberated iodine with *0.1 M sodium thiosulphate*, using 1 ml of *starch solution R* as indicator. Carry out a blank test.

1 ml of *0.02 M potassium bromate* is equivalent to 4.10 mg of H_3PO_3.

Store in an airtight container.

Methacrylic acid. $C_4H_6O_2$. (M_r 86.1). *1101800*. [79-41-4].
2-Methylprop-2-enoic acid.
A colourless liquid.

n_D^{20}: about 1.431.
bp: about 160 °C.
mp: about 16 °C.

Methanesulphonic acid. CH_4O_3S. (M_r 96.1). *1053100*.
[75-75-2].
A clear, colourless liquid, solidifying at about 20 °C, miscible with water, slightly soluble in toluene, practically insoluble in hexane.
d_{20}^{20}: about 1.48.
n_D^{20}: about 1.430.

Methanol. CH_4O. (M_r 32.04). *1053200*. [67-56-1].
A clear, colourless, flammable liquid, miscible with water and with alcohol.
d_{20}^{20}: 0.791 to 0.793.
bp: 64 °C to 65 °C.

Methanol R1. *1053201*.
Complies with the requirements prescribed for *methanol R* and the following additional requirement.

Minimum transmittance (2.2.25), determined using *water R* as compensation liquid:

20 per cent at 210 nm,

50 per cent at 220 nm,

75 per cent at 230 nm,

95 per cent at 250 nm,

98 per cent at 260 nm and at higher wavelengths.

Methanol R2. *1053202*.
Methanol R2 used in liquid chromatography complies with the following additional requirements.

Contains not less than 99.8 per cent of CH_4O (M_r 32.04).

Absorbance (2.2.25). The absorbance at 225 nm using *water R* as the compensation liquid is not more than 0.17.

Methanol, hydrochloric. *1053203*.
Dilute 1.0 ml of *hydrochloric acid R1* to 100.0 ml with *methanol R*.

Methanol, aldehyde-free. *1053300*.
Dissolve 25 g of *iodine R* in 1 litre of *methanol R* and pour the solution, with constant stirring, into 400 ml of *1 M sodium hydroxide*. Add 150 ml of *water R* and allow to stand for 16h. Filter. Boil under a reflux condenser until the odour of iodoform disappears. Distil the solution by fractional distillation.

Contains not more than 0.001 per cent of aldehydes and ketones.

Methanol, anhydrous. *1053400*. [67-56-1].
Treat 1000 ml of *methanol R* with 5 g of *magnesium R*. If necessary initiate the reaction by adding 0.1 ml of *mercuric chloride solution R*. When the evolution of gas has ceased, distil the liquid and collect the distillate in a dry container protected from moisture.
Water (2.5.12). Not more than 0.3 g/l.

DL-Methionine. *1129400*. [59-51-8].
See *DL-Methionine (0624)*.

L-Methionine. *1053500*. [63-68-3].
See *Methionine (1027)*.

(RS)-Methotrexate. *1120200*. [60388-53-6].
(RS)-2-[4-[[(2,4-diaminopteridin-6-yl)methyl]methyl-lamino]benzoylamino]pentanedioic acid.
Contains not less than 96.0 per cent of $C_{20}H_{22}N_8O_5$.
mp: about 195 °C.

Methoxychlor. $C_{16}H_{15}Cl_3O_2$. (M_r 345.7). *1129300*. [72-43-5].
1,1-(2,2,2-Trichloroethylidene)-bis(4-methoxybenzene).
Practically insoluble in water, freely soluble in most organic solvents.
bp: about 346 °C.
mp: 78 °C to 86 °C.
A suitable certified reference solution (10 ng/µl in iso-octane) may be used.

trans-2-Methoxycinnamaldehyde. $C_{10}H_{10}O_2$. (M_r 162.2). *1129500*. [60125-24-8].
mp: 44 °C to 46 °C.
trans-2-Methoxycinnamaldehyde used in gas chromatography complies with the following additional test.

Assay. Examine by gas chromatography *(2.2.28)* as prescribed in the monograph on *Cassia oil (1496)*.

The content is not less than 96.0 per cent, calculated by the normalisation procedure.

Methoxyphenylacetic acid. $C_9H_{10}O_3$. (M_r 166.2). *1053600*.
[7021-09-2]. (RS)-2-Methoxy-2-phenylacetic acid.
A white, crystalline powder or white or almost white crystals, sparingly soluble in water, freely soluble in alcohol and in ether.
mp: about 70 °C.
Store in a cool place.

Methoxyphenylacetic reagent. *1053601*.
Dissolve 2.7 g of *methoxyphenylacetic acid R* in 6 ml of *tetramethylammonium hydroxide solution R* and add 20 ml of *ethanol R*.

Store in a polyethylene container.

Methyl acetate. $C_3H_6O_2$. (M_r 74.1). *1053700*. [79-20-9].
A clear, colourless liquid, soluble in water, miscible with alcohol.
d_{20}^{20}: about 0.933.
n_D^{20}: about 1.361
bp: 56 °C to 58 °C.

4-Methylaminophenol sulphate. $C_{14}H_{20}N_2O_6S$. (M_r 344.4). *1053800*. [55-55-0].
Colourless crystals, very soluble in water, slightly soluble in alcohol, practically insoluble in ether.
mp: about 260 °C.

Methyl anthranilate. $C_8H_9NO_2$. (M_r 151.2). *1107300*.
[134-20-3]. Methyl 2-aminobenzoate.
Colourless crystals or a colourless or yellowish liquid, soluble in water, freely soluble in alcohol and in ether.
bp: 134 °C to 136 °C.
mp: 24 °C to 25 °C.
Methyl anthranilate used in gas chromatography complies with the following additional test.

Assay. Examine by gas chromatography *(2.2.28)* as prescribed in the monograph on *Bitter-orange-flower oil (1175)*, using the substance to be examined as the test solution. The area of the principal peak is not less than 95.0 per cent of the total area of the peaks.

Methyl arachidate. $C_{21}H_{42}O_2$. (M_r 326.6). *1053900*.
[1120-28-1]. Methyl eicosanoate.
Contains not less than 98.0 per cent of $C_{21}H_{42}O_2$, determined by gas chromatography *(2.4.22)*.

A white or yellow, crystalline mass, soluble in alcohol and in light petroleum.
mp: about 46 °C.

Methyl behenate. $C_{23}H_{46}O_2$. (M_r 354.6). *1107500*. [929-77-1]. Methyl docosanoate.
mp: 54 °C to 55 °C.

Methylbenzothiazolone hydrazone hydrochloride.
$C_8H_{10}ClN_3S,H_2O$. (M_r 233.7). *1055300*. [38894-11-0].
3-Methylbenzothiazol-2(3*H*)-one hydrazone hydrochloride monohydrate.
An almost white or yellowish, crystalline powder.
mp: about 270 °C.
Suitability for determination of aldehydes. To 2 ml of *aldehyde-free methanol R* add 60 µl of a 1 g/l solution of *propionaldehyde R* in *aldehyde-free methanol R* and 5 ml of a 4 g/l solution of methylbenzothiazolone hydrazone hydrochloride. Mix. Allow to stand for 30 min. Prepare a blank omitting the propionaldehyde solution. Add 25.0 ml of a 2 g/l solution of *ferric chloride R* to the test solution and to the blank, dilute to 100.0 ml with *acetone R* and mix. The absorbance (*2.2.25*) of the test solution, measured at 660 nm using the blank as compensation liquid, is not less than 0.62.

2-Methylbutane. C_5H_{12}. (M_r 72.2). *1099500*. [78-78-4].
Isopentane.
Contains not less than 99.5 per cent of C_5H_{12}.

A very flammable colourless liquid.
d_{20}^{20}: about 0.621.
n_D^{20}: about 1.354.
bp: about 29 °C.
Water (2.5.12). Not more than 0.02 per cent.

Residue on evaporation. Not more than 0.0003 per cent.

Minimum transmittance (2.2.25), determined using *water R* as compensation liquid:

50 per cent at 210 nm,

85 per cent at 220 nm,

98 per cent at 240 nm and at higher wavelengths.

2-Methylbut-2-ene. C_5H_{10}. (M_r 70.1). *1055400*. [513-35-9].
A very flammable liquid, practically insoluble in water, miscible with alcohol and with ether.
bp: 37.5 °C to 38.5 °C.

Methyl caprate. *1054000*.
See *Methyl decanoate R*.

Methyl caproate. $C_7H_{14}O_2$. (M_r 130.2). *1120300*. [106-70-7].
Methyl hexanoate.
d_{20}^{20}: about 0.885.
n_D^{20}: about 1.405.
bp: 150 °C to 151 °C.

Methyl caprylate. $C_9H_{18}O_2$. (M_r 158.2). *1120400*. [111-11-5].
Methyl octanoate.
d_{20}^{20}: about 0.876.
n_D^{20}: about 1.417.
bp: 193 °C to 194 °C.

Methylcellulose 450. *1055500*. [9004-67-5].
See *Methylcellulose (0345)*.
The nominal viscosity is 450 mPa·s

Methyl cinnamate. $C_{10}H_{10}O_2$. (M_r 162.2). *1099400*. [103-26-4].
Colourless crystals practically insoluble in water, soluble in alcohol and in ether.
n_D^{20}: about 1.56.
bp: about 260 °C.
mp: 34 °C to 36 °C.

Methyl decanoate. $C_{11}H_{22}O_2$. (M_r 186.3). *1054000*. [110-42-9]. Methyl *n*-decanoate.
Contains not less than 99.0 per cent of $C_{11}H_{22}O_2$.

A clear, colourless or yellow liquid, soluble in light petroleum.
d_{20}^{20}: 0.871 to 0.876.
n_D^{20}: 1.425 to 1.426.
Foreign substances. Examine by gas chromatography (*2.2.28*), injecting equal volumes of each of the following:
(I) a 0.02 g/l solution of the substance to be examined in *carbon disulphide R*, (II) a 2 g/l solution of the substance to be examined in *carbon disulphide R*, and (III) *carbon disulphide R*. Carry out the chromatographic procedure under the conditions of the test for butylated hydroxytoluene prescribed in the monograph on *Wool fat (0134)*. The total area of any peaks, apart from the solvent peak and the principal peak, in the chromatogram obtained with solution (II) is less than the area of the principal peak in the chromatogram obtained with solution (I).

3-*O*-Methyldopamine hydrochloride. $C_9H_{14}ClNO_2$.
(M_r 203.7). *1055600*. [1477-68-5]. 4-(2-Aminoethyl)-2-methoxyphenol hydrochloride.
mp: 213 °C to 215 °C.
Chromatography. Examine as prescribed in the monograph on *Dopamine hydrochloride (0664)*, applying 10 µl of a 0.075 g/l solution in *methanol R*. The chromatogram obtained shows only one principal spot.

4-*O*-Methyldopamine hydrochloride. $C_9H_{14}ClNO_2$.
(M_r 203.7). *1055700*. [645-33-0]. 5-(2-Aminoethyl)-2-methoxyphenol hydrochloride.
mp: 207 °C to 208 °C.
Chromatography. Examine as prescribed in the monograph on *Dopamine hydrochloride (0664)*, applying 10 µl of a 0.075 g/l solution in *methanol R*. The chromatogram obtained shows only one principal spot.

Methylenebisacrylamide. $C_7H_{10}N_2O_2$. (M_r 154.2). *1056000*.
[110-26-9]. *N,N*′-Methylenebispropenamide.
A fine, white or almost white powder, slightly soluble in water, soluble in alcohol.
mp: It melts with decomposition at a temperature above 300 °C.

Methylene blue. $C_{16}H_{18}ClN_3S,xH_2O$. (M_r 319.9 for the anhydrous substance). *1055800*. [7220-79-3].
Schultz No. 1038.
Colour Index No. 52015.
3,7-Dimethylaminophenothiazin-5-ium chloride.
It occurs in different hydrated forms and may contain up to 22 per cent of water. A dark-green or bronze, crystalline powder, freely soluble in water, soluble in alcohol.

Methylene chloride. CH_2Cl_2. (M_r 84.9). *1055900*. [75-09-2].
Dichloromethane.
A colourless liquid, sparingly soluble in water, miscible with alcohol and with ether.
bp: 39 °C to 42 °C.
Methylene chloride used in fluorimetry complies with the following additional requirement.

Fluorescence. Under irradiation at 365 nm, the fluorescence (*2.2.21*) measured at 460 nm in a 1 cm cell is not more intense than that of a solution containing 0.002 ppm of *quinine R* in *0.5 M sulphuric acid* measured in the same conditions.

Methylene chloride, acidified. *1055901*.
To 100 ml of *methylene chloride R* add 10 ml of *hydrochloric acid R*, shake, allow to stand and separate the two layers. Use the lower layer.

Methyl eicosenoate. $C_{21}H_{40}O_2$. (M_r 324.5). *1120500*.
[2390-09-2]. (11*Z*)-eicos-11-enoate.

Methyl erucate. $C_{23}H_{44}O_2$. (M_r 352.6). *1146100*. [1120-34-9].
Methyl *cis*-13-docosenoate.

d_{20}^{20}: about 0.871.

n_D^{20}: about 1.456.

3-_O_-Methylestrone. $C_{19}H_{24}O_2$. (M_r 284.4). *1137000*.
[1624-62-0]. 3-Methoxy-1,3,5(10)-estratrien-17-one.
White to yellowish-white powder.

$[\alpha]_D^{20}$: about + 157.

mp: about 173 °C.

Methyl ethyl ketone. C_4H_8O. (M_r 72.1). *1054100*. [78-93-3].
Ethyl methyl ketone. 2-Butanone.
A clear, colourless, flammable liquid, very soluble in water,
miscible with alcohol and with ether.

d_{20}^{20}: about 0.81.

bp: 79 °C to 80 °C.

Methyl green. $C_{26}H_{33}Cl_2N_3$. (M_r 458.5). *1054200*.
[7114-03-6].
Schultz No. 788.
Colour Index No. 42585.
4-[[4-(Dimethyl-amino)phenyl][4-(dimethyliminio)cyclohexa-
2,5-dienylidene]-methylphenyl]trimethylammonium
dichloride.
Green powder, soluble in water, soluble in sulphuric acid
giving a yellow solution turning green on dilution with water.

> **Methyl green-iodomercurate paper.** *1054201*.
> Immerse thin strips of suitable filter paper in a 40 g/l
> solution of *methyl green R* and allow to dry in air.
> Immerse the strips for 1 h in a solution containing
> 140 g/l of *potassium iodide R* and 200 g/l of *mercuric
> iodide R*. Wash with *distilled water R* until the washings
> are practically colourless and allow to dry in air.
> Store protected from light and use within 48 h.

1-Methylimidazole. $C_4H_6N_2$. (M_r 82.1). *1139700*. [616-47-7].
1-Methyl-1*H*-imidazole.
Colourless or slightly yellowish liquid.

n_D^{20}: about 1.495.

bp: 195 °C to 197 °C.

Store in an airtight container, protected from light.

2-Methylimidazole. $C_4H_6N_2$. (M_r 82.1). *1143400*. [693-98-1].
White, crystalline powder.

mp: about 145 °C.

Methyl isobutyl ketone. $C_6H_{12}O$. (M_r 100.2). *1054300*.
[108-10-1]. 4-Methyl-2-pentanone.
A clear, colourless liquid, slightly soluble in water, miscible
with most organic solvents.

d_{20}^{20}: about 0.80.

bp: about 115 °C.

Distillation range (2.2.11). Distil 100 ml. The range of
temperature of distillation from 1 ml to 95 ml of distillate
does not exceed 4.0 °C.

Residue on evaporation. Not more than 0.01 per cent,
determined by evaporating on a water-bath and drying at
100 °C to 105 °C.

> **Methyl isobutyl ketone R1.** *1054301*.
> Shake 50 ml of freshly distilled *methyl isobutyl ketone R*
> with 0.5 ml of *hydrochloric acid R1* for 1 min. Allow the
> phases to separate and discard the lower phase. Prepare
> immediately before use.

> **Methyl isobutyl ketone R3.** *1054302*.
> Complies with the requirements for *methyl isobutyl
> ketone R* and with the following limits:
> Chromium: maximum 0.02 ppm.
> Copper: maximum 0.02 ppm.
> Lead: maximum 0.1 ppm.
> Nickel: maximum 0.02 ppm.

Tin: maximum 0.1 ppm.

Methyl laurate. $C_{13}H_{26}O_2$. (M_r 214.4). *1054400*. [111-82-0].
Methyl dodecanoate.
Contains not less than 98.0 per cent of $C_{13}H_{26}O_2$, determined
by gas chromatography (*2.4.22*).
A colourless or yellow liquid, soluble in alcohol and in light
petroleum.

d_{20}^{20}: about 0.87.

n_D^{20}: about 1.431.

mp: about 5 °C.

Methyl lignocerate. $C_{25}H_{50}O_2$. (M_r 382.7). *1120600*.
[2442-49-1]. Methyl tetracosanoate.
Flakes.

mp: about 58 °C.

Methyl linoleate. $C_{19}H_{34}O_2$. (M_r 294.5). *1120700*. [112-63-0].
Methyl (9*Z*,12*Z*)-octadeca-9,12-dienoate.

d_{20}^{20}: about 0.888.

n_D^{20}: about 1.466.

bp: 207 °C to 208 °C.

Methyl linolenate. $C_{19}H_{32}O_2$. (M_r 292.5). *1120800*.
[301-00-8]. Methyl (9*Z*,12*Z*,15*Z*)-octadeca-9,12,15-trienoate.

d_{20}^{20}: about 0.901.

n_D^{20}: about 1.471.

bp: about 207 °C.

Methyl margarate. $C_{18}H_{36}O_2$. (M_r 284.5). *1120900*.
[1731-92-6]. Methyl heptadecanoate.
White or almost white powder.

mp: 32 °C to 34 °C.

*Methyl margarate used in the assay of total fatty acids in
Saw palmetto fruit (1848) complies with the following
additional requirement.*

Assay. Examine by gas chromatography (*2.2.28*) as
prescribed in the monograph on *Saw palmetto fruit (1848)*.
The content of methyl margarate is not less than 97 per cent,
calculated by the normalisation procedure.

Methyl methacrylate. $C_5H_8O_2$. (M_r 100.1). *1054500*.
[80-62-6]. Methyl 2-methylprop-2-enoate.
A colourless liquid.

n_D^{20}: about 1.414.

bp: about 100 °C.

mp: about −48 °C.

It contains a suitable stabilising reagent.

Methyl myristate. $C_{15}H_{30}O_2$. (M_r 242.4). *1054600*.
[124-10-7]. Methyl tetradecanoate.
Contains not less than 98.0 per cent of $C_{15}H_{30}O_2$, determined
by gas chromatography (*2.4.22*).
A colourless or slightly yellow liquid, soluble in alcohol and
in light petroleum.

d_{20}^{20}: about 0.87.

n_D^{20}: about 1.437.

mp: about 20 °C.

2-Methyl-5-nitroimidazole. $C_4H_5N_3O_2$. (M_r 127.1). *1056100*.
[88054-22-2].
White to light yellow powder.

mp: 252 °C to 254 °C.

Contains not less than 98.0 per cent of $C_4H_5N_3O_2$.

Methyl oleate. $C_{19}H_{36}O_2$. (M_r 296.4). *1054700*. [112-62-9].
Methyl (*Z*)-octadec-9-enoate.
Contains not less than 98.0 per cent of $C_{19}H_{36}O_2$, determined
by gas chromatography (*2.4.22*).
A colourless or slightly yellow liquid, soluble in alcohol and
in light petroleum.

d_{20}^{20}: about 0.88.

---

n_D^{20}: about 1.452.

Methyl orange. $C_{14}H_{14}N_3NaO_3S$. (M_r 327.3). *1054800*.
[547-58-0].
Schultz No. 176.
Colour Index No. 13025.
Sodium 4'-(dimethylamino)azobenzene-4-sulphonate.
An orange-yellow, crystalline powder, slightly soluble in
water, practically insoluble in alcohol.

> **Methyl orange mixed solution.** *1054801*.
> Dissolve 20 mg of *methyl orange R* and 0.1 g of
> *bromocresol green R* in 1 ml of *0.2 M sodium hydroxide*
> and dilute to 100 ml with *water R*.
>
> *Colour change.* pH 3.0 (orange) to pH 4.4 (olive-green).

> **Methyl orange solution.** *1054802*.
> Dissolve 0.1 g of *methyl orange R* in 80 ml of *water R*
> and dilute to 100 ml with *alcohol R*.
>
> *Test for sensitivity.* A mixture of 0.1 ml of the methyl
> orange solution and 100 ml of *carbon dioxide-free
> water R* is yellow. Not more than 0.1 ml of *0.1 M
> hydrochloric acid* is required to change the colour to red.
>
> *Colour change.* pH 3.0 (red) to pH 4.4 (yellow).

Methyl palmitate. $C_{17}H_{34}O_2$. (M_r 270.5). *1054900*.
[112-39-0]. Methyl hexadecanoate.
Contains not less than 98.0 per cent of $C_{17}H_{34}O_2$, determined
by gas chromatography (*2.4.22*).

A white or yellow, crystalline mass, soluble in alcohol and in
light petroleum.
mp: about 30 °C.

Methyl palmitoleate. $C_{17}H_{32}O_2$. (M_r 268.4). *1121000*.
[1120-25-8]. Methyl (9Z)-hexadec-9-enoate.
d_{20}^{20}: about 0.876.
n_D^{20}: about 1.451.

Methyl parahydroxybenzoate. *1055000*. [99-76-3].
See *Methyl parahydroxybenzoate (0409)*.

Methyl pelargonate. $C_{10}H_{20}O_2$. (M_r 172.3). *1143500*.
[1731-84-6]. Methyl nonanoate.
Clear, colourless liquid.
d_4^{20}: about 0.873.
n_D^{20}: about 1.422.
bp: 91 °C to 92 °C.
*Methyl pelargonate used in the assay of total fatty acids
in Saw palmetto fruit (1848) complies with the following
additional requirement.*

Assay. Examine by gas chromatography (*2.2.28*) as
prescribed in the monograph on *Saw palmetto fruit (1848)*.

The content of methyl pelargonate is not less than 98 per
cent, calculated by the normalisation procedure.

3-Methylpentan-2-one. $C_6H_{12}O$. (M_r 100.2). *1141100*.
[565-61-7].
Colourless, flammable liquid.
d_{20}^{20}: about 0.815.
n_D^{20}: about 1.400.
bp: about 118 °C

4-Methylpentan-2-ol. $C_6H_{14}O$. (M_r 102.2). *1114300*.
[108-11-2].
A clear, colourless, volatile liquid.
d_4^{20}: : about 0.802.
n_D^{20}: about 1.411.
bp: about 132 °C.

Methylphenyloxazolylbenzene. $C_{26}H_{20}N_2O_2$. (M_r 392.5).
1056200. [3073-87-8]. 1,4-Bis[2-(4-methyl-5-phenyl)oxa-
zolyl]benzene.
A fine, greenish-yellow powder with a blue fluorescence or
small crystals, soluble in alcohol, sparingly soluble in xylene.
mp: about 233 °C.
*Methylphenyloxazolylbenzene used for liquid scintillation
is of a suitable analytical grade.*

1-Methyl-4-phenyl-1,2,3,6-tetrahydropyridine. $C_{12}H_{15}N$.
(173.3). *1137100*. [28289-54-5]. MPTP.
A white or almost white, crystalline powder, slightly soluble
in water.
mp: about 41 °C.

Methylpiperazine. $C_5H_{12}N_2$. (M_r 100.2). *1056300*.
[74879-18-8]. 1-Methylpiperazine.
A colourless liquid, miscible with water and with alcohol.
d_{20}^{20}: about 0.90.
n_D^{20}: about 1.466.
bp: about 138 °C.

4-(4-Methylpiperidino)pyridine. $C_{11}H_{16}N_2$. (M_r 176.3).
1114400. [80965-30-6].
A clear liquid.
n_D^{20}: about 1.565.

2-Methylpropanol. $C_4H_{10}O$. (M_r 74.1). *1056400*. [78-83-1].
Isobutyl alcohol. 2-Methylpropan-1-ol.
A clear colourless liquid, soluble in water, miscible with
alcohol and with ether.
d_{20}^{20}: about 0.80.
n_D^{15}: 1.397 to 1.399.
bp: about 107 °C.
Distillation range (2.2.11). Not less than 96 per cent distils
between 107 °C and 109 °C.

2-Methyl-2-propanol. $C_4H_{10}O$. (M_r 74.1). *1056500*. [75-65-0].
1,1-Dimethyl ethyl alcohol. *tert*-Butyl alcohol.
A clear, colourless liquid or crystalline mass, soluble in
water, miscible with alcohol and with ether.
Freezing point (2.2.18). About 25 °C.

Distillation range (2.2.11). Not less than 95 per cent distils
between 81 °C and 83 °C.

Methyl red. $C_{15}H_{15}N_3O_2$. (M_r 269.3). *1055100*. [493-52-7].
Schultz No. 250.
Colour Index No. 13020.
2-(4-Dimethylamino-phenylazo)benzoic acid.
A dark-red powder or violet crystals, practically insoluble
in water, soluble in alcohol.

> **Methyl red mixed solution.** *1055101*.
> Dissolve 0.1 g of *methyl red R* and 50 mg of *methylene
> blue R* in 100 ml of *alcohol R*.
>
> *Colour change.* pH 5.2 (red-violet) to pH 5.6 (green).

> **Methyl red solution.** *1055102*.
> Dissolve 50 mg in a mixture of 1.86 ml of *0.1 M sodium
> hydroxide* and 50 ml of *alcohol R* and dilute to 100 ml
> with *water R*.
>
> *Test for sensitivity.* To 0.1 ml of the methyl red solution
> add 100 ml of *carbon dioxide-free water R* and 0.05 ml of
> *0.02 M hydrochloric acid*. The solution is red. Not more
> than 0.1 ml of *0.02 M sodium hydroxide* is required to
> change the colour to yellow.
>
> *Colour change.* pH 4.4 (red) to pH 6.0 (yellow).

Methyl salicylate. *1146200*. [119-36-8].
See *Methyl salicylate (0230)*

Methyl stearate. $C_{19}H_{38}O_2$. (M_r 298.5). *1055200*. [112-61-8]. Methyl octadecanoate.

Contains not less than 98.0 per cent of $C_{19}H_{38}O_2$, determined by gas chromatography (*2.4.22*).

A white or yellow, crystalline mass, soluble in alcohol and in light petroleum.
mp: about 38 °C.

Methyl tricosanoate. $C_{24}H_{48}O_2$. (M_r 368.6). *1111500*. [2433-97-8]. Tricosanoic acid methyl ester.
Contains not less than 99.0 per cent of $C_{24}H_{48}O_2$.

White crystals, practically insoluble in water, soluble in hexane.
mp: 55 °C to 56 °C.

Methyl tridecanoate. $C_{14}H_{28}O_2$. (M_r 228.4). *1121100*. [1731-88-0].
A colourless or slightly yellow liquid, soluble in alcohol and in light petroleum.
d_{20}^{20}: about 0.86.
n_D^{20}: about 1.441.
mp: about 6 °C.

N-Methyltrimethylsilyl-trifluoroacetamide.
$C_6H_{12}F_3NOSi$. (M_r 199.3). *1129600*. [24589-78-4].
2,2,2-Trifluoro-N-methyl-N-(trimethylsilyl)acetamide.
n_D^{20}: about 1.380.
bp: 130 °C to 132 °C.

Minocycline hydrochloride. *1146300*.
See *Minocycline hydrochloride (1030)*.

Molecular sieve. *1056600*.
Molecular sieve composed of sodium aluminosilicate. It is available as beads with a pore size of 0.4 nm and with a diameter of 2 mm.

Molecular sieve for chromatography. *1129700*.
A molecular sieve composed of sodium aluminosilicate. The pore size is indicated after the name of the reagent in the tests where it is used. If necessary, the particle size is also indicated.

Molybdovanadic reagent. *1056700*.
In a 150 ml beaker, mix 4 g of finely powdered *ammonium molybdate R* and 0.1 g of finely powdered *ammonium vanadate R*. Add 70 ml of *water R* and grind the particles using a glass rod. A clear solution is obtained within a few minutes. Add 20 ml of *nitric acid R* and dilute to 100 ml with *water R*.

Monodocosahexaenoin. $C_{25}H_{38}O_4$. (M_r 402.6). *1143600*. [124516-13-8]. Monoglyceride of docosahexaenoic acid (C22:6). Glycerol monodocosahexaenoate.
(*all-Z*)-Docosa-4,7,10,13,16,19-hexaenoic acid, monoester with propane-1,2,3-triol.
The reagent from Nu-Chek Prep, Inc. has been found suitable.

Mordant black 11. $C_{20}H_{12}N_3NaO_7S$. (M_r 461.4). *1056800*. [1787-61-7].
Schultz No. 241.
Colour Index No. 14645.
Sodium 2-hydroxy-1-[(1-hydroxynaphth-2-yl)azo]-6-nitronaphthalene-4-sulphonate. Eriochrome black.
A brownish-black powder, soluble in water and in alcohol.
Store in an airtight container, protected from light.

Mordant black 11 triturate. *1056801*.
Mix 1 g of *mordant black 11 R* with 99 g of *sodium chloride R*.
Test for sensitivity. Dissolve 50 mg in 100 ml of *water R*. The solution is brownish-violet. On addition of 0.3 ml of *dilute ammonia R1* the solution turns blue. On the subsequent addition of 0.1 ml of a 10 g/l solution of *magnesium sulphate R*, it turns violet.

Store in an airtight container, protected from light.

Morphine hydrochloride. *1056900*.
See *Morphine hydrochloride (0097)*.

Morpholine. C_4H_9NO. (M_r 87.1). *1057000*. [110-91-8].
Tetrahydro-1,4-oxazine.
A colourless, hygroscopic liquid, flammable, soluble in water and in alcohol.
d_{20}^{20}: about 1.01.
Distillation range (2.2.11). Not less than 95 per cent distils between 126 °C and 130 °C.

Store in an airtight container.

Morpholine for chromatography. *1057001*.
It complies with the requirements of *morpholine R* and with the following requirement:
Contains not less than 99.5 per cent of C_4H_9NO.

Murexide. $C_8H_8N_6O_6,H_2O$. (M_r 302.2). *1137200*.
5,5′-Nitrilobis(pyrimidine-2,4,6(1*H*,3*H*,5*H*)-trione) monoammonium salt.
Brownish-red crystalline powder, sparingly soluble in cold water, soluble in hot water, practically insoluble in alcohol, soluble in solutions of potassium hydroxide or sodium hydroxide giving a blue colour.

Myosmine. $C_9H_{10}N_2$. (M_r 146.2). *1121200*. [532-12-7].
3-(4,5-Dihydro-3*H*-pyrrol-2-yl)pyridine.
Colourless crystals.
mp: about 45 °C.

β-Myrcene. $C_{10}H_{16}$. (M_r 136.2). *1114500*. [123-35-3].
7-Methyl-3-methylenocta-1,6-diene.
An oily liquid with a pleasant odour, practically insoluble in water, miscible with alcohol, soluble in ether and in glacial acetic acid. It dissolves in solutions of alkali hydroxides.
d_4^{20}: about 0.794.
n_D^{20}: about 1.470.
βMyrcene used in gas chromatography complies with the following additional test.

Assay. Examine by gas chromatography (*2.2.28*) as prescribed in the monograph on *Peppermint oil (0405)*.

Test solution. The substance to be examined.

The area of the principal peak is not less than 90.0 per cent of the area of all the peaks in the chromatogram obtained.

Myristic acid. $C_{14}H_{28}O_2$. (M_r 228.4). *1143700*. [544-63-8].
Tetradecanoic acid.
Colourless or white flakes.
mp: about 58.5 °C.
Myristic acid used in the assay of total fatty acids in Saw palmetto fruit (1848) complies with the following additional requirement.

Assay. Examine by gas chromatography (*2.2.28*) as prescribed in the monograph on *Saw palmetto fruit (1848)*.

The content of myristic acid is not less than 97 per cent, calculated by the normalisation procedure.

Myristicine. $C_{11}H_{12}O_3$. (M_r 192.2). *1099600.* [607-91-0].
5-Allyl-1-methoxy-2,3-methylenedioxybenzene.
4-Methoxy-6-(prop-2-enyl)-1,3-benzodioxole.
An oily colourless liquid, practically insoluble in water, slightly soluble in ethanol, soluble in ether, miscible with toluene and with xylene.
d_{20}^{20}: about 1.144.
n_D^{20}: about 1.540.
bp: 276 °C to 277 °C.
mp: about 173 °C.
Chromatography. Examined as prescribed in the monograph on *Star anise (1153)*, the chromatogram obtained shows only one principal spot.

Myristicine used in gas chromatography complies with the following additional test.

Assay. Examine by gas chromatography *(2.2.28)* under the conditions prescribed in the monograph on *Nutmeg oil (1552)*.

The content is not less than 95.0 per cent, calculated by the normalisation procedure.

Store in a cool place, protected from light.

Myristyl alcohol. $C_{14}H_{30}O$. (M_r 214.4). *1121300.* [112-72-1].
1-Tetradecanol.
d_{20}^{20}: about 0.823.
mp: 38 °C to 40 °C.

Naphthalene. $C_{10}H_8$. (M_r 128.2). *1057100.* [91-20-3].
White crystals, practically insoluble in water, freely soluble in ether, soluble in alcohol.
mp: about 80 °C.
Naphthalene used for liquid scintillation is of a suitable analytical grade.

Naphtharson. $C_{16}H_{11}AsN_2Na_2O_{10}S_2$. ($M_r$ 576.3). *1121400.* [132-33-2]. Thorin. Disodium 4-[(2-arsonophenyl)azo]-3-hydroxynaphthalene-2,7-disulphonate.
A red powder, soluble in water.

> **Naphtharson solution.** *1121401.*
> A 0.58 g/l solution.
> *Test for sensitivity.* To 50 ml of *alcohol R*, add 20 ml of *water R*, 1 ml of *0.05 M sulphuric acid* and 1 ml of the naphtharson solution. Titrate with *0.025 M barium perchlorate*; the colour changes from orange-yellow to orange-pink.
>
> Store protected from light and use within one week.

α-Naphthol. $C_{10}H_8O$. (M_r 144.2). *1057300.* [90-15-3].
1-Naphthol.
A white, crystalline powder or colourless or white crystals, darkening on exposure to light, slightly soluble in water, freely soluble in alcohol, and in ether.
mp: about 95 °C.
Store protected from light.

> **α-Naphthol solution.** *1057301.*
> Dissolve 0.10 g of α-naphthol R in 3 ml of a 150 g/l solution of *sodium hydroxide R* and dilute to 100 ml with *water R*. Prepare immediately before use.

β-Naphthol. $C_{10}H_8O$. (M_r 144.2). *1057400.* [135-19-3].
2-Naphthol.
White or slightly pink plates or crystals, very slightly soluble in water, very soluble in alcohol.
mp: about 122 °C.
Store protected from light.

β-Naphthol solution. *1057401.*
Dissolve 5 g of freshly recrystallised β-naphthol R in 40 ml of *dilute sodium hydroxide solution R* and dilute to 100 ml with *water R*. Prepare immediately before use.

β-Naphthol solution R1. *1057402.*
Dissolve 3.0 mg of *β-naphthol R* in 50 ml of *sulphuric acid R* and dilute to 100.0 ml with the same acid. Use the recently prepared solution.

Naptholbenzein. $C_{27}H_{20}O_3$. (M_r 392.5). *1057600.*
[6948-88-5]. α-Naptholbenzein. Phenylbis(4-hydroxy-naphthyl)methanol.
A brownish-red powder or shiny brownish-black crystals, practically insoluble in water, soluble in alcohol and in glacial acetic acid.

> **Naptholbenzein solution.** *1057601.*
> A 2 g/l solution in *anhydrous acetic acid R*.
> *Test for sensitivity.* To 50 ml of *glacial acetic acid R* add 0.25 ml of the naptholbenzein solution. The solution is brownish-yellow. Not more than 0.05 ml of *0.1 M perchloric acid* is required to change the colour to green.

Naphthol yellow. $C_{10}H_5N_2NaO_5$. (M_r 256.2). *1136600.*
2,4-Dinitro-1-naphthol, sodium salt.
Orange-yellow powder or crystals, freely soluble in water, slightly soluble in ethanol.

Naphthol yellow S. $C_{10}H_4N_2Na_2O_8S$. (M_r 358.2). *1143800.*
[846-70-8].
Colour Index No. 10316.
8-Hydroxy-5,7-dinitro-2-naphthalenesulphonic acid disodium salt. Disodium 5,7-dinitro-8-oxidonaphthalene-2-sulphonate.
Yellow or orange-yellow powder, freely soluble in water.

Naphthylamine. $C_{10}H_9N$. (M_r 143.2). *1057700.* [134-32-7].
1-Naphthylamine.
A white, crystalline powder, turning pink on exposure to light and air, slightly soluble in water, freely soluble in alcohol and in ether.
mp: about 51 °C.
Store protected from light.

Naphthylethylenediamine dihydrochloride.
$C_{12}H_{16}Cl_2N_2$. (M_r 259.2). *1057800.* [1465-25-4].
N-(1-Naphthyl)ethylene-diamine dihydrochloride.
It may contain methanol of crystallisation.
A white to yellowish-white powder, soluble in water, slightly soluble in alcohol.

> **Naphthylethylenediamine dihydrochloride solution.** *1057801.*
> Dissolve 0.1 g of *naphthylethylenediamine dihydrochloride R* in *water R* and dilute to 100 ml with the same solvent. Prepare immediately before use.

Naringin. $C_{27}H_{32}O_{14}$. (M_r 580.5). *1137300.*
[10236-47-2]. 7-[[2-*O*-(6-Deoxy-α-L-mannopyranosyl)-β-D-glucopyranosyl]oxy]-5-hydroxy-2-(4-hydroxyphenyl)-2,3-dihydro-4*H*–chromen-4-one.
A white or almost white crystalline powder, slightly soluble in water, soluble in methanol and in dimethylformamide.
mp: about 171 °C.
Absorbance (2.2.25). Naringin dissolved in a 5 g/l solution of *dimethylformamide R* in *methanol R* shows an absorption maximum at 283 nm.

***trans*-Nerolidol.** $C_{15}H_{26}O$. (M_r 222.4). *1107900.* [40716-66-3].
3,7,11-Trimethyldodeca-1,6,10-trien-3-ol.
A slightly yellow liquid, slight odour of lily and lily of the valley, practically insoluble in water and in glycerol, miscible with alcohol.

d_{20}^{20}: about 0.876.
n_D^{20}: about 1.479.
bp$_{12}$: 145 °C to 146 °C.
trans-Nerolidol used in gas chromatography complies with the following additional test.

Assay. Examine by gas chromatography (*2.2.28*) as prescribed in the monograph on *Bitter-orange-flower oil (1175)*, using the substance to be examined as the test solution. The area of the principal peak is not less than 90.0 per cent of the total area of the peaks.

Neryl acetate. $C_{12}H_{20}O_2$. (M_r 196.3). *1108000.* [141-12-8].
(Z)-3,7-Dimethylocta-2,6-dienyl acetate.
A colourless, oily liquid.
d_{20}^{20}: about 0.907.
n_D^{20}: about 1.460.
bp$_{25}$: 134 °C.
Neryl acetate used in gas chromatography complies with the following additional test.

Assay. Examine by gas chromatography (*2.2.28*) as prescribed in the monograph on *Bitter-orange-flower oil (1175)*, using the substance to be examined as the test solution. The area of the principal peak is not less than 93.0 per cent of the total area of the peaks.

Nickel-aluminium alloy. *1058100.*
Contains 48 per cent to 52 per cent of aluminium (Al, A_r 26.98) and 48 per cent to 52 per cent of nickel (Ni, A_r 58.70).
Before use, reduce to a fine powder (180).

It is practically insoluble in water and soluble in mineral acids.

Nickel-aluminium alloy (halogen-free). *1118100.*
Contains 48 per cent to 52 per cent of aluminium (Al, A_r 26.98) and 48 per cent to 52 per cent of nickel (Ni, A_r 58.71).
A fine, grey powder, practically insoluble in water, soluble in mineral acids with formation of salts.

Chlorides. Not more than 10 ppm. Dissolve 2.00 g in 40 ml of *nitric acid R*. Evaporate the solution nearly to dryness, dissolve the residue in *water R* and dilute to 20.0 ml with the same solvent. To one half-aliquot of the solution, add 1.0 ml of *0.1 M silver nitrate*. Filter after 15 min and add 0.25 ml of sodium chloride solution (containing 40 µg of chlorides per millilitre) to the filtrate. After 5 min the solution is more opalescent than a mixture of the second half-aliquot of the solution with 1.0 ml of *0.1 M silver nitrate*.

Nickel chloride. $NiCl_2$. (M_r 129.6). *1057900.* [7718-54-9].
Nickel chloride, anhydrous.
A yellow, crystalline powder, very soluble in water, soluble in alcohol. It sublimes in the absence of air and readily absorbs ammonia. The aqueous solution is acid.

Nickel sulphate. $NiSO_4,7H_2O$. (M_r 280.9). *1058000.*
[10101-98-1]. Nickel sulphate heptahydrate.
A green, crystalline powder or crystals, freely soluble in water, slightly soluble in alcohol.

Nicotinamide-adenine dinucleotide. $C_{21}H_{27}N_7O_{14}P_2$. (M_r 663). *1108100.* [53-84-9]. NAD$^+$.
A white powder, very hygroscopic, freely soluble in water.

Nicotinamide-adenine dinucleotide solution. *1108101.*
Dissolve 40 mg of *nicotinamide-adenine dinucleotide R* in *water R* and dilute to 10 ml with the same solvent. Prepare immediately before use.

Nile blue A. $C_{20}H_{21}N_3O_5S$. (M_r 415.5). *1058200.* [3625-57-8].
Schultz No. 1029.
Colour Index No. 51180.
5-Amino-9-(diethylamino)benzo[a]phenoxazinylium hydrogen sulphate.
A green, crystalline powder with a bronze lustre, sparingly soluble in alcohol, in glacial acetic acid and in pyridine.
A 0.005 g/l solution in *alcohol (50 per cent V/V) R* shows an absorption maximum (*2.2.25*) at 640 nm.

Nile blue A solution. *1058201.*
A 10 g/l solution in *anhydrous acetic acid R*.
Test for sensitivity. To 50 ml of *anhydrous acetic acid R* add 0.25 ml of the Nile blue A solution. The solution is blue. On the addition of 0.1 ml of *0.1 M perchloric acid*, the colour changes to blue-green.

Colour change. pH 9.0 (blue) to pH 13.0 (red).

Ninhydrin. $C_9H_4O_3,H_2O$. (M_r 178.1). *1058300.* [485-47-2].
1,2,3-Indanetrione monohydrate.
A white or very pale yellow, crystalline powder, soluble in water and in alcohol, slightly soluble in ether.
Store protected from light.

Ninhydrin and stannous chloride reagent. *1058301.*
Dissolve 0.2 g of *ninhydrin R* in 4 ml of hot *water R*, add 5 ml of a 1.6 g/l solution of *stannous chloride R*, allow to stand for 30 min, then filter and store at a temperature of 2 °C to 8 °C. Immediately before use dilute 2.5 ml of the solution with 5 ml of *water R* and 45 ml of *2-propanol R*.

Ninhydrin and stannous chloride reagent R1. *1058302.*
Dissolve 4 g of *ninhydrin R* in 100 ml of *ethylene glycol monomethyl ether R*. Shake gently with 1 g of *cation exchange resin R* (300 µm to 840 µm) and filter (solution a). Dissolve 0.16 g of *stannous chloride R* in 100 ml of *buffer solution pH 5.5 R* (solution b). Immediately before use, mix equal volumes of each solution.

Ninhydrin solution. *1058303.*
A 2 g/l solution of *Ninhydrin R* in a mixture of 5 volumes of *dilute acetic acid R* and 95 volumes of *butanol R*.

Ninhydrin solution R1. *1058304.*
Dissolve 1.0 g of *ninhydrin R* in 50 ml of *alcohol R* and add 10 ml of *glacial acetic acid R*.

Ninhydrin solution R2. *1058305.*
Dissolve 3 g of *ninhydrin R* in 100 ml of a 45.5 g/l solution of *sodium metabisulphite R*.

Ninhydrin solution R3. *1058306.*
A 4 g/l solution in a mixture of 5 volumes of *anhydrous acetic acid R* and 95 volumes of *butanol R*.

Nitrazepam. *1143900.* [146-22-5].
See *Nitrazepam (0415)*.

Nitric acid. HNO_3. (M_r 63.0). *1058400.* [7697-37-2].
Contains not less than 63.0 per cent *m/m* and not more than 70.0 per cent *m/m* of HNO_3.

A clear, colourless or almost colourless liquid, miscible with water.
d_{20}^{20}: 1.384 to 1.416.
A 10 g/l solution is strongly acid and gives the reaction of nitrates (*2.3.1*).

Appearance. Nitric acid is clear (*2.2.1*) and not more intensely coloured than reference solution Y_6 (*Method II, 2.2.2*).

Chlorides (*2.4.4*). To 5 g add 10 ml of *water R* and 0.3 ml of *silver nitrate solution R2* and allow to stand for 2 min protected from light. Any opalescence is not more intense than that of a standard prepared in the same manner using 13 ml of *water R*, 0.5 ml of *nitric acid R*, 0.5 ml of *chloride standard solution (5 ppm Cl) R* and 0.3 ml of *silver nitrate solution R2* (0.5 ppm).

Sulphates (*2.4.13*). Evaporate 10 g to dryness with 0.2 g of *sodium carbonate R*. Dissolve the residue in 15 ml of *distilled water R*. The solution complies with the limit test for sulphates (2 ppm). Prepare the standard using a mixture of 2 ml of *sulphate standard solution (10 ppm SO_4) R* and 13 ml of *distilled water R*.

Arsenic (*2.4.2*). Gently heat 50 g with 0.5 ml of *sulphuric acid R* until white fumes begin to evolve. To the residue add 1 ml of a 100 g/l solution of *hydroxylamine hydrochloride R* and dilute to 2 ml with *water R*. The solution complies with limit test A for arsenic (0.02 ppm). Prepare the standard using 1.0 ml of *arsenic standard solution (1 ppm As) R*.

Heavy metals (*2.4.8*). Dilute 10 ml of the solution prepared for the limit test for iron to 20 ml with *water R*. 12 ml of the solution complies with limit test A for heavy metals (2 ppm). Prepare the standard using *lead standard solution (2 ppm Pb) R*.

Iron (*2.4.9*). Dissolve the residue from the determination of sulphated ash in 1 ml of *dilute hydrochloric acid R* and dilute to 50 ml with *water R*. 5 ml of the solution diluted to 10 ml with *water R* complies with the limit test for iron (1 ppm).

Sulphated ash. Carefully evaporate 100 g to dryness. Moisten the residue with a few drops of *sulphuric acid R* and heat to dull red. The residue does not exceed 0.001 per cent.

Assay. To 1.50 g add about 50 ml of *water R* and titrate with *1 M sodium hydroxide*, using 0.1 ml of *methyl red solution R* as indicator.

1 ml of *1 M sodium hydroxide* is equivalent to 63.0 mg of HNO_3.

Store protected from light.

Nitric acid, cadmium- and lead-free. *1058401.*
Complies with the requirements prescribed for Nitric acid R and with the following additional test.

Test solution. To 100 g add 0.1 g of *anhydrous sodium carbonate R* and evaporate to dryness. Dissolve the residue in *water R* heating slightly, and dilute to 50.0 ml with the same solvent.

Cadmium. Not more than 0.1 ppm of cadmium (Cd) determined by atomic absorption spectrometry (*Method II, 2.2.23*) measuring the absorbance at 228.8 nm using a cadmium hollow-cathode lamp and an air-acetylene or air-propane flame.

Lead. Not more than 0.1 ppm of lead (Pb) determined by atomic absorption spectrometry (*Method II, 2.2.23*) measuring the absorbance at 283.3 nm or 217.0 nm using a lead hollow-cathode lamp and an air-acetylene flame.

Nitric acid, dilute. *1058402.*
Contains about 125 g/l of HNO_3 (M_r 63.0).
Dilute 20 g of *nitric acid R* to 100 ml with *water R*.

Nitric acid, heavy metal-free. *1058404.*
Complies with the requirements prescribed for *nitric acid R* and with the following maximum contents of heavy metals:

As: 0.005 ppm;
Cd: 0.005 ppm;

Cu: 0.001 ppm;
Fe: 0.02 ppm;
Hg: 0.002 ppm;
Ni: 0.005 ppm;
Pb: 0.001 ppm;
Zn: 0.01 ppm.

Nitric acid, lead-free. *1058403.*
Complies with the requirements prescribed for *Nitric acid R* and with the following additional test:

To 100 g add 0.1 g of *anhydrous sodium carbonate R* and evaporate to dryness. Dissolve the residue in *water R*, heating slightly, and dilute to 50.0 ml with the same solvent. Determine the lead content by atomic absorption spectrometry (*Method II, 2.2.23*) measuring the absorbance at 283.3 nm or 217.0 nm using a lead hollow-cathode lamp and an air-acetylene flame. It contains not more than 0.1 ppm of lead (Pb).

Nitric acid, fuming. *1058500.* [52583-42-3].
A clear, slightly yellowish liquid, fuming on contact with air. d_{20}^{20}: about 1.5.

Nitrilotriacetic acid. $C_6H_9NO_6$. (M_r 191.1). *1137400.* [139-13-9].
White crystalline powder, insoluble in water and in most organic solvents.
mp: about 240 °C, with decomposition.

Nitroaniline. $C_6H_6N_2O_2$. (M_r 138.1). *1058600.* [100-01-6]. 4-Nitroaniline.
A bright yellow, crystalline powder, very slightly soluble in water, sparingly soluble in boiling water, soluble in alcohol and in ether, forms water-soluble salts with strong mineral acids.
mp: about 147 °C.

Nitrobenzaldehyde. $C_7H_5NO_3$. (M_r 151.1). *1058700.* [552-89-6]. 2-Nitrobenzaldehyde.
Yellow needles, slightly soluble in water, freely soluble in alcohol, soluble in ether, volatile in steam.
mp: about 42 °C.

Nitrobenzaldehyde paper. *1058701.*
Dissolve 0.2 g of *nitrobenzaldehyde R* in 10 ml of a 200 g/l solution of *sodium hydroxide R*. Use the solution within 1 h. Immerse the lower half of a slow filter paper strip 10 cm long and 0.8 cm to 1 cm wide. Absorb the excess reagent between two sheets of filter paper. Use within a few minutes of preparation.

Nitrobenzaldehyde solution. *1058702.*
Add 0.12 g of powdered *nitrobenzaldehyde R* to 10 ml of *dilute sodium hydroxide solution R*; allow to stand for 10 min shaking frequently and filter. Prepare immediately before use.

Nitrobenzene. $C_6H_5NO_2$. (M_r 123.1). *1058800.* [98-95-3].
A colourless or very slightly yellow liquid, practically insoluble in water, miscible with alcohol and with ether.
bp: about 211 °C.
Dinitrobenzene. To 0.1 ml add 5 ml of *acetone R*, 5 ml of *water R* and 5 ml of *strong sodium hydroxide solution R*. Shake and allow to stand. The upper layer is almost colourless.

4-Nitrobenzoic acid. $C_7H_5NO_4$. (M_r 167.1). *1144000.* [62-23-7].
Yellow crystals.
mp: about 240 °C.

Nitrobenzoyl chloride. $C_7H_4ClNO_3$. (M_r 185.6). *1058900*. [122-04-3]. 4-Nitrobenzoyl chloride.
Yellow crystals or a crystalline mass, decomposing in moist air, completely soluble in sodium hydroxide solution giving a yellowish-orange colour.
mp: about 72 °C.

Nitrobenzyl chloride. $C_7H_6ClNO_2$. (M_r 171.6). *1059000*. [100-14-1]. 4-Nitrobenzyl chloride.
Pale-yellow crystals, lachrymatory, practically insoluble in water, very soluble in alcohol and in ether.

4-(4-Nitrobenzyl)pyridine. $C_{12}H_{10}N_2O_2$. (M_r 214.2). *1101900*. [1083-48-3].
Yellow powder.
mp: about 70 °C.

Nitrochromic reagent. *1059100*.
Dissolve 0.7 g of *potassium dichromate R* in *nitric acid R* and dilute to 100 ml with the same acid.

Nitroethane. $C_2H_5NO_2$. (M_r 75.1). *1059200*. [79-24-3].
A clear, oily, colourless liquid.
bp: about 114 °C.

Nitrofurantoin. *1099700*. [67-20-9].
See *Nitrofurantoin (0101)*.

(5-Nitro-2-furyl)methylene diacetate. $C_9H_9NO_7$. (M_r 243.2). *1099800*. [92-55-7]. Nitrofurfural diacetate.
5-Nitrofurfurylidene diacetate.
Yellow crystals.
mp: about 90 °C.

Nitrogen. N_2. (M_r 28.01). *1059300*. [7727-37-9].
Nitrogen, washed and dried.

Nitrogen R1. *1059400*.
Contains not less than 99.999 per cent V/V of N_2.
Carbon monoxide: less than 5 ppm.
Oxygen: less than 5 ppm.

Nitrogen for chromatography. *1059500*.
Contains not less than 99.95 per cent V/V of N_2.

Nitrogen gas mixture. *1136900*.
Nitrogen R containing 1 per cent V/V of each of the following gases: *carbon dioxide R2, carbon monoxide R1* and *oxygen R1*.

Nitrogen monoxide. NO. (M_r 30.01). *1108300*.
Contains not less than 98.0 per cent V/V of NO.

Nitrogen, oxygen-free. *1059600*.
Nitrogen R which has been freed from oxygen by passing it through *alkaline pyrogallol solution R*.

Nitromethane. CH_3NO_2. (M_r 61.0). *1059700*. [75-52-5].
A clear, colourless, oily liquid, slightly soluble in water, miscible with alcohol and with ether.
d_{20}^{20}: 1.132 to 1.134.
n_D^{20}: 1.381 to 1.383.
Distillation range (2.2.11). Not less than 95 per cent distils between 100 °C and 103 °C.

Nitro-molybdovanadic reagent. *1060100*.
Solution I. Dissolve 10 g of *ammonium molybdate R* in *water R*, add 1 ml of *ammonia R* and dilute to 100 ml with *water R*.
Solution II. Dissolve 2.5 g of *ammonium vanadate R* in hot *water R*, add 14 ml of *nitric acid R* and dilute to 500 ml with *water R*.
To 96 ml of *nitric acid R* add 100 ml of solution I and 100 ml of solution II and dilute to 500 ml with *water R*.

4-Nitrophenol. $C_6H_5NO_3$. (M_r 139.1). *1146400*. [100-02-7].
p-Nitrophenol.
Contains not less than 95 per cent of $C_6H_5NO_3$.
Colourless or slightly yellow powder, sparingly soluble in water and in methanol.
mp: about 114 °C.

***N*-Nitrosodiethanolamine.** $C_4H_{10}N_2O_3$. (M_r 134.1). *1129800*. [1116-54-7]. 2,2′-(Nitrosoimino)diethanol.
A yellow liquid, miscible with ethanol.
n_D^{20}: about 1.485.
bp: about 125 °C.

Nitrosodipropylamine. $C_6H_{14}N_2O$. (M_r 130.2). *1099900*. [621-64-7]. Dipropylnitrosamine.
Liquid, soluble in ethanol, in ether and in strong acids.
d_{20}^{20}: about 0.915.
bp: about 78 °C.
Appropriate grade for chemiluminescence determination.

Nitrosodipropylamine solution. *1099901*.
Inject 78.62 g of *ethanol R* through the septum of a vial containing *nitrosodipropylamine R*. Dilute 1/100 in *ethanol R* and place 0.5 ml aliquots in crimp-sealed vials.
Store in the dark at 5 °C.

Nitrotetrazolium blue. $C_{40}H_{30}Cl_2N_{10}O_6$. ($M_r$ 818). *1060000*. [298-83-9]. 3,3′-(3,3′-Dimethoxy-4,4′-diphenylene)di[2-(4-nitrophenyl)-5-phenyl-2*H*-tetrazolium] dichloride.
p-Nitro-tetrazolium blue.
Crystals, soluble in methanol, giving a clear, yellow solution.
mp: about 189 °C, with decomposition.

Nitrous oxide. N_2O. (M_r 44.01). *1108500*.
Contains not less than 99.99 per cent V/V of N_2O.
Nitrogen monoxide: less than 1 ppm.
Carbon monoxide: less than 1 ppm.

Nonylamine. $C_9H_{21}N$. (M_r 143.3). *1139800*. [120-20-9].
1-Aminononane.
Corrosive, colourless, clear liquid.
d_4^{20}: about 0.788.
n_D^{20}: about 1.433.

Nordazepam. $C_{15}H_{11}ClN_2O$. (M_r 270.7). *1060200*. [340-57-8].
7-Chloro-2,3-dihydro-5-phenyl-1*H*-1,4-benzodiazepin-2-one.
A white or pale yellow, crystalline powder, practically insoluble in water, slightly soluble in alcohol.
mp: about 216 °C.

DL-Norleucine. $C_6H_{13}NO_2$. (M_r 131.2). *1060300*. [616-06-8].
(*RS*)-2-Aminohexanoic acid.
Shiny crystals, sparingly soluble in water and in alcohol, soluble in acids.

Noscapine hydrochloride. *1060500*. [912-60-7].
See *Noscapine hydrochloride (0515)*.

Octadecyl [3-[3,5-bis(1,1-dimethylethyl)-4-hydroxyphenyl]-propionate]. $C_{35}H_{62}O_3$. (M_r 530.9). *1060600*. [2082-79-3].
Octadecyl 3-(3,5-di-*tert*-butyl-4-hydroxyphenyl)propionate.
A white or slightly yellowish, crystalline powder, practically insoluble in water, very soluble in acetone and in hexane, slightly soluble in methanol.
mp: 49 °C to 55 °C.

Octanol. $C_8H_{18}O$. (M_r 130.2). *1060700*. [111-87-5].
1-Octanol. Caprylic alcohol.
A colourless liquid, insoluble in water, miscible with alcohol and with ether.
d_{20}^{20}: about 0.828.
bp: about 195 °C.

4. Reagents

3-Octanone. $C_8H_{16}O$. (M_r 128.2). *1114600.* [106-68-3].
Ethylpentylketone.
A colourless liquid with a characteristic odour.
d_{20}^{20}: about 0.822.
n_D^{20}: about 1.415.
bp: about 167 °C.

3-Octanone used in gas chromatography complies with the following additional test.

Assay. Examine by gas chromatography (*2.2.28*) as prescribed in the monograph on *Lavender oil (1338).*

Test solution. The substance to be examined.

The area of the principal peak is not less than 98.0 per cent of the area of all the peaks in the chromatogram obtained.

Octoxinol 10. $C_{34}H_{62}O_{11}$ (average). (M_r 647). *1060800.* [9002-93-1]. α-[4-(1,1,3,3-Tetramethylbutyl)phenyl]-ω-hydroxypoly-(oxyethylene).
A clear, pale-yellow, viscous liquid, miscible with water, with acetone and with alcohol, soluble in toluene.
Store in an airtight container.

Oleamide. $C_{18}H_{35}NO$. (M_r 281.5). *1060900.*
(Z)-Octadec-9-enoamide.
Yellowish or white powder or granules, practically insoluble in water, very soluble in methylene chloride, soluble in ethanol.
mp: about 80 °C.

Oleic acid. $C_{18}H_{34}O_2$. (M_r 282.5). *1144100.* [112-80-1].
(9Z)-Octadec-9-enoic acid.
Clear, colourless liquid, practically insoluble in water.
d_4^{20}: about 0.891.
n_D^{20}: about 1.459.
mp: 13 °C to 14 °C.

Oleic acid used in the assay of total fatty acids in Saw palmetto fruit (1848) complies with the following additional requirement.

Assay. Examine by gas chromatography (*2.2.28*) as prescribed in the monograph on *Saw palmetto fruit (1848).*

The content of oleic acid is not less than 98 per cent, calculated by the normalisation procedure.

Olive oil. *1061000.* [8001-25-0].
See *Olive oil, virgin (0518).*

Oracet blue 2R. $C_{20}H_{14}N_2O_2$. (M_r 314.3). *1061100.* [4395-65-7].
Colour Index No. 61110.
1-Amino-4-(phenylamino)anthracene-9,10-dione.
mp: about 194 °C.

Orcinol. $C_7H_8O_2,H_2O$. (M_r 142.2). *1108700.* [6153-39-5].
5-Methylbenzene-1,3-diol monohydrate.
A crystalline powder, sensitive to light.
bp: about 290 °C.
mp: 58 °C to 61 °C.

Organosilica polymer, amorphous, octadecylsilyl. *1144200.* [75−05−8].
Synthetic, spherical hybrid particles, containing both inorganic (silica) and organic (organosiloxanes) components, chemically modified at the surface by trifunctionally bonded octadecylsilyl groups.

Osmium tetroxide. OsO_4. (M_r 254.2). *1061200.* [20816-12-0].
Light-yellow needles or a yellow, crystalline mass, hygroscopic, light sensitive, soluble in water, in alcohol and in ether.
Store in an airtight container.

Osmium tetroxide solution. *1061201.*
A 2.5 g/l solution in *0.05 M sulphuric acid.*

Oxalic acid. $C_2H_2O_4,2H_2O$. (M_r 126.1). *1061400.* [6153-56-6].
Ethanedioic acid dihydrate.
White crystals, soluble in water, freely soluble in alcohol.

Oxalic acid and sulphuric acid solution. *1061401.*
A 50 g/l solution of *oxalic acid R* in a cooled mixture of equal volumes of *sulphuric acid R* and *water R.*

Oxazepam. *1144300.* [604-75-1].
See *Oxazepam (0778).*

Ox brain, acetone-dried. *1061300.*
Cut into small pieces a fresh ox brain previously freed from vascular and connective tissue. Place in *acetone R* for preliminary dehydration. Complete the dehydration by pounding in a mortar 30 g of this material with successive quantities, each of 75 ml, of *acetone R* until a dry powder is obtained after filtration. Dry at 37 °C for 2 h or until the odour of acetone is no longer present.

2,2′-Oxybis(*N,N*-dimethylethylamine). $C_8H_{20}N_2O$. (M_r 160.3). *1141200.* [3033-62-3]. bis(2-Dimethylaminoethyl) ether.
Colourless, corrosive liquid.
d_{20}^{20}: about 0.85.
n_D^{20}: about 1.430.

Oxygen. O_2. (M_r 32.00). *1108800.*
Contains not less than 99 per cent *V/V* of O_2.
Nitrogen and argon: less than 100 ppm.
Carbon dioxide: less than 10 ppm.
Carbon monoxide: less than 5 ppm.

Oxygen R1. O_2. (M_r 32.00). *1137600.*
Contains not less than 99 per cent *V/V* of O_2.

Oxytetracycline hydrochloride. *1146500.*
See *Oxytetracycline hydrochloride (0198).*

Palladium. Pd. (A_r 106.4). *1114700.* [7440-05-3].
Grey white metal, soluble in hydrochloric acid.

Palladium chloride. $PdCl_2$. (M_r 177.3). *1061500.* [7647-10-1].
Red crystals.
mp: 678 °C to 680 °C.

Palladium chloride solution. *1061501.*
Dissolve 1 g of *palladium chloride R* in 10 ml of warm *hydrochloric acid R*. Dilute the solution to 250 ml with a mixture of equal volumes of *dilute hydrochloric acid R* and *water R*. Dilute this solution immediately before use with 2 volumes of *water R.*

Palmitic acid. $C_{16}H_{32}O_2$. (M_r 256.4). *1061600.* [57-10-3].
Hexadecanoic acid.
White, crystalline scales, practically insoluble in water, freely soluble in hot alcohol.
mp: about 63 °C.
Chromatography. Examine as prescribed in the monograph on *Chloramphenicol palmitate (0473).* The chromatogram shows only one principal spot.

Palmitic acid used in the assay of total fatty acids in Saw palmetto fruit (1848) complies with the following additional requirement.

Assay. Examine by gas chromatography (*2.2.28*) as prescribed in the monograph on *Saw palmetto fruit (1848).*

The content of palmitic acid is not less than 98 per cent, calculated by the normalisation procedure.

Palmitoleic acid. $C_{16}H_{30}O_2$. (M_r 254.4). *1144400*. [373-49-9]. (9Z)-Hexadec-9-enoic acid.
Clear, colourless liquid.
bp: about 162 °C.
Palmitoleic acid used in the assay of total fatty acids in Saw palmetto fruit (1848) complies with the following additional requirement.

Assay. Examine by gas chromatography (*2.2.28*) as prescribed in the monograph on *Saw palmetto fruit (1848)*.

The content of palmitoleic acid is not less than 98 per cent, calculated by the normalisation procedure.

Pancreas powder. *1061700*.
See *Pancreas powder (0350)*.

Papaverine hydrochloride. *1061800*. [61-25-6].
See *Papaverine hydrochloride (0102)*.

Paracetamol. *1061900*. [103-90-2].
See *Paracetamol (0049)*.

Paracetamol, 4-aminophenol-free. *1061901*.
Recrystallise *paracetamol R* from *water R* and dry *in vacuo* at 70 °C; repeat the procedure until the product complies with the following test: dissolve 5 g of the dried substance in a mixture of equal volumes of *methanol R* and *water R* and dilute to 100 ml with the same mixture of solvents. Add 1 ml of a freshly prepared solution containing 10 g/l of *sodium nitroprusside R* and 10 g/l of *anhydrous sodium carbonate R*, mix and allow to stand for 30 min protected from light. No blue or green colour is produced.

Paraffin, liquid. *1062000*. [8042-47-5].
See *Liquid paraffin (0239)*.

Paraffin, white soft. *1062100*.
A semi-liquid mixture of hydrocarbons obtained from petroleum and bleached, practically insoluble in water and in alcohol, soluble in ether and in *light petroleum R1*, the solution sometimes showing a slight opalescence.

Pararosaniline hydrochloride. $C_{19}H_{18}ClN_3$. (M_r 323.8). *1062200*. [569-61-9].
Schultz No. 779.
Colour Index No. 42500.
4-[bis(4-Aminophenyl)methylene]cyclohexa-2,5-dieniminium chloride.
A bluish-red, crystalline powder, slightly soluble in water, soluble in ethanol, practically insoluble in ether. Solutions in water and ethanol are deep-red; solutions in sulphuric acid and in hydrochloric acid are yellow.
mp: about 270 °C, with decomposition.

Decolorised pararosaniline solution. *1062201*.
To 0.1 g of *pararosaniline hydrochloride R* in a ground-glass-stoppered flask add 60 ml of *water R* and a solution of 1.0 g of *anhydrous sodium sulphite R* or 2.0 g of *sodium sulphite R* or 0.75 g of *sodium metabisulphite R* in 10 ml of *water R*. Slowly and with stirring add 6 ml of *dilute hydrochloric acid R*, stopper the flask and continue stirring until dissolution is complete. Dilute to 100 ml with *water R*. Allow to stand for 12 h before use.

Store protected from light.

Parthenolide. $C_{15}H_{20}O_3$. (M_r 248.3). *1129900*. [20554-84-1].
(4E)-(1aR,7aS,10aS,10bS)-1a,5-Dimethyl-8-methylene-2,3,6,7,7a,8,10a,10b-octahydro-oxireno[9,10]cyclodeca[1,2-b]furan-9(1aH)-one. (E)-(5S,6S)-4,5-Epoxygermacra-1(10),11(13)-dieno-12(6)-lactone.
A white, crystalline powder, very slightly soluble in water, very soluble in methylene chloride, soluble in methanol.
$[\alpha]_D^{22}$: −71.4, determined on a 2.2 g/l solution in *methylene chloride R*.
mp: 115 °C to 116 °C.

Absorbance (2.2.25). A 0.01 g/l solution in *alcohol R* shows an absorption maximum at 214 nm.

Assay. Examine by liquid chromatography (*2.2.29*), as prescribed in the monograph on *Feverfew (1516)*, at the concentration of the reference solution. The content of parthenolide is not less than 90 per cent calculated by the normalisation procedure.

Penicillinase solution. *1062300*.
Dissolve 10 g of casein hydrolysate, 2.72 g of *potassium dihydrogen phosphate R* and 5.88 g of *sodium citrate R* in 200 ml of *water R*, adjust to pH 7.2 with a 200 g/l solution of *sodium hydroxide R* and dilute to 1000 ml with *water R*. Dissolve 0.41 g of *magnesium sulphate R* in 5 ml of *water R* and add 1 ml of a 1.6 g/l solution of *ferrous ammonium sulphate R* and sufficient *water R* to produce 10 ml. Sterilise both solutions by heating in an autoclave, cool, mix, distribute in shallow layers in conical flasks and inoculate with *Bacillus cereus* (NCTC 9946). Allow the flasks to stand at 18 °C to 37 °C until growth is apparent and then maintain at 35 °C to 37 °C for 16 h, shaking constantly to ensure maximum aeration. Centrifuge and sterilise the supernatant liquid by filtration through a membrane filter. 1.0 ml of penicillinase solution contains not less than 0.4 microkatals (corresponding to the hydrolysis of not less than 500 mg of benzylpenicillin to benzylpenicilloic acid per hour) at 30 °C and pH 7, provided that the concentration of benzylpenicillin does not fall below the level necessary for enzyme saturation.
The Michaelis constant for benzylpenicillin of the penicillinase in penicillinase solution is approximately 12 µg/ml.

Sterility (2.6.1). It complies with the test for sterility.

Store at a temperature between 0 °C and 2 °C and use within 2 to 3 days. When freeze-dried and kept in sealed ampoules, it may be stored for several months.

Pentaerythrityl tetrakis[3-(3,5-di(1,1-dimethylethyl)-4-hydroxyphenyl)propionate]. $C_{73}H_{108}O_{12}$. (M_r 1178). *1062400*. [6683-19-8]. Pentaerythrityl tetrakis[3-(3,5-di-*tert*-butyl-4-hydroxyphenyl) propionate]. 2,2′-bis(Hydroxymethyl)propane-1,3-diol tetrakis[3-[3,5-di(1,1-dimethylethyl)-4-hydroxyphenyl]]propionate.
A white to slightly yellow, crystalline powder, practically insoluble in water, very soluble in acetone, soluble in methanol, slightly soluble in hexane.
mp: 110 °C to 125 °C.
α-form: 120 °C to 125 °C.
β-form: 110 °C to 115 °C.

Pentane. C_5H_{12}. (M_r 72.2). *1062500*. [109-66-0].
A clear, colourless, flammable liquid, very slightly soluble in water, miscible with acetone, with ethanol and with ether.
d_{20}^{20}: about 0.63.
n_D^{20}: about 1.359.
bp: about 36 °C.
Pentane used in spectrophotometry complies with the following additional requirement.
Minimum transmittance (2.2.25), determined using *water R* as compensation liquid:

20 per cent at 200 nm,

50 per cent at 210 nm,

85 per cent at 220 nm,

93 per cent at 230 nm,

98 per cent at 240 nm.

Pentanol. $C_5H_{12}O$. (M_r 88.1). *1062600*. [71-41-0]. 1-Pentanol.
Colourless liquid, sparingly soluble in water, miscible with alcohol and with ether.
n_D^{20}: about 1.410.
bp: about 137 °C.

***tert*-Pentyl alcohol.** $C_5H_{12}O$. (M_r 88.1). *1062700*. [75-85-4].
tert-Amyl alcohol. 2-Methyl-2-butanol.
A volatile, flammable liquid, freely soluble in water, miscible with alcohol, with ether and with glycerol.
d_{20}^{20}: about 0.81.
Distillation range (2.2.11). Not less than 95 per cent distils between 100 °C and 104 °C.

Store protected from light.

Pepsin powder. *1062800*. [9001-75-6].
See *Pepsin powder (0682)*.

Perchloric acid. $HClO_4$. (M_r 100.5). *1062900*. [7601-90-3].
Contains not less than 70.0 per cent *m/m* and not more than 73.0 per cent *m/m* of $HClO_4$.

A clear, colourless liquid, miscible with water.
d_{20}^{20}: about 1.7.
Assay. To 2.50 g add 50 ml of *water R* and titrate with *1 M sodium hydroxide*, using 0.1 ml of *methyl red solution R* as indicator.

1 ml of *1 M sodium hydroxide* is equivalent to 100.5 mg of $HClO_4$.

> **Perchloric acid solution.** *1062901*.
> Dilute 8.5 ml of *perchloric acid R* to 100 ml with *water R*.

Periodic acetic acid solution. *1063000*.
Dissolve 0.446 g of *sodium periodate R* in 2.5 ml of a 25 per cent *V/V* solution of *sulphuric acid R*. Dilute to 100.0 ml with *glacial acetic acid R*.

Periodic acid. H_5IO_6. (M_r 227.9). *1108900*. [10450-60-9].
Crystals, freely soluble in water and soluble in alcohol.
mp: about 122 °C.

Permethrin. $C_{21}H_{20}Cl_2O_3$. (M_r 391.3). *1130000*. [52645-53-1].
mp: 34 °C to 35 °C.
A suitable certified reference solution (10 ng/µl in cyclohexane) may be used.

Perylene. $C_{20}H_{12}$. (M_r 252.3). *1130100*. [198-55-0].
Dibenz(de,kl)anthracene.
Orange powder.
mp: about 279 °C.

Petroleum, light. *1063100*. [8032-32-4].
A clear, colourless, flammable liquid without fluorescence, practically insoluble in water, miscible with alcohol.
d_{20}^{20}: 0.661 to 0.664.
Distillation range (2.2.11). 50 °C to 70 °C.

> **Petroleum, light R1.** *1063101*.
> Complies with the requirements prescribed for *light petroleum R*, with the following modifications:
> d_{20}^{20}: 0.630 to 0.656.
> *Distillation range (2.2.11)*. 40 °C to 60 °C.
>
> It does not become cloudy at 0 °C.

> **Petroleum, light R2.** *1063102*.
> Complies with the requirements prescribed for *light petroleum R*, with the following modifications:
> d_{20}^{20}: 0.620 to 0.630.
> *Distillation range (2.2.11)*. 30 °C to 40 °C.
>
> It does not become cloudy at 0 °C.

> **Petroleum, light R3.** *1063103*.
> Complies with the requirements prescribed for *light petroleum R*, with the following modifications:
> d_{20}^{20}: 0.659 to 0.671.
> *Distillation range (2.2.11)*. 40 °C to 80 °C.

α-Phellandrene. $C_{10}H_{16}$. (M_r 136.2). *1130400*.
[4221-98-1]. (*R*)-5-Isopropyl-2-methyl-cyclohexa-1,3-diene.
(−)-p-Mentha-1,5-diene.
d_{20}^{20}: about 0.839.
n_D^{20}: about 1.471.
$[\alpha]_D^{20}$: about −217.
bp: 171 °C to 174 °C.

α-Phellandrene used in gas chromatography complies with the following additional test.

Assay. Examine by gas chromatography (2.2.28) as prescribed in the monograph on *Eucalyptus oil (0390)* using the substance to be examined as the test solution.

The area of the principal peak is not less than 98.0 per cent of the total area of the peaks.

Phenanthrene. $C_{14}H_{10}$. (M_r 178.2). *1063200*. [85-01-8].
White crystals, practically insoluble in water, freely soluble in ether, sparingly soluble in alcohol.
mp: about 100 °C.

Phenanthroline hydrochloride. $C_{12}H_9ClN_2,H_2O$. (M_r 234.7).
1063300. [3829-86-5]. 1,10-Phenanthroline hydrochloride monohydrate.
A white or almost white powder, freely soluble in water, soluble in alcohol.
mp: about 215 °C, with decomposition.

Phenazone. *1063400*. [60-80-0].
See *Phenazone (0421)*.

Phenol. *1063500*. [108-95-2].
See *Phenol (0631)*.

Phenolphthalein. $C_{20}H_{14}O_4$. (M_r 318.3). *1063700*. [77-09-8].
3,3-bis(4-Hydroxyphenyl)-3*H*-isobenzofuran-1-one.
A white to yellowish-white powder, practically insoluble in water, soluble in alcohol.

> **Phenolphthalein paper.** *1063704*.
> Immerse strips of filter paper for a few minutes in *phenolphthalein solution R*. Allow to dry.

> **Phenolphthalein solution.** *1063702*.
>
> Dissolve 0.1 g of *phenolphthalein R* in 80 ml of *alcohol R* and dilute to 100 ml with *water R*.
>
> *Test for sensitivity*. To 0.1 ml of the phenolphthalein solution add 100 ml of *carbon dioxide-free water R*. The solution is colourless. Not more than 0.2 ml of *0.02 M sodium hydroxide* is required to change the colour to pink.
>
> *Colour change.* pH 8.2 (colourless) to pH 10.0 (red).

> **Phenolphthalein solution R1.** *1063703*.
> A 10 g/l solution in *alcohol R*.

Phenol red. *1063600*. [143-74-8].
Bright red or dark red, crystalline powder, very slightly soluble in water, slightly soluble in alcohol.

Phenol red solution. *1063601.*

Dissolve 0.1 g of *phenol red R* in a mixture of 2.82 ml of *0.1 M sodium hydroxide* and 20 ml of *alcohol R* and dilute to 100 ml with *water R*.

Test for sensitivity. Add 0.1 ml of the phenol red solution to 100 ml of *carbon dioxide-free water R*. The solution is yellow. Not more than 0.1 ml of *0.02 M sodium hydroxide* is required to change the colour to reddish-violet.

Colour change. pH 6.8 (yellow) to pH 8.4 (reddish-violet).

Phenol red solution R2. *1063603.*

Solution I. Dissolve 33 mg of *phenol red R* in 1.5 ml of *dilute sodium hydroxide solution R* and dilute to 100 ml with *water R*.

Solution II. Dissolve 25 mg of *ammonium sulphate R* in 235 ml of *water R*; add 105 ml of *dilute sodium hydroxide solution R* and 135 ml of *dilute acetic acid R*.

Add 25 ml of solution I to solution II. If necessary, adjust the pH of the mixture to 4.7.

Phenol red solution R3. *1063604.*

Solution I. Dissolve 33 mg of *phenol red R* in 1.5 ml of *dilute sodium hydroxide solution R* and dilute to 50 ml with *water R*.

Solution II. Dissolve 50 mg of *ammonium sulphate R* in 235 ml of *water R*; add 105 ml of *dilute sodium hydroxide solution R* and 135 ml of *dilute acetic acid R*.

Add 25 ml of solution I to solution II; if necessary, adjust the pH of the mixture to 4.7.

Phenoxyacetic acid. $C_8H_8O_3$. (M_r 152.1). *1063800.* [122-59-8]. 2-Phenoxyethanoic acid.

Almost white crystals, sparingly soluble in water, freely soluble in alcohol, in ether and in glacial acetic acid.

mp: about 98 °C.

Chromatography. Examine as prescribed in the monograph on *Phenoxymethylpenicillin (0148)*; the chromatogram shows only one principal spot.

Phenoxybenzamine hydrochloride. $C_{18}H_{23}Cl_2NO$. (M_r 340.3). *1063900.* *N*-(2-Chloroethyl)-*N*-(1-methyl-2-phenoxyethyl)-benzylamine hydrochloride.

Contains not less than 97.0 per cent and not more than the equivalent of 103.0 per cent of $C_{18}H_{23}Cl_2NO$, calculated with reference to the dried substance.

A white or almost white, crystalline powder, sparingly soluble in water, freely soluble in alcohol.

mp: about 138 °C.

Loss on drying (2.2.32). Not more than 0.5 per cent, determined by drying over *diphosphorus pentoxide R* at a pressure not exceeding 670 Pa for 24 h.

Assay. Dissolve 0.500 g in 50.0 ml of *ethanol-free chloroform R* and extract with three quantities, each of 20 ml, of *0.01 M hydrochloric acid*. Discard the acid extracts, filter the chloroform layer through cotton and dilute 5.0 ml of the filtrate to 500.0 ml with *ethanol-free chloroform R*. Measure the absorbance of the resulting solution in a closed cell at the maximum at 272 nm.

Calculate the content of $C_{18}H_{23}Cl_2NO$, taking the specific absorbance to be 56.3.

Store protected from light.

Phenoxyethanol. $C_8H_{10}O_2$. (M_r 138.2). *1064000.* [122-99-6]. 2-Phenoxyethanol.

A clear, colourless, oily liquid, slightly soluble in water, freely soluble in alcohol and in ether.

d_{20}^{20}: about 1.11.

n_D^{20}: about 1.537.

Freezing point (2.2.18). Not lower than 12 °C.

Phenylalanine. *1064100.* [63-91-2].

See *Phenylalanine (0782)*.

***p*-Phenylenediamine dihydrochloride.** $C_6H_{10}Cl_2N_2$. (M_r 181.1). *1064200.* [615-28-1]. 1,4-Diaminobenzene dihydrochloride.

A crystalline powder or white or slightly coloured crystals, turning reddish on exposure to air, freely soluble in water, slightly soluble in alcohol and in ether.

α-Phenylglycine. $C_8H_9NO_2$. (M_r 151.2). *1064300.* [2835-06-5]. (*RS*)-2-Amino-2-phenylacetic acid.

D-Phenylglycine. $C_8H_9NO_2$. (M_r 151.2). *1144500.* [875-74-1]. (2*R*)-2-Amino-2-phenylacetic acid.

Contains not less than 99 per cent of $C_8H_9NO_2$.

White or almost white, crystalline powder.

Phenylhydrazine hydrochloride. $C_6H_9ClN_2$. (M_r 144.6). *1064500.* [59-88-1].

A white or almost white, crystalline powder, becoming brown on exposure to air, soluble in water and in alcohol.

mp: about 245 °C, with decomposition.

Store protected from light.

Phenylhydrazine hydrochloride solution. *1064501.*

Dissolve 0.9 g of *phenylhydrazine hydrochloride R* in 50 ml of *water R*. Decolorise with *activated charcoal R* and filter. To the filtrate add 30 ml of *hydrochloric acid R* and dilute to 250 ml with *water R*.

Phenylhydrazine-sulphuric acid solution. *1064502.*

Dissolve 65 mg of *phenylhydrazine hydrochloride R*, previously recrystallised from *alcohol (85 per cent V/V) R*, in a mixture of 80 volumes of *water R* and 170 volumes of *sulphuric acid R* and dilute to 100 ml with the same mixture of solvents. Prepare immediately before use.

Phenyl isothiocyanate. C_7H_5NS. (M_r 135.2). *1121500.* [103-72-0].

A liquid, insoluble in water, soluble in alcohol.

d_{20}^{20}: about 1.13.

n_D^{20}: about 1.65.

bp: about 221 °C.

mp: about −21 °C.

Use a grade suitable for protein sequencing.

1-Phenylpiperazine. $C_{10}H_{14}N_2$. (M_r 162.2). *1130500.* [92-54-6].

Slightly viscous, yellow liquid, not miscible with water.

d_4^{20}: about 1.07.

n_D^{20}: about 1.588.

Phloroglucinol. $C_6H_6O_3,2H_2O$. (M_r 162.1). *1064600.* [6099-90-7]. Benzene-1,3,5-triol.

White or yellowish crystals, slightly soluble in water, soluble in alcohol.

mp: about 223 °C (instantaneous method).

Phloroglucinol solution. *1064601.*

To 1 ml of a 100 g/l solution of *phloroglucinol R* in *alcohol R*, add 9 ml of *hydrochloric acid R*.

Store protected from light.

Phosalone. $C_{12}H_{15}ClNO_4PS_2$. (M_r 367.8). *1130200.* [2310-17-0].

mp: 45 °C to 48 °C.

A suitable certified reference solution (10 ng/µl in iso-octane) may be used.

Phospholipids. *1064800.*

Wash a quantity of human or bovine brain, well separated from the meninges and blood vessels and liquidise in a suitable apparatus. Weigh 1000 g to 1300 g of the liquidised substance and measure the volume (*V* ml). Extract with three quantities, each of *4V* ml, of *acetone R*, filter under reduced pressure and dry the residue at 37 °C for 18 h. Extract the residue with two quantities, each of *2V* ml, of a mixture of 2 volumes of *light petroleum R2* and 3 volumes of *light petroleum R1*, filtering each extract on a filter paper previously moistened with the mixture of solvents. Combine the extracts and evaporate to dryness at 45 °C at a pressure not exceeding 670 Pa. Dissolve the residue in 0.2*V* ml of *ether R* and allow to stand at 4 °C until a deposit forms. Centrifuge and evaporate the clear supernatant liquid under low pressure to a volume of 100 ml per kilogram of the liquidised substance and weigh. Allow to stand at 4 °C until a precipitate forms (12 h to 24 h) and centrifuge. Add to the clear supernatant liquid five times its volume of *acetone R*, centrifuge and reject the supernatant liquid. Dry the precipitate.

Store it in a desiccator under vacuum protected from light.

Phosphomolybdic acid. $12MoO_3,H_3PO_4,xH_2O$. *1064900.* [51429-74-4].

Orange-yellow, fine crystals, freely soluble in water, soluble in alcohol and in ether.

Phosphomolybdic acid solution. *1064901.*

Dissolve 4 g of *phosphomolybdic acid R* in *water R* and dilute to 40 ml with the same solvent. Add cautiously and with cooling 60 ml of *sulphuric acid R*. Prepare immediately before use.

Phosphomolybdotungstic reagent. *1065000.*

Dissolve 100 g of *sodium tungstate R* and 25 g of *sodium molybdate R* in 700 ml of *water R*. Add 100 ml of *hydrochloric acid R* and 50 ml of *phosphoric acid R*. Heat the mixture under a reflux condenser in a glass apparatus for 10 h. Add 150 g of *lithium sulphate R*, 50 ml of *water R* and a few drops of *bromine R*. Boil to remove the excess of bromine (15 min), allow to cool, dilute to 1000 ml with *water R* and filter. The reagent should be yellow in colour. If it acquires a greenish tint, it is unsatisfactory for use but may be regenerated by boiling with a few drops of *bromine R*. Care must be taken to remove the excess of bromine by boiling.

Store at 2 °C to 8 °C.

Phosphomolybdotungstic reagent, dilute. *1065001.*

To 1 volume of *phosphomolybdotungstic reagent R* add 2 volumes of *water R*.

Phosphoric acid. *1065100.* [7664-38-2].

See *Concentrated phosphoric acid (0004)*.

Phosphoric acid, dilute. *1065101.*

See *Dilute phosphoric acid (0005)*.

Phosphoric acid, dilute R1. *1065102.*

Dilute 93 ml of *dilute phosphoric acid R* to 1000 ml with *water R*.

Phosphorous acid. H_3PO_3. (*M_r* 82.0). *1130600.* [13598-36-2].

White, very hygroscopic and deliquescent crystalline mass; slowly oxidised by oxygen (air) to H_3PO_4.

Unstable, orthorhombic crystals, soluble in water, in alcohol and in a mixture of 3 volumes of ether and 1 volume of alcohol.

d_4^{21}: 1.651.

mp: about 73 °C.

Phosphotungstic acid solution. *1065200.*

Heat under a reflux condenser for 3 h, 10 g of *sodium tungstate R* with 8 ml of *phosphoric acid R* and 75 ml of *water R*. Allow to cool and dilute to 100 ml with *water R*.

Phthalaldehyde. $C_8H_6O_2$. (*M_r* 134.1). *1065300.* [643-79-8].

Benzene-1,2-dicarboxaldehyde.

A yellow, crystalline powder.

mp: about 55 °C.

Store protected from light and air.

Phthalaldehyde reagent. *1065301.*

Dissolve 2.47 g of *boric acid R* in 75 ml of *water R*, adjust to pH 10.4 using a 450 g/l solution of *potassium hydroxide R* and dilute to 100 ml with *water R*. Dissolve 1.0 g of *phthalaldehyde R* in 5 ml of *methanol R*, add 95 ml of the boric acid solution and 2 ml of *thioglycollic acid R* and adjust to pH 10.4 with a 450 g/l solution of *potassium hydroxide R*.

Store protected from light and use within 3 days.

Phthalazine. $C_8H_6N_2$. (*M_r* 130.1). *1065400.* [253-52-1].

Pale yellow crystals, freely soluble in water, soluble in ethanol, in ethyl acetate and in methanol, sparingly soluble in ether.

mp: 89 °C to 92 °C.

Phthalein purple. $C_{32}H_{32}N_2O_{12},xH_2O$. (*M_r* 637, anhydrous substance). *1065500.* [2411-89-4].

Metalphthalein. 2,2′,2″,2‴-[*o*-Cresolphthalein-3′,3″-bis(methylenenitrilo)]tetra-acetic acid. (1,3-Dihydro-3-oxo-isobenzofuran-1-ylidene)bis[(6-hydroxy-5-methyl-3,1-phenylene)bis(methyleneimino)diacetic acid].

A yellowish-white to brownish powder, practically insoluble in water, soluble in alcohol. The product may be found in commerce in the form of the sodium salt: a yellowish-white to pink powder, soluble in water, practically insoluble in alcohol.

Test for sensitivity. Dissolve 10 mg in 1 ml of *concentrated ammonia R* and dilute to 100 ml with *water R*. To 5 ml of the solution add 95 ml of *water R*, 4 ml of *concentrated ammonia R*, 50 ml of *alcohol R* and 0.1 ml of *0.1 M barium chloride*. The solution is blue-violet. Add 0.15 ml of *0.1 M sodium edetate*. The solution becomes colourless.

Phthalic acid. $C_8H_6O_4$. (*M_r* 166.1). *1065600.* [88-99-3].

Benzene-1,2-dicarboxylic acid.

A white, crystalline powder, soluble in hot water and in alcohol.

Phthalic anhydride. $C_8H_4O_3$. (*M_r* 148.1). *1065700.* [85-44-9].

Isobenzofuran-1,3-dione.

Contains not less than 99.0 per cent of $C_8H_4O_3$.

White flakes.

mp: 130 °C to 132 °C.

Assay. Dissolve 2.000 g in 100 ml of *water R* and boil under a reflux condenser for 30 min. Cool and titrate with *1 M sodium hydroxide*, using *phenolphthalein solution R* as indicator.

1 ml of *1 M sodium hydroxide* is equivalent to 74.05 mg of $C_8H_4O_3$.

Phthalic anhydride solution. *1065701.*

Dissolve 42 g of *phthalic anhydride R* in 300 ml of *anhydrous pyridine R*. Allow to stand for 16 h.

Store protected from light and use within 1 week.

Picein. $C_{14}H_{18}O_7$. (*M_r* 298.3). *1130700.* [530-14-3].

1-[4-(β-D-Glucopyranosyloxy)phenyl]ethanone.

p-(Acetylphenyl)-β-D-glucopyranoside.

mp: 194 °C to 195 °C.

Picric acid. $C_6H_3N_3O_7$. (M_r 229.1). *1065800.* [88-89-1].
2,4,6-Trinitrophenol.
Yellow prisms or plates, soluble in water and in alcohol.
Store moistened with *water R*.

Picric acid solution. *1065801.*
A 10 g/l solution.

Picric acid solution R1. *1065802.*
Prepare 100 ml of a saturated solution of *picric acid R* and add 0.25 ml of *strong sodium hydroxide solution R*.

α-Pinene. $C_{10}H_{16}$. (M_r 136.2). *1130800.* [7785-70-8].
(1R,5R)-2,6,6-Trimethylbicyclo[3.1.1]hept-2-ene.
A liquid not miscible with water.
d_{20}^{20}: about 0.859.
n_D^{20}: about 1.466.
bp: 154 °C to 156 °C.

α-Pinene used in gas chromatography complies with the following additional test.

Assay. Examine by gas chromatography (*2.2.28*) as prescribed in the monograph on *Bitter-orange-flower oil (1175)* using the substance to be examined as the test solution.

The area of the principal peak is not less than 99.0 per cent of the total area of the peaks.

β-Pinene. $C_{10}H_{16}$. (M_r 136.2). *1109000.* [19902-08-0].
6,6-Dimethyl-2-methylenebicyclo[*3.1.1*]heptane.
A colourless, oily liquid, odour reminiscent of turpentine, practically insoluble in water, miscible with alcohol, and with ether.
d_{20}^{20}: about 0.867.
n_D^{20}: about 1.474.
bp: 164 °C to 166 °C.
β-Pinene used in gas chromatography complies with the following additional test.

Assay. Examine by gas chromatography (*2.2.28*) as prescribed in the monograph on *Bitter-orange-flower oil (1175)*, using the substance to be examined as the test solution. The area of the principal peak is not less than 99.0 per cent of the total area of the peaks.

Piperazine hydrate. *1065900.* [142-63-2].
See *Piperazine hydrate (0425)*.

Piperidine. $C_5H_{11}N$. (M_r 85.2). *1066000.* [110-89-4].
Hexahydropyridine.
A colourless to slightly yellow, alkaline liquid, miscible with water, with alcohol, with ether and with light petroleum.
bp: about 106 °C.

Pirimiphos-ethyl. $C_{13}H_{24}N_3O_3PS$. (M_r 333.4). *1130300.*
[23505-41-1].
mp: 15 °C to 18 °C.
A suitable certified reference solution (10 ng/μl in cyclohexane) may be used.

Plasma, platelet-poor. *1066100.*
Withdraw 45 ml of human blood into a 50 ml plastic syringe containing 5 ml of a sterile 38 g/l solution of *sodium citrate R*. Without delay, centrifuge at 1500 *g* at 4 °C for 30 min. Remove the upper two-thirds of the supernatant plasma using a plastic syringe and without delay centrifuge at 3500 *g* at 4 °C for 30 min. Remove the upper two-thirds of the liquid and freeze it rapidly in suitable amounts in plastic tubes at or below −40 °C. Use plastic or silicone-treated equipment.

Plasma substrate. *1066200.*
Separate the plasma from human or bovine blood collected into one-ninth its volume of a 38 g/l solution of *sodium citrate R*, or into two-sevenths its volume of a solution containing 20 g/l of *disodium hydrogen citrate R* and 25 g/l of *glucose R*. With the former, prepare the substrate on the day of collection of the blood. With the latter, prepare within two days of collection of the blood.

Store at −20 °C.

Plasma substrate R1. *1066201.*

Use water-repellent equipment (made from materials such as suitable plastics or suitably silicone-treated glass) for taking and handling blood.

Collect a suitable volume of blood from each of at least five sheep; a 285 ml volume of blood collected into 15 ml of anticoagulant solution is suitable but smaller volumes may be collected, taking the blood, either from a live animal or at the time of slaughter, using a needle attached to a suitable cannula which is long enough to reach the bottom of the collecting vessel. Discarding the first few millilitres and collecting only free-flowing blood, collect the blood in a sufficient quantity of an anticoagulant solution containing 8.7 g of *sodium citrate R* and 4 mg of *aprotinin R* per 100 ml of *water R* to give a final ratio of blood to anticoagulant solution of 19 to 1. During and immediately after collection, swirl the flask gently to ensure mixing but do not allow frothing to occur. When collection is complete, close the flask and cool to 10 °C to 15 °C. When cold, pool the contents of all the flasks with the exception of any that show obvious haemolysis or clots and keep the pooled blood at 10 °C to 15 °C.

As soon as possible and within 4 h of collection, centrifuge the pooled blood at 1000 *g* to 2000 *g* at 10 °C to 15 °C for 30 min. Separate the supernatant liquid and centrifuge it at 5000 *g* for 30 min. (Faster centrifugation, for example 20 000 *g* for 30 min, may be used if necessary to clarify the plasma, but filtration procedures should not be used.) Separate the supernatant liquid and, without delay, mix thoroughly and distribute the plasma substrate into small stoppered containers in portions sufficient for a complete heparin assay (for example 10 ml to 30 ml). Without delay, rapidly cool to a temperature below −70 °C (for example by immersing the containers into liquid nitrogen) and store at a temperature below −30 °C.

The plasma is suitable for use as plasma substrate in the assay for heparin if, under the conditions of the assay, it gives a clotting time appropriate to the method of detection used and if it provides reproducible, steep log dose-response curves.

When required for use, thaw a portion of the plasma substrate in a water-bath at 37 °C, gently swirling until thawing is complete; once thawed it should be kept at 10 °C to 20 °C and used without delay. The thawed plasma substrate may be lightly centrifuged if necessary; filtration procedures should not be used.

Plasma substrate R2. *1066202.*
Prepare from human blood containing less than 1 per cent of the normal amount of factor IX. Collect the blood into one-ninth its volume of a 38 g/l solution of *sodium citrate R*.

Store in small amounts in plastic tubes at a temperature of −30 °C or lower.

Plasma substrate R3. *1066203.*

Prepare from human blood containing less than 1 per cent of the normal amount of factor XI. Collect the blood into one-ninth its volume of a 38 g/l solution of *sodium citrate R*.

Store in small amounts in plastic tubes at a temperature of −30 °C or lower.

Plasma substrate deficient in factor V. *1066300.*
Use preferably a plasma which is congenitally deficient, or prepare it as follows: separate the plasma from human blood collected into one tenth of its volume of a 13.4 g/l solution of *sodium oxalate R*. Incubate at 37 °C for 24 h to 36 h. The coagulation time determined by the method described for *coagulation factor V solution R* should be 70 s to 100 s. If the coagulation time is less than 70 s, incubate again for 12 h to 24 h.

Store in small quantities at a temperature of −20 °C or lower.

Plasminogen, human. *1109100.* [9001-91-6].
A substance present in blood that may be activated to plasmin, an enzyme that lyses fibrin in blood clots.

Platelet substitute. *1066400.*

To 0.5 g to 1 g of *phospholipid R* add 20 ml of *acetone R* and allow to stand for 2 h with frequent shaking. Centrifuge for 2 min and discard the supernatant liquid. Dry the residue using a water pump, mix with 20 ml of *chloroform R* and shake for 2 h. Filter under vacuum and suspend the residue obtained in 5 ml to 10 ml of a 9 g/l solution of *sodium chloride R*.

For use in the assay of factor IX, prepare a dilution in a 9 g/l solution of *sodium chloride R* that will give coagulation time differences between consecutive dilutions of the reference preparation of about 10 s.

Store the diluted suspensions at −30 °C and use within 6 weeks.

Poly[(cyanopropyl)methylphenylmethylsiloxane]. *1066500.*
See *poly[(cyanopropyl)(methyl)][(phenyl)(methyl)]siloxane R*.

Poly[(cyanopropyl)(methyl)][(phenyl)(methyl)]siloxane. *1066500.*
Contains 25 per cent of cyanopropyl groups, 25 per cent of phenyl groups and 50 per cent of methyl groups. (Average relative molecular mass 8000).

A very viscous liquid (viscosity about 9000 mPa·s).
d_{25}^{25}: about 1.10.
n_D^{25}: about 1.502.

Poly[(cyanopropyl)(phenyl)][dimethyl]siloxane. *1114800.*
Stationary phase for gas chromatography. Contains 6 per cent of (cyanopropyl)(phenyl) groups and 94 per cent of dimethyl groups.

Poly(cyanopropyl)(phenylmethyl)siloxane. *1066600.*
Contains 90 per cent of cyanopropylgroups and 10 per cent of phenylmethyl groups.

Stationary phase for gas chromatography.

Poly(cyanopropyl)(7)(phenyl)(7)(methyl)(86)siloxane. *1109200.*
Polysiloxane substituted with 7 per cent of cyanopropyl groups, 7 per cent of phenyl groups and 86 per cent of dimethyl groups.

Stationary phase for gas chromatography.

Poly(cyanopropyl)siloxane. *1066700.*
Polysiloxane substituted with 100 per cent of cyanopropyl groups.

Poly(dimethyl)(diphenyl)(divinyl)siloxane. *1100000.*
Contains 94 per cent of methyl groups, 5 per cent of phenyl groups and 1 per cent of vinyl groups. SE54.

Stationary phase for gas chromatography.

Poly(dimethyl)(diphenyl)siloxane. *1066900.*
Contains 95 per cent of methyl groups and 5 per cent of phenyl groups. DB-5, SE52.

Stationary phase for gas chromatography.

Poly(dimethyl)siloxane. *1066800.*
Silicone gum rubber (methyl). Organosilicon polymer with the appearance of a semi-liquid, colourless gum.

The intrinsic viscosity, determined as follows is about 115 ml·g⁻¹. Weigh 1.5 g, 1 g and 0.3 g of the substance to be examined to the nearest 0.1 mg, into 100 ml volumetric flasks. Add 40 ml to 50 ml of *toluene R*, shake until the substance is completely dissolved and dilute to 100.0 ml with the same solvent. Determine the viscosity (*2.2.9*) of each solution. Determine the viscosity of *toluene R* under the same conditions. Reduce the concentration of each solution by half by diluting with *toluene R*. Determine the viscosity of these solutions.

c = concentration in grams per 100 ml,

t_1 = flow time of the solution to be examined,

t_2 = flow time of toluene,

η_1 = viscosity of the solution to be examined in millipascal seconds,

η_2 = viscosity of toluene in millipascal seconds,

d_1 = relative density of the solution to be examined,

d_2 = relative density of toluene.

To obtain the relative densities use the following data:

Concentration (g/100 ml)	Relative Density (d_1)
0 - 0.5	1.000
0.5 - 1.25	1.001
1.25 - 2.20	1.002
2.20 - 2.75	1.003
2.75 - 3.20	1.004
3.20 - 3.75	1.005
3.75 - 4.50	1.006

The specific viscosity is obtained from the equation:

$$\eta_{sp} = \frac{\eta_1 - \eta_2}{\eta_2} = \frac{t_1 d_1}{t_2 d_2} - 1$$

and the reduced viscosity from:

$$\eta_{red} = \frac{\eta_{sp}}{c}$$

The intrinsic viscosity (η) is obtained by extrapolating the preceding equation to $c = 0$. This is done by plotting the curve η_{sp}/c or log η_{sp}/c as a function of c. Extrapolation to $c = 0$ gives η. The intrinsic viscosity is expressed in millilitres per gram; the value obtained must therefore be multiplied by 100.

The infrared absorption spectrum (*2.2.24*) obtained by applying the substance, if necessary dispersed in a few drops of *carbon tetrachloride R*, to a sodium chloride plate, does not show absorption at 3053 cm^{-1}, corresponding to vinyl groups.

Loss on drying (*2.2.32*). Not more than 2.0 per cent, determined on 1.000 g by drying *in vacuo* at 350 °C for 15 min. Not more than 0.8 per cent, determined on 2.000 g by drying at 200 °C for 2 h.

Polyether hydroxylated gel for chromatography. *1067000.* Gel with a small particle size having a hydrophilic surface with hydroxyl groups. It has an exclusion limit for dextran of relative molecular mass 2×10^5 to 2.5×10^6.

Polyethyleneglycol adipate. $(C_8H_{12}O_4)_n$. (M_r $(172.2)_n$). *1067700.*
A white, wax-like mass, practically insoluble in water, soluble in chloroform.
mp: about 43 °C.

Polyethyleneglycol succinate. $(C_6H_8O_4)_n$. (M_r $(144.1)_n$). *1067800.*
A white, crystalline powder, practically insoluble in water, soluble in chloroform.
mp: about 102 °C.

Polymethylphenylsiloxane. *1067900.*
Contains 50 per cent of methyl groups and 50 per cent of phenyl groups. (Average relative molecular mass 4000).

A very viscous liquid (viscosity about 1300 mPa·s). Stationary phase for gas chromatography.
d_{25}^{25}: about 1.09.
n_D^{25}: about 1.540.

Poly[methyl(95)phenyl(5)]siloxane. *1068000.*
See *Poly(dimethyl)(diphenyl)siloxane R*.

Poly[methyl(94)phenyl(5)vinyl(1)]siloxane. *1068100.*
See *Poly(dimethyl)(diphenyl)(divinyl)siloxane R*.

Polyoxyethylated castor oil. *1068200.*
A light yellow liquid. It becomes clear above 26 °C.

Polysorbate 20. *1068300.* [9005-64-5].
See *Polysorbate 20 (0426)*.

Polysorbate 80. *1068400.* [9005-65-6].
See *Polysorbate 80 (0428)*.

Polystyrene 900-1000. *1112200.* [9003-53-6].
Organic standard used for calibration in gas chromatography.

M_w: about 950.

M_w/M_n: 1.10.

Potassium bicarbonate. *1069900.* [298-14-6].
See *potassium hydrogen carbonate R*.

   Potassium bicarbonate solution, saturated methanolic. *1069901.*
   See *potassium hydrogen carbonate solution, saturated methanolic R*.

Potassium bromate. KBrO$_3$. (M_r 167.0). *1068700.* [7758-01-2].
White granular powder or crystals, soluble in water, slightly soluble in alcohol.

Potassium bromide. *1068800.* [7758-02-3]. See *Potassium bromide (0184)*.
Potassium bromide used for infrared absorption spectrophotometry (2.2.24) also complies with the following requirement.
A disc 2 mm thick prepared from the substance previously dried at 250 °C for 1 h, has a substantially flat baseline over the range 4000 cm^{-1} to 620 cm^{-1}. It exhibits no maxima with absorbance greater than 0.02 above the baseline, except maxima for water at 3440 cm^{-1} and 1630 cm^{-1}.

Potassium carbonate. K$_2$CO$_3$. (M_r 138.2). *1068900.* [584-08-7]. Dipotassium carbonate.
A white, granular powder, hygroscopic, very soluble in water, practically insoluble in ethanol.
Store in an airtight container.

Potassium chlorate. KClO$_3$. (M_r 122.6). *1069000.* [3811-04-9].
A white powder, granules or crystals, soluble in water.

Potassium chloride. *1069100.* [7447-40-7]. See *Potassium chloride (0185)*.
Potassium chloride used for infrared absorption spectrophotometry (2.2.24) also complies with the following requirement.
A disc 2 mm thick, prepared from the substance previously dried at 250 °C for 1 h, has a substantially flat baseline over the range 4000 cm^{-1} to 620 cm^{-1}. It exhibits no maxima with absorbance greater than 0.02 above the baseline, except maxima for water at 3440 cm^{-1} and 1630 cm^{-1}.

   Potassium chloride, 0.1 M. *1069101.*
   A solution of *potassium chloride R* containing the equivalent of 7.46 g of KCl in 1000.0 ml.

Potassium chromate. K$_2$CrO$_4$. (M_r 194.2). *1069200.* [7789-00-6]. Dipotassium chromate.
Yellow crystals, freely soluble in water.

   Potassium chromate solution. *1069201.*
   A 50 g/l solution.

Potassium citrate. *1069300.* [6100-05-6].
See *Potassium citrate (0400)*.

Potassium cyanide. KCN. (M_r 65.1). *1069400.* [151-50-8].
A white, crystalline powder or white mass or granules, freely soluble in water, slightly soluble in alcohol.

   Potassium cyanide solution. *1069401.*
   A 100 g/l solution.

   Potassium cyanide solution, lead-free. *1069402.*
   Dissolve 10 g of *potassium cyanide R* in 90 ml of *water R*, add 2 ml of *strong hydrogen peroxide solution R* diluted 1 to 5. Allow to stand for 24 h, dilute to 100 ml with *water R* and filter.

   The solution complies with the following test: take 10 ml of the solution, add 10 ml of *water R* and 10 ml of *hydrogen sulphide solution R*. No colour is evolved even after addition of 5 ml of *dilute hydrochloric acid R*.

Potassium dichromate. K$_2$Cr$_2$O$_7$. (M_r 294.2). *1069500.* [7778-50-9]. Dipotassium dichromate.
Potassium dichromate used for the calibration of spectrophotometers (*2.2.25*) contains not less than 99.9 per cent of K$_2$Cr$_2$O$_7$, calculated with reference to the substance dried at 130 °C.

Orange-red crystals, soluble in water, practically insoluble in alcohol.

Assay. Dissolve 1.000 g in *water R* and dilute to 250.0 ml with the same solvent. To 50.0 ml of this solution add a freshly prepared solution of 4 g of *potassium iodide R*, 2 g of *sodium hydrogen carbonate R* and 6 ml of *hydrochloric acid R* in 100 ml of *water R* in a 500 ml flask. Stopper the flask and allow to stand protected from light for 5 min. Titrate with *0.1 M sodium thiosulphate*, using 1 ml of *iodide-free starch solution R* as indicator.

1 ml of *0.1 M sodium thiosulphate* is equivalent to 4.903 mg of $K_2Cr_2O_7$.

Potassium dichromate solution. *1069501.*
A 106 g/l solution.

Potassium dichromate solution R1. *1069502.*
A 5 g/l solution.

Potassium dihydrogen phosphate. *1069600.* [7778-77-0].
See *Potassium dihydrogen phosphate (0920).*

Potassium dihydrogen phosphate, 0.2 M. *1069601.*
A solution of *potassium dihydrogen phosphate R* containing the equivalent of 27.22 g of KH_2PO_4 in 1000.0 ml.

Potassium ferricyanide. $K_3[Fe(CN)_6]$. (M_r 329.3). *1069700.* [13746-66-2]. Potassium hexacyanoferrate(III).
Red crystals, freely soluble in water.

Potassium ferricyanide solution. *1069701.*
Wash 5 g of *potassium ferricyanide R* with a little *water R*, dissolve and dilute to 100 ml with *water R*. Prepare immediately before use.

Potassium ferrocyanide. $K_4[Fe(CN)_6],3H_2O$. (M_r 422.4). *1069800.* [14459-95-1]. Potassium hexacyanoferrate(II).
Transparent yellow crystals, freely soluble in water, practically insoluble in alcohol.

Potassium ferrocyanide solution. *1069801.*
A 53 g/l solution.

Potassium fluoride. KF. (M_r 58.1). *1137800.* [7789-23-3].
Colourless crystals or white crystalline powder, deliquescent, soluble in water, practically insoluble in alcohol.

Potassium hydrogen carbonate. $KHCO_3$. (M_r 100.1). *1069900.* [298-14-6]. Potassium bicarbonate.
Transparent, colourless crystals, freely soluble in water, practically insoluble in alcohol.

Potassium hydrogen carbonate solution, saturated methanolic. *1069901.*
Dissolve 0.1 g of *potassium hydrogen carbonate R* in 0.4 ml of *water R*, heating on water-bath. Add 25 ml of *methanol R* and swirl, keeping the solution on the water-bath until dissolution is complete. Use a freshly prepared solution.

Potassium hydrogen phthalate. $C_8H_5KO_4$. (M_r 204.2). *1070000.* [877-24-7]. Potassium hydrogen benzene-1,2-dicarboxylate.
White crystals, soluble in water, slightly soluble in alcohol.

Potassium hydrogen phthalate, 0.2 M. *1070001.*
A solution of *potassium hydrogen phthalate R* containing the equivalent of 40.84 g of $C_8H_5KO_4$ in 1000.0 ml.

Potassium hydrogen sulphate. $KHSO_4$. (M_r 136.2). *1070100.* [7646-93-7].
Colourless, transparent, hygroscopic crystals, freely soluble in water giving a strongly acid solution.
Store in an airtight container.

Potassium hydrogen tartrate. $C_4H_5KO_6$. (M_r 188.2). *1070200.* [868-14-1]. Potassium hydrogen (2R,3R)-2,3-dihydroxybutane-1,4-dioate.
A white, crystalline powder or colourless, slightly opaque crystals, slightly soluble in water, soluble in boiling water, practically insoluble in alcohol.

Potassium hydroxide. *1070300.* [1310-58-3].
See *Potassium hydroxide (0840).*

Potassium hydroxide, alcoholic 2 M. *1070301.*
Dissolve 12 g of *potassium hydroxide R* in 10 ml of *water R* and dilute to 100 ml with *alcohol R*.

Potassium hydroxide in alcohol (10 per cent V/V), 0.5 M. *1070302.*
Dissolve 28 g of *potassium hydroxide R* in 100 ml of *alcohol R* and dilute to 1000 ml with *water R*.

Potassium hydroxide solution, alcoholic. *1070303.*
Dissolve 3 g of *potassium hydroxide R* in 5 ml of *water R* and dilute to 100 ml with *aldehyde-free alcohol R*. Decant the clear solution. The solution should be almost colourless.

Potassium hydroxide solution, alcoholic R1. *1070304.*
Dissolve 6.6 g of *potassium hydroxide R* in 50 ml of *water R* and dilute to 1000 ml with *ethanol R*.

Potassium iodate. KIO_3. (M_r 214.0). *1070400.* [7758-05-6].
A white, crystalline powder, soluble in water.

Potassium iodide. *1070500.* [7681-11-0].
See *Potassium iodide (0186).*

Potassium iodide and starch solution. *1070501.*
Dissolve 0.75 g of *potassium iodide R* in 100 ml of *water R*. Heat to boiling and add whilst stirring a solution of 0.5 g of *soluble starch R* in 35 ml of *water R*. Boil for 2 min and allow to cool.

Test for sensitivity. A mixture of 15 ml of the potassium iodide and starch solution, 0.05 ml of *glacial acetic acid R* and 0.3 ml of *iodine solution R2* is blue.

Potassium iodide solution. *1070502.*
A 166 g/l solution.

Potassium iodide solution, iodinated. *1070503.*
Dissolve 2 g of *iodine R* and 4 g of *potassium iodide R* in 10 ml of *water R*. When solution is complete dilute to 100 ml with *water R*.

Potassium iodide solution, saturated. *1070504.*
A saturated solution of *potassium iodide R* in *carbon dioxide-free water R*. Make sure the solution remains saturated as indicated by the presence of undissolved crystals.

Test by adding to 0.5 ml of the saturated potassium iodide solution 30 ml of a mixture of 2 volumes of *chloroform R* and 3 volumes of *glacial acetic acid R*, as well as 0.1 ml of *starch solution R*. Any blue colour formed should be discharged by the addition of 0.05 ml of *0.1 M sodium thiosulphate*.

Store protected from light.

Potassium iodobismuthate solution. *1070600.*
To 0.85 g of *bismuth subnitrate R* add 40 ml of *water R*, 10 ml of *glacial acetic acid R* and 20 ml of a 400 g/l solution of *potassium iodide R*.

Potassium iodobismuthate solution R1. *1070601.*
Dissolve 100 g of *tartaric acid R* in 400 ml of *water R*
and add 8.5 g of *bismuth subnitrate R*. Shake for 1 h, add
200 ml of a 400 g/l solution of *potassium iodide R* and
shake well. Allow to stand for 24 h and filter.
Store protected from light.

Potassium iodobismuthate solution R2. *1070602.*
Stock solution. Suspend 1.7 g of *bismuth subnitrate R*
and 20 g of *tartaric acid R* in 40 ml of *water R*. To the
suspension add 40 ml of a 400 g/l solution of *potassium
iodide R* and stir for 1 h. Filter. The solution may be kept
for several days in brown bottles.
Spray solution. Mix immediately before use 5 ml of the
stock solution with 15 ml of *water R*.

Potassium iodobismuthate solution R3. *1070604.*
Dissolve 0.17 g of *bismuth subnitrate R* in a mixture of
2 ml of *glacial acetic acid R* and 18 ml of *water R*. Add
4 g of *potassium iodide R*, 1 g of *iodine R* and dilute to
100 ml with *dilute sulphuric acid R*.

Potassium iodobismuthate solution R4. *1070605.*
Dissolve 1.7 g of *bismuth subnitrate R* in 20 ml of *glacial
acetic acid R*. Add 80 ml of *distilled water R*, 100 ml of a
400 g/l solution of *potassium iodide R*, 200 ml of *glacial
acetic acid R* and dilute to 1000 ml with *distilled water R*.
Mix 2 volumes of this solution with 1 volume of a 200 g/l
solution of *barium chloride R*.

Potassium iodobismuthate solution, dilute. *1070603.*
Dissolve 100 g of *tartaric acid R* in 500 ml of *water R* and
add 50 ml of *potassium iodobismuthate solution R1*.
Store protected from light.

Potassium nitrate. KNO_3. (M_r 101.1). *1070700.* [7757-79-1].
Colourless crystals, very soluble in water.

Potassium periodate. KIO_4. (M_r 230.0). *1070800.*
[7790-21-8].
A white, crystalline powder or colourless crystals, soluble in
water.

Potassium ferriperiodate solution. *1070801.*
Dissolve 1 g of *potassium periodate R* in 5 ml of a freshly
prepared 120 g/l solution of *potassium hydroxide R*. Add
20 ml of *water R* and 1.5 ml of *ferric chloride solution R1*.
Dilute to 50 ml with a freshly prepared 120 g/l solution
of *potassium hydroxide R*.

Potassium permanganate. *1070900.* [7722-64-7].
See *Potassium permanganate (0121)*.

Potassium permanganate and phosphoric acid solution.
1070901.
Dissolve 3 g of *potassium permanganate R* in a mixture
of 15 ml of *phosphoric acid R* and 70 ml of *water R*.
Dilute to 100 ml with *water R*.

Potassium permanganate solution. *1070902.*
A 30 g/l solution.

Potassium perrhenate. $KReO_4$. (M_r 289.3). *1071000.*
[10466-65-6].
A white, crystalline powder, soluble in water, slightly soluble
in alcohol, in methanol and in propylene glycol.

Potassium persulphate. $K_2S_2O_8$. (M_r 270.3). *1071100.*
[7727-21-1]. Dipotassium peroxodisulphate.
Colourless crystals or a white, crystalline powder, sparingly
soluble in water, practically insoluble in alcohol. Aqueous
solutions decompose at room temperature and more rapidly
on warming.
Store in a cool place.

Potassium plumbite solution. *1071200.*
Dissolve 1.7 g of *lead acetate R*, 3.4 g of *potassium citrate R*
and 50 g of *potassium hydroxide R* in *water R* and dilute to
100 ml with the same solvent.

Potassium pyroantimonate. $KSb(OH)_6$. (M_r 262.9).
1071300. [12208-13-8]. Potassium hexahydroxoantimoniate.
White crystals or a white, crystalline powder, sparingly
soluble in water.

Potassium pyroantimonate solution. *1071301.*
Dissolve 2 g of *potassium pyroantimonate R* in 95 ml of
hot *water R*. Cool quickly and add a solution containing
2.5 g of *potassium hydroxide R* in 50 ml of *water R* and
1 ml of *dilute sodium hydroxide solution R*. Allow to
stand for 24 h, filter and dilute to 150 ml with *water R*.

Potassium tartrate. $C_4H_4K_2O_6, {}^1/_2 H_2O$. ($M_r$
235.3). *1071400.* [921-53-9]. Dipotassium
(2R,3R)-2,3-dihydroxybutane-1,4-dioate hemihydrate.
White, granular powder or crystals, very soluble in water,
very slightly soluble in alcohol.

Potassium tetraiodomercurate solution. *1071500.*
Dissolve 1.35 g of *mercuric chloride R* in 50 ml of *water R*.
Add 5 g of *potassium iodide R* and dilute to 100 ml with
water R.

Potassium tetraiodomercurate solution, alkaline. *1071600.*
Dissolve 11 g of *potassium iodide R* and 15 g of *mercuric
iodide R* in *water R* and dilute to 100 ml with the same
solvent. Immediately before use, mix 1 volume of this
solution with an equal volume of a 250 g/l solution of
sodium hydroxide R.

Potassium tetraoxalate. $C_4H_3KO_8, 2H_2O$. (M_r 254.2).
1071700. [6100-20-5].
A white, crystalline powder, sparingly soluble in water,
soluble in boiling water, slightly soluble in alcohol.

Potassium thiocyanate. KSCN. (M_r 97.2). *1071800.*
[333-20-0].
Colourless crystals, deliquescent, very soluble in water and
in alcohol.
Store in an airtight container.

Potassium thiocyanate solution. *1071801.*
A 97 g/l solution.

Povidone. *1068500.* [9003-39-8].
See *Povidone (0685)*.

Procaine hydrochloride. *1109400.*
See *Procaine hydrochloride (0050)*.

Propanol. C_3H_8O. (M_r 60.1). *1072000.* [71-23-8]. 1-Propanol.
A clear colourless liquid, miscible with water and with
alcohol.
d_{20}^{20}: about 0.802 to 0.806.
bp: about 97.2 °C.
Distillation range (2.2.11). Not less than 95 per cent distils
between 96 °C and 99 °C.

2-Propanol. C_3H_8O. (M_r 60.1). *1072100.* [67-63-0]. Isopropyl
alcohol.
A clear, colourless, flammable liquid, miscible with water
and with alcohol.
d_{20}^{20}: about 0.785.
bp: 81 °C to 83 °C.

2-Propanol R1. *1072101.*
Complies with the requirements prescribed for
2-propanol R and with the following requirements:

n_D^{20}: about 1.378.

Water (*2.5.12*). Not more than 0.05 per cent, determined on 10 g.

Minimum transmittance (*2.2.25*), determined using *water R* as compensation liquid:

25 per cent at 210 nm,

55 per cent at 220 nm,

75 per cent at 230 nm,

95 per cent at 250 nm,

98 per cent at 260 nm.

Propanolamine. C_3H_9NO. (M_r 75.1). *1072200.* [156-87-6].
3-Amino-1-propanol.
A clear, colourless, viscous liquid.
d_{20}^{20}: about 0.99.
n_D^{20}: about 1.461.
mp: about 11 °C.

Propetamphos. $C_{10}H_{20}NO_4PS$. (M_r 281.3). *1130900.*
[31218-83-4].
A suitable certified reference solution (10 ng/µl in cyclohexane) may be used.

Propionaldehyde. C_3H_6O. (M_r 58.1). *1072300.* [123-38-6].
Propanal.
A liquid freely soluble in water, miscible with alcohol and with ether.
d_{20}^{20}: about 0.81.
n_D^{20}: about 1.365.
bp: about 49 °C.
mp: about −81 °C.

Propionic acid. $C_3H_6O_2$. (M_r 74.1). *1072400.* [79-09-4].
An oily liquid, soluble in alcohol and in ether, miscible with water.
d_{20}^{20}: about 0.993.
n_D^{20}: about 1.387.
bp: about 141 °C.
mp: about −21 °C.

Propionic anhydride. $C_6H_{10}O_3$. (M_r 130.1). *1072500.*
[123-62-6].
A clear, colourless liquid, soluble in alcohol and in ether.
d_{20}^{20}: about 1.01.
bp: about 167 °C.

Propionic anhydride reagent. *1072501.*

Dissolve 1 g of *toluenesulphonic acid R* in 30 ml of *glacial acetic acid R*, add 5 ml of *propionic anhydride R* and allow to stand for at least 15 min before use.

Use within 24 h of preparation.

Propyl acetate. $C_5H_{10}O_2$. (M_r 102.1). *1072600.* [109-60-4].
d_{20}^{20}: about 0.888.
bp: about 102 °C.
mp: about −95 °C.

Propyl parahydroxybenzoate. *1072700.* [94-13-3].
See *Propyl parahydroxybenzoate (0431)*.

D-Prolyl-L-phenylalanyl-L-arginine 4-nitroanilide dihydrochloride. $C_{26}H_{36}Cl_2N_8O_5$. (M_r 612). *1072800.*

Propylene glycol. *1072900.* [57-55-6].
See *Propylene glycol (0430)*.

Propylene oxide. C_3H_6O. (M_r 58.1). *1121800.* [75-56-9].
Colourless liquid, miscible with alcohol.

Protamine sulphate. *1073000.* [53597-25-4 (salmine) 9007-31-2 (clupeine)].
See *Protamine sulphate (0569)*.

Pteroic acid. $C_{14}H_{12}N_6O_3$. (M_r 312.3). *1144600.*
[119-24-4]. 4-[[(2-Amino-4-oxo-1,4-dihydropteridin-6-yl)methyl]amino]benzoic acid.
Crystals, soluble in solutions of alkali hydroxides.

Pulegone. $C_{10}H_{16}O$. (M_r 152.2). *1073100.* [89-82-7].
(*R*)-2-Isopropylidene-5-methylcyclohexanone.
(+)-*p*-Menth-4-en-3-one.
An oily, colourless liquid, practically insoluble in water, miscible with alcohol and with ether.
d_{15}^{20}: about 0.936.
n_D^{20}: 1.485 to 1.489.
$[\alpha]_D^{20}$: + 19.5 to + 22.5.
bp: 222 °C to 224 °C.

Pulegone used in gas chromatography complies with the following additional test.

Assay. Examine by gas chromatography (*2.2.28*) as prescribed in the monograph on *Peppermint oil (0405)* using the substance to be examined as the test solution.

The area of the principal peak is not less than 98.0 per cent of the total area of the peaks.

Putrescine. $C_4H_{12}N_2$. (M_r 88.15). *1137900.* [110−60−1].
1,4-Butanediamine. Tetramethylenediamine.
A colourless oily liquid, very soluble in water. Strong piperidine-like odour.
bp: about 159 °C.
mp: about 23 °C.

Pyridine. C_5H_5N. (M_r 79.1). *1073200.* [110-86-1].
A clear, colourless liquid, hygroscopic, miscible with water and with alcohol.
bp: about 115 °C.
Store in an airtight container.

Pyridine, anhydrous. *1073300.* [110-86-1].
Dry *pyridine R* over *anhydrous sodium carbonate R*. Filter and distil.
Water (*2.5.12*). Not more than 0.01 per cent *m/m*.

Pyrid-2-ylamine. $C_5H_6N_2$. (M_r 94.1). *1073400.* [504-29-0].
2-Aminopyridine.
Large crystals soluble in water, in alcohol and in ether.
bp: about 210 °C.
mp: about 58 °C.

Pyridylazonaphthol. $C_{15}H_{11}N_3O$. (M_r 249.3). *1073500.*
[85-85-8]. 1-(2-Pyridylazo)-2-naphthol.
A brick-red powder, practically insoluble in water, soluble in alcohol, in methanol and in hot dilute alkali solutions.
mp: about 138 °C.

Pyridylazonaphthol solution. *1073501.*

A 1 g/l solution in *ethanol R*.

Test for sensitivity. To 50 ml of *water R* add 10 ml of *acetate buffer solution pH 4.4 R*, 0.10 ml of *0.02 M sodium edetate* and 0.25 ml of the pyridylazonaphthol solution. After addition of 0.15 ml of a 5 g/l solution of *copper sulphate R*, the colour changes from light yellow to violet.

4-(2-Pyridylazo)resorcinol monosodium salt. $C_{11}H_8N_3NaO_2$, H_2O. (M_r 255.2). *1131500.* [16593-81-0].
Orange crystalline powder.

Pyrocatechol. $C_6H_6O_2$. (M_r 110.1). *1073600.* [120-80-9].
Benzene-1,2-diol.
Colourless or slightly yellow crystals, soluble in water, in acetone, in alcohol and in ether.
mp: about 102 °C.
Store protected from light.

Pyrogallol. $C_6H_6O_3$. (M_r 126.1). *1073700*. [87-66-1].
Benzene-1,2,3-triol.
White crystals, becoming brownish on exposure to air and light, very soluble in water, in alcohol and in ether, slightly soluble in carbon disulphide. On exposure to air, aqueous solutions, and more rapidly alkaline solutions, become brown owing to the absorption of oxygen.
mp: about 131 °C.
Store protected from light.

> **Pyrogallol solution, alkaline.** *1073701*.
> Dissolve 0.5 g of *pyrogallol R* in 2 ml of *carbon dioxide-free water R*. Dissolve 12 g of *potassium hydroxide R* in 8 ml of *carbon dioxide-free water R*. Mix the two solutions immediately before use.

2-Pyrrolidone. C_4H_7NO. (M_r 85.1). *1138000*. [616-45-5].
Pyrrolidin-2-one.
Liquid above 25 °C, miscible with water, with ethanol and with ethyl acetate.
d_4^{25}: 1.116.

Pyruvic acid. $C_3H_4O_3$. (M_r 88.1). *1109300*. [127-17-3].
2-Oxopropanoic acid.
A yellowish liquid, miscible with water, with ethanol and with ether.
d_{20}^{20}: about 1.267.
n_D^{20}: about 1.413.
bp: about 165 °C.

Quercetin dihydrate. $C_{15}H_{10}O_7,2H_2O$. (M_r 338.2). *1138100*.
2-(3,4-Dihydroxyphenyl)-3,5,7-trihydroxy-4*H*-1-benzopyran-4-one.
Yellow crystals or yellowish powder, practically insoluble in water, soluble in acetone and in methanol.

Water (*2.5.12*): not more than 12.0 per cent, determined on 0.100 g.

Assay. Examine by liquid chromatography (*2.2.29*) as prescribed in the monograph on *Ginkgo leaf (1828)*.

The content is not less than 90 per cent (anhydrous substance) calculated by the normalisation procedure.

Store protected from light.

Quercitrin. $C_{21}H_{20}O_{11}$. (M_r 448.4). *1138200*.
[522-12-3]. Quercetin 3-L-rhamnopyranoside.
3-[(6-Deoxy-α-L-mannopyranosyl)oxy]-2-(3,4-dihydroxyphenyl)-5,7-dihydroxy-4*H*-1-benzopyran-4-one.
Quercitroside.
Yellow crystals, practically insoluble in cold water, soluble in alcohol.
mp: 176 °C to 179 °C.

Chromatography. Examine as prescribed in the monograph on *Goldenrod (1892)* applying 20 µl of the solution. After spraying, the chromatogram shows a yellowish-brown fluorescent zone with an R_f of about 0.6.

Store at a temperature of 2 °C to 8 °C.

Quinaldine red. $C_{21}H_{23}IN_2$. (M_r 430.3). *1073800*. [117-92-0].
2-[2-[4-(Dimethylamino)phenyl]ethenyl]-1-ethylquinolinium iodide.
Dark bluish-black powder, sparingly soluble in water, freely soluble in alcohol.

> **Quinaldine red solution.** *1073801*.
> Dissolve 0.1 g of *quinaldine red R* in *methanol R* and dilute to 100 ml with the same solvent.
>
> *Colour change.* pH 1.4 (colourless) to pH 3.2 (red).

Quinhydrone. $C_{12}H_{10}O_4$. (M_r 218.2). *1073900*. [106-34-3].
Equimolecular compound of 1,4-benzoquinone and hydroquinone.
Dark green, lustrous crystals or a crystalline powder, slightly soluble in water, sparingly soluble in hot water, soluble in alcohol, in concentrated ammonia and in ether.
mp: about 170 °C.

Quinidine. $C_{20}H_{24}N_2O_2$. (M_r 324.4). *1074000*. [56-54-2].
(*S*)-(6-Methoxyquinol-4-yl)[(2*R*,4*S*,5*R*)-5-vinylquinuclidin-2-yl]methanol.
White crystals, very slightly soluble in water, sparingly soluble in alcohol, slightly soluble in ether and in methanol.
$[\alpha]_D^{20}$: about + 260, determined on a 10 g/l solution in *ethanol R*.
mp: about 172 °C.
Store protected from light.

Quinidine sulphate. *1109500*. [6591-63-5].
See *Quinidine sulphate (0017)*.

Quinine. $C_{20}H_{24}N_2O_2$. (M_r 324.4). *1074100*. [130-95-0].
(*R*)-(6-Methoxyquinol-4-yl)[(2*S*,4*S*,5*R*)-5-vinylquinuclidin-2-yl]methanol.
A white, microcrystalline powder, very slightly soluble in water, slightly soluble in boiling water, very soluble in ethanol, soluble in ether.
$[\alpha]_D^{20}$: about − 167, determined on a 10 g/l solution in *ethanol R*.
mp: about 175 °C.
Store protected from light.

Quinine hydrochloride. *1074200*. [6119-47-7].
See *Quinine hydrochloride (0018)*.

Quinine sulphate. *1074300*. [6119-70-6].
See *Quinine sulphate (0019)*.

Rabbit erythrocyte suspension. *1074500*.
Prepare a 1.6 per cent *V/V* suspension of rabbit erythrocytes as follows: defibrinate 15 ml of freshly drawn rabbit blood by shaking with glass beads, centrifuge at 2000 *g* for 10 min and wash the erythrocytes with three quantities, each of 30 ml, of a 9 g/l solution of *sodium chloride R*. Dilute 1.6 ml of the suspension of erythrocytes to 100 ml with a mixture of 1 volume of *phosphate buffer solution pH 7.2 R* and 9 volumes of a 9 g/l solution of *sodium chloride R*.

Raclopride tartrate. $C_{19}H_{26}Cl_2N_2O_9$. (M_r 497.3). *1144700*.
[98185-20-7]. Raclopride L-tartrate.
A white solid, sensitive to light, soluble in water.
$[\alpha]_D^{25}$: + 0.3, determined on a 3 g/l solution.
mp: about 141 °C.

Rapeseed oil. *1074600*.
See *Rapeseed oil, refined (1369)*.

Reducing mixture. *1074700*.
Grind the substances added in the following order to obtain a homogeneous mixture: 20 mg of *potassium bromide R*, 0.5 g of *hydrazine sulphate R* and 5 g of *sodium chloride R*.

Resin for reversed-phase ion chromatography. *1131100*.
A neutral, macroporous, high specific surface area with a non-polar character resin consisting of polymer lattice of polystyrene cross-linked with divinylbenzene.

Resin, weak cationic. *1096000*.
See *weak cationic resin R*.

Resorcinol. *1074800*. [108-46-3].
See *Resorcinol (0290)*.

Resorcinol reagent. *1074801.*

To 80 ml of *hydrochloric acid R1* add 10 ml of a 20 g/l solution of *resorcinol R* and 0.25 ml of a 25 g/l solution of *copper sulphate R* and dilute to 100.0 ml with *water R*. Prepare the solution at least 4 h before use.

Store at 2 °C to 8 °C and use within 1 week.

Rhamnose. $C_6H_{12}O_5,H_2O$. (M_r 182.2). *1074900.* [6155-35-7]. L-(+)-Rhamnose. 6-Deoxy-L-mannose.
A white, crystalline powder, freely soluble in water.
$[\alpha]_D^{20}$: + 7.8 to + 8.3, determined on a 50 g/l solution in *water R* containing about 0.05 per cent of NH_3.

Rhaponticin. $C_{21}H_{24}O_9$. (M_r 420.4). *1075000.* [155-58-8]. 3-Hydroxy-5-[2-(3-hydroxy-4-methoxyphenyl)ethenyl]phenyl β-D-glucopyranoside.
A yellowish-grey, crystalline powder, soluble in alcohol and in methanol.
Chromatography. Examine as prescribed in the monograph on *Rhubarb (0291)*; the chromatogram shows only one principal spot.

Rhodamine B. $C_{28}H_{31}ClN_2O_3$. (M_r 479.0). *1075100.* [81-88-9]. Schultz No. 864.
Colour Index No. 45170.
[9-(2-Carboxyphen-yl)-6-(diethylamino)-3*H*-xanthen-3-ylidene]diethylammonium chloride.
Green crystals or reddish-violet powder, very soluble in water and in alcohol.

Ribose. $C_5H_{10}O_5$. (M_r 150.1). *1109600.* [50-69-1]. D-Ribose.
Soluble in water, slightly soluble in alcohol.
mp: 88 °C to 92 °C.

Ricinoleic acid. $C_{18}H_{34}O_3$. (M_r 298.5). *1100100.* [141-22-0]. 12-Hydroxyoleic acid.
A yellow or yellowish-brown viscous liquid, consisting of a mixture of fatty acids obtained by the hydrolysis of castor oil, practically insoluble in water, very soluble in ethanol, soluble in ether.
d_{20}^{20}: about 0.942.
n_D^{20}: about 1.472.
mp: about 285 °C, with decomposition.

Rosmarinic acid. $C_{18}H_{16}O_8$. (M_r 360.3). *1138300.* [20283-92-5].
mp: 170 °C to 174 °C.

Ruscogenins. *1141300.*

Mixture of neoruscogenin ($C_{27}H_{40}O_4$; M_r 428.6) and ruscogenin ($C_{27}H_{42}O_4$; M_r 430.6).

White powder, very slightly soluble in water, soluble in alcohol.

Ruscogenins used in liquid chromatography complies with the following additional requirement.

Assay. Examine by liquid chromatography (*2.2.29*) as prescribed in the monograph on *Butcher's broom (1847)*. The content is not less than 90 per cent of ruscogenins of which at least 60 per cent consists of neoruscogenin, calculated by the normalisation procedure.

The reagent from Vinyals laboratory has been found suitable.

Ruthenium red. [(NH₃)₅RuORu(NH₃)₄ORu(NH₃)₅]Cl₆,4H₂O. (M_r 858). *1075200.* [11103-72-3].
A brownish-red powder, soluble in water.

Ruthenium red solution. *1075201.*
A 0.8 g/l solution in *lead acetate solution R*.

Rutin. $C_{27}H_{30}O_{16},3H_2O$. (M_r 665). *1075300.* [153-18-4].
Rutoside. 3-(*O*-6-Deoxy-α-L-mannopyranosyl-(1→6)-β-D-glucopyranosyloxy)-2-(3,4-dihydroxyphenyl)-5,7-dihydroxy-4*H*-chromen-4-one.
A yellow, crystalline powder, darkening in light, very slightly soluble in water, soluble in about 400 parts of boiling water, slightly soluble in alcohol, practically insoluble in ether, soluble in solutions of the alkali hydroxides and in ammonia.
mp: about 210 °C, with decomposition.
A solution in *alcohol R* shows two absorption maxima (*2.2.25*), at 259 nm and 362 nm.

Store protected from light.

Sabinene. $C_{10}H_{16}$. (M_r 136.2). *1109700.* [2009-00-9].
Thuj-4(10)-ene. 4-Methylene-1-isopropylbicyclo[3.1.0]hexane.
A colourless, oily liquid.
d_{25}^{25}: about 0.843.
n_D^{20}: about 1.468.
bp: 163 °C to 165 °C.

Sabinene used in gas chromatography complies with the following additional test.

Assay. Examine by gas chromatography (*2.2.28*) as prescribed in the monograph on *Bitter-orange-flower oil (1175)*, using the substance to be examined as the test solution.

The area of the principal peak is not less than 99.0 per cent of the total area of the peaks.

Saccharin sodium. *1131400.* [128-44-9].
See *Saccharin sodium (0787)*.

Safrole. $C_{10}H_{10}O_2$. (M_r 162.2). *1131200.* [94-59-7]. 5-(Prop-2-enyl)-1,3-benzodioxole. 4-Allyl-1,2-(methylenedioxy)benzene.
A colourless or slightly yellow, oily liquid, with the odour of sassafras, insoluble in water, very soluble in alcohol, miscible with hexane.
d_{20}^{20}: 1.095 to 1.096.
n_D^{20}: 1.537 to 1.538.
bp: 232 °C to 234 °C.

Freezing point: about 11 °C.

Safrole used in gas chromatography complies with the following additional test.

Assay. Examine by gas chromatography (*2.2.28*) as prescribed in the monograph on *Cinnamon bark oil, Ceylon (1501)*.

The content is not less than 96.0 per cent, calculated by the normalisation procedure.

Salicin. $C_{13}H_{18}O_7$. (M_r 286.3). *1131300.* [138-52-3].
2-(Hydroxymethyl)phenyl-β-D-glucopyranoside. Salicoside.
$[\alpha]_D^{20}$: −62.5 ± 2.
mp: 199 °C to 201 °C.
Assay. Examine by liquid chromatography (*2.2.29*) as prescribed in the monograph on *Willow bark (1583)* at the concentration of the reference solution. The content is not less than 99.0 per cent calculated by the normalisation procedure.

Salicylaldehyde. $C_7H_6O_2$. (M_r 122.1). *1075400.* [90-02-8].
2-Hydroxybenzaldehyde.
A clear, colourless, oily liquid.
d_{20}^{20}: about 1.167.
n_D^{20}: about 1.574.
bp: about 196 °C.
mp: about −7 °C.

Salicylaldehyde azine. $C_{14}H_{12}N_2O_2$. (M_r 240.3). *1075500*.
2,2′-Azinodimethyldiphenol.
Dissolve 0.30 g of *hydrazine sulphate R* in 5 ml of *water R*, add 1 ml of *glacial acetic acid R* and 2 ml of a freshly prepared 20 per cent *V/V* solution of *salicylaldehyde R* in *2-propanol R*. Mix, allow to stand until a yellow precipite is formed. Shake with two quantities, each of 15 ml, of *methylene chloride R*. Combine the organic layers and dry over *anhydrous sodium sulphate R*. Decant or filter the solution and evaporate to dryness. Recrystallise from a mixture of 40 volumes of *methanol R* and 60 volumes of *toluene R* with cooling. Dry the crystals *in vacuo*.
mp: about 213 °C.
Chromatography. Examine as prescribed in the test for hydrazine in the monograph on *Povidone (0685)*; the chromatogram shows only one principal spot.

Salicylic acid. *1075600*. [69-72-7].
See *Salicylic acid (0366)*.

Sand. *1075800*.
White or slightly greyish grains of silica with a particle size between 150 µm and 300 µm.

Santonin. $C_{15}H_{18}O_3$. (M_r 246.3). *1122000*. [481-06-1].
(-)-α-Santonin. 3,5a,9-Trimethyl-3a,5,5a,9b-tetrahydro-3*H*,4*H*-naphtho[1,2]furan-2,8-dione.
Colourless, shiny crystals colouring yellow in light, very slightly soluble in water, freely soluble in hot ethanol, sparingly soluble in ethanol.
$[\alpha]_D^{18}$: −173 in ethanol.
mp: 174 °C to 176 °C.
Chromatography. Examine as prescribed in identification test C in the monograph on *Arnica flower (1391)*, the chromatogram obtained with 10 µl of the solution shows a quenching zone with an R_f value of about 0.5. Spray with *anisaldehyde solution R* and examine while heating at 105 °C for 5 min to 10 min. In daylight the quenching zone is at first a yellow zone that quickly changes to a violet-red zone.

Sclareol. $C_{20}H_{36}O_2$. (M_r 308.5). *1139900*. [515-03-7].
(1*R*,2*R*,4a*S*,8a*S*)-1-[(3*R*)-3-Hydroxy-3-methylpent-4-enyl]-2,5,5,8a-tetramethyldecahydronaphthalen-2-ol.
Odourless crystals.
$[\alpha]_D^{20}$: 6.7, in solution in ethanol.
$bp_{19\,mm}$: 218 °C to 220 °C.
mp: 96 °C to 98 °C.

Sclareol used in the chromatographic profile test in the monograph on Clary sage oil (1850) complies with the following additional test.

Assay. Examine by gas chromatography (*2.2.28*) as prescribed in the monograph on *Clary sage oil (1850)*.

The content of sclareol is not less than 97 per cent, calculated by the normalisation procedure.

SDS-PAGE running buffer. *1114900*.
Dissolve 151.4 g of *tris(hydroxymethyl)aminomethane R*, 721.0 g of *glycine R* and 50.0 g of *sodium lauryl sulphate R* in *water R* and dilute to 5000 ml with the same solvent. Immediately before use, dilute to 10 times its volume with *water R* and mix. Measure the pH (*2.2.3*) of the diluted solution. The pH is between 8.1 and 8.8.

SDS-PAGE sample buffer (concentrated). *1115000*.
Dissolve 1.89 g of *tris(hydroxymethyl)aminomethane R*, 5.0 g of *sodium lauryl sulphate R* and 50 mg of *bromophenol blue R* in *water R*. Add 25.0 ml of *glycerol R* and dilute to 100 ml with *water R*. Adjust the pH to 6.8 with *hydrochloric acid R*, and dilute to 125 ml with *water R*.

SDS-PAGE sample buffer for reducing conditions (concentrated). *1122100*.
Dissolve 3.78 g of *tris(hydroxymethyl)aminomethane R*, 10.0 g of *sodium dodecyl sulphate R* and 100 mg of *bromophenol blue R* in *water R*. Add 50.0 ml of *glycerol R* and dilute to 200 ml with *water R*. Add 25.0 ml of *2-mercaptoethanol R*. Adjust to pH 6.8 (*2.2.3*) with *hydrochloric acid R*, and dilute to 250.0 ml with *water R*.

Alternatively, dithiothreitol may be used as reducing agent instead of 2-mercaptoethanol. In this case prepare the sample buffer as follows: dissolve 3.78 g of *tris(hydroxymethyl)aminomethane R*, 10.0 g of *sodium dodecyl sulphate R* and 100 mg of *bromophenol blue R* in *water R*. Add 50.0 ml of *glycerol R* and dilute to 200 ml with *water R*. Adjust to pH 6.8 (*2.2.3*) with *hydrochloric acid R*, and dilute to 250.0 ml with *water R*. Immediately before use, add *dithiothreitol R* to a final concentration of 100 mM.

Selenious acid. H_2SeO_3. (M_r 129.0). *1100200*. [7783-00-8].
Deliquescent crystals, freely soluble in water.
Store in an airtight container.

Selenium. Se. (A_r 79.0). *1075900*. [7782-49-2].
A brown-red to black powder or granules, practically insoluble in water and in alcohol, soluble in nitric acid.
mp: about 220 °C.

Serine. *1076000*. [56-45-1].
See *Serine (0788)*.

Sialic acid. *1001100*. [131-48-6].
See *N-acetylneuraminic acid R*.

Silica gel, anhydrous. *1076100*. [112926-00-8].
Partly dehydrated polymerised, amorphous silicic acid, absorbing at 20 °C about 30 per cent of its mass of water. It contains cobalt chloride as indicator. Practically insoluble in water, partly soluble in solutions of sodium hydroxide.

Silica gel for chromatography. *1076900*.
A very finely divided (3 µm-10 µm) silica gel. The particle size is indicated after the name of the reagent in the tests where it is used.

A fine, white, homogeneous powder, practically insoluble in water and in alcohol.

Silica gel for chromatography, aminohexadecylsilyl. *1138400*.

A very finely divided (3-10 µm) silica gel with a fine particle size chemically modified at the surface by the bonding of aminohexadecylsilyl groups. The particle size is indicated after the name of the reagent in the test where it is used.

A fine, white, homogeneous powder, practically insoluble in water and in alcohol.

Silica gel for chromatography, aminopropylmethylsilyl. *1102400*.
Silica gel with a fine particle size (between 3 µm and 10 µm), chemically modified by bonding aminopropylmethylsilyl groups on the surface. The particle size is indicated after the name of the reagent in the tests where it is used.

A fine, white, homogeneous powder, practically insoluble in water and in alcohol.

Silica gel for chromatography, aminopropylsilyl. *1077000*.
Silica gel with a fine particle size (between 3 µm and 10 µm), chemically modified by bonding aminopropylsilyl groups on the surface. The particle size is indicated after the name of the reagent in the tests where it is used.

A fine, white, homogeneous powder, practically insoluble in water and in alcohol.

Silica gel for chromatography, amylose derivative of. *1109800.*

A very finely divided (10 µm) silica gel, chemically modified at the surface by the bonding of an amylose derivative. The particle size is indicated after the name of the reagent in the test where it is used.

A fine, white, homogenous powder, practically insoluble in water and in alcohol.

Silica gel for chromatography, butylsilyl. *1076200.*

A very finely divided silica gel (3 µm-10 µm), chemically modified at the surface by the bonding of butylsilyl groups. The particle size is indicated after the name of the reagent in the tests where it is used.

A fine, white, homogeneous powder, practically insoluble in water and in alcohol.

Spheroidal silica: 30 nm.

Pore volume: 0.6 cm^3/g.

Specific surface area: 80 m^2/g.

Silica gel for chromatography, cyanosilyl. *1109900.*

A very finely divided silica gel chemically modified at the surface by the bonding of cyanosilyl groups. The particle size is indicated after the name of reagent in the tests where it is used.

A fine, white, homogeneous powder, practically insoluble in water and in alcohol.

Silica gel for chromatography, di-isobutyloctadecylsilyl. *1140000.*

A very finely divided silica gel chemically modified at the surface by the bonding of di-isobutyloctadecylsilyl groups. The particle size is indicated after the name of the reagent in the tests where it is used.

Silica gel for chromatography, dimethyloctadecylsilyl. *1115100.*

A very finely divided silica gel (3 µm-10 µm), chemically modified at the surface by the bonding of dimethyloctadecylsilyl groups. The particle size is indicated after the name of the reagent in the tests where it is used.

A fine, white, homogeneous powder, practically insoluble in water and in alcohol. Irregular particle size.

Specific surface area: 300 m^2/g.

Silica gel for chromatography, diol. *1110000.*

Spherical silica particles to which dihydroxypropyl groups are bonded. Pore size 10 nm.

Silica gel for chromatography, hexylsilyl. *1077100.*

A very finely divided (3 µm-10 µm) silica gel, chemically modified at the surface by the bonding of hexylsilyl groups. The particle size is indicated after the name of the reagent in the tests where it is used.

A fine, white, homogeneous powder, practically insoluble in water and in alcohol.

Silica gel for chromatography, human albumin coated. *1138500.*

A very finely divided (3 µm to 10 µm) silica gel, chemically modified at the surface by the bonding of human albumin. The particle size is indicated after the name of the reagent in the tests where it is used.

A white, fine, homogeneous powder.

Silica gel for chromatography, hydrophilic. *1077200.*

A very finely divided (3 µm-10 µm) silica gel whose surface has been modified to provide hydrophilic characteristics. The particle size may be stated after the name of the reagent in the tests where it is used.

Silica gel for chromatography, nitrile. *1077300.*

A very finely divided silica gel, chemically modified at the surface by the bonding of cyanopropylsilyl groups. The particle size is indicated after the name of the reagent in the test where it is used.

A fine white, homogenous powder, practically insoluble in water, in alcohol and in ether.

Silica gel for chromatography, nitrile R1. *1077400.*

A very finely divided silica gel consisting of porous, spherical particles with chemically bonded nitrile groups. The particle size is indicated after the name of the reagent in the test where it is used.

A fine, white, homogeneous powder, practically insoluble in water, in alcohol and in ether.

Silica gel for chromatography, nitrile R2. *1119500.*

Ultrapure silica gel, chemically modified at the surface by the introduction of cyanopropylsilyl groups. Less than 20 ppm of metals. The particle size is indicated after the name of the reagent in the tests where it is used.

A fine white, homogenous powder, practically insoluble in water and in alcohol.

Silica gel for chromatography, octadecanoylaminopropylsilyl. *1115200.*

A very finely divided (3 µm-10 µm) silica gel, chemically modified at the surface by the bonding of aminopropylsilyl groups which are acylated with octadecanoyl groups. The particle size is indicated after the name of the reagent in the tests where it is used.

A fine, white, homogeneous powder, practically insoluble in water and in alcohol.

Silica gel for chromatography, octadecylsilyl. *1077500.*

A very finely divided (3 µm-10 µm) silica gel, chemically modified at the surface by the bonding of octadecylsilyl groups. The particle size is indicated after the name of the reagent in the tests where it is used.

A fine, white, homogeneous powder, practically insoluble in water and in alcohol.

Silica gel for chromatography, octadecylsilyl R1. *1110100.*

A very finely divided ultrapure silica gel, chemically modified at the surface by the bonding of octadecylsilyl groups. The particle size, the pore size and the carbon loading are indicated after the name of the reagent in the tests where it is used. Less than 20 ppm of metals.

Silica gel for chromatography, octadecylsilyl R2. *1115300.*

A very finely divided (15 nm pore size) ultrapure silica gel, chemically modified at the surface by the bonding of octadecylsilyl groups (20 per cent carbon load), optimised for the analysis of polycyclic aromatic hydrocarbons. The particle size is indicated after the name of the reagent in the tests where it is used.

A fine, white, homogeneous powder, practically insoluble in water and in alcohol.

Silica gel for chromatography, octadecylsilyl, base-deactivated. *1077600.*

A very finely divided (3 µm-10 µm) silica gel, pretreated before the bonding of octadecylsilyl groups by careful washing and hydrolysing most of the superficial siloxane bridges to minimise the interaction with basic components. The particle size is indicated after the name of the reagent in the tests where it is used.

A fine, white, homogeneous powder, practically insoluble in water and in alcohol.

Silica gel for chromatography, octadecylsilyl, end-capped. *1115400.*

A very finely divided (3 µm-10 µm) silica gel, chemically modified at the surface by the bonding of octadecylsilyl groups. To minimise any interaction with basic compounds it is carefully end-capped to cover most of the remaining silanol groups. The particle size is indicated after the name of the reagent in the tests where it is used.

A fine, white, homogenous powder, practically insoluble in water and in alcohol.

Silica gel for chromatography, octadecylsilyl, end-capped, base-deactivated. *1108600.*

A very finely divided (3 µm-10 µm) silica gel with a pore size of 10 nm and a carbon loading of 16 per cent, pre-treated before the bonding of octadecylsilyl groups by washing and hydrolysing most of the superficial siloxane bridges. To further minimise any interaction with basic compounds it is carefully end-capped to cover most of the remaining silanol groups. The particle size is indicated after the name of the reagent in the test where it is used.

A fine, white, homogeneous powder, practically insoluble in water and in alcohol.

Silica gel for chromatography, octylsilyl. *1077700.*

A very finely divided (3 µm-10 µm) silica gel, chemically modified at the surface by the bonding of octylsilyl groups. The particle size is indicated after the name of the reagent in the tests where it is used.

A fine, white, homogeneous powder, practically insoluble in water and in alcohol.

Silica gel for chromatography, octylsilyl R1. *1077701.*

A very finely divided (3 µm-10 µm) silica gel, chemically modified at the surface by the bonding of octylsilyl and methyl groups (double bonded phase). The particle size is indicated after the name of the reagent in the tests where it is used.

A fine, white, homogeneous powder, practically insoluble in water and in alcohol.

Silica gel for chromatography, octylsilyl R2. *1077702.*

Ultrapure very finely divided (10 nm pore size) silica gel, chemically modified at the surface by the bonding of octylsilyl groups (19 per cent carbon load). Less than 20 ppm of metals.

Silica gel for chromatography, octylsilyl, base-deactivated. *1131600.*

A very finely divided (3 µm-10 µm) silica gel, pretreated before the bonding of octylsilyl groups by careful washing and hydrolysing most of the superficial siloxane bridges to minimise the interaction with basic components. The particle size is indicated after the name of the reagent in the tests where it is used.

A fine, white, homogeneous powder, practically insoluble in water and in alcohol.

Silica gel for chromatography, octylsilyl, end-capped. *1119600.*

A very finely divided (3 µm-10 µm) silica gel, chemically modified at the surface by the bonding of octylsilyl groups. To minimise any interaction with basic compounds, it is carefully end-capped to cover most of the remaining silanol groups. The particle size is indicated after the name of the reagent in the tests where it is used.

A fine, white, homogeneous powder, practically insoluble in water and in alcohol.

Silica gel for chromatography, phenylsilyl. *1110200.*

A very finely divided (5 µm-10 µm) silica gel, chemically modified at the surface by the bonding of phenyl groups.

Silica gel for chromatography, phenylsilyl R1. *1075700.*

A very finely divided silica gel (5 µm), chemically modified at the surface by the bonding of phenyl groups. The particle size is indicated after the name of the reagent in the tests where it is used.

A fine, white, homogeneous powder, practically insoluble in water, in alcohol and in methylene chloride.

Spheroidal silica: 8 nm.

Specific surface area: 180 m^2/g.

Carbon loading: 5.5 per cent.

Silica gel for chromatography, strong-anion-exchange. *1077800.*

A very finely divided (3 µm-10 µm) silica gel, chemically modified at the surface by the bonding of quaternary ammonium groups. The particle size is indicated after the name of the reagent in the tests where it is used.

A fine, white, homogeneous powder, practically insoluble in water and in alcohol.

pH limit of use: 2 to 8.

Silica gel for chromatography, trimethylsilyl. *1115500.*

A very finely divided (3 µm-10 µm) silica gel, chemically modified at the surface by the bonding of trimethylsilyl groups. The particle size is indicated after the name of the reagent in the tests where it is used.

A fine, white, homogeneous powder, practically insoluble in water and in alcohol.

Silica gel for size-exclusion chromatography. *1077900.*

A very finely divided silica gel (10 µm) with a very hydrophilic surface. The average diameter of the pores is about 30 nm. It is compatible with aqueous solutions between pH 2 and 8 and with organic solvents. It is suitable for the separation of proteins with relative molecular masses of 1×10^3 to 3×10^5.

Silica gel G. *1076300.* [112926-00-8].

Contains about 13 per cent of calcium sulphate hemihydrate.

A fine, white, homogeneous powder with a particle size of about 15 µm.

Calcium sulphate content. Place 0.25 g in a ground-glass stoppered flask, add 3 ml of *dilute hydrochloric acid R* and 100 ml of *water R* and shake vigorously for 30 min. Filter through a sintered-glass filter and wash the residue. Carry out on the combined filtrate and washings the complexometric assay of calcium (*2.5.11*).

1 ml of *0.1 M sodium edetate* is equivalent to 14.51 mg of $CaSO_4, ^1/_2 H_2O$.

pH (2.2.3). Shake 1 g for 5 min with 10 ml of *carbon dioxide-free water R*. The pH of the suspension is about 7.

Silica gel GF$_{254}$. *1076400.* [112926-00-8].

Contains about 13 per cent of calcium sulphate hemihydrate and about 1.5 per cent of a fluorescent indicator having an optimal intensity at 254 nm.

A fine, white, homogeneous powder with a particle size of about 15 µm.

Calcium sulphate content. Determine by the method prescribed for *silica gel G R.*

General Notices (1) apply to all monographs and other texts

pH (2.2.3). Complies with the test prescribed for *silica gel G R*.

Fluorescence. Examine by thin-layer chromatography (*2.2.27*) using *silica gel G R* as the coating substance. Apply separately to the plate at ten points increasing volumes from 1 µl to 10 µl of a 1 g/l solution of *benzoic acid R* in a mixture of 10 volumes of *anhydrous formic acid R* and 90 volumes of *2-propanol R*. Develop over a path of 10 cm with the same mixture of solvents. After evaporating the solvents examine the chromatogram in ultraviolet light at 254 nm. The benzoic acid appears as dark spots on a fluorescent background in the upper third of the chromatogram for quantities of 2 µg and greater.

Silica gel H. *1076500*. [112926-00-8].
A fine, white, homogeneous powder with a particle size of about 15 µm.
pH (2.2.3). Complies with the test prescribed for *silica gel G R*.

Silica gel H, silanised. *1076600*.
Preparation of a thin layer. See *silanised silica gel HF$_{254}$R*.
A fine, white homogeneous powder which, after being shaken with water, floats on the surface because of its water-repellent properties.
Chromatographic separation. Complies with the test prescribed for *silanised silica gel HF$_{254}$R*.

Silica gel HF$_{254}$. *1076700*.
Contains about 1.5 per cent of a fluorescent indicator having an optimal intensity at 254 nm.
A fine, white, homogeneous powder with a particle size of about 15 µm.
pH (2.3.3). Complies with the test prescribed for *silica gel G R*.
Fluorescence. Complies with the test prescribed for *silica gel GF$_{254}$R*.

Silica gel HF$_{254}$, silanised. *1076800*.
Contains about 1.5 per cent of a fluorescent indicator having an optimal intensity at 254 nm.
A fine, white, homogeneous powder which, after shaking with water, floats on the surface because of its water-repellent properties.
Preparation of a thin layer. Vigorously shake 30 g for 2 min with 60 ml of a mixture of 1 volume of *methanol R* and 2 volumes of *water R*. Coat carefully cleaned plates with a layer 0.25 mm thick using a spreading device. Allow the coated plates to dry in air and then heat in an oven at 100 °C to 105 °C for 30 min.
Chromatographic separation. Introduce 0.1 g each of *methyl laurate R, methyl myristate R, methyl palmitate R* and *methyl stearate R* into a 250 ml conical flask. Add 40 ml of *alcoholic potassium hydroxide solution R* and heat under a reflux condenser on a water-bath for 1 h. Allow to cool, transfer the solution to a separating funnel by means of 100 ml of *water R*, acidify (pH 2 to 3) with *dilute hydrochloric acid R* and shake with three quantities, each of 10 ml of *chloroform R*. Dry the combined chloroform extracts over *anhydrous sodium sulphate R*, filter and evaporate to dryness on a water-bath. Dissolve the residue in 50 ml of *chloroform R*. Examine by thin-layer chromatography (*2.2.27*), using silanised silica gel HF$_{254}$ as the coating substance. Apply to the plate at each of three separate points 10 µl of the chloroformic solution. Develop over a path of 14 cm with a mixture of 10 volumes of *glacial acetic acid R*, 25 volumes of *water R* and 65 volumes of *dioxan R*. Dry the plate at 120 °C for 30 min. Allow to cool, spray with a 35 g/l solution of *phosphomolybdic acid R* in *2-propanol R* and

heat at 150 °C until the spots become visible. Treat the plate with ammonia vapour until the background is white. The chromatograms show four clearly separated, well-defined spots.

Silica gel OC for chiral separations. *1146800*.
A very finely divided silica gel for chromatography (5 µm) coated with the following derivative:

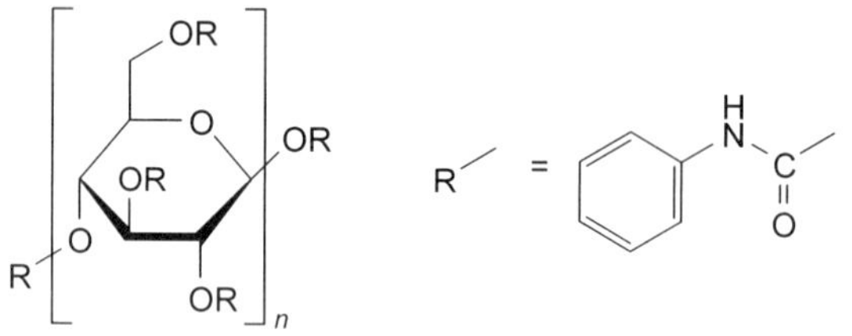

Silica gel OD for chiral separations. *1110300*.
A very finely divided silica gel for chromatography (5 µm) coated with the following derivative:

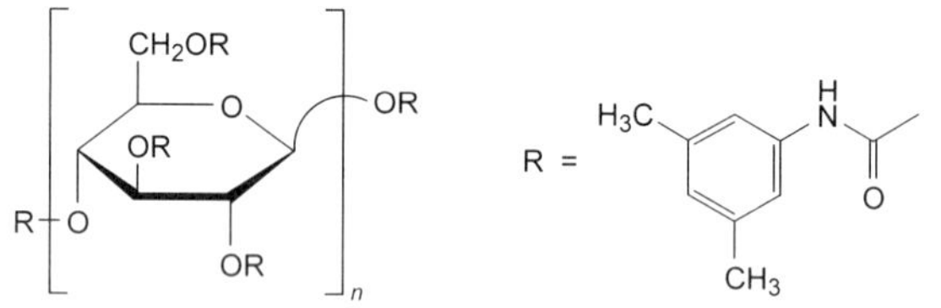

Silicotungstic acid. $H_4SiW_{12}O_{40}, xH_2O$. *1078000*. [11130-20-4].
White or yellowish-white crystals, deliquescent, very soluble in water and in alcohol.
Store in an airtight container.

Silver diethyldithiocarbamate. $C_5H_{10}AgNS_2$. (M_r 256.1). *1110400*. [1470-61-7].
A pale-yellow or greyish-yellow powder, practically insoluble in water, soluble in pyridine.
It may be prepared as follows. Dissolve 1.7 g of *silver nitrate R* in 100 ml of *water R*. Separately dissolve 2.3 g of *sodium diethyldithiocarbamate R* in 100 ml of *water R*. Cool both solutions to 10 °C, then mix and while stirring collect the yellow precipitate on a sintered-glass filter and wash with 200 ml of cold *water R*. Dry the precipitate *in vacuo* for 2 h to 3 h.
Silver diethyldithiocarbamate may be used provided it has not changed in colour or developed a strong odour.

Silver manganese paper. *1078200*.
Immerse strips of slow filter paper into a solution containing 8.5 g/l of *manganese sulphate R* and 8.5 g/l of *silver nitrate R*. Maintain for a few minutes and allow to dry over *diphosphorus pentoxide R* protected from acid and alkaline vapours.

Silver nitrate. *1078300*. [7761-88-8].
See *Silver nitrate (0009)*.

Silver nitrate reagent. *1078305*.
To a mixture of 3 ml of *concentrated ammonia R* and 40 ml of *1 M sodium hydroxide*, add 8 ml of a 200 g/l solution of *silver nitrate R*, dropwise, with stirring. Dilute to 200 ml with *water R*.

Silver nitrate solution R1. *1078301*.
A 42.5 g/l solution.
Store protected from light.

Silver nitrate solution R2. *1078302*.
A 17 g/l solution.
Store protected from light.

Silver nitrate solution, ammoniacal. *1078303.*
Dissolve 2.5 g of *silver nitrate R* in 80 ml of *water R* and
add *dilute ammonia R1* dropwise until the precipitate
has dissolved. Dilute to 100 ml with *water R*. Prepare
immediately before use.

Silver nitrate solution in pyridine. *1078304.*
An 85 g/l solution in *pyridine R.*

Store protected from light.

Silver oxide. Ag_2O. (M_r 231.7). *1078400.* [20667-12-3].
Disilver oxide.
A brownish-black powder, practically insoluble in water and
in alcohol, freely soluble in dilute nitric acid and in ammonia.
Store protected from light.

Sinensetin. $C_{20}H_{20}O_7$. (M_r 372.4). *1110500.* [2306-27-6].
3′,4′,5,6,7-Pentamethoxyflavone.
A white, crystalline powder, practically insoluble in water,
soluble in alcohol.
mp: about 177 °C.

Absorbance (2.2.25). A solution in *methanol R* shows 3
absorption maxima, at 243 nm, 268 nm and 330 nm.

Assay. Examine by liquid chromatography (*2.2.29*) as
prescribed in the monograph on *Java tea (1229).*

The content is not less than 95 per cent, calculated by the
normalisation procedure.

Sitostanol. $C_{29}H_{52}O$. (M_r 416.7). *1140100.* [19466-47-8].
Contains not less than 95.0 per cent of $C_{29}H_{52}O$.

β-Sitosterol. $C_{29}H_{50}O$. (M_r 414.7). *1140200.* [83-46-5].
Stigmast-5-en-3β-ol. 22,23-Dihydrostigmasterol.

A white powder, practically insoluble in water, sparingly
soluble in tetrahydrofuran.

Contains not less than 75.0 per cent *m/m* of $C_{29}H_{50}O$,
calculated with reference to the dried substance.

Assay. Gas chromatography (*2.2.28*), as prescribed in the
monograph on *Phytosterol (1911).*

Test solution. Dissolve 0.100 g of the substance to be
examined in *tetrahydrofuran R* and dilute to 10.0 ml
with the same solvent. Introduce 100 µl of this solution
into a suitable 3 ml flask and evaporate to dryness under
nitrogen R. To the residue add 100 µl of a freshly prepared
mixture of 50 µl of *1-methylimidazole R* and 1.0 ml of
heptafluoro-N-methyl-N-(trimethylsilyl)butanamide R. Close
the flask tightly and heat at 100 °C for 15 min. Allow to cool.

Inject 1 µl of the test solution.

Sodium. Na. (A_r 22.99). *1078500.* [7440-23-5].
A metal whose freshly cut surface is bright silver-grey.
It rapidly tarnishes in contact with air and is oxidised
completely to sodium hydroxide and converted to sodium
carbonate. It reacts violently with water, yielding hydrogen
and a solution of sodium hydroxide; soluble in anhydrous
methanol, yielding hydrogen and a solution of sodium
methoxide; practically insoluble in ether and light petroleum.
Store under light petroleum or liquid paraffin.

Sodium acetate. *1078600.* [6131-90-4].
See *Sodium acetate (0411).*

Sodium acetate, anhydrous. $C_2H_3NaO_2$. (M_r 82.0). *1078700.*
[127-09-3].
Colourless crystals or granules, very soluble in water,
sparingly soluble in alcohol.
Loss on drying (2.2.32). Not more than 2.0 per cent,
determined by drying in an oven at 100 °C to 105 °C.

Sodium ascorbate solution. *1078800.* [134-03-2].
Dissolve 3.5 g of *ascorbic acid R* in 20 ml of *1 M sodium
hydroxide*. Prepare immediately before use.

Sodium azide. NaN_3. (M_r 65.0). *1078900.* [26628-22-8].
A white, crystalline powder or crystals, freely soluble in
water, slightly soluble in alcohol, practically insoluble in
ether.

Sodium bicarbonate. *1081300.* [144-55-8].
See *sodium hydrogen carbonate R.*

Sodium bismuthate. $NaBiO_3$. (M_r 280.0). *1079000.*
[12232-99-4].
Contains not less than 85.0 per cent of $NaBiO_3$.

A yellow or yellowish-brown powder, slowly decomposing
when moist or at a high temperature, practically insoluble
in cold water.

Assay. Suspend 0.200 g in 10 ml of a 200 g/l solution
of *potassium iodide R* and add 20 ml of *dilute sulphuric
acid R*. Using 1 ml of *starch solution R* as indicator, titrate
with *0.1 M sodium thiosulphate* until an orange colour is
obtained.

1 ml of *0.1 M sodium thiosulphate* is equivalent to 14.00 mg
of $NaBiO_3$.

Sodium butanesulphonate. $C_4H_9NaO_3S$. (M_r 160.2).
1115600. [2386-54-1].
A white, crystalline powder, soluble in water.
mp: greater than 300 °C.

Sodium carbonate. *1079200.* [6132-02-1].
See *Sodium carbonate decahydrate (0191).*

Sodium carbonate, anhydrous. Na_2CO_3. (M_r 106.0).
1079300. [497-19-8]. Disodium carbonate.
A white powder, hygroscopic, freely soluble in water.
When heated to about 300 °C it loses not more than 1 per
cent of its mass.

Store in an airtight container.

Sodium carbonate solution. *1079301.*
A 106 g/l solution of *anhydrous sodium carbonate R.*

Sodium carbonate solution R1. *1079302.*
A 20 g/l solution of *anhydrous sodium carbonate R* in
0.1 M sodium hydroxide.

Sodium carbonate solution R2. *1079303.*
A 40 g/l solution of *anhydrous sodium carbonate R* in
0.2 M sodium hydroxide.

Sodium carbonate monohydrate. Na_2CO_3,H_2O. *1131700.*
[5968-11-6].
See *Sodium carbonate monohydrate (0192).*

Sodium cetostearyl sulphate. *1079400.*
See *Sodium cetostearyl sulphate (0847).*

Sodium chloride. *1079500.* [7647-14-5].
See *Sodium chloride (0193).*

Sodium chloride solution. *1079502.*
A 20 per cent *m/m* solution.

Sodium chloride solution, saturated. *1079503.*
Mix 1 part of *sodium chloride R* with 2 parts of *water R*,
shake from time to time and allow to stand. Before use,
decant the solution from any undissolved substance and
filter, if necessary.

Sodium citrate. *1079600.* [6132-04-3].
See *Sodium citrate (0412).*

Sodium cobaltinitrite. $Na_3[Co(NO_2)_6]$. (M_r 403.9). *1079700*. [13600-98-1]. Trisodium hexanitrocobaltate(III).
Orange-yellow powder, freely soluble in water, slightly soluble in alcohol.

Sodium cobaltinitrite solution. *1079701*.
A 100 g/l solution. Prepare immediately before use.

Sodium decanesulphonate. $C_{10}H_{21}NaO_3S$. (M_r 244.3). *1079800*. [13419-61-9].
Crystalline powder or flakes, white or almost white, freely soluble in water, soluble in methanol.

Sodium decyl sulphate. $C_{10}H_{21}NaO_4S$. (M_r 260.3). *1138600*. [142-87-0].
Contains not less than 95.0 per cent of $C_{10}H_{21}NaO_4S$.
White or almost white powder, freely soluble in water.

Sodium deoxycholate. $C_{24}H_{39}NaO_4$. (M_r 414.6). *1131800*. [302-95-4]. Sodium 3α,12α-dihydroxy-5β-cholan-24-oate.

Sodium deoxyribonucleate. (About 85 per cent has a relative molecular mass of 2×10^7 or greater). *1079900*. [73049-39-5].
A white, fibrous preparation obtained from calf thymus.
Test for suitability. Dissolve 10 mg in *imidazole buffer solution pH 6.5 R* and dilute to 10.0 ml with the same buffer solution (solution a). Dilute 2.0 ml of solution (a) to 50.0 ml with *imidazole buffer solution pH 6.5 R*. The absorbance (*2.2.25*) of the solution, measured at 260 nm, is 0.4 to 0.8.
To 0.5 ml of solution (a) add 0.5 ml of *imidazole buffer solution pH 6.5 R* and 3 ml of perchloric acid (25 g/l $HClO_4$). A precipitate is formed. Centrifuge. The absorbance of the supernatant liquid, measured at 260 nm using a mixture of 1 ml of *imidazole buffer solution pH 6.5 R* and 3 ml of perchloric acid (25 g/l $HClO_4$) as compensation liquid, is not greater than 0.3.
In each of two tubes, place 0.5 ml of solution (a) and 0.5 ml of a solution of a reference preparation of streptodornase containing 10 IU/ml in *imidazole buffer solution pH 6.5 R*. To one tube add immediately 3 ml of perchloric acid (25 g/l $HClO_4$). A precipitate is formed. Centrifuge and collect the supernatant liquid (a). Heat the other tube at 37 °C for 15 min and add 3 ml of perchloric acid (25 g/l $HClO_4$). Centrifuge and collect the supernatant liquid (b). The absorbance of supernatant liquid (b), measured at 260 nm with reference to supernatant liquid (a) is not less than 0.15.

Sodium diethyldithiocarbamate. $C_5H_{10}NNaS_2,3H_2O$. (M_r 225.3). *1080000*. [20624-25-3].
White or colourless crystals, freely soluble in water, soluble in alcohol. The aqueous solution is colourless.

Sodium dihydrogen phosphate. *1080100*. [13472-35-0].
See *Sodium dihydrogen phosphate dihydrate (0194)*.

Sodium dihydrogen phosphate, anhydrous. NaH_2PO_4. (M_r 120.0). *1080200*. [7558-80-7].
White powder, hygroscopic.
Store in an airtight container.

Sodium dihydrogen phosphate monohydrate.
NaH_2PO4,H_2O. (M_r 138.0). *1080300*. [10049-21-5].
White, slightly deliquescent crystals or granules, freely soluble in water, practically insoluble in alcohol.
Store in an airtight container.

Sodium dithionite. $Na_2S_2O_4$. (M_r 174.1). *1080400*. [7775-14-6].
White or greyish-white, crystalline powder, oxidises in air, very soluble in water, slightly soluble in alcohol.
Store in an airtight container.

Sodium dodecyl sulphate. *1080500*. [151-21-3].
See *Sodium laurilsulfate (0098)* except for the content which should be not less than 99.0 per cent.

Sodium edetate. *1080600*. [6381-92-6].
See *Disodium edetate (0232)*.

Sodium fluoresceinate. $C_{20}H_{10}Na_2O_5$. (M_r 376.3). *1080700*. [518-47-8].
Schultz No. 880.
Colour Index No. 45350.
Fluorescein sodium. Disodium 2-(3-oxo-6-oxido-3H-xanthen-9-yl)benzoate.
An orange-red powder, freely soluble in water. Aqueous solutions display an intense yellowish-green fluorescence.

Sodium fluoride. *1080800*. [7681-49-4].
See *Sodium fluoride (0514)*.

Sodium formate. $CHNaO_2$. (M_r 68.0). *1122200*. [141-53-7].
Sodium methanoate.
White, crystalline powder or deliquescent granules, soluble in water and in glycerol, slightly soluble in alcohol.
mp: about 253 °C.

Sodium glucuronate. $C_6H_9NaO_7,H_2O$. (M_r 234.1). *1080900*.
Sodium D-glucuronate monohydrate.
$[\alpha]_D^{20}$: about + 21.5, determined on a 20 g/l solution.

Sodium heptanesulphonate. $C_7H_{15}NaO_3S$. (M_r 202.3). *1081000*. [22767-50-6].
A white or almost white, crystalline mass, freely soluble in water, soluble in methanol.

Sodium heptanesulphonate monohydrate. $C_7H_{15}NaO_3S,H_2O$. (M_r 220.3). *1081100*.
Contains not less than 96 per cent of $C_7H_{15}NaO_3S$, calculated with reference to the anhydrous substance.
A white, crystalline powder, soluble in water, very slightly soluble in ethanol, practically insoluble in ether.
Water (2.5.12). Not more than 8 per cent, determined on 0.300 g.
Assay. Dissolve 0.150 g in 50 ml of *anhydrous acetic acid R*. Titrate with *0.1 M perchloric acid*, determining the end-point potentiometrically (*2.2.20*).
1 ml of *0.1 M perchloric acid* is equivalent to 20.22 mg of $C_7H_{15}NaO_3S$.

Sodium hexanesulphonate. $C_6H_{13}NaO_3S$. (M_r 188.2). *1081200*. [2832-45-3].
A white or almost white powder, freely soluble in water.

Sodium hydrogen carbonate. *1081300*. [144-55-8].
See *Sodium hydrogen carbonate (0195)*.

Sodium hydrogen carbonate solution. *1081301*.
A 42 g/l solution.

Sodium hydrogen sulphate. $NaHSO_4$. (M_r 120.1). *1131900*. [7681-38-1]. Sodium bisulphate.
Freely soluble in water, very soluble in boiling water. It decomposes in alcohol into sodium sulphate and free sulphuric acid.
mp: about 315 °C.

Sodium hydrogensulphite. $NaHO_3S$. (M_r 104.1). *1115700*. [7631-90-5].
A white, crystalline powder, freely soluble in water, sparingly soluble in alcohol.
On exposure to air, some sulphur dioxide is lost and the substance is gradually oxidised to sulphate.

Sodium hydroxide. *1081400*. [1310-73-2].
See *Sodium hydroxide (0677)*.

Sodium hydroxide solution. *1081401.*
Dissolve 20.0 g of *sodium hydroxide R* in *water R* and dilute to 100.0 ml with the same solvent. Verify the concentration by titration with *1 M hydrochloric acid*, using *methyl orange solution R* as indicator, and adjust if necessary to 200 g/l.

Sodium hydroxide solution, carbonate-free. *1081406.*
Dissolve *sodium hydroxide R* in *carbon dioxide-free water R* to give a concentration of 500 g/l and allow to stand. Decant the clear supernatant liquid, taking precautions to avoid the introduction of carbon dioxide.

Sodium hydroxide solution, dilute. *1081402.*
Dissolve 8.5 g of *sodium hydroxide R* in *water R* and dilute to 100 ml with the same solvent.

Sodium hydroxide solution, methanolic. *1081403.*
Dissolve 40 mg of *sodium hydroxide R* in 50 ml of *water R*. Cool and add 50 ml of *methanol R*.

Sodium hydroxide solution, methanolic R1. *1081405.*
Dissolve 200 mg of *sodium hydroxide R* in 50 ml of *water R*. Cool and add 50 ml of *methanol R*.

Sodium hydroxide solution, strong. *1081404.*
Dissolve 42 g of *sodium hydroxide R* in *water R* and dilute to 100 ml with the same solvent.

Sodium hypobromite solution. *1081500.*
In a bath of iced water mix 20 ml of *strong sodium hydroxide solution R* and 500 ml of *water R*, add 5 ml of *bromine solution R* and stir gently until solution is complete. Prepare immediately before use.

Sodium hypochlorite solution, strong. *1081600.*
Contains not less than 25 g/l and not more than 30 g/l of active chlorine.

A yellowish liquid with an alkaline reaction.

Assay. Introduce into a flask, successively, 50 ml of *water R*, 1 g of *potassium iodide R* and 12.5 ml of *dilute acetic acid R*. Dilute 10.0 ml of the substance to be examined to 100.0 ml with *water R*. Introduce 10.0 ml of this solution into the flask and titrate with *0.1 M sodium thiosulphate*, using 1 ml of *starch solution R* as indicator.

1 ml of *0.1 M sodium thiosulphate* is equivalent to 3.546 mg of active chlorine.

Store protected from light.

Sodium hypophosphite. NaH_2PO_2,H_2O. (M_r 106.0). *1081700.* [10039-56-2]. Sodium phosphinate monohydrate.
A white, crystalline powder or colourless crystals, hygroscopic, freely soluble in water, soluble in alcohol.
Store in an airtight container.

Sodium iodide. *1081800.* [7681-82-5].
See *Sodium iodide (0196)*.

Sodium laurilsulfate. *1081900.* [151-21-3].
See *Sodium laurilsulfate (0098)*.

Sodium lauryl sulphate. *1081900.* [151-21-3].
See *Sodium laurilsulfate R*.

Sodium laurylsulphonate for chromatography.
$C_{12}H_{25}NaO_3S$. (M_r 272.4). *1132000.* [2386-53-0].
White or almost white powder or crystals, freely soluble in water.
Absorbance (*2.2.25*):
$A_{1\,cm}^{5\%}$: about 0.05 at 210 nm,
$A_{1\,cm}^{5\%}$: about 0.03 at 220 nm,
$A_{1\,cm}^{5\%}$: about 0.02 at 230 nm,

$A_{1\,cm}^{5\%}$: about 0.02 at 500 nm,
determined in *water R*.

Sodium metabisulphite. *1082000.* [7681-57-4].
See *Sodium metabisulphite (0849)*.

Sodium methanesulphonate. CH_3SO_3Na. (M_r 118.1). *1082100.* [2386-57-4].
A white, crystalline powder, hygroscopic.
Store in an airtight container.

Sodium molybdate. $Na_2MoO_4,2H_2O$. (M_r 242.0). *1082200.* [10102-40-6]. Disodium molybdate dihydrate.
A white, crystalline powder or colourless crystals, freely soluble in water.

Sodium naphthoquinonesulphonate. $C_{10}H_5NaO_5S$. (M_r 260.2). *1082300.* [521-24-4]. Sodium 1,2-naphthoquinone-4-sulphonate.
A yellow to orange-yellow, crystalline powder, freely soluble in water, practically insoluble in alcohol.

Sodium nitrate. $NaNO_3$. (M_r 85.0). *1082400.* [7631-99-4].
White powder or granules or colourless, transparent crystals, deliquescent in moist air, freely soluble in water, slightly soluble in alcohol.
Store in an airtight container.

Sodium nitrite. $NaNO_2$. (M_r 69.0). *1082500.* [7632-00-0].
Contains not less than 97.0 per cent of $NaNO_2$.
A white, granular powder or a slightly yellow, crystalline powder, freely soluble in water.
Assay. Dissolve 0.100 g in 50 ml of *water R*. Add 50.0 ml of *0.02 M potassium permanganate* and 15 ml of *dilute sulphuric acid R*. Add 3 g of *potassium iodide R*. Titrate with *0.1 M sodium thiosulphate*, using 1.0 ml of *starch solution R* added towards the end of the titration as indicator.
1 ml of *0.02 M potassium permanganate* is equivalent to 3.450 mg of $NaNO_2$.

Sodium nitrite solution. *1082501.*
A 100 g/l solution. Prepare immediately before use.

Sodium nitroprusside. $Na_2[Fe(CN)_5(NO)],2H_2O$. (M_r 298.0). *1082600.* [13755-38-9]. Sodium pentacyano-nitrosylferrate(III) dihydrate.
Reddish-brown powder or crystals, freely soluble in water, slightly soluble in alcohol.

Sodium octanesulphonate. $C_8H_{17}NaO_3S$. (M_r 216.3). *1082700.* [5324-84-5].
Contains not less than 98.0 per cent of $C_8H_{17}NaO_3S$.
White or almost white, crystalline powder or flakes, freely soluble in water, soluble in methanol.
Absorbance. The absorbance (*2.2.25*) of a 54 g/l solution measured at 200 nm is not greater than 0.10 and that measured at 250 nm is not greater than 0.01.

Sodium octyl sulphate. $C_8H_{17}NaO_4S$. (M_r 232.3). *1082800.* [142-31-4].
White or almost white, crystalline powder or flakes, freely soluble in water, soluble in methanol.

Sodium oxalate. $C_2Na_2O_4$. (M_r 134.0). *1082900.* [62-76-0].
A white, crystalline powder, soluble in water, practically insoluble in alcohol and in ether.

Sodium pentanesulphonate. $C_5H_{11}NaO_3S$. (M_r 174.2). *1083000.* [22767-49-3].
A white, crystalline solid, soluble in water.

Sodium pentanesulphonate monohydrate. $C_5H_{11}NaO_3S,H_2O$. (M_r 192.2). *1132100.*
A white crystalline solid, soluble in water.

4. Reagents

Sodium perchlorate. $NaClO_4,H_2O$. (M_r 140.5). *1083100*. [7791-07-3].
Contains not less than 99.0 per cent of $NaClO_4,H_2O$.
White, deliquescent crystals, very soluble in water.
Store in a well-closed container.

Sodium periodate. $NaIO_4$. (M_r 213.9). *1083200*. [7790-28-5].
Sodium metaperiodate.
Contains not less than 99.0 per cent of $NaIO_4$.
A white, crystalline powder or white crystals, soluble in water and in mineral acids.

    Sodium periodate solution. *1083201*.
    Dissolve 1.07 g of *sodium periodate R* in *water R*, add 5 ml of *dilute sulphuric acid R* and dilute to 100.0 ml with *water R*. Use a freshly prepared solution.

Sodium phosphite pentahydrate. $Na_2HPO_3,5H_2O$. (M_r 216.0). *1132200*. [13517-23-2].
A white, crystalline powder, hygroscopic, freely soluble in water.
Store in an airtight container.

Sodium picrate solution, alkaline. *1083300*.
Mix 20 ml of *picric acid solution R* and 10 ml of a 50 g/l solution of *sodium hydroxide R* and dilute to 100 ml with *water R*.

Use within 2 days of preparation.

Sodium potassium tartrate. $C_4H_4KNaO_6,4H_2O$. (M_r 282.2). *1083500*. [6381-59-5].
Colourless, prismatic crystals, very soluble in water.

Sodium pyrophosphate. $Na_4P_2O_7,10H_2O$. (M_r 446.1). *1083600*. [13472-36-1]. Tetrasodium diphosphate decahydrate.
Colourless, slightly efflorescent crystals, freely soluble in water.

Sodium rhodizonate. $C_6Na_2O_6$. (M_r 214.0). *1122300*. [523-21-7]. [(3,4,5,6-Tetraoxocyclohex-1-en-1,2-ylene)dioxy]disodium.
Violet crystals, soluble in water with an orange-yellow colour. Solutions are unstable and must be prepared on the day of use.

Sodium salicylate. *1083700*. [54-21-7].
See *Sodium salicylate (0413)*.

Sodium sulphate, anhydrous. *1083800*. [7757-82-6].
Ignite at 600 °C to 700 °C anhydrous sodium sulphate complying with the requirements prescribed in the monograph on *Anhydrous sodium sulphate (0099)*.
Loss on drying (*2.2.32*). Not more than 0.5 per cent, determined by drying in an oven at 130 °C.

Sodium sulphate decahydrate. $Na_2SO_4,10H_2O$. (M_r 322.2). *1132300*. [7727-73-3].
See *Sodium sulphate decahydrate (0100)*.

Sodium sulphide. $Na_2S,9H_2O$. (M_r 240.2). *1083900*. [1313-84-4]. Disodium sulphide nonahydrate.
Colourless, rapidly yellowing crystals, deliquescent, very soluble in water.
Store in an airtight container.

    Sodium sulphide solution. *1083901*.
    Dissolve 12 g of *sodium sulphide R* with heating in 45 ml of a mixture of 10 volumes of *water R* and 29 volumes of *glycerol (85 per cent) R*, allow to cool and dilute to 100 ml with the same mixture of solvents.
    The solution should be colourless.

Sodium sulphite. *1084000*. [10102-15-5].
See *Sodium sulphite heptahydrate (0776)*.

Sodium sulphite, anhydrous. *1084100*. [7757-83-7].
See *Anhydrous sodium sulphite (0775)*.

Sodium tartrate. $C_4H_4Na_2O_6,2H_2O$. (M_r 230.1). *1084200*. [6106-24-7]. Disodium (2R,3R)-2,3-dihydroxybutanedioate dihydrate.
White crystals or granules, very soluble in water, practically insoluble in alcohol.

Sodium tetradeuteriodimethylsilapentanoate.
$C_6H_9{}^2H_4NaO_2Si$. (M_r 172.3). *1084300*. TSP. Sodium (2,2,3,3-tetradeuterio)-4,4-dimethyl-4-silapentanoate.
The degree of deuteration is not less than 99 per cent.
A white, crystalline powder, freely soluble in water, in ethanol and in methanol.
mp: about 300 °C.
Water and deuterium oxide: not more than 0.5 per cent.

Sodium tetrahydroborate. $NaBH_4$. (M_r 37.83). *1146900*. [16940-66-2].
Hygroscopic crystals, freely soluble in water, soluble in ethanol.

Sodium tetraphenylborate. $NaB(C_6H_5)_4$. (M_r 342.2). *1084400*. [143-66-8].
A white or slightly yellowish, bulky powder, freely soluble in water and in acetone.

    Sodium tetraphenylborate solution. *1084401*.
    Filter before use if necessary.
    A 10 g/l solution.
    Use within 1 week.

Sodium thioglycollate. $C_2H_3NaO_2S$. (M_r 114.1). *1084500*. [367-51-1]. Sodium mercaptoacetate.
White, granular powder or crystals, hygroscopic, freely soluble in water and in methanol, slightly soluble in alcohol.
Store in an airtight container.

Sodium thiosulphate. *1084600*. [10102-17-7].
See *Sodium thiosulphate (0414)*.

Sodium tungstate. $Na_2WO_4,2H_2O$. (M_r 329.9). *1084700*. [10213-10-2]. Disodium tungstate dihydrate.
A white, crystalline powder or colourless crystals, freely soluble in water forming a clear solution, practically insoluble in alcohol.

Sorbitol. *1084800*. [50-70-4].
See *Sorbitol (0435)*.

Squalane. $C_{30}H_{62}$. (M_r 422.8). *1084900*. [111-01-3]. 2,6,10,15,19,23-Hexamethyltetracosane.
A colourless, oily liquid, freely soluble in ether and in fatty oils, slightly soluble in acetone, in alcohol, in glacial acetic acid and in methanol.
d_{20}^{20}: 0.811 to 0.813.
n_D^{20}: 1.451 to 1.453.

Stannous chloride. $SnCl_2,2H_2O$. (M_r 225.6). *1085000*. [10025-69-1]. Tin dichloride dihydrate.
Contains not less than 97.0 per cent of $SnCl_2,2H_2O$.
Colourless crystals, very soluble in water, freely soluble in alcohol, in glacial acetic acid and in dilute and concentrated hydrochloric acid.
Assay. Dissolve 0.500 g in 15 ml of *hydrochloric acid R* in a ground-glass-stoppered flask. Add 10 ml of *water R* and 5 ml of *chloroform R*. Titrate rapidly with *0.05 M potassium iodate* until the chloroform layer is colourless.

1 ml of *0.05 M potassium iodate* is equivalent to 22.56 mg of $SnCl_2,2H_2O$.

Stannous chloride solution. *1085001.*
Heat 20 g of *tin R* with 85 ml of *hydrochloric acid R* until no more hydrogen is released. Allow to cool.
Store the solution over an excess of *tin R*, protected from air.

Stannous chloride solution R1. *1085002.*
Immediately before use, dilute 1 volume of *stannous chloride solution R* with 10 volumes of *dilute hydrochloric acid R*.

Stannous chloride solution R2. *1085003.*
To 8 g of *stannous chloride R* add 100 ml of a 20 per cent *V/V* solution of *hydrochloric acid R*. Shake until dissolved, heating, if necessary, on a water-bath at 50 °C. Pass a current of *nitrogen R* for 15 min. Prepare immediately before use.

Standard solution for the micro determination of water. *1147300.*
Commercially available standard solution for the coulometric titration of water, containing a certified content of water in a suitable solvent.

***Staphylococcus aureus* strain V8 protease. Type XVII-B.** *1115800.* [66676-43-5].
Microbial extracellular proteolytic enzyme. A lyophilised powder containing 500 units to 1000 units per milligram of solid.

Starch, soluble. *1085100.* [9005-84-9].
A white powder.
Prepare a 20 g/l solution in hot *water R*. The solution is at most slightly opalescent and remains fluid on cooling.

Starch iodate paper. *1085101.*
Immerse strips of filter paper in 100 ml of *iodide-free starch solution R* containing 0.1 g of *potassium iodate R*. Drain and allow to dry protected from light.

Starch iodide paper. *1085106.*
Immerse strips of filter paper in 100 ml of *starch solution R* containing 0.5 g of *potassium iodide R*. Drain and allow to dry protected from light.
Test for sensitivity. Mix 0.05 ml of *0.1 M sodium nitrite* with 4 ml of *hydrochloric acid R* and dilute to 100 ml with *water R*. Apply one drop of the solution to starch iodide paper; a blue spot appears.

Starch solution. *1085103.*
Triturate 1.0 g of *soluble starch R* with 5 ml of *water R* and whilst stirring pour the mixture into 100 ml of boiling *water R* containing 10 mg of *mercuric iodide R*.
Carry out the test for sensitivity each time the reagent is used.
Test for sensitivity. To a mixture of 1 ml of the starch solution and 20 ml of *water R*, add about 50 mg of *potassium iodide R* and 0.05 ml of *iodine solution R1* is blue.

Starch solution, iodide-free. *1085104.*
Prepare the solution as prescribed for *starch solution R* omitting the mercuric iodide. Prepare immediately before use.

Starch solution R1. *1085105.*
Mix 1 g of *soluble starch R* and a small amount of cold *water R*. Add this mixture, while stirring, to 200 ml of boiling *water R*. Add 250 mg of *salicylic acid R* and boil for 3 min. Immediately remove from the heat and cool.

If long storage is required, the solution shall be stored at 4 °C to 10 °C. A fresh starch solution shall be prepared when the end-point of the titration from blue to colourless fails to be sharp. If stored under refrigeration, the starch solution is stable for about 2 to 3 weeks.
Test for sensitivity. A mixture of 2 ml of *starch solution R1*, 20 ml of *water R*, about 50 mg of *potassium iodide R* and 0.05 ml of *iodine solution R1* is blue.

Starch solution R2. *1085107.*
Triturate 1.0 g of *soluble starch R* with 5 ml of *water R* and whilst stirring pour the mixture into 100 ml of boiling *water R*. Use a freshly prepared solution.
Test for sensitivity. To a mixture of 1 ml of the starch solution and 20 ml of *water R*, add about 50 mg of *potassium iodide R* and 0.05 ml of *iodine solution R1*. The solution is blue.

Stearic acid. $C_{18}H_{36}O_2$. (M_r 284.5). *1085200.* [57-11-4].
Octadecanoic acid.
White powder or flakes, greasy to the touch, practically insoluble in water, soluble in hot alcohol.
mp: about 70 °C.
Stearic acid used in the assay of total fatty acids in Saw palmetto fruit (1848) complies with the following additional requirement.
Assay. Examine by gas chromatography (*2.2.28*) as prescribed in the monograph on *Saw palmetto fruit (1848)*.
The content of stearic acid is not less than 98 per cent, calculated by the normalisation procedure.

Stigmasterol. $C_{29}H_{48}O$. (M_r 412.7). *1141400.*
[83-48-7]. (22*E*)-Stigmasta-5,22-dien-3β-ol.
(22*E*)-24-Ethylcholesta-5,22-dien-3β-ol.
White powder, insoluble in water.
mp: about 170 °C.
$[\alpha]_D^{22}$: about − 51 (*c* = 2 in chloroform).

Streptomycin sulphate. *1085300.* [3810-74-0].
See *Streptomycin sulphate (0053)*.

Strongly acidic ion-exchange resin. *1085400.*
See *ion-exchange resin, strongly acidic R*.

Strontium carbonate. $SrCO_3$. (M_r 147.6). *1122700.*
[1633-05-2].
A white, crystalline powder.
Contains not less than 99.5 per cent of $SrCO_3$.

Styrene-divinylbenzene copolymer. *1085500.*
Porous, rigid, cross-linked polymer beads. Several grades are available with different sizes of beads. The size range of the beads is specified after the name of the reagent in the tests where it is used.

Succinic acid. $C_4H_6O_4$. (M_r 118.1). *1085600.* [110-15-6].
Butanedioic acid.
A white, crystalline powder or colourless crystals, soluble in water and in alcohol.
mp: 184 °C to 187 °C.

Sucrose. *1085700.* [57-50-1].
See *Sucrose (0204)*.
When sucrose is used for controlling the polarimeter, it must be kept dry in a sealed ampoule.

Sudan orange. $C_{16}H_{12}N_2O$. (M_r 248.3). *1110700.* [842-07-9].
Colour Index No. 12055.
1-(Phenylazo)naphthalen-2-ol. Sudan I.
An orange-red powder, practically insoluble in water, soluble in methylene chloride.
mp: about 131 °C.

Sudan red G. $C_{17}H_{14}N_2O_2$. (M_r 278.3). *1085800*.
Schultz No. 149.
Colour Index No. 12150.
Solvent Red 1. 1-[(2-Methoxyphenyl)azo]naphtalen-2-ol.
A reddish-brown powder, practically insoluble in water.
Chromatography. Examine by thin-layer chromatography
(*2.2.27*) using *silica gel G R* as the coating substance. Apply
10 µl of a 0.1 g/l solution in *methylene chloride R* and
develop over a path of 10 cm with the same solvent. The
chromatogram shows only one principal spot.

Sulfanilamide. $C_6H_8N_2O_2S$. (M_r 172.2). *1086100*. [63-74-1].
4-Aminobenzenesulphonamide.
A white powder, slightly soluble in water, freely soluble in
boiling water, in acetone, in dilute acids and in solutions of
the alkali hydroxides, sparingly soluble in alcohol, in ether
and in light petroleum.
mp: about 165 °C.

Sulphamic acid. H_3NO_3S. (M_r 97.1). *1085900*. [5329-14-6].
White crystalline powder or crystals, freely soluble in water,
sparingly soluble in acetone, in alcohol and in methanol,
practically insoluble in ether.
mp: about 205 °C, with decomposition.

Sulphan blue. $C_{27}H_{31}N_2NaO_6S_2$. (M_r 566.6). *1086000*.
[129-17-9].
Schultz No. 769.
Colour Index No. 42045.
Acid Blue 1. Patent Blue VF. Disulphine blue.
Blue VS. Sodium [[[(4-diethylamino)phenyl](2,4-
disulphonatophenyl)methylene]cyclohexa-2,5-dien-1-
ylidene]diethylammonium.
A violet powder, soluble in water. Dilute solutions are blue
and turn yellow on the addition of concentrated hydrochloric
acid.

Sulphanilic acid. $C_6H_7NO_3S$. (M_r 173.2). *1086200*.
[121-57-3]. 4-Aminobenzenesulphonic acid.
Colourless crystals, sparingly soluble in water, practically
insoluble in alcohol.

>   **Sulphanilic acid solution.** *1086203*.
>   Dissolve 0.33 g of *sulphanilic acid R* in 75 ml of *water R*
>   heating gently if necessary and dilute to 100 ml with
>   *glacial acetic acid R*.

>   **Sulphanilic acid solution R1.** *1086201*.
>   Dissolve 0.5 g of *sulphanilic acid R* in a mixture of 75 ml
>   of *dilute acetic acid R* and 75 ml of *water R*.

>   **Sulphanilic acid solution, diazotised.** *1086202*.
>   Dissolve, with warming, 0.9 g of *sulphanilic acid R* in
>   9 ml of *hydrochloric acid R*, and dilute to 100 ml with
>   *water R*. Cool 10 ml of this solution in iced water and add
>   10 ml of an ice-cold 4.5 per cent *m/V* solution of *sodium
>   nitrite R*. Allow to stand at 0 °C for 15 min (if stored at
>   this temperature, the solution is stable for 3 days) and
>   immediately before use add 20 ml of a 10 per cent *m/V*
>   solution of *sodium carbonate R*.

Sulfathiazole. $C_9H_9N_3O_2S_2$. (M_r 255.3). *1086300*. [72-14-0].
4-Amino-*N*-(thiazol-2-yl)benzenesulphonamide.
White or yellowish-white powder or crystals, very slightly
soluble in water, soluble in acetone, slightly soluble in
alcohol. It dissolves in dilute mineral acids and in solutions
of alkali hydroxides and carbonates.
mp: about 200 °C.

Sulphomolybdic reagent R2. *1086400*.
Dissolve about 50 mg of *ammonium molybdate R* in 10 ml
of *sulphuric acid R*.

Sulphomolybdic reagent R3. *1086500*.
Dissolve with heating 2.5 g of *ammonium molybdate R* in
20 ml of *water R*. Dilute 28 ml of *sulphuric acid R* in 50 ml
of *water R*, then cool. Mix the two solutions and dilute to
100 ml with *water R*.

Store in a polyethylene container.

Sulphosalicylic acid. $C_7H_6O_6S,2H_2O$. (M_r 254.2). *1086600*.
[5965-83-3]. 2-Hydroxy-5-sulphobenzoic acid.
A white, crystalline powder or crystals, very soluble in water
and in alcohol, soluble in ether.
mp: about 109 °C.

Sulphur. *1110800*.
See *Sulphur for external use (0953)*.

Sulphur dioxide. SO_2. (M_r 64.1). *1086700*. [7446-09-5].
Sulphurous anhydride.
A colourless gas. When compressed it is a colourless liquid.

Sulphur dioxide R1. SO_2. (M_r 64.1). *1110900*.
Contains not less than 99.9 per cent *V/V* of SO_2.

Sulphuric acid. H_2SO_4. (M_r 98.1). *1086800*. [7664-93-9].
Contains not less than 95.0 per cent *m/m* and not more than
97.0 per cent *m/m* of H_2SO_4.
A colourless, caustic liquid with an oily consistency, highly
hygroscopic, miscible with water and with alcohol producing
intense heat.
d_{20}^{20}: 1.834 to 1.837.
A 10 g/l solution is strongly acid and gives the reactions of
sulphates (*2.3.1*).
Appearance. It is clear (*2.2.1*) and colourless (*Method II,
2.2.2*).
Oxidisable substances. Pour 20 g cautiously, with cooling,
into 40 ml of *water R*. Add 0.5 ml of *0.002 M potassium
permanganate*. The violet colour persists for at least 5 min.
Chlorides. Pour 10 g, carefully and while cooling, into 10 ml
of *water R* and after cooling dilute to 20 ml with the same
solvent. Add 0.5 ml of *silver nitrate solution R2*. Allow to
stand for 2 min protected from bright light. The solution is
not more opalescent than a standard prepared at the same
time using a mixture of 1 ml of *chloride standard solution
(5 ppm Cl) R*, 19 ml of *water R* and 0.5 ml of *silver nitrate
solution R2* (0.5 ppm).
Nitrates. Pour 50 g or 27.2 ml, carefully and while cooling,
into 15 ml of *water R*. Add 0.2 ml of a freshly prepared 50 g/l
solution of *brucine R* in *glacial acetic acid R*. After 5 min
any colour is less intense than that of a reference mixture
prepared in the same manner and containing 12.5 ml of
water R, 50 g of *nitrogen-free sulphuric acid R*, 2.5 ml
of *nitrate standard solution (10 ppm NO_3) R* and 0.2 ml
of a 50 g/l solution of *brucine R* in *glacial acetic acid R*
(0.5 ppm).
Ammonium. Pour 2.5 g, carefully and while cooling, into
water R and dilute to 20 ml with the same solvent. Cool,
and add dropwise 10 ml of a 200 g/l solution of *sodium
hydroxide R*, followed by 1 ml of *alkaline potassium
tetraiodomercurate solution R*. The colour of the solution
is less intense than that of a mixture of 5 ml of *ammonium
standard solution (1 ppm NH_4) R*, 15 ml of *water R*, 10 ml
of a 200 g/l solution of *sodium hydroxide R* and 1 ml of
alkaline potassium tetraiodomercurate solution R (2 ppm).
Arsenic (2.4.2). To 50 g add 3 ml of *nitric acid R* and
evaporate carefully until the volume is reduced to about
10 ml. Cool, add to the residue 20 ml of *water R* and
concentrate to 5 ml. The solution complies with limit test A
for arsenic (0.02 ppm). Prepare the standard using 1.0 ml of
arsenic standard solution (1 ppm As) R.

Heavy metals (2.4.8). Dilute 10 ml of the solution obtained in the test for iron to 20 ml with *water R*. 12 ml of the solution complies with limit test A for heavy metals (2 ppm). Prepare the standard using *lead standard solution (2 ppm Pb) R*.

Iron (2.4.9). Dissolve the residue on ignition with slight heating in 1 ml of *dilute hydrochloric acid R* and dilute to 50.0 ml with *water R*. 5 ml of the solution diluted to 10 ml with *water R* complies with the limit test for iron (1 ppm).

Residue on ignition. Not more than 0.001 per cent, determined on 100 g by evaporating cautiously in a small crucible over a naked flame and igniting the residue to redness.

Assay. Weigh accurately a ground-glass-stoppered flask containing 30 ml of *water R*, introduce 0.8 ml of the sulphuric acid, cool and weigh again. Titrate with *1 M sodium hydroxide*, using 0.1 ml of *methyl red solution R* as indicator.

1 ml of *1 M sodium hydroxide* is equivalent to 49.04 mg of H_2SO_4.

Store in a ground-glass-stoppered container made of glass or other inert material.

Sulphuric acid, alcoholic, 2.5 M. *1086801.*
Carefully and with constant cooling, stir 14 ml of *sulphuric acid R* into 60 ml of *ethanol R*. Allow to cool and dilute to 100 ml with *ethanol R*. Prepare immediately before use.

Sulphuric acid, alcoholic, 0.25 M. *1086802.*
Dilute 10 ml of *2.5 M alcoholic sulphuric acid R* to 100 ml with *ethanol R*. Prepare immediately before use.

Sulphuric acid, alcoholic solution of. *1086803.*
Carefully and with constant cooling, stir 20 ml of *sulphuric acid R* into 60 ml of *alcohol R*. Allow to cool and dilute to 100 ml with *alcohol R*. Prepare immediately before use.

Sulphuric acid, dilute. *1086804.*
Contains 98 g/l of H_2SO_4.

Add 5.5 ml of *sulphuric acid R* to 60 ml of *water R*, allow to cool and dilute to 100 ml with the same solvent.

Assay. Into a ground-glass-stoppered flask containing 30 ml of *water R*, introduce 10.0 ml of the dilute sulphuric acid. Titrate with *1 M sodium hydroxide*, using 0.1 ml of *methyl red solution R* as indicator.

1 ml of *1 M sodium hydroxide* is equivalent to 49.04 mg of H_2SO_4.

Sulphuric acid-formaldehyde reagent. *1086805.*
Mix 2 ml of *formaldehyde solution R* with 100 ml of *sulphuric acid R*.

Sulphuric acid, heavy metal-free. *1086807.*
Complies with the requirements prescribed for *sulphuric acid R* and with the following maximum contents of heavy metals:

As: 0.005 ppm;

Cd: 0.002 ppm;

Cu: 0.001 ppm;

Fe: 0.05 ppm;

Hg: 0.005 ppm;

Ni: 0.002 ppm;

Pb: 0.001 ppm;

Zn: 0.005 ppm.

Sulphuric acid, nitrogen-free. *1086806.*
Complies with the requirements prescribed for *sulphuric acid R* and with the following additional test.

Nitrates. To 5 ml of *water R* add carefully 45 ml of the sulphuric acid, allow to cool to 40 °C and add 8 mg of *diphenylbenzidine R*. The solution is faint pink or very pale blue.

Sunflower oil. *1086900.*
See *Sunflower oil, refined (1371).*

Tagatose. $C_6H_{12}O_6$. (M_r 180.16). *1111000.* [87-81-0].
D-*lyxo*-Hexulose.
White powder.
$[\alpha]_D^{20}$: −2.3 (21.9 g/l solution in *water R*).
mp: 134 °C to 135 °C.

Talc. *1087000.* [14807-96-6].
See *Talc (0438).*

Tannic acid. *1087100.* [1401-55-4].
Yellowish to light-brown, glistening scales or amorphous powder, very soluble in water, freely soluble in alcohol, soluble in acetone, practically insoluble in ether.
Store protected from light.

Tartaric acid. *1087200.* [87-69-4].
See *Tartaric acid (0460).*

Tecnazene. $C_6HCl_4NO_2$. (M_r 260.9). *1132400.* [117-18-0].
bp: about 304 °C.
mp: 99 °C to 100 °C.
A suitable certified reference solution (10 ng/µl in cyclohexane) may be used.

α-Terpinene. $C_{10}H_{16}$. (M_r 136.2). *1140300.* [99-86-5].
1-Isopropyl-4-methylcyclohexa-1,3-diene.
Clear, almost colourless liquid.
d_4^{20}: about 0.837.
n_D^{20}: about 1.478.
bp: about 174 °C.
α-Terpinene used in gas chromatography complies with the following additional test.

Assay. Examine by gas chromatography (2.2.28) as prescribed in the monograph on *Tea tree oil (1837).*

The content is not less than 95 per cent, calculated by the normalisation procedure.

γ-Terpinene. $C_{10}H_{16}$. (M_r 136.2). *1115900.* [99-85-4].
1-Isopropyl-4-methylcyclohexa-1,4-diene.
An oily liquid.
d_4^{15}: about 0.850.
n_D^{15}: 1.474 to 1.475.
bp: 183 °C to 186 °C.
γ-Terpinene used in gas chromatography complies with the following additional test.

Assay. Examine by gas chromatography (2.2.28) as prescribed in the monograph *Peppermint oil (0405).*

Test solution. The substance to be examined.

The area of the principal peak is not less than 93.0 per cent of the area of all the peaks in the chromatogram obtained.

Terpinen-4-ol. $C_{10}H_{18}O$. (M_r 154.2). *1116000.*
[562-74-3]. 4-Methyl-1-(1-methylethyl)cyclohex-3-en-1-ol.
p-Menth-1-en-4-ol.
An oily, colourless liquid.
d_{20}^{20}: about 0.934.
n_D^{20}: about 1.477.
bp: 209 °C to 212 °C.
Terpinen-4-ol used in gas chromatography complies with the following additional test.

Assay. Examine by gas chromatography (2.2.28) as prescribed in the monograph on *Lavender oil (1338).*

Test solution. The substance to be examined.

The area of the principal peak is not less than 98.0 per cent of the area of all the peaks in the chromatogram obtained.

α-Terpineol. $C_{10}H_{18}O$. (M_r 154.2). *1087300*. [98-55-5]. (*RS*)-2-(4-Methylcyclohex-3-enyl)-2-propanol. Colourless crystals, practically insoluble in water, soluble in alcohol and in ether.
d_{20}^{20}: about 0.935.
n_D^{20}: about 1.483.
$[\alpha]_D^{20}$: about 92.5.
mp: about 35 °C.

It may contain 1 to 3 per cent of β-terpineol.

α-Terpineol used in gas chromatography complies with the following test.

Assay. Examine by gas chromatography (*2.2.28*) under the conditions described in the monograph on *Anise oil (0804)*.

Test solution. A 100 g/l solution in *hexane R*.

The area of the principal peak is not less than 97.0 per cent of the total area of the peaks. Disregard the peak due to hexane.

Terpinolene. $C_{10}H_{16}$. (M_r 136.2). *1140400*. [586-62-9]. *p*-Mentha-1,4(8)-diene. 4-Isopropylidene-1-methylcyclohexene. Clear, almost colourless liquid.
d_4^{20}: about 0.863.
n_D^{20}: about 1.488.
bp: about 184 °C.
Terpinolene used in gas chromatography complies with the following additional test.

Assay. Examine by gas chromatography (*2.2.28*) as prescribed in the monograph on *Tea tree oil (1837)*.

The content is not less than 90 per cent, calculated by the normalisation procedure.

Testosterone. *1116100*. [58-22-0].
See *Testosterone (1373)*.

Testosterone propionate. *1087400*. [57-85-2].
See *Testosterone propionate (0297)*.

Tetrabutylammonium bromide. $C_{16}H_{36}BrN$. (M_r 322.4). *1087500*. [1643-19-2].
White or almost white crystals.
mp: 102 °C to 104 °C.

Tetrabutylammonium dihydrogen phosphate. $C_{16}H_{38}NO_4P$. (M_r 339.5). *1087600*. [5574-97-0].
White powder, hygroscopic.
pH (*2.2.3*). A 170 g/l solution has a pH of about 7.5.
Absorbance (*2.2.25*). About 0.10 determined at 210 nm using a 170 g/l solution.
Store in an airtight container.

Tetrabutylammonium hydrogen sulphate. $C_{16}H_{37}NO_4S$. (M_r 339.5). *1087700*. [32503-27-8].
A crystalline powder or colourless crystals, freely soluble in water and in methanol.
mp: 169 °C to 173 °C.
Absorbance (*2.2.25*). The absorbance of a 50 g/l solution, at wavelengths from 240 nm to 300 nm, is not greater than 0.05.

Tetrabutylammonium hydrogen sulphate R1. *1087701*.
Complies with the requirements prescribed for *tetrabutylammonium hydrogen sulphate R* and with the following additional requirement:
Absorbance (*2.2.25*). The absorbance of a 50 g/l solution, at wavelengths from 215 nm to 300 nm, is not greater than 0.02.

Tetrabutylammonium hydroxide. $C_{16}H_{37}NO,30H_2O$. (M_r 800). *1087800*. [2052-49-5].
Contains not less than 98.0 per cent of $C_{16}H_{37}NO,30H_2O$.

White or almost white crystals, soluble in water.

Assay. Dissolve 1.000 g in 100 ml of *water R*. Titrate immediately with *0.1 M hydrochloric acid* determining the end-point potentiometrically (*2.2.20*). Carry out a blank titration.

1 ml of *0.1 M hydrochloric acid* is equivalent to 80.0 mg $C_{16}H_{37}NO,30H_2O$.

Tetrabutylammonium hydroxide solution (104 g/l). *1087801*. [2052-49-5].
A solution containing 104 g/l of $C_{16}H_{37}NO$ (M_r 259.5), prepared by dilution of a suitable reagent grade.

Tetrabutylammonium hydroxide solution (400 g/l). *1087802*. [2052-49-5].
A solution containing 400 g/l of $C_{16}H_{37}NO$ M_r 259.5) of a suitable grade.

Tetrabutylammonium iodide. $C_{16}H_{36}IN$. (M_r 369.4). *1087900*. [311-28-4].
Contains not less than 98.0 per cent of $C_{16}H_{36}IN$.

White or slightly coloured, crystalline powder or crystals, soluble in alcohol.

Sulphated ash (*2.4.14*). Not more than 0.02 per cent.

Assay. Dissolve 1.200 g in 30 ml of *water R*. Add 50.0 ml of *0.1 M silver nitrate* and 5 ml of *dilute nitric acid R*. Titrate the excess of silver nitrate with *0.1 M ammonium thiocyanate*, using 2 ml of *ferric ammonium sulphate solution R2* as indicator.

1 ml of *0.1 M silver nitrate* is equivalent to 36.94 mg of $C_{16}H_{36}IN$.

Tetrachloroethane. $C_2H_2Cl_4$. (M_r 167.9). *1088000*. [79-34-5]. 1,1,2,2-Tetrachloroethane.
A clear, colourless liquid, slightly soluble in water, miscible with alcohol and with ether.
d_{20}^{20}: about 1.59.
n_D^{20}: about 1.495.
Distillation range (*2.2.11*). Not less than 95 per cent distils between 145 °C and 147 °C.

Tetrachlorvinphos. $C_{10}H_9Cl_4O_4P$. (M_r 366.0). *1132500*. [22248-79-9].
mp: about 95 °C.
A suitable certified reference solution (10 ng/μl in iso-octane) may be used.

Tetracos-15-enoic acid methyl ester. $C_{25}H_{48}O_2$. (M_r 380.7). *1144800*. [2733-88-2]. 15-Tetracosaenoic acid methyl ester. Methyl tetracos-15-enoate. Nervonic acid methyl ester.
Contains not less than 99.0 per cent of $C_{25}H_{48}O_2$, determined by gas chromatography.
Liquid.

Tetracycline hydrochloride. *1147000*.
See *Tetracycline hydrochloride (0210)*.

Tetradecane. $C_{14}H_{30}$. (M_r 198.4). *1088200*. [629-59-4]. *n*-Tetradecane.
Contains not less than 99.5 per cent m/m of $C_{14}H_{30}$.

A colourless liquid.
d_{20}^{20}: about 0.76.
n_D^{20}: about 1.429.
bp: about 252 °C.
mp: about −5 °C.

Tetradecylammonium bromide. $C_{40}H_{84}BrN$. (M_r 659). *1088300*. [14937-42-9]. Tetrakis(decyl)ammonium bromide. A white or slightly coloured, crystalline powder or crystals. mp: 88 °C to 89 °C.

Tetraethylammonium hydrogen sulphate. $C_8H_{21}NO_4S$. (M_r 227.3). *1116200*. [16873-13-5]. Hygroscopic powder. mp: about 245 °C.

Tetraethylammonium hydroxide solution. $C_8H_{21}NO$. (M_r 147.3). *1100300*. [77-98-5]. A 200 g/l aqueous solution, colourless liquid, strongly alkaline. d_{20}^{20}: about 1.01. n_D^{20}: about 1.372. *HPLC grade.*

Tetraethylene pentamine. $C_8H_{23}N_5$. (M_r 189.3). *1102000*. [112-57-2]. 3,6,9-Triazaundecan-1,11-diamine. Colourless liquid, soluble in acetone. n_D^{20}: about 1.506. Store protected from humidity and heat.

Tetraheptylammonium bromide. $C_{28}H_{60}BrN$. (M_r 490.7). *1088400*. [4368-51-8]. A white or slightly coloured, crystalline powder or crystals. mp: 89 °C to 91 °C.

Tetrahexylammonium hydrogen sulphate. $C_{24}H_{53}NO_4S$. (M_r 451.8). *1116300*. [32503-34-7]. *N,N,N*-Trihexylhexan-1-aminium hydrogen sulphate. White crystals. mp: 100 °C to 102 °C.

Tetrahydrofuran. C_4H_8O. (M_r 72.1). *1088500*. [109-99-9]. Tetramethylene oxide. A clear, colourless, flammable liquid, miscible with water, with alcohol and with ether. d_{20}^{20}: about 0.89.

Do not distil if the tetrahydrofuran does not comply with the test for peroxides.

Peroxides. Place 8 ml of *potassium iodide and starch solution R* in a 12 ml ground-glass-stoppered cylinder about 1.5 cm in diameter. Fill completely with the substance to be examined, shake vigorously and allow to stand protected from light for 30 min. No colour is produced.

Tetrahydrofuran used in spectrophotometry complies with the following additional requirement.

Minimum transmittance (2.2.25), determined using *water R* as compensation liquid:

20 per cent at 255 nm,

80 per cent at 270 nm,

98 per cent at 310 nm.

Tetrahydrofuran for chromatography R. *1147100*. It complies with the requirements of *tetrahydrofuran R* and with the following requirements: d_4^{20} = 0.8892. bp: about 66 °C. Contains not less than 99.8 per cent of C_4H_8O.

Tetramethylammonium chloride. $C_4H_{12}ClN$. (M_r 109.6). *1100400*. [75-57-0]. Colourless crystals, soluble in water and in alcohol. mp: about 300 °C, with decomposition.

Tetramethylammonium hydrogen sulphate. $C_4H_{13}NO_4S$. (M_r 171.2). *1116400*. [80526-82-5]. Hygroscopic powder. mp: about 295 °C.

Tetramethylammonium hydroxide. $C_4H_{13}NO,5H_2O$. (M_r 181.2). *1122800*. [10424-65-4]. Tetramethylammonium hydroxide pentahydrate. Suitable grade for HPLC.

Tetramethylammonium hydroxide solution. *1088600*. [75-59-2].

Contains not less than 10.0 per cent *m/m* of $C_4H_{13}NO$. (M_r 91.2).

A clear, colourless or very pale yellow liquid, miscible with water and with alcohol.

Assay. To 1.000 g add 50 ml of *water R* and titrate with *0.05 M sulphuric acid*, using 0.1 ml of *methyl red solution R* as indicator.

1 ml of *0.05 M sulphuric acid* is equivalent to 9.12 mg of $C_4H_{13}NO$.

> **Tetramethylammonium hydroxide solution, dilute.** *1088601*.
> Dilute 10 ml of *tetramethylammonium hydroxide solution R* to 100 ml with *aldehyde-free alcohol R*. Prepare immediately before use.

Tetramethylbenzidine. $C_{16}H_{20}N_2$. (M_r 240.3). *1132600*. [54827-17-7]. 3,3',5,5'-Tetramethylbiphenyl-4,4'-diamine. A powder, practically insoluble in water, very soluble in methanol. mp: about 169 °C.

1,1,3,3-Tetramethylbutylamine. $C_8H_{19}N$. (M_r 129.3). *1141500*. [107-45-9]. 2-Amino-2,4,4-trimethylpentane. Clear, colourless liquid. d_{20}^{20}: about 0.805. n_D^{20}: about 1.424. bp: about 140 °C.

Tetramethyldiaminodiphenylmethane. $C_{17}H_{22}N_2$. (M_r 254.4). *1088700*. [101-61-1]. 4,4'-Methylenebis-(*N,N*-dimethylaniline). White to bluish-white crystals or leaflets, practically insoluble in water, slightly soluble in alcohol, soluble in mineral acids, freely soluble in ether. mp: about 90 °C.

> **Tetramethyldiaminodiphenylmethane reagent.** *1088701*.
>
> *Solution A.* Dissolve 2.5 g of *tetramethyldiaminodiphenylmethane R* in 10 ml of *glacial acetic acid R* and add 50 ml of *water R*.
>
> *Solution B.* Dissolve 5 g of *potassium iodide R* in 100 ml of *water R*.
>
> *Solution C.* Dissolve 0.30 g of *ninhydrin R* in 10 ml of *glacial acetic acid R* and add 90 ml of *water R*.
>
> Mix solution A, solution B and 1.5 ml of solution C.

Tetramethylethylenediamine. $C_6H_{16}N_2$. (M_r 116.2). *1088800*. [110-18-9]. *N,N,N',N'*-Tetramethylethylenediamine. A colourless liquid, miscible with water, with alcohol and with ether. d_{20}^{20}: about 0.78. n_D^{20}: about 1.418. bp: about 121 °C.

Tetramethylsilane. $C_4H_{12}Si$. (M_r 88.2). *1088900*. [75-76-3]. TMS. A clear, colourless liquid, very slightly soluble in water, soluble in acetone and in alcohol. d_{20}^{20}: about 0.64.

n_D^{20}: about 1.358.
bp: about 26 °C.

Tetramethylsilane used in nuclear magnetic resonance spectrometry complies with the following additional requirement.

In the nuclear magnetic resonance spectrum of an approximately 10 per cent V/V solution of the tetramethylsilane in *deuterated chloroform R*, the intensity of any foreign signal, excluding those due to spinning side bands and to chloroform, is not greater than the intensity of the C-13 satellite signals located at a distance of 59.1 Hz on each side of the principal signal of tetramethylsilane.

Tetrazolium blue. $C_{40}H_{32}Cl_2N_8O_2$. (M_r 728). *1089000*. [1871-22-3]. 3,3'-(3,3'-Dimethoxy[1,1'-biphenyl]-4,4'-diyl)bis[2,5-diphenyl-2H-tetrazolium] dichloride.
Yellow crystals, slightly soluble in water, freely soluble in alcohol and in methanol, practically insoluble in acetone and in ether.
mp: about 245 °C, with decomposition.

Thallous sulphate. Tl_2SO_4. (M_r 504.8). *1089100*. [7446-18-6]. Dithallium sulphate.
White, rhomboid prisms, slightly soluble in water, practically insoluble in alcohol.

Thebaine. $C_{19}H_{21}NO_3$. (M_r 311.4). *1089200*. [115-37-7]. (5R,9R,13S)-4,5-Epoxy-3,6-dimethoxy-9a-methylmorphina-6,8-diene.
A white or pale yellow, crystalline powder, very slightly soluble in water, soluble in hot ethanol and in toluene, slightly soluble in ether.
mp: about 193 °C.
Chromatography (2.2.27). Examine as prescribed in identification test B in the monograph on *Raw opium (0777)*, applying to the plate as a band (20 mm × 3 mm) 20 μl of a 0.5 g/l solution. The chromatogram obtained shows an orange-red or red principal band with an R_f of about 0.5.

Theobromine. *1138800*. [83-67-0].
See *Theobromine (0298)*.

Theophylline. *1089300*. [58-55-9].
See *Theophylline (0299)*.

Thiamazole. $C_4H_6N_2S$. (M_r 114.2). *1089400*. [60-56-0]. Methimazole. 1-Methyl-1H-imidazole-2-thiol.
A white or almost white, crystalline powder, freely soluble in water, soluble in alcohol and in methylene chloride, sparingly soluble in ether.
mp: about 145 °C.

2-(2-Thienyl)acetic acid. $C_6H_6O_2S$. (M_r 142.1). *1089500*. [1918-77-0].
A brown powder.
mp: about 65 °C.

Thioacetamide. C_2H_5NS. (M_r 75.1). *1089600*. [62-55-5].
A crystalline powder or colourless crystals, freely soluble in water and in alcohol.
mp: about 113 °C.

> **Thioacetamide reagent.** *1089601*.
> To 0.2 ml of *thioacetamide solution R* add 1 ml of a mixture of 5 ml of *water R*, 15 ml of *1 M sodium hydroxide* and 20 ml of *glycerol (85 per cent) R*. Heat in a water-bath for 20 s. Prepare immediately before use.

> **Thioacetamide solution.** *1089602*.
> A 40 g/l solution.

Thiobarbituric acid. $C_4H_4N_2O_2S$. (M_r 144.2). *1111200*. [504-17-6]. 4,6-Dihydroxy-2-sulfanylpyrimidine.

Thiodiethylene glycol. $C_4H_{10}O_2S$. (M_r 122.2). *1122900*. [111-48-8]. Di(2-hydroxyethyl) sulphide.
A colourless or yellow, viscous liquid. It contains at least 99.0 per cent of $C_4H_{10}O_2S$.
d_{20}^{20}: about 1.18.

Thioglycollic acid. $C_2H_4O_2S$. (M_r 92.1). *1089700*. [68-11-1]. 2-Mercaptoacetic acid.
A colourless liquid, miscible with water, soluble in alcohol.

Thiomersal. $C_9H_9HgNaO_2S$. (M_r 404.8). *1089800*. [54-64-8]. Sodium mercurothiolate. Sodium 2-[(ethylmercurio)thio]benzoate.
A light, yellowish-white, crystalline powder, very soluble in water, freely soluble in alcohol, practically insoluble in ether.

Thiourea. CH_4N_2S. (M_r 76.1). *1089900*. [62-56-6].
White, crystalline powder or crystals, soluble in water and in alcohol.
mp: about 178 °C.

Threonine. *1090000*. [72-19-5].
See *Threonine (1049)*.

Thrombin, bovine. *1090200*. [9002-04-4].
A preparation of the enzyme, obtained from bovine plasma, that converts fibrinogen into fibrin.

A yellowish-white powder.
Store at a temperature below 0 °C.

Thrombin, human. *1090100*. [9002-04-4].

Dried human thrombin. A preparation of the enzyme which converts human fibrinogen into fibrin. It is obtained from liquid human plasma and may be prepared by precipitation with suitable salts and organic solvents under controlled conditions of pH, ionic strength and temperature.

A yellowish-white powder, freely soluble in a 9 g/l solution of sodium chloride forming a cloudy, pale yellow solution. Store in a sealed, sterile container under nitrogen, protected from light, at a temperature below 25 °C.

> **Thrombin solution, human.** *1090101*.
> Reconstitute *human thrombin R* as directed by the manufacturer and dilute with *tris(hydroxymethyl)aminomethane sodium chloride buffer solution pH 7.4 R* to 5 IU/ml.

Thromboplastin. *1090300*.
Extract 1.5 g of *acetone-dried ox brain R* with 60 ml of *water R* at 50 °C for 10 min to 15 min, centrifuge at 1500 r/min for 2 min and decant the supernatant liquid. The extract retains its activity for several days when stored in a refrigerator. It may contain 3 g/l of *cresol R* as an antimicrobial preservative.

Thujone. $C_{10}H_{16}O$. (M_r 152.2). *1116500*. [546-80-5]. 4-Methyl-1-(1-methylethyl)bicyclo[3.1.0]hexan-3-one.
A colourless or almost colourless liquid, practically insoluble in water, soluble in alcohol and in many other organic solvents.
d_{20}^{20}: about 0.925.
n_D^{20}: about 1.455.
$[\alpha]_D^{20}$: about − 15.
bp: about 200 °C.

Thymine. $C_5H_6N_2O_2$. (M_r 126.1). *1090400*. [65-71-4]. 5-Methylpyrimidine-2,4(1H,3H)-dione.
Short needles or plates, slightly soluble in cold water, soluble in hot water. It dissolves in dilute solution of alkali hydroxides.

Thymol. *1090500.* [89-83-8]. See *Thymol (0791).*

Thymol used in gas chromatography complies with the following additional test.

Assay. Examine by gas chromatography (*2.2.28*) as prescribed in the monograph *Peppermint oil (0405).*

Test solution. Dissolve 0.1 g in about 10 ml of *acetone R.*

The area of the principal peak is not less than 95.0 per cent of the area of all the peaks in the chromatogram obtained (disregard the peak due to acetone).

Thymol blue. $C_{27}H_{30}O_5S$. (M_r 466.6). *1090600.* [76-61-9]. Thymolsulphonphthalein. 4,4'-(3H-2,1-Benzoxathiol-3-ylidene)bis(2-isopropyl-5-methylphenol) S,S-dioxide. A brownish-green to greenish-blue, crystalline powder, slightly soluble in water, soluble in alcohol and in dilute solutions of alkali hydroxides.

Thymol blue solution. *1090601.*

Dissolve 0.1 g of *thymol blue R* in a mixture of 2.15 ml of *0.1 M sodium hydroxide* and 20 ml of *alcohol R* and dilute to 100 ml with *water R.*

Test for sensitivity. To 0.1 ml of the thymol blue solution add 100 ml of *carbon dioxide-free water R* and 0.2 ml of *0.02 M sodium hydroxide.* The solution is blue. Not more than 0.15 ml of *0.02 M hydrochloric acid* is required to change the colour to yellow.

Colour change. pH 1.2 (red) to pH 2.8 (yellow); pH 8.0 (olive-green) to pH 9.6 (blue).

Thymolphthalein. $C_{28}H_{30}O_4$. (M_r 430.5). *1090700.* [125-20-2]. 3,3-bis(4-Hydroxy-5-isopropyl-2-methylphenyl)-3H-isobenzo-furan-1-one. A white or yellowish-white powder, practically insoluble in water, soluble in alcohol and in dilute solutions of alkali hydroxides.

Thymolphthalein solution. *1090701.*

A 1 g/l solution in *alcohol R.*

Test for sensitivity. To 0.2 ml of the thymolphthalein solution add 100 ml of *carbon dioxide-free water R.* The solution is colourless. Not more than 0.05 ml of *0.1 M sodium hydroxide* is required to change the colour to blue.

Colour change. pH 9.3 (colourless) to pH 10.5 (blue).

Tin. Sn. (A_r 118.7). *1090800.* [7440-31-5]. Silvery-white granules, soluble in hydrochloric acid with release of hydrogen.
Arsenic (2.4.2). 0.1 g complies with limit test A (10 ppm).

Titan yellow. $C_{28}H_{19}N_5Na_2O_6S_4$. ($M_r$ 696). *1090900.* [1829-00-1]. Schultz No. 280. Colour Index No. 19540. Thiazol yellow. Disodium 2,2'-[(1-triazene-1,3-diyl)di-4,1-phenylene]bis-[6-methylbenzothiazole-7-sulphonate]. A yellowish-brown powder, freely soluble in water and in alcohol.

Titan yellow paper. *1090901.*
Immerse strips of filter paper in *titan yellow solution R* and leave for a few minutes. Allow to dry at room temperature.

Titan yellow solution. *1090902.*
A 0.5 g/l solution.
Test for sensitivity. To 0.1 ml of the titan yellow solution add 10 ml of *water R,* 0.2 ml of *magnesium standard solution (10 ppm Mg) R* and 1.0 ml of *1 M sodium hydroxide.* A distinct pink colour is visible by comparison with a reference solution prepared in a similar manner omitting the magnesium.

Titanium. Ti. (A_r 47.88). *1091000.* [7440-32-6]. Contains not less than 99 per cent of Ti.
Metal powder, fine wire (diameter not more than 0.5 mm), sponge.
mp: about 1668 °C.
Density: about 4.507 g/cm³.

Titanium dioxide. *1117900.* [13463-67-7]. See *Titanium dioxide (0150).*

Titanium trichloride. $TiCl_3$. (M_r 154.3). *1091200.* [7705-07-9]. Titanium(III) chloride. Reddish-violet crystals, deliquescent, soluble in water and in alcohol, practically insoluble in ether.
mp: about 440 °C.
Store in an airtight container.

Titanium trichloride solution. *1091201.*
d_{20}^{20}: about 1.19.
A 150 g/l solution in hydrochloric acid (100 g/l HCl).

Titanium trichloride-sulphuric acid reagent. *1091202.*
Carefully mix 20 ml of *titanium trichloride solution R* with 13 ml of *sulphuric acid R.* Add sufficient *strong hydrogen peroxide solution R* to give a yellow colour. Heat until white fumes are evolved. Allow to cool. Dilute with *water R* and repeat the evaporation and addition of *water R* until a colourless solution is obtained. Dilute to 100 ml with *water R.*

TLC octadecylsilyl silica gel F$_{254}$ plate R. *1146600.*
Support of glass, metal or plastic coated with a layer of octadecylsilyl silica gel.
It contains a fluorescent indicator having a maximum absorbance in ultraviolet light at 254 nm.

TLC performance test solution. *1116600.*
Prepare a mixture of 1.0 ml of each of the following solutions and dilute to 10.0 ml with *acetone R:* a 0.5 g/l solution of *Sudan red G R* in *toluene R,* a 0.5 g/l solution of *methyl orange R* in *ethanol R* prepared immediately before use, a 0.5 g/l solution of *bromocresol green R* in *acetone R* and a 0.25 g/l solution of *methyl red R* in *acetone R.*

TLC silica gel plate. *1116700.*
Support of glass, metal or plastic, coated with a layer of silica gel of a suitable thickness and particle size (usually 2 μm to 10 μm for fine particle size (High Performance Thin-Layer Chromatography, HPTLC) plates and 5 μm to 40 μm for normal TLC plates). If necessary, the particle size is indicated after the name of the reagent in the tests where it is used.
The plate may contain an organic binder.

Chromatographic separation. Apply to the plate an appropriate volume (10 μl for a normal TLC plate and 1 μl to 2 μl for a fine particle size plate) of *TLC performance test solution R.* Develop over a pathlength two-thirds of the plate height, using a mixture of 20 volumes of *methanol R* and 80 volumes of *toluene R.* The plate is not satisfactory, unless the chromatogram shows four clearly separated spots, the spot of bromocresol green with an R_f value less than 0.15, the spot of methyl orange with an R_f value in the range of 0.1 to 0.25, the spot of methyl red with an R_f value in the range of 0.35 to 0.55 and the spot of Sudan red G with an R_f value in the range of 0.75 to 0.98.

TLC silica gel F$_{254}$ plate. *1116800.*
It complies with the requirements prescribed for *TLC silica gel plate R* with the following modification.

It contains a fluorescent indicator having a maximum absorbance at 254 nm.

Fluorescence suppression. Apply separately to the plate at five points increasing volumes (1 µl to 10 µl for normal TLC plates and 0.2 µl to 2 µl for fine particle size plates) of a 1 g/l solution of *benzoic acid R* in a mixture of 15 volumes of *ethanol R* and 85 volumes of *cyclohexane R*. Develop over a pathlength half of the plate height with the same mixture of solvents. After evaporating the solvents examine the chromatogram in ultraviolet light at 254 nm. For normal TLC plates the benzoic acid appears as dark spots on a fluorescent background approximately in the middle of the chromatogram for quantities of 2 µg and greater. For fine particle size plates the benzoic acid appears as dark spots on a fluorescent background approximately in the middle of the chromatogram for quantities of 0.2 µg and greater.

TLC silica gel F$_{254}$, silanised plate. *1117200.*
It complies with the requirements prescribed for *TLC silica gel silanised plate R* with the following modification.

It contains a fluorescent indicator having a maximum absorbance at 254 nm.

TLC silica gel G plate. *1116900.*
It complies with the requirements prescribed for *TLC silica gel plate R* with the following modification.

It contains calcium sulphate hemihydrate as binder.

TLC silica gel GF$_{254}$ plate. *1117000.*
It complies with the requirements prescribed for *TLC silica gel plate R* with the following modifications.

It contains calcium sulphate hemihydrate as binder and a fluorescent indicator having a maximum absorbance at 254 nm.

Fluorescence suppression. Complies with the test prescribed for *TLC silica gel F$_{254}$ plate R*.

TLC silica gel plate for chiral separations, octadecylsilyl. *1137700.*
Support of glass, metal or plastic, coated with a layer of octadecylsilyl silica gel, impregnated with Cu^{2+} ions and enantiomerically pure hydroxyproline. The plate may contain an organic binder.

TLC silica gel, silanised plate. *1117100.*
Support of glass, metal or plastic, coated with a layer of silanised silica gel of a suitable thickness and particle size (usually 2 µm to 10 µm for fine particle size (High Performance Thin-Layer Chromatography, HPTLC) plates and 5 µm to 40 µm for normal TLC plates). If necessary, the particle size is indicated after the name of the reagent in the tests where it is used.

The plate may contain an organic binder.

Chromatographic separation. Introduce 0.1 g each of *methyl laurate R, methyl myristate R, methyl palmitate R* and *methyl stearate R* into a 250 ml conical flask. Add 40 ml of *alcoholic potassium hydroxide solution R* and heat under a reflux condenser on a water-bath for 1 h. Allow to cool, transfer the solution to a separating funnel by means of 100 ml of *water R*, acidify (pH 2 to 3) with *dilute hydrochloric acid R* and shake with three quantitites each of 10 ml of *methylene chloride R*. Dry the combined methylene chloride extracts over *anhydrous sodium sulphate R*, filter and evaporate to dryness on a water-bath. Dissolve the residue in 50 ml of *methylene chloride R*. Examine by thin-layer chromatography (*2.2.27*), using *silanised TLC silica gel plate R*. Apply an appropriate quantity (about 10 µl for normal TLC plates and about 1 µl to 2 µl for fine particle size plates) of the methylene chloride solution at each of three separate points. Develop over a pathlength two-thirds of the plate height with a mixture of 10 volumes of *glacial acetic acid R*, 25 volumes of *water R* and 65 volumes of *dioxan R*. Dry the plate at 120 °C for 30 min. Allow to cool, spray with a 35 g/l solution of *phosphomolybdic acid R* in *2-propanol R* and heat at 150 °C until the spots become visible. Treat the plate with ammonia vapour until the background is white. The chromatograms show four clearly separated, well-defined spots.

***o*-Tolidine.** C$_{14}$H$_{16}$N$_2$. (*M$_r$* 212.3). *1123000.* [119-93-7]. 3,3′-Dimethylbenzidine.
Contains not less than 97.0 per cent of C$_{14}$H$_{16}$N$_2$.
A light brownish, crystalline power.
mp: about 130 °C.

> ***o*-Tolidine solution.** *1123001.*
> Dissolve 0.16 g of *o-tolidine R* in 30.0 ml of *glacial acetic acid R*, add 1.0 g of *potassium iodide R* and dilute to 500.0 ml with *water R*.

Toluene. C$_7$H$_8$. (*M$_r$* 92.1). *1091300.* [108-88-3]. Methylbenzene.
A clear, colourless, flammable liquid, very slightly soluble in water, miscible with alcohol.
d_{20}^{20}: 0.865 to 0.870.
bp: about 110 °C.

> **Toluene, sulphur-free.** *1091301.*
> Complies with the requirements prescribed for *toluene R* and with the following additional requirements:
> *Sulphur compounds.* To 10 ml add 1 ml of *ethanol R* and 3 ml of *potassium plumbite solution R* and boil under a reflux condenser for 15 min. Allow to stand for 5 min. No darkening is produced in the aqueous layer.
> *Thiophen-related substances.* Shake 2 ml with 5 ml of *isatin reagent R* for 5 min and allow to stand for 15 min. No blue colour is produced in the lower layer.

Toluenesulphonamide. C$_7$H$_9$NO$_2$S. (*M$_r$* 171.2). *1091500.* [70-55-3]. 4-Methylbenzenesulphonamide. *p*-Toluenesulphonamide.
A white, crystalline powder, slightly soluble in water and in ether, soluble in alcohol and in solutions of alkali hydroxides.
mp: about 136 °C.
Chromatography. Examine as prescribed in the monograph on *Tolbutamide (0304)*; the chromatogram shows only one principal spot.

***o*-Toluenesulphonamide.** C$_7$H$_9$NO$_2$S. (*M$_r$* 171.2). *1091400.* [88-19-7]. 2-Methylbenzenesulphonamide.
A white, crystalline powder, slightly soluble in water and in ether, soluble in alcohol and in solutions of alkali hydroxides.
mp: about 156 °C.

***p*-Toluenesulphonamide.** *1091500.* [70-55-3].
See *toluenesulphonamide R*.

Toluenesulphonic acid. C$_7$H$_8$O$_3$S,H$_2$O. (*M$_r$* 190.2). *1091600.* [6192-52-5]. 4-Methylbenzenesulphonic acid.
Contains not less than 87.0 per cent of C$_7$H$_8$O$_3$S.
A white, crystalline powder or crystals, freely soluble in water, soluble in alcohol and in ether.

***o*-Toluidine.** C$_7$H$_9$N. (*M$_r$* 107.2). *1091700.* [95-53-4]. 2-Methylaniline.
A pale-yellow liquid becoming reddish-brown on exposure to air and light, slightly soluble in water, soluble in alcohol and in dilute acids.
d_{20}^{20}: about 1.01.
n_D^{20}: about 1.569.
bp: about 200 °C.
Store in an airtight container, protected from light.

o-Toluidine hydrochloride. $C_7H_{10}ClN$. (M_r 143.6). *1117300*. [636-21-5]. 2-Methylaniline hydrochloride. 2-Methylbenzenamine hydrochloride.
It contains not less than 98.0 per cent of $C_7H_{10}ClN$.
mp: 215 °C to 217 °C.

p-Toluidine. C_7H_9N. (M_r 107.2). *1091800*. [106-49-0].
4-Methylaniline.
Lustrous plates or flakes, slightly soluble in water, freely soluble in acetone and in alcohol, soluble in ether.
mp: about 44 °C.

Toluidine blue. $C_{15}H_{16}ClN_3S$. (M_r 305.8). *1091900*. [92-31-9].
Schultz No. 1041.
Colour Index No. 52040.
Toluidine Blue O. 3-Amino-7-dimethylamino-2-methylphenothiazin-5-ium chloride.
A dark-green powder, soluble in water, slightly soluble in alcohol.

Tosylarginine methyl ester hydrochloride.
$C_{14}H_{23}ClN_4O_4S$. (M_r 378.9). *1092000*. [1784-03-8].
N-Tosyl-L-arginine methyl ester hydrochloride. Ethyl (*S*)-5-guanidino-2-(4-methylbenzene-sulphonamido)valerate hydrochloride.
$[\alpha]_D^{20}$: − 12 to − 16, determined on a 40 g/l solution.
mp: about 145 °C.

Tosylarginine methyl ester hydrochloride solution. *1092001*.
To 98.5 mg of *tosylarginine methyl ester hydrochloride R* add 5 ml of *tris(hydroxymethyl)aminomethane buffer solution pH 8.1 R* and shake to dissolve. Add 2.5 ml of *methyl red mixed solution R* and dilute to 25.0 ml with *water R*.

Tosyl-lysyl-chloromethane hydrochloride.
$C_{14}H_{22}Cl_2N_2O_3S$. (M_r 369.3). *1092100*. [4238-41-9].
N-Tosyl-L-lysyl-chloromethane hydrochloride. (3*S*)-7-Amino-1-chloro-3-(4-methylbenzenesulphonamido)heptan-2-one hydrochloride.
$[\alpha]_D^{20}$: −7 to −9, determined on a 20 g/l solution.
mp: about 155 °C, with decomposition.
$A_{1\,cm}^{1\%}$: 310 to 340, determined at 230 nm using a solution in *water R*.

Tosylphenylalanylchloromethane. $C_{17}H_{18}ClNO_3S$. (M_r 351.9). *1092200*. [402-71-1]. *N*-Tosyl-L-phenylalanylchloromethane.
$[\alpha]_D^{20}$: −85 to −89, determined on a 10 g/l solution in *alcohol R*.
mp: about 105 °C.
$A_{1\,cm}^{1\%}$: 290 to 320, determined at 228.5 nm in *alcohol R*.

Toxaphene. *1132800*. [8001-35-2].
A mixture of polychloro derivatives.
mp: 65 °C to 90 °C.
A suitable certified reference solution (10 ng/μl in iso-octane) may be used.

Tragacanth. *1092300*. [9000-65-1].
See *Tragacanth (0532)*.

Triacetin. $C_9H_{14}O_6$. (M_r 218.2). *1092400*. [102-76-1].
Propane-1,2,3-triyl triacetate.
An almost clear, colourless to yellowish liquid, soluble in water, miscible with alcohol and with ether.
d_{20}^{20}: about 1.16.
n_D^{20}: about 1.43.
bp: about 260 °C.

Triamcinolone. $C_{21}H_{27}FO_6$. (M_r 394.4). *1111300*. [124-94-7].
9-Fluoro-11β,16α,17,21-tetrahydroxypregna-1,4-diene-3,20-dione.
A crystalline powder.
mp: 262 °C to 263 °C.

Triamcinolone acetonide. *1133100*. [76-25-5].
See *Triamcinolone acetonide (0533)*.

Trichlorethylene. *1102100*.
See *Trichloroethylene R*.

Trichloroacetic acid. $C_2HCl_3O_2$. (M_r 163.4). *1092500*. [76-03-9].
Colourless crystals or a crystalline mass, very deliquescent, very soluble in water and in alcohol.
Store in an airtight container.

Trichloroacetic acid solution. *1092501*.
Dissolve 40.0 g of *trichloroacetic acid R* in *water R* and dilute to 1000.0 ml with the same solvent. Verify the concentration by titration with *0.1 M sodium hydroxide* and adjust if necessary to 40 ± 1 g/l.

1,1,1-Trichloroethane. $C_2H_3Cl_3$. (M_r 133.4). *1092600*. [71-55-6]. Methylchloroform.
A non-flammable liquid, practically insoluble in water, soluble in acetone, in ether and in methanol.
d_{20}^{20}: about 1.34.
n_D^{20}: about 1.438.
bp: about 74 °C.

Trichloroethylene. C_2HCl_3. (M_r 131.4). *1102100*. [79-01-6].
A colourless liquid, practically insoluble in water, miscible with alcohol and with ether.
d_{20}^{20}: about 1.46.
n_D^{20}: about 1.477.

Trichlorotrifluoroethane. $C_2Cl_3F_3$. (M_r 187.4). *1092700*. [76-13-1]. 1,1,2-Trichloro-1,2,2-trifluoroethane.
A colourless, volatile liquid, practically insoluble in water, miscible with acetone and with ether.
d_{20}^{20}: about 1.58.
Distillation range (2.2.11). Not less than 98 per cent distils between 47 °C and 48 °C.

Tricine. $C_6H_{13}NO_5$. (M_r 179.2). *1138900*. [5704-04-1].
N-[2-Hydroxy-1,1-bis(hydroxymethyl)ethyl]glycine.
Use electrophoresis-grade reagent.
mp: about 183 °C.

Tricosane. $C_{23}H_{48}$. (M_r 324.6). *1092800*. [638-67-5].
White crystals, practically insoluble in water, soluble in ether and in hexane.
n_D^{20}: about 1.447.
mp: about 48 °C.

Tridocosahexaenoin. $C_{69}H_{98}O_6$. (M_r 1023.5). *1144900*. [124596-98-1]. Triglyceride of docosahexaenoic acid (C22:6). Glycerol tridocosahexaenoate. Propane-1,2,3-triyl tri-(*all-Z*)-docosa-4,7,10,13,16,19-hexaenoate.
The reagent from Nu-Chek Prep, Inc. has been found suitable.

Triethanolamine. *1092900*. [102-71-6].
See *Trolamine (1577)*.

Triethylamine. $C_6H_{15}N$. (M_r 101.2). *1093000*. [121-44-8].
N,*N*-Diethylethanamine.
A colourless liquid, slightly soluble in water at a temperature below 18.7 °C, miscible with alcohol and ether.
d_{20}^{20}: about 0.727.
n_D^{20}: about 1.401.
bp: about 90 °C.

Triethylenediamine. $C_6H_{12}N_2$. (M_r 112.2). *1093100*.
1,4-Diazabicyclo[2.2.2]octane.
Crystals, very hygroscopic, sublimes readily at room temperature, freely soluble in water, in acetone and in ethanol.
bp: about 174 °C.
mp: about 158 °C.
Store in an airtight container.

Triethyl phosphonoformate. $C_7H_{15}O_5P$. (M_r 210.2). *1132900*. [1474-78-8]. Ethyl (diethoxyphosphoryl)formate.
Colourless liquid.
$bp_{12\,mm}$: about 135 °C.

Trifluoroacetic acid. $C_2HF_3O_2$. (M_r 114.0). *1093200*. [76-05-1].
Contains not less than 99 per cent of $C_2HF_3O_2$.
Liquid, miscible with acetone, with alcohol and with ether.
d_{20}^{20}: about 1.53.
bp: about 72 °C.
Use a grade suitable for protein sequencing.
Store in an airtight container.

Trifluoroacetic anhydride. $C_4F_6O_3$. (M_r 210.0). *1093300*. [407-25-0].
Colourless liquid.
d_{20}^{20}: about 1.5.

Trigonelline hydrochloride. $C_7H_8ClNO_2$. (M_r 173.6). *1117400*. [6138-41-6]. 3-Carboxy-1-methylpyridinium chloride. Nicotinic acid N-methylbetaine hydrochloride.
A crystalline powder, very soluble in water, soluble in alcohol, practically insoluble in ether.
mp: about 258 °C.

Trimethylpentane. C_8H_{18}. (M_r 114.2). *1093400*. [540-84-1].
Iso-octane. 2,2,4-Trimethylpentane.
A colourless, flammable liquid, practically insoluble in water, soluble in ethanol.
d_{20}^{20}: 0.691 to 0.696.
n_D^{20}: 1.391 to 1.393.
Distillation range (2.2.11). Not less than 95 per cent distils between 98 °C and 100 °C.

Trimethylpentane used in spectrophotometry complies with the following additional requirement.

Minimum transmittance (2.2.25), determined using *water R* as compensation liquid: 98 per cent from 250 nm to 420 nm.

> **Trimethylpentane R1.** *1093401*.
> Complies with the requirements prescribed for *trimethylpentane R* with the following modification.
> *Absorbance (2.2.25).* Not more than 0.07 from 220 nm to 360 nm, determined using *water R* as the compensation liquid.

N,O-bis(Trimethylsilyl)acetamide. $C_8H_{21}NOSi_2$. (M_r 203.4). *1093600*. [10416-59-8].
Colourless liquid.
d_{20}^{20}: about 0.83.

N-Trimethylsilylimidazole. $C_6H_{12}N_2Si$. (M_r 140.3). *1100500*. [18156-74-6]. 1-Trimethylsilylimidazole.
A colourless, hygroscopic liquid.
d_{20}^{20}: about 0.96.
n_D^{20}: about 1.48.
Store in an airtight container.

N,O-bis(Trimethylsilyl)trifluoroacetamide. $C_8H_{18}F_3NOSi_2$. (M_r 257.4). *1133200*. [25561-30-2]. BSTFA.
Colourless liquid.
d_{20}^{20}: about 0.97.

n_D^{20}: about 1.38.
bp_{12mm}: about 40 °C

Trimethylsulphonium hydroxide. $C_3H_{10}OS$. (M_r 94.2). *1145000*. [17287-03-5].
d_4^{20}: about 0.81.

2,4,6-Trinitrobenzene sulphonic acid. $C_6H_3N_3O_9S,3H_2O$. (M_r 347.2). *1117500*. [2508-19-2].
A white, crystalline powder, soluble in water.
mp: 190 °C to 195 °C.

Triphenylmethanol. $C_{19}H_{16}O$. (M_r 260.3). *1093700*. [76-84-6]. Triphenylcarbinol.
Colourless crystals, practically insoluble in water, freely soluble in alcohol.

Triphenyltetrazolium chloride. $C_{19}H_{15}ClN_4$. (M_r 334.8). *1093800*. [298-96-4]. 2,3,5-Triphenyl-$2H$-tetrazolium chloride.
Contains not less than 98.0 per cent of $C_{19}H_{15}ClN_4$. A pale or dull-yellow powder, soluble in water, in acetone and in alcohol, practically insoluble in ether.
mp: about 240 °C, with decomposition.
Assay. Dissolve 1.000 g in a mixture of 5 ml of *dilute nitric acid R* and 45 ml of *water R*. Add 50.0 ml of *0.1 M silver nitrate* and heat to boiling. Allow to cool, add 3 ml of *dibutyl phthalate R*, shake vigorously and titrate with *0.1 M ammonium thiocyanate*, using 2 ml of *ferric ammonium sulphate solution R2* as indicator.
1 ml of *0.1 M silver nitrate* is equivalent to 33.48 mg of $C_{19}H_{15}ClN_4$.
Store protected from light.

> **Triphenyltetrazolium chloride solution.** *1093801*.
> A 5 g/l solution in *aldehyde-free alcohol R*. Store protected from light.

Triscyanoethoxypropane. $C_{12}H_7N_3O_3$. (M_r 251.3). *1093900*.
1,2,3-Tris(2-cyanoethoxy)propane.
A viscous, brown-yellow liquid, soluble in methanol. Used as a stationary phase in gas chromatography.
d_{20}^{20}: about 1.11.
Viscosity(2.2.9). about 172 mPa·s.

1,3,5-Tris[3,5-di(1,1-dimethylethyl)-4-hydroxybenzyl]-1,3,5-triazine-2,4,6($1H,3H,5H$)-trione. $C_{48}H_{69}O_6N_3$. (M_r 784.1). *1094000*. [27676-62-6].
A white, crystalline powder.
mp: 218 °C to 222 °C.

Tris[2,4-di(1,1-dimethylethyl)phenyl] phosphite.
$C_{42}H_{63}O_3P$. (M_r 647). *1094100*. [31570-04-4].
White powder.
mp: 182 °C to 186 °C.

Tris(hydroxymethyl)aminomethane. *1094200*. [77-86-1].
See *Trometamol (1053)*.

> **Tris(hydroxymethyl)aminomethane solution.** *1094201*.
> A solution containing the equivalent of 24.22 g of $C_4H_{11}NO_3$ in 1000.0 ml.

> **Tris(hydroxymethyl)aminomethane solution R1.** *1094202*.
> Dissolve 60.6 mg of *tris(hydroxymethyl)aminomethane R* and 0.234 g of *sodium chloride R* in *water R* and dilute to 100 ml with the same solvent.
> Store at 2 °C to 8 °C and use within 3 days.

Trisodium phosphate dodecahydrate. $Na_3PO_4,12H_2O$. (M_r 380.1). *1094300*. [10101-89-0].
Colourless or white crystals, freely soluble in water.

Trypsin. *1094500.* [9002-07-7].
A proteolytic enzyme obtained by activation of trypsinogen extracted from the pancreas of beef (*Bos taurus* L.).
A white, crystalline or amorphous powder, sparingly soluble in water.

Trypsin for peptide mapping. *1094600.* [9002-07-7].
Trypsin of high purity treated to eliminate chymotryptic activity.

Tryptophan. $C_{11}H_{12}N_2O_2$. (M_r 204.2). *1094700.* [73-22-3].
A white or yellowish-white, crystalline powder or colourless crystals, slightly soluble in water, very slightly soluble in alcohol, practically insoluble in ether.
$[\alpha]_D^{20}$: about -30, determined on a 10 g/l solution.

Tyramine. $C_8H_{11}NO$. (M_r 137.2). *1117600.* [51-67-2].
4-(2-Aminoethyl)phenol.
Crystals, sparingly soluble in water, soluble in boiling ethanol.
mp: 164 °C to 165 °C.

Tyrosine. $C_9H_{11}NO_3$. (M_r 181.2). *1094800.* [60-18-4].
2-Amino-3-(4-hydroxyphenyl)propionic acid.
A white, crystalline powder or colourless or white crystals, slightly soluble in water, practically insoluble in acetone, in ethanol and in ether, soluble in dilute hydrochloric acid and in solutions of alkali hydroxides.
Chromatography. Examine as prescribed in the monograph on *Levodopa (0038)*; the chromatogram shows only one principal spot.

Umbelliferone. $C_9H_6O_3$. (M_r 162.1). *1137500.* [93-35-6].
7-Hydroxycoumarin. 7-Hydroxy-2*H*-1-benzopyran-2-one.
Needles from water.
mp: 225 °C to 228 °C.

Urea. *1095000.* [57-13-6].
See *Urea (0743)*.

Uridine. $C_9H_{12}N_2O_6$. (M_r 244.2). *1095100.* [58-96-8].
1-β-D-Ribofuranosyluracil.
A white or almost white, crystalline powder, soluble in water.
mp: about 165 °C.

Ursolic acid. $C_{30}H_{48}O_3$. (M_r 456.7). *1141600.* [77-52-1].
(3β)-3-Hydroxyurs-12-en-28-oic acid.
White powder, practically insoluble in water, sparingly soluble in methanol, slightly soluble in alcohol.
$[\alpha]_D^{21}$: about 67.50 (10 g/l solution in a 56.1 g/l solution of *potassium hydroxide R* in *alcohol R*).
mp: 285 °C to 288 °C.

Valeric acid. $C_5H_{10}O_2$. (M_r 102.1). *1095200.* [109-52-4].
Pentanoic acid.
A colourless liquid, soluble in water, freely soluble in alcohol and in ether.
d_{20}^{20}: about 0.94.
n_D^{20}: about 1.409.
bp: about 186 °C.

Vanillin. *1095300.* [121-33-5].
See *Vanillin (0747)*.

　　Vanillin reagent. *1095301.*
　　Carefully add, dropwise, 2 ml of *sulphuric acid R* to 100 ml of a 10 g/l solution of *vanillin R* in *alcohol R*.

　　Use within 48 h of preparation.

　　Vanillin solution, phosphoric. *1095302.*
　　Dissolve 1.0 g of *vanillin R* in 25 ml of *alcohol R*. Add 25 ml of *water R* and 35 ml of *phosphoric acid R*.

Verbenone. $C_{10}H_{14}O$. (M_r 150.2). *1140500.* [1196-01-6].
(1*S*,5*S*)-4,6,6-Trimethylbicyclo[3.1.1]hept-3-en-2-one.
Oil with a characteristic odour, practically insoluble in water, miscible with organic solvents.
d_{20}^{20}: about 0.978.
n_D^{18}: about 1.49.
$[\alpha]_D^{18}$: about + 249.6.
bp: 227 °C to 228 °C.
mp: about 6.5 °C.
Verbenone used in gas chromatography complies with the following additional test.

Assay. Examine by gas chromatography (2.2.28) as prescribed in the monograph on *Rosemary oil (1846)*.

The content is not less than 99 per cent, calculated by the normalisation procedure.

Vinyl acetate. $C_4H_6O_2$. (M_r 86,10). *1111800.* [108-05-4].
Ethenyl acetate.
d_{20}^{20}: about 0.930.
bp: about 72 °C.

Vinyl chloride. C_2H_3Cl. (M_r 62.5). *1095400.* [75-01-4].
A colourless gas, slightly soluble in organic solvents.

Vinyl polymer, octadecylsilyl, for chromatography. *1121600.*
Spherical particles (5 μm) of a vinyl alcohol copolymer bonded to an octadecylsilane. Carbon content of 17 per cent.

2-Vinylpyridine. C_7H_7N. (M_r 105.1). *1102200.* [100-69-6].
A yellow liquid, miscible in water.
d_{20}^{20}: about 0.97.
n_D^{20}: about 1.549.

1-Vinylpyrrolidin-2-one. C_6H_9NO. (M_r 111.1). *1111900.*
[88-12-0]. 1-Ethenylpyrrolidin-2-one.
Contains not less than 99.0 per cent of C_6H_9NO.

A clear colourless liquid.

Water (2.5.12). Not more than 0.1 per cent, determined on 2.5 g. Use as the solvent, a mixture of 50 ml of *anhydrous methanol R* and 10 ml of *butyrolactone R*.

Assay. Examine by gas chromatography (2.2.28).

The chromatography may be carried out using

— a fused-silica column 30 m long and 0.5 mm in internal diameter the inner wall of which is coated with a 1.0 μm layer of *macrogol 20 000 R*,

— *helium for chromatography R* as the carrier gas,

— a flame-ionisation detector,

maintaining the temperature of the injection port at 190 °C and programming the temperature of the column as follows: maintain the temperature at 80 °C for 1 min and then increase it to 190 °C at a rate of 10 °C per minute. Maintain at 190 °C for 15 min. Inject 0.3 μl of the substance to be examined and adjust the flow rate of the carrier gas so that the retention time of the peak corresponding to 1-vinylpyrrolidin-2-one is about 17 min. Determine the content of C_6H_9NO by internal normalisation.

Vitexin. $C_{21}H_{20}O_{11}$. (M_r 448.4). *1133300.* [3681-93-4].
Apigenin-8-C-glucoside.
Yellow powder.
Store in an airtight container, protected from light.

Water. *1095500.* [7732-18-5].
See *Purified water (0008)*.

Water, ammonium-free. *1095501.* [7732-18-5].
To 100 ml of *water R* add 0.1 ml of *sulphuric acid R*.
Distil using the apparatus described for the determination
of *Distillation range* (*2.2.11*). Reject the first 10 ml and
collect the following 50 ml.

Water, carbon dioxide-free. *1095502.* [7732-18-5].
Water R which has been boiled for a few minutes and
protected from the atmosphere during cooling and
storage.

Water for chromatography. *1095503.* [7732-18-5].
Deionised *water R* with a resistivity of not less than
0.18 Mohm·m.

Water, distilled. *1095504.* [7732-18-5].
Water R prepared by distillation.

Water for injections. *1095505.* [7732-18-5].
See *Water for injections (0169)*.

Water, nitrate-free. *1095506.* [7732-18-5].
To 100 ml of *water R* add a few milligrams of *potassium
permanganate R* and of *barium hydroxide R*. Distil
using the apparatus described for the determination of
Distillation range (*2.2.11*). Reject the first 10 ml and
collect the following 50 ml.

Water, particle-free. *1095507.* [7732-18-5].
Filter *water R* through a membrane with a pore size of
0.22 µm.

Weak cationic resin. *1096000.*

Polymethacrylic resin, slightly acid, with carboxyl groups
present in a protonated form.

Particle size: 75 µm to 160 µm.

pH limits of use: 5 to 14.

Maximum temperature of use: 120 °C.

Xanthydrol. $C_{13}H_{10}O_2$. (M_r 198.2). *1096100.* [90-46-0].
9-Xanthenol.

Contains not less than 90.0 per cent of $C_{13}H_{10}O_2$.

A white to pale-yellow powder, very slightly soluble in water,
soluble in alcohol, in ether and in glacial acetic acid.

It is also available as a methanolic solution containing 90 g/l
to 110 g/l of xanthydrol.

mp: about 123 °C.

Assay. In a 250 ml flask dissolve 0.300 g in 3 ml of
methanol R or use 3.0 ml of solution. Add 50 ml of *glacial
acetic acid R* and, dropwise with shaking, 25 ml of a 20 g/l
solution of *urea R*. Allow to stand for 12 h, collect the
precipitate on a sintered-glass filter (16), wash with 20 ml of
alcohol R, dry in an oven at 100 °C to 105 °C and weigh.

1 g of precipitate is equivalent to 0.9429 g of xanthydrol.

Store protected from light. If a methanolic solution is
used, store in small sealed ampoules and filter before use
if necessary.

Xanthydrol R1. *1096101.*
Complies with the requirements prescribed for
xanthydrol R and with the following requirement.

Contains not less than 98.0 per cent of $C_{13}H_{10}O_2$.

Xanthydrol solution. *1096102.*
To 0.1 ml of a 100 g/l solution of *xanthydrol R* in
methanol R add 100 ml of *anhydrous acetic acid R* and
1 ml of *hydrochloric acid R*. Allow to stand for 24 h
before using.

Xylene. C_8H_{10}. (M_r 106.2). *1096200.* [1330-20-7].
Mixture of isomers. A clear, colourless, flammable liquid,
practically insoluble in water, miscible with alcohol and with
ether.
d_{20}^{20}: about 0.867.
n_D^{20}: about 1.497.
bp: about 138 °C.

***m*-Xylene.** C_8H_{10}. (M_r 106.2). *1117700.* [108-38-3].
1,3-Dimethylbenzene.
A clear, colourless, flammable liquid, practically insoluble in
water, miscible with alcohol and with ether.
d_{20}^{20}: about 0.884.
n_D^{20}: about 1.497.
bp: about 139 °C.
mp: about −47 °C.

***o*-Xylene.** C_8H_{10}. (M_r 106.2). *1100600.* [95-47-6].
1,2-Dimethylbenzene.
A clear, colourless, flammable liquid, practically insoluble in
water, miscible with alcohol and with ether.
d_{20}^{20}: about 0.881.
n_D^{20}: about 1.505.
bp: about 144 °C.
mp: about 25 °C.

Xylenol orange. $C_{31}H_{28}N_2Na_4O_{13}S$. ($M_r$ 761). *1096300.* [3618-
43-7]. Tetrasodium 3,3′-(3*H*-2,1-benzoxathiol-3-ylidene)bis[(6-
hydroxy-5-methyl-3,1-phenylene)methyleneiminobisacetate]
S,S-dioxide.
A reddish-brown crystalline powder, soluble in water.

Xylenol orange triturate. *1096301.*

Triturate 1 part of *xylenol orange R* with 99 parts of
potassium nitrate R.

Test for sensitivity. To 50 ml of *water R* add 1 ml
of *dilute acetic acid R*, 50 mg of the xylenol orange
triturate and 0.05 ml of *lead nitrate solution R*. Add
hexamethylenetetramine R until the colour changes
from yellow to violet-red. After addition of 0.1 ml of *0.1 M
sodium edetate* the colour changes to yellow.

Xylose. *1096400.* [58-86-6].
See *Xylose (1278)*.

Zinc. Zn. (A_r 65.4). *1096500.* [7440-66-6].
Contains not less than 99.5 per cent of Zn.

Silver-white cylinders, granules, pellets or filings with a blue
sheen.

Arsenic (*2.4.2*). 5.0 g complies with limit test A (0.2 ppm).
Dissolve in a mixture of the 15 ml of *hydrochloric acid R*
and 25 ml of *water R* prescribed.

Zinc, activated. *1096501.*

Place the zinc cylinders or pellets to be activated in a
conical flask and add a sufficient quantity of a 50 ppm
solution of *chloroplatinic acid R* to cover the metal.
Allow the metal to remain in contact with the solution for
10 min, wash, drain and dry immediately.

Arsenic. To 5 g of the activated zinc add 15 ml of
hydrochloric acid R, 25 ml of *water R*, 0.1 ml of *stannous
chloride solution R* and 5 ml of *potassium iodide
solution R*. Treat as described in limit test A for arsenic
(*2.4.2*). No stain is produced on the *mercuric bromide
paper R*.

Activity. Repeat the test for arsenic using the same
reagents and adding a solution containing 1 µg of arsenic.
An appreciable stain appears on the *mercuric bromide
paper R*.

Zinc acetate. $(C_2H_3O_2)_2Zn,2H_2O$. (M_r 219.5). *1102300*. [5970-45-6]. Zinc acetate dihydrate.
Bright white crystals, slightly efflorescent, freely soluble in water, soluble in alcohol. It loses its crystallisation water at 100 °C.
d_{20}^{20}: about 1.735.
mp: about 237 °C.

> **Zinc acetate solution.** *1102301*.
> Mix 600 ml of *water R* with 150 ml of *glacial acetic acid R*, 54.9 g of *zinc acetate R* and stir to dissolve. Continue stirring while adding 150 ml of *concentrated ammonia R*. Cool to room temperature and adjust with *ammonia R* to pH 6.4. Dilute the mixture to 1 litre with *water R*.

Zinc chloride. *1096600*. [7646-85-7].
See *Zinc chloride (0110)*.

> **Zinc chloride-formic acid solution.** *1096601*.
> Dissolve 20 g of *zinc chloride R* in 80 g of an 850 g/l solution of *anhydrous formic acid R*.

> **Zinc chloride solution, iodinated.** *1096602*.
> Dissolve 20 g of *zinc chloride R* and 6.5 g of *potassium iodide R* in 10.5 ml of *water R*. Add 0.5 g of *iodine R* and shake for 15 min. Filter if necessary.
> Store protected from light.

Zinc iodide and starch solution. *1096502*.
To a solution of 2 g of *zinc chloride R* in 10 ml of *water R* add 0.4 g of *soluble starch R* and heat until the starch has dissolved. After cooling to room temperature add 1.0 ml of a colourless solution containing 0.10 g *zinc R* as filings and 0.2 g of *iodine R* in *water R*. Dilute the solution to 100 ml with *water R* and filter. Store protected from light.

Test for sensitivity. Dilute 0.05 ml of *sodium nitrite solution R* to 50 ml with *water R*. To 5 ml of this solution add 0.1 ml of *dilute sulphuric acid R* and 0.05 ml of the zinc iodide and starch solution and mix. The solution becomes blue.

Zinc oxide. *1096700*. [1314-13-2].
See *Zinc oxide (0252)*.

Zinc powder. Zn. (A_r 65.4). *1096800*. [7440-66-6].
Contains not less than 90.0 per cent of Zn (A_r 65.4).

A very fine, grey powder, soluble in *dilute hydrochloric acid R*.

Zinc sulphate. *1097000*. [7446-20-0].
See *Zinc sulphate (0111)*.

Zirconyl chloride. A basic salt corresponding approximately to the formula $ZrCl_2O, 8H_2O$. *1097100*. [15461-27-5].
Contains not less than 96.0 per cent of $ZrCl_2O,8H_2O$.

White or almost white, crystalline powder or crystals, freely soluble in water and in alcohol.
Assay. Dissolve 0.600 g in a mixture of 5 ml of *nitric acid R* and 50 ml of *water R*. Add 50.0 ml of *0.1 M silver nitrate* and 3 ml of *dibutyl phthalate R* and shake. Using 2 ml of *ferric ammonium sulphate solution R2* as indicator, titrate with *0.1 M ammonium thiocyanate* until a reddish-yellow colour is obtained.

1 ml of *0.1 M silver nitrate* is equivalent to 16.11 mg of $ZrCl_2O,8H_2O$.

Zirconyl nitrate. A basic salt corresponding approximately to the formula $ZrO(NO_3)_2,2H_2O$. *1097200*. [14985-18-3].
A white powder or crystals, hygroscopic, soluble in water. The aqueous solution is a clear or at most slightly opalescent liquid.
Store in an airtight container.

> **Zirconyl nitrate solution.** *1097201*.
> A 1 g/l solution in a mixture of 40 ml of *water R* and 60 ml of *hydrochloric acid R*.

4.1.2. STANDARD SOLUTIONS FOR LIMIT TESTS

Acetaldehyde standard solution (100 ppm C_2H_4O). *5000100*.
Dissolve 1.0 g of *acetaldehyde R* in *2-propanol R* and dilute to 100.0 ml with the same solvent. Dilute 5.0 ml of the solution to 500.0 ml with *2-propanol R*. Prepare immediately before use.

Acetaldehyde standard solution (100 ppm C_2H_4O) R1. *5000101*.
Dissolve 1.0 g of *acetaldehyde R* in *water R* and dilute to 100.0 ml with the same solvent. Dilute 5.0 ml of the solution to 500.0 ml with *water R*. Prepare immediately before use.

Aluminium standard solution (200 ppm Al). *5000200*.
Dissolve in *water R* a quantity of *aluminium potassium sulphate R* equivalent to 0.352 g of $AlK(SO_4)_2,12H_2O$. Add 10 ml of *dilute sulphuric acid R* and dilute to 100.0 ml with *water R*.

Aluminium standard solution (100 ppm Al). *5000203*.
Immediately before use, dilute with *water R* to 10 times its volume a solution containing 8.947 g of *aluminium chloride R* in 1000.0 ml of *water R*.

Aluminium standard solution (10 ppm Al). *5000201*.
Immediately before use, dilute with *water R* to 100 times its volume in a solution containing *aluminium nitrate R* equivalent to 1.39 g of $Al(NO_3)_3,9H_2O$ in 100.0 ml.

Aluminium standard solution (2 ppm Al). *5000202*.
Immediately before use, dilute with *water R* to 100 times its volume a solution containing *aluminium potassium sulphate R* equivalent to 0.352 g of $AlK(SO_4)_2,12H_2O$ and 10 ml of *dilute sulphuric acid R* in 100.0 ml.

Ammonium standard solution (100 ppm NH_4). *5000300*.
Immediately before use, dilute to 25 ml with *water R* 10 ml of a solution containing *ammonium chloride R* equivalent to 0.741 g of NH_4Cl in 1000 ml.

Ammonium standard solution (2.5 ppm NH_4). *5000301*.
Immediately before use, dilute with *water R* to 100 times its volume a solution containing *ammonium chloride R* equivalent to 0.741 g of NH_4Cl in 1000.0 ml.

Ammonium standard solution (1 ppm NH_4). *5000302*.
Immediately before use, dilute ammonium standard solution (2.5 ppm NH_4) R to 2.5 times its volume with *water R*.

Antimony standard solution (100 ppm Sb). *5000401*.
Dissolve *antimony potassium tartrate R* equivalent to 0.274 g of $C_4H_4KO_7Sb,^1/_2H_2O$ in 500 ml of *1M hydrochloric acid* and dilute the clear solution to 1000 ml with *water R*.

Antimony standard solution (1 ppm Sb). *5000400*.
Dissolve *antimony potassium tartrate R* equivalent to 0.274 g of $C_4H_4KO_7Sb,^1/_2H_2O$ in 20 ml of *hydrochloric acid R1* and dilute the clear solution to 100.0 ml with *water R*. To 10.0 ml of this solution add 200 ml of

hydrochloric acid R1 and dilute to 1000.0 ml with *water R*. To 100.0 ml of this solution add 300 ml of *hydrochloric acid R1* and dilute to 1000.0 ml with *water R*. Prepare the dilute solutions immediately before use.

Arsenic standard solution (10 ppm As). *5000500.*
Immediately before use, dilute with *water R* to 100 times its volume a solution prepared by dissolving *arsenious trioxide R* equivalent to 0.330 g of As_2O_3 in 5 ml of *dilute sodium hydroxide solution R* and diluting to 250.0 ml with *water R*.

Arsenic standard solution (1 ppm As). *5000501.*
Immediately before use, dilute *arsenic standard solution (10 ppm As) R* to 10 times its volume with *water R*.

Arsenic standard solution (0.1 ppm As). *5000502.*
Immediately before use, dilute *arsenic standard solution (1 ppm As) R* to 10 times its volume with *water R*.

Barium standard solution (50 ppm Ba). *5000600.*
Immediately before use, dilute with *distilled water R* to 20 times its volume a solution in *distilled water R* containing *barium chloride R* equivalent to 0.178 g of $BaCl_2,2H_2O$ in 100.0 ml.

Cadmium standard solution (0.1 per cent Cd). *5000700.*
Dissolve *cadmium R* equivalent to 0.100 g of Cd in the smallest necessary amount of a mixture of equal volumes of *hydrochloric acid R* and *water R* and dilute to 100.0 ml with a 1 per cent *V/V* solution of *hydrochloric acid R*.

Cadmium standard solution (10 ppm Cd) . *5000701.*
Immediately before use, dilute *cadmium standard solution (0.1 per cent Cd) R* to 100 times its volume with a 1 per cent *V/V* solution of *hydrochloric acid R*.

Calcium standard solution (400 ppm Ca). *5000800.*
Immediately before use, dilute with *distilled water R* to 10 times its volume a solution in *distilled water R* containing *calcium carbonate R* equivalent to 1.000 g of $CaCO_3$ and 23 ml of *1 M hydrochloric acid* in 100.0 ml.

Calcium standard solution (100 ppm Ca). *5000801.*
Immediately before use, dilute with *distilled water R* to 10 times its volume a solution in *distilled water R* containing *calcium carbonate R* equivalent to 0.624 g of $CaCO_3$ and 3 ml of *acetic acid R* in 250.0 ml.

Calcium standard solution (100 ppm Ca) R1. *5000804.*
Immediately before use, dilute with *water R* to 10 times its volume a solution containing *anhydrous calcium chloride R* equivalent to 2.769 g of $CaCl_2$ in 1000.0 ml of *dilute hydrochloric acid R*.

Calcium standard solution (100 ppm Ca), alcoholic. *5000802.*
Immediately before use, dilute with *alcohol R* to 10 times its volume a solution in *distilled water R* containing *calcium carbonate R* equivalent to 2.50 g of $CaCO_3$ and 12 ml of *acetic acid R* in 1000.0 ml.

Calcium standard solution (10 ppm Ca). *5000803.*
Immediately before use, dilute with *distilled water R* to 100 times its volume a solution in *distilled water R* containing *calcium carbonate R* equivalent to 0.624 g of $CaCO_3$ and 3 ml of *acetic acid R* in 250.0 ml.

Chloride standard solution (50 ppm Cl). *5004100.*
Immediately before use, dilute with *water R* to 10 times its volume a solution containing *sodium chloride R* equivalent to 0.824 g of NaCl in 1000.0 ml.

Chloride standard solution (8 ppm Cl). *5000900.*
Immediately before use, dilute with *water R* to 100 times its volume a solution containing *sodium chloride R* equivalent to 1.32 g of NaCl in 1000.0 ml.

Chloride standard solution (5 ppm Cl). *5000901.*
Immediately before use, dilute with *water R* to 100 times its volume a solution containing *sodium chloride R* equivalent to 0.824 g of NaCl in 1000.0 ml.

Chromium liposoluble standard solution (1000 ppm Cr). *5004600.*
A chromium (metal) organic compound in an oil.
The reagent CONOSTAN standard, available, for example, from SPIN − 91965 Courtaboeuf Cedex − France (info@spin.fr) has been found suitable.

Chromium standard solution (0.1 per cent Cr). *5001002.*
Dissolve *potassium dichromate R* equivalent to 2.83 g of $K_2Cr_2O_7$ in *water R* and dilute to 1000.0 ml with the same solvent.

Chromium standard solution (100 ppm Cr). *5001000.*
Dissolve *potassium dichromate R* equivalent to 0.283 g of $K_2Cr_2O_7$ in *water R* and dilute to 1000.0 ml with the same solvent.

Chromium standard solution (0.1 ppm Cr). *5001001.*
Immediately before use, dilute *chromium standard solution (100 ppm Cr) R* to 1000 times its volume with *water R*.

Cobalt standard solution (100 ppm Co). *5004300.*
Dissolve *cobalt nitrate R* equivalent to 0.494 g of $Co(NO_3)_2,6H_2O$ in 500 ml of *1M nitric acid* and dilute the clear solution to 1000 ml with *water R*.

Copper liposoluble standard solution (1000 ppm Cu). *5004700.*
A copper (metal) organic compound in an oil.
The reagent CONOSTAN standard, available, for example, from SPIN − 91965 Courtaboeuf Cedex − France (info@spin.fr) has been found suitable.

Copper standard solution (0.1 per cent Cu). *5001100.*
Dissolve *copper sulphate R* equivalent to 0.393 g of $CuSO_4,5H_2O$ in *water R* and dilute to 100.0 ml with the same solvent.

Copper standard solution (10 ppm Cu). *5001101.*
Immediately before use, dilute *copper standard solution (0.1 per cent Cu) R* to 100 times its volume with *water R*.

Copper standard solution (0.1 ppm Cu). *5001102.*
Immediately before use, dilute *copper standard solution (10 ppm Cu) R* to 100 times its volume with *water R*.

Ferrocyanide standard solution (100 ppm Fe(CN)₆). *5001200.*
Immediately before use, dilute with *water R* to 10 times its volume a solution containing *potassium ferrocyanide R* equivalent to 0.20 g of $K_4Fe(CN)_6,3H_2O$ in 100.0 ml.

Ferricyanide standard solution (50 ppm Fe(CN)₆). *5001300.*
Immediately before use, dilute with *water R* to 100 times its volume a solution containing *potassium ferricyanide R* equivalent to 0.78 g of $K_3Fe(CN)_6$ in 100.0 ml.

Fluoride standard solution (10 ppm F). *5001400.*
Dissolve in *water R sodium fluoride R* previously dried at 300 °C for 12 h, equivalent to 0.442 g of NaF, and dilute to 1000.0 ml with the same solvent (1 ml = 0.2 mg F). Store in a polyethylene container. Immediately before use, dilute the solution to 20 times its volume with *water R*.

Fluoride standard solution (1 ppm F). *5001401.*
Immediately before use, dilute *fluoride standard solution (10 ppm F) R* to 10 times its volume with *water R*.

Formaldehyde standard solution (5 ppm CH_2O). *5001500.*
Immediately before use, dilute with *water R* to 200 times its volume a solution containing 1.0 g of CH_2O per litre prepared from *formaldehyde solution R*.

Germanium standard solution (100 ppm Ge). *5004400.*
Dissolve *ammonium hexafluorogermanate (IV) R* equivalent to 0.307 g of $(NH_4)_2GeF_6$ in a 0.01 per cent V/V solution of *hydrofluoric acid R*. Dilute the clear solution to 1000 ml with *water R*.

Glyoxal standard solution (20 ppm $C_2H_2O_2$). *5003700.*
In a 100 ml graduated flask weigh a quantity of *glyoxal solution R* corresponding to 0.200 g of $C_2H_2O_2$ and make up to volume with *ethanol R*. Immediately before use dilute the solution to 100 times its volume with the same solvent.

Iodide standard solution (10 ppm I). *5003800.*
Immediately before use, dilute with *water R* to 100 times its volume a solution containing *potassium iodide R* equivalent to 0.131 g of KI in 100.0 ml.

Iron standard solution (0.1 per cent Fe). *5001605.*
Dissolve 0.100 g of Fe in the smallest amount necessary of a mixture of equal volumes of *hydrochloric acid R* and *water R* and dilute to 100.0 ml with *water R*.

Iron standard solution (250 ppm Fe). *5001606.*
Immediately before use, dilute with *water R* to 40 times its volume a solution containing 4.840 g of *ferric chloride R* in a 150 g/l solution of *hydrochloric acid R* diluted to 100.0 ml.

Iron standard solution (20 ppm Fe). *5001600.*
Immediately before use, dilute with *water R* to 10 times its volume a solution containing *ferric ammonium sulphate R* equivalent to 0.863 g of $FeNH_4(SO_4)_2,12H_2O$ and 25 ml of *dilute sulphuric acid R* in 500.0 ml.

Iron standard solution (10 ppm Fe). *5001601.*
Immediately before use, dilute with *water R* to 100 times its volume a solution containing *ferrous ammonium sulphate R* equivalent to 7.022 g of $Fe(NH_4)_2(SO_4)_2,6H_2O$ and 25 ml of *dilute sulphuric acid R* in 1000.0 ml.

Iron standard solution (8 ppm Fe). *5001602.*
Immediately before use, dilute with *water R* to 10 times its volume a solution containing 80 mg of *iron R* and 50 ml of *hydrochloric acid R* (220 g/l HCl) in 1000.0 ml.

Iron standard solution (2 ppm Fe). *5001603.*
Immediately before use, dilute *iron standard solution (20 ppm Fe) R* to 10 times its volume with *water R*.

Iron standard solution (1 ppm Fe). *5001604.*
Immediately before use, dilute *iron standard solution (20 ppm Fe) R* to 20 times its volume with *water R*.

Lead liposoluble standard solution (1000 ppm Pb). *5004800.*
A lead (metal) organic compound in an oil.

The reagent CONOSTAN standard, available, for example, from SPIN – 91965 Courtaboeuf Cedex – France (info@spin.fr) has been found suitable.

Lead standard solution (0.1 per cent Pb). *5001700.*
Dissolve *lead nitrate R* equivalent to 0.400 g of $Pb(NO_3)_2$ in *water R* and dilute to 250.0 ml with the same solvent.

Lead standard solution (100 ppm Pb). *5001701.*
Immediately before use, dilute *lead standard solution (0.1 per cent Pb) R* to 10 times its volume with *water R*.

Lead standard solution (10 ppm Pb). *5001702.*
Immediately before use, dilute *lead standard solution (100 ppm Pb) R* to 10 times its volume with *water R*.

Lead standard solution (10 ppm Pb) R1. *5001706.*
Immediately before use, dilute with *water R* to 10 times its volume a solution containing 0.160 g of *lead nitrate R* in 100 ml of *water R*, to which is added 1 ml of *lead-free nitric acid R* and dilute to 1000.0 ml.

Lead standard solution (2 ppm Pb). *5001703.*
Immediately before use, dilute *lead standard solution (10 ppm Pb) R* to 5 times its volume with *water R*.

Lead standard solution (1 ppm Pb). *5001704.*
Immediately before use, dilute *lead standard solution (10 ppm Pb) R* to 10 times its volume with *water R*.

Lead standard solution (0.1 ppm Pb). *5001705.*
Immediately before use, dilute *lead standard solution (1 ppm Pb) R* to 10 times its volume with *water R*.

Magnesium standard solution (100 ppm Mg). *5001800.*
Immediately before use, dilute with *water R* to 10 times its volume a solution containing *magnesium sulphate R* equivalent to 1.010 g of $MgSO_4,7H_2O$ in 100.0 ml.

Magnesium standard solution (10 ppm Mg). *5001801.*
Immediately before use, dilute magnesium standard solution (100 ppm Mg) R to 10 times its volume with *water R*.

Magnesium standard solution (10 ppm Mg) R1. *5001802.*
Immediately before use, dilute with *water R* to 100 times its volume a solution containing 8.365 g of *magnesium chloride R* in 1000.0 ml of *dilute hydrochloric acid R*.

Manganese standard solution (100 ppm Mn). *5004500.*
Dissolve *manganese sulphate R* equivalent to 0.308 g of $MnSO_4,H_2O$ in 500 ml of *1M nitric acid* and dilute the clear solution to 1000 ml with *water R*.

Mercury standard solution (1000 ppm Hg). *5001900.*
Dissolve *mercuric chloride R* equivalent to 1.354 g of $HgCl_2$ in 50 ml of *dilute nitric acid R* and dilute to 1000.0 ml with *water R*.

Mercury standard solution (10 ppm Hg). *5001901.*
Immediately before use, dilute with water to 100 times its volume a solution containing *mercuric chloride R* equivalent to 0.338 g of $HgCl_2$ in 250.0 ml.

Nickel liposoluble standard solution (1000 ppm Ni). *5004900.*
A nickel (metal) organic compound in an oil.

The reagent CONOSTAN standard, available, for example, from SPIN – 91965 Courtaboeuf Cedex – France (info@spin.fr) has been found suitable.

Nickel standard solution (10 ppm Ni). *5002000.*
Immediately before use, dilute with *water R* to 100 times its volume a solution containing *nickel sulphate R* equivalent to 4.78 g of $NiSO_4,7H_2O$ in 1000.0 ml.

Nickel standard solution (0.2 ppm Ni). *5002002.*
Immediately before use, dilute *nickel standard solution (10 ppm Ni) R* to 50 times its volume with *water R*.

Nickel standard solution (0.1 ppm Ni). *5002001.*
Immediately before use, dilute *nickel standard solution (10 ppm Ni) R* to 100 times its volume with *water R*.

Nitrate standard solution (100 ppm NO_3). *5002100.*
Immediately before use, dilute with *water R* to 10 times its volume a solution containing *potassium nitrate R* equivalent to 0.815 g of KNO_3 in 500.0 ml.

Nitrate standard solution (10 ppm NO₃). *5002101.*
Immediately before use, dilute *nitrate standard solution (100 ppm NO₃) R* to 10 times its volume with *water R*.

Nitrate standard solution (2 ppm NO₃). *5002102.*
Immediately before use, dilute *nitrate standard solution (10 ppm NO₃) R* to 5 times its volume with *water R*.

Palladium standard solution (500 ppm Pd). *5003600.*
Dissolve 50.0 mg of *palladium R* in 9 ml of *hydrochloric acid R* and dilute to 100.0 ml with *water R*.

Palladium standard solution (20 ppm Pd). *5003602.*
Dissolve 0.333 g of *palladium chloride R* in 2 ml of warm *hydrochloric acid R*. Dilute the solution to 1000.0 ml with a mixture of equal volumes of *dilute hydrochloric acid R* and *water R*. Immediately before use dilute to 10 times its volume with *water R*.

Palladium standard solution (0.5 ppm Pd). *5003601.*
Dilute *palladium standard solution (500 ppm Pd) R* with a mixture of 0.3 volumes of *nitric acid R* and 99.7 volumes of *water R*.

Phosphate standard solution (200 ppm PO₄). *5004200.*
Dissolve *potassium dihydrogen phosphate R* equivalent to 0.286 g of KH_2PO_4 in *water R* and dilute to 1000.0 ml with the same solvent.

Phosphate standard solution (5 ppm PO₄). *5002200.*
Immediately before use, dilute with *water R* to 100 times its volume a solution containing *potassium dihydrogen phosphate R* equivalent to 0.716 g of KH_2PO_4 in 1000.0 ml.

Platinum standard solution (30 ppm Pt). *5002300.*
Immediately before use, dilute with *1 M hydrochloric acid* to 10 times its volume a solution containing 80 mg of *chloroplatinic acid R* in 100.0 ml of *1 M hydrochloric acid*.

Potassium standard solution (600 ppm K). *5005100.*
Immediately before use, dilute with *water R* to 20 times its volume a solution containing *dipotassium sulphate R* equivalent to 2.676 g of K_2SO_4 in 100.0 ml.

Potassium standard solution (100 ppm K). *5002400.*
Immediately before use, dilute with *water R* to 20 times its volume a solution containing *dipotassium sulphate R* equivalent to 0.446 g of K_2SO_4 in 100.0 ml.

Potassium standard solution (20 ppm K). *5002401.*
Immediately before use, dilute *potassium standard solution (100 ppm K) R* to 5 times its volume with *water R*.

Selenium standard solution (100 ppm Se). *5002500.*
Dissolve 0.100 g of *selenium R* in 2 ml of *nitric acid R*. Evaporate to dryness. Take up the residue in 2 ml of *water R* and evaporate to dryness; carry out three times. Dissolve the residue in 50 ml of *dilute hydrochloric acid R* and dilute to 1000.0 ml with the same acid.

Selenium standard solution (1 ppm Se). *5002501.*
Immediately before use, dilute with *water R* to 40 times its volume a solution containing *selenious acid R* equivalent to 6.54 mg of H_2SeO_3 in 100.0 ml.

Silver standard solution (5 ppm Ag). *5002600.*
Immediately before use, dilute with *water R* to 100 times its volume a solution containing *silver nitrate R* equivalent to 0.790 g of $AgNO_3$ in 1000.0 ml.

Sodium standard solution (200 ppm Na). *5002700.*
Immediately before use, dilute with *water R* to 10 times its volume a solution containing *sodium chloride R* equivalent to 0.509 g of $NaCl$ in 100.0 ml.

Sodium standard solution (50 ppm Na). *5002701.*
Dilute the *sodium standard solution (200 ppm Na) R* to four times its volume with *water R*.

Strontium standard solution (1.0 per cent Sr). *5003900.*
Cover with *water R*, *strontium carbonate R* equivalent to 1.6849 g of $SrCO_3$. Cautiously add *hydrochloric acid R* until all the solid has dissolved and there is no sign of further effervescence. Dilute to 100.0 ml with *water R*.

Sulphate standard solution (100 ppm SO₄). *5002802.*
Immediately before use, dilute with *distilled water R* to 10 times its volume a solution in *distilled water R* containing *dipotassium sulphate R* equivalent to 0.181 g of K_2SO_4 in 100.0 ml.

Sulphate standard solution (10 ppm SO₄). *5002800.*
Immediately before use, dilute with *distilled water R* to 100 times its volume a solution in *distilled water R* containing *dipotassium sulphate R* equivalent to 0.181 g of K_2SO_4 in 100.0 ml.

Sulphate standard solution (10 ppm SO₄) R1. *5002801.*
Immediately before use, dilute with *alcohol (30 per cent V/V) R* to 100 times its volume a solution containing *dipotassium sulphate R* equivalent to 0.181 g of K_2SO_4 in 100.0 ml of *alcohol (30 per cent V/V) R*.

Sulphite standard solution (1.5 ppm SO₂). *5002900.*
Dissolve *sodium metabisulphite R* equivalent to 0.152 g of $Na_2S_2O_5$ in *water R* and dilute to 100.0 ml with the same solvent. Dilute 5.0 ml of this solution to 100.0 ml with *water R*. To 3.0 ml of the resulting solution, add 4.0 ml of *0.1 M sodium hydroxide* and dilute to 100.0 ml with *water R*.

Thallium standard solution (10 ppm Tl). *5003000.*
Dissolve *thallous sulphate R* equivalent to 0.1235 g of Tl_2SO_4 in a 9 g/l solution of *sodium chloride R* and dilute to 1000.0 ml with the same solution. Dilute 10.0 ml of the solution to 100.0 ml with the 9 g/l solution of *sodium chloride R*.

Tin liposoluble standard solution (1000 ppm Sn). *5005000.*
A tin metal organic compound in an oil.

The reagent CONOSTAN standard, available, for example, from SPIN − 91965 Courtaboeuf Cedex − France (info@spin.fr) has been found suitable.

Tin standard solution (5 ppm Sn). *5003100.*
Dissolve *tin R* equivalent to 0.500 g of Sn in a mixture of 5 ml of *water R* and 25 ml of *hydrochloric acid R* and dilute to 1000.0 ml with *water R*. Dilute the solution to 100 times its volume with a 2.5 per cent *V/V* solution of *hydrochloric acid R* immediately before use.

Tin standard solution (0.1 ppm Sn). *5003101.*
Immediately before use, dilute *tin standard solution (5 ppm Sn) R* to 50 times its volume with *water R*.

Titanium standard solution (100 ppm Ti). *5003200.*
Dissolve 100.0 mg of *titanium R* in 100 ml of *hydrochloric acid R* diluted to 150 ml with *water R*, heating if necessary. Allow to cool and dilute to 1000 ml with *water R*.

Vanadium standard solution (1 g/l V). *5003300.*
Dissolve in *water R ammonium vanadate R* equivalent to 0.230 g of NH_4VO_3 and dilute to 100.0 ml with the same solvent.

Zinc standard solution (5 mg/ml Zn). *5003400.*
Dissolve 3.15 g of *zinc oxide R* in 15 ml of *hydrochloric acid R* and dilute to 500.0 ml with *water R*.

Zinc standard solution (100 ppm Zn). *5003401.*
Immediately before use, dilute with *water R* to 10 times its volume a solution containing *zinc sulphate R* equivalent to 0.440 g of $ZnSO_4,7H_2O$ and 1 ml of *acetic acid R* in 100.0 ml.

Zinc standard solution (10 ppm Zn). *5003402.*
Immediately before use, dilute *zinc standard solution (100 ppm Zn) R* to 10 times its volume with *water R*.

Zinc standard solution (5 ppm Zn). *5003403.*
Immediately before use, dilute *zinc standard solution (100 ppm Zn) R* to 20 times its volume with *water R*.

Zirconium standard solution (1 g/l Zr). *5003500.*
Dissolve *zirconyl nitrate R* equivalent to 0.293 g of $ZrO(NO_3)_2,2H_2O$ in a mixture of 2 volumes of *hydrochloric acid R* and 8 volumes of *water R* and dilute to 100.0 ml with the same mixture of solvents.

4.1.3. BUFFER SOLUTIONS

Buffered acetone solution. *4000100.*
Dissolve 8.15 g of *sodium acetate R* and 42 g of *sodium chloride R* in *water R*, add 68 ml of *0.1 M hydrochloric acid* and 150 ml of *acetone R* and dilute to 500 ml with *water R*.

Buffer solution pH 2.0. *4000200.*
Dissolve 6.57 g of *potassium chloride R* in *water R* and add 119.0 ml of *0.1 M hydrochloric acid*. Dilute to 1000.0 ml with *water R*.

Phosphate buffer solution pH 2.0. *4007900.*
Dissolve 8.95 g of *disodium hydrogen phosphate R* and 3.40 g of *potassium dihydrogen phosphate R* in *water R* and dilute to 1000.0 ml with the same solvent. If necessary adjust the pH (*2.2.3*) with *phosphoric acid R*.

Sulphate buffer solution pH 2.0. *4008900.*
Dissolve 132.1 g of *ammonium sulphate R* in *water R* and dilute to 500.0 ml with the same solvent (Solution I). Carefully and with constant cooling stir 14 ml of sulphuric acid R into about 400 ml of *water R*; allow to cool and dilute to 500.0 ml with *water R* (Solution II). Mix equal volumes of solutions I and II. Adjust the pH (*2.2.3*) if necessary.

Buffer solution pH 2.2. *4010500.*
Mix of 6.7 ml of *phosphoric acid R* with 50.0 ml of a 4 per cent solution of *dilute sodium hydroxide solution R* and dilute to 1000.0 ml with *water R*.

Buffer solution pH 2.5. *4000300.*
Dissolve 100 g of *potassium dihydrogen phosphate R* in 800 ml of *water R*; adjust to pH 2.5 (*2.2.3*) with *hydrochloric acid R* and dilute to 1000.0 ml with *water R*.

Buffer solution pH 2.5 R1. *4000400.*
To 4.9 g of *dilute phosphoric acid R* add 250 ml of *water R*. Adjust the pH (*2.2.3*) with *dilute sodium hydroxide solution R* and dilute to 500.0 ml with *water R*.

Phosphate buffer solution pH 2.8. *4010600.*
Dissolve 7.8 g of *sodium dihydrogen phosphate R* in 900 ml of *water R*, adjust to pH 2.8 (*2.2.3*) with *phosphoric acid R* and dilute to 1000 ml with the same solvent.

Buffer solution pH 3.0. *4008000.*
Dissolve 21.0 g of *citric acid R* in 200 ml of *1 M sodium hydroxide* and dilute to 1000 ml with *water R*. Dilute 40.3 ml of this solution to 100.0 ml with *0.1 M hydrochloric acid*.

Phosphate buffer solution pH 3.0. *4000500.*
Mix 0.7 ml of *phosphoric acid R* with 100 ml of *water R*. Dilute to 900 ml with the same solvent. Adjust to pH 3.0 (*2.2.3*) with *strong sodium hydroxide solution R* and dilute to 1000 ml with *water R*.

0.1 M Phosphate buffer solution pH 3.0. *4011500.*
Dissolve 12.0 g of *anhydrous sodium dihydrogen phosphate R* in *water R*, adjust the pH (*2.2.3*) with *dilute phosphoric acid R1* and dilute to 1000 ml with *water R*.

Phosphate buffer solution pH 3.0 R1. *4010000.*
Dissolve 3.40 g of *potassium dihydrogen phosphate R* in 900 ml of *water R*. Adjust to pH 3.0 (*2.2.3*) with *phosphoric acid R* and dilute to 1000.0 ml with *water R*.

Phosphate buffer solution pH 3.2. *4008100.*
To 900 ml of a 4 g/l solution of *sodium dihydrogen phosphate R*, add 100 ml of a 2.5 g/l solution of *phosphoric acid R*. Adjust the pH (*2.2.3*) if necessary.

Phosphate buffer solution pH 3.2 R1. *4008500.*
Adjust a 35.8 g/l solution of *disodium hydrogen phosphate R* to pH 3.2 (*2.2.3*) with *dilute phosphoric acid R*. Dilute 100.0 ml of the solution to 2000.0 ml with *water R*.

Buffer solution pH 3.5. *4000600.*
Dissolve 25.0 g of *ammonium acetate R* in 25 ml of *water R* and add 38.0 ml of *hydrochloric acid R1*. Adjust the pH (*2.2.3*) if necessary with *dilute hydrochloric acid R* or *dilute ammonia R1*. Dilute to 100.0 ml with *water R*.

Phosphate buffer solution pH 3.5. *4000700.*
Dissolve 68.0 g of *potassium dihydrogen phosphate R* in *water R* and dilute to 1000.0 ml with the same solvent. Adjust the pH (*2.2.3*) with *phosphoric acid R*.

Buffer solution pH 3.6. *4000800.*
To 250.0 ml of *0.2 M potassium hydrogen phthalate R* add 11.94 ml of *0.2 M hydrochloric acid*. Dilute to 1000.0 ml with *water R*.

Buffer solution pH 3.7. *4000900.*
To 15.0 ml of *acetic acid R* add 60 ml of *alcohol R* and 20 ml of *water R*. Adjust to pH 3.7 (*2.2.3*) by the addition of *ammonia R*. Dilute to 100.0 ml with *water R*.

Buffered copper sulphate solution pH 4.0. *4001000.*
Dissolve 0.25 g of *copper sulphate R* and 4.5 g of *ammonium acetate R* in *dilute acetic acid R* and dilute to 100.0 ml with the same solvent.

Acetate buffer solution pH 4.4. *4001100.*
Dissolve 136 g of *sodium acetate R* and 77 g of *ammonium acetate R* in *water R* and dilute to 1000.0 ml with the same solvent; add 250.0 ml of *glacial acetic acid R* and mix.

Phthalate buffer solution pH 4.4. *4001200.*
Dissolve 2.042 g of *potassium hydrogen phthalate R* in 50 ml of *water R*, add 7.5 ml of *0.2 M sodium hydroxide* and dilute to 200.0 ml with *water R*.

0.05 M Phosphate buffer solution pH 4.5. *4009000.*
Dissolve 6.80 g of *potassium dihydrogen phosphate R* in 1000.0 ml of *water R*. The pH (*2.2.3*) of the solution is 4.5.

Sodium acetate buffer solution pH 4.5. *4010100.*
Dissolve 63 g of *anhydrous sodium acetate R* in *water R*, add 90 ml *acetic acid R* and adjust to pH 4.5, and dilute to 1000 ml with *water R*.

Acetate buffer solution pH 4.6. *4001400.*
Dissolve 5.4 g of *sodium acetate R* in 50 ml of *water R*, add 2.4 g of *glacial acetic acid R* and dilute to 100.0 ml with *water R*. Adjust the pH (*2.2.3*) if necessary.

Succinate buffer solution pH 4.6. *4001500.*

Disssolve 11.8 g of *succinic acid R* in a mixture of 600 ml of *water R* and 82 ml of *1 M sodium hydroxide* and dilute to 1000.0 ml with *water R*.

Acetate buffer solution pH 4.7. *4001600.*

Dissolve 136.1 g of *sodium acetate R* in 500 ml of *water R*. Mix 250 ml of this solution with 250 ml of *dilute acetic acid R*. Shake twice with a freshly prepared, filtered, 0.1 g/l solution of *dithizone R* in *chloroform R*. Shake with *carbon tetrachloride R* until the extract is colourless. Filter the aqueous layer to remove traces of carbon tetrachloride.

Acetate buffer solution pH 5.0. *4009100.*

To 120 ml of a 6 g/l solution of *glacial acetic acid R* add 100 ml of *0.1 M potassium hydroxide* and about 250 ml of *water R*. Mix. Adjust the pH to 5.0 with a 6 g/l solution of *acetic acid R* or with *0.1 M potassium hydroxide* and dilute to 1000.0 ml with *water R*.

Citrate buffer solution pH 5.0. *4010700.*

Prepare a solution containing 20.1 g/l of *citric acid R* and 8.0 g/l of *sodium hydroxide R*. Adjust the pH with *dilute hydrochloric acid R*.

Phosphate buffer solution pH 5.0. *4011300.*

Dissolve 2.72 g of *potassium dihydrogen phosphate R* in 800 ml of *water R*. Adjust the pH (*2.2.3*) with *1 M potassium hydroxide* and dilute to 1000 ml with *water R*.

Buffer solution pH 5.2. *4001700.*

Dissolve 1.02 g of *potassium hydrogen phthalate R* in 30.0 ml of *0.1 M sodium hydroxide*. Dilute to 100.0 ml with *water R*.

Acetate-edetate buffer solution pH 5.5. *4001900.*

Dissolve 250 g of *ammonium acetate R* and 15 g *sodium edetate R* in 400 ml of *water R* and add 125 ml of *glacial acetic acid R*.

Buffer solution pH 5.5. *4001800.*

Dissolve 54.4 g of *sodium acetate R* in 50 ml of *water R*, heating to 35 °C if necessary. After cooling, slowly add 10 ml of *anhydrous acetic acid R*. Shake and dilute to 100.0 ml with *water R*.

Phosphate buffer solution pH 5.5. *4002000.*

Solution I. Dissolve 13.61 g of *potassium dihydrogen phosphate R* in *water R* and dilute to 1000.0 ml with the same solvent.

Solution II. Dissolve 35.81 g of *disodium hydrogen phosphate R* in *water R* and dilute to 1000.0 ml with the same solvent.

Mix 96.4 ml of solution I and 3.6 ml of solution II.

Phosphate-citrate buffer solution pH 5.5. *4008700.*

Mix 56.85 ml of a 28.4 g/l solution of *anhydrous disodium hydrogen phosphate R* and 43.15 ml of a 21 g/l solution of *citric acid R*.

Phosphate buffer solution pH 5.6. *4011200.*

Solution I. Dissolve 0.908 g of *potassium dihydrogen phosphate R* in *water R* and dilute to 100.0 ml with the same solvent.

Solution II. Dissolve 1.161 g of *dipotassium hydrogen phosphate R* in *water R* and dilute to 100.0 ml with the same solvent.

Mix 94.4 ml of solution I and 5.6 ml of solution II. If necessary, adjust to pH 5.6 (*2.2.3*) using solution I or solution II.

Phosphate buffer solution pH 5.8. *4002100.*

Dissolve 1.19 g of *disodium hydrogen phosphate dihydrate R* and 8.25 g of *potassium dihydrogen phosphate R* in *water R* and dilute to 1000.0 ml with the same solvent.

Acetate buffer solution pH 6.0. *4002200.*

Dissolve 100 g of *ammonium acetate R* in 300 ml of *water R*, add 4.1 ml of *glacial acetic acid R*, adjust the pH (*2.2.3*) if necessary using *ammonia R* or *acetic acid R* and dilute to 500.0 ml with *water R*.

Diethylammonium phosphate buffer solution pH 6.0. *4002300.*

Dilute 68 ml of *phosphoric acid R* to 500 ml with *water R*. To 25 ml of this solution add 450 ml of *water R* and 6 ml of *diethylamine R*, adjust to pH 6 ± 0.05 (*2.2.3*), if necessary, using *diethylamine R* or *phosphoric acid R* and dilute to 500.0 ml with *water R*.

Phosphate buffer solution pH 6.0. *4002400.*

Mix 63.2 ml of a 71.5 g/l solution of *disodium hydrogen phosphate R* and 36.8 ml of a 21 g/l solution of *citric acid R*.

Phosphate buffer solution pH 6.0 R1. *4002500.*

Dissolve 6.8 g of *sodium dihydrogen phosphate R* in *water R* and dilute to 1000.0 ml with *water R*. Adjust the pH (*2.2.3*) with *strong sodium hydroxide solution R*.

Phosphate buffer solution pH 6.0 R2. *4002600.*

To 250.0 ml of *0.2 M potassium dihydrogen phosphate R* add 28.5 ml of *0.2 M sodium hydroxide* and dilute to 1000.0 ml with *water R*.

Phosphate buffer solution pH 6.4. *4002800.*

Dissolve 2.5 g of *disodium hydrogen phosphate R*, 2.5 g of *sodium dihydrogen phosphate R* and 8.2 g of *sodium chloride R* in 950 ml of *water R*. Adjust the pH (*2.2.3*) of the solution to 6.4 with *1 M sodium hydroxide* or *1 M hydrochloric acid*, if necessary. Dilute to 1000.0 ml with *water R*.

0.5 M Phthalate buffer solution pH 6.4. *4009200.*

Dissolve 100 g of *potassium hydrogen phthalate R* in *water R* and dilute to 1000.0 ml with the same solvent. Adjust the pH (*2.2.3*) if necessary, using *strong sodium hydroxide solution R*.

Buffer solution pH 6.5. *4002900.*

Dissolve 60.5 g of *disodium hydrogen phosphate R* and 46 g of *potassium dihydrogen phosphate R* in *water R*. Add 100 ml of *0.02 M sodium edetate* and 20 mg of *mercuric chloride R* and dilute to 1000.0 ml with *water R*.

Imidazole buffer solution pH 6.5. *4003000.*

Dissolve 6.81 g of *imidazole R* and 1.23 g of *magnesium sulphate R* in 752 ml of *0.1 M hydrochloric acid*. Adjust the pH (*2.2.3*) if necessary and dilute to 1000.0 ml with *water R*.

0.1 M phosphate buffer solution pH 6.5. *4010800.*

Dissolve 13.80 g of *sodium dihydrogen phosphate monohydrate R* in 900 ml of *distilled water R*. Adjust the pH (*2.2.3*) using a 400 g/l solution of *sodium hydroxide R*. Dilute to 1000 ml with *distilled water R*.

Buffer solution pH 6.6. *4003100.*

To 250.0 ml of *0.2 M potassium dihydrogen phosphate R* add 89.0 ml of *0.2 M sodium hydroxide*. Dilute to 1000.0 ml with *water R*.

Phosphate buffered saline pH 6.8. *4003200.*

Dissolve 1.0 g of *potassium dihydrogen phosphate R*, 2.0 g of *dipotassium hydrogen phosphate R* and 8.5 g of *sodium chloride R* in 900 ml of *water R*, adjust the pH (*2.2.3*) if necessary and dilute to 1000.0 ml with the same solvent.

See the information section on general monographs (cover pages)

Phosphate buffer solution pH 6.8. *4003300.*
Mix 77.3 ml of a 71.5 g/l solution of *disodium hydrogen phosphate R* with 22.7 ml of a 21 g/l solution of *citric acid R*.

Phosphate buffer solution pH 6.8 R1. *4003400.*
To 51.0 ml of a 27.2 g/l solution of *potassium dihydrogen phosphate R* add 49.0 ml of a 71.6 g/l solution of *disodium hydrogen phosphate R*. Adjust the pH (*2.2.3*) if necessary. Store at 2 °C to 8 °C.

1 M tris-hydrochloride buffer solution pH 6.8. *4009300.*
Dissolve 60.6 g of *tris(hydroxymethyl)aminomethane R* in 400 ml of *water R*. Adjust the pH (*2.2.3*) with *hydrochloric acid R* and dilute to 500.0 ml with *water R*.

Buffer solution pH 7.0. *4003500.*
To 1000 ml of a solution containing 18 g/l of *disodium hydrogen phosphate R* and 23 g/l of *sodium chloride R* add sufficient (about 280 ml) of a solution containing 7.8 g/l of *sodium dihydrogen phosphate R* and 23 g/l of *sodium chloride R* to adjust the pH (*2.2.3*). Dissolve in the solution sufficient *sodium azide R* to give a 0.2 g/l solution.

Maleate buffer solution pH 7.0. *4003600.*
Dissolve 10.0 g of *sodium chloride R*, 6.06 g of *tris(hydroxymethyl)aminomethane R* and 4.90 g of *maleic anhydride R* in 900 ml of *water R*. Adjust the pH (*2.2.3*) using a 170 g/l solution of *sodium hydroxide R*. Dilute to 1000.0 ml with *water R*.

Store at 2 °C to 8 °C and use within 3 days.

Phosphate buffer solution pH 7.0. *4003700.*
Mix 82.4 ml of a 71.5 g/l solution of *disodium hydrogen phosphate R* with 17.6 ml of a 21 g/l solution of *citric acid R*.

0.025 M Phosphate buffer solution pH 7.0. *4009400.*
Mix 1 volume of *0.063 M phosphate buffer solution pH 7.0 R* with 1.5 volumes of *water R*.

0.03 M Phosphate buffer solution pH 7.0. *4010300.*
Dissolve 5.2 g of *dipotassium hydrogen phosphate R* in 900 ml of *water for chromatography R*. Adjust the solution to pH 7.0 ± 0.1 using *phosphoric acid R* and dilute to 1000 ml with *water for chromatography R*.

0.063 M Phosphate buffer solution pH 7.0. *4009500.*
Dissolve 5.18 g of *anhydrous disodium hydrogen phosphate R* and 3.65 g of *sodium dihydrogen phosphate monohydrate R* in 950 ml of *water R* and adjust the pH (*2.2.3*) with *phosphoric acid R*; dilute to 1000.0 ml with *water R*.

0.067 M Phosphate buffer solution pH 7.0. *4003800.*
Solution I. Dissolve 0.908 g of *potassium dihydrogen phosphate R* in *water R* and dilute to 100.0 ml with the same solvent.

Solution II. Dissolve 2.38 g of *disodium hydrogen phosphate R* in *water R* and dilute to 100.0 ml with the same solvent.

Mix 38.9 ml of solution I and 61.1 ml of solution II. Adjust the pH (*2.2.3*) if necessary.

0.1 M Phosphate buffer solution pH 7.0. *4008200.*
Dissolve 1.361 g of *potassium dihydrogen phosphate R* in *water R* and dilute to 100.0 ml with the same solvent. Adjust the pH (*2.2.3*) using a 35 g/l solution of *disodium hydrogen phosphate R*.

Phosphate buffer solution pH 7.0 R1. *4003900.*
Mix 250.0 ml of *0.2 M potassium dihydrogen phosphate R* and 148.2 ml of a 8 g/l solution of *sodium hydroxide R*, adjust the pH (*2.2.3*) if necessary. Dilute to 1000.0 ml with *water R*.

Phosphate buffer solution pH 7.0 R2. *4004000.*
Mix 50.0 ml of a 136 g/l solution of *potassium dihydrogen phosphate R* with 29.5 ml of *1 M sodium hydroxide* and dilute to 100.0 ml with *water R*. Adjust the pH (*2.2.3*) to 7.0 ± 0.1.

Phosphate buffer solution pH 7.0 R3. *4008600.*
Dissolve 5 g of *potassium dihydrogen phosphate R* and 11 g of *dipotassium hydrogen phosphate R* in 900 ml of *water R*. Adjust to pH 7.0 (*2.2.3*) with *dilute phosphoric acid R* or *dilute sodium hydroxide solution R*. Dilute to 1000 ml with *water R* and mix.

Phosphate buffer solution pH 7.0 R4. *4010200.*
Dissolve 28.4 g of *anhydrous disodium hydrogen phosphate R* and 18.2 g of *potassium dihydrogen phosphate R* in *water R* and dilute to 500 ml with the same solvent.

Phosphate buffer solution pH 7.0 R5. *4011400.*
Dissolve 28.4 g of *anhydrous disodium hydrogen phosphate R* in 800 ml of *water R*. Adjust the pH (*2.2.3*) using a 30 per cent *m/m* solution of *phosphoric acid R* and dilute to 1000 ml with *water R*.

Tetrabutylammonium buffer solution pH 7.0. *4010900.*
Dissolve 6.16 g of *ammonium acetate R* in a mixture of 15 ml of *tetrabutylammonium hydroxide solution (400 g/l) R* and 185 ml of *water R*. Adjust the pH (*2.2.3*) with *nitric acid R*.

Buffered salt solution pH 7.2. *4004300.*
Dissolve in *water R* 8.0 g of *sodium chloride R*, 0.2 g of *potassium chloride R*, 0.1 g of *anhydrous calcium chloride R*, 0.1 g of *magnesium chloride R*, 3.18 g of *disodium hydrogen phosphate R* and 0.2 g of *potassium dihydrogen phosphate R* and dilute to 1000.0 ml with *water R*.

Buffer solution pH 7.2. *4004100.*
To 250.0 ml of *0.2 M potassium dihydrogen phosphate R* add 175.0 ml of *0.2 M sodium hydroxide*. Dilute to 1000.0 ml with *water R*. Adjust the pH (*2.2.3*) if necessary.

Phosphate-albumin buffered saline pH 7.2. *4004400.*
Dissolve 10.75 g of *disodium hydrogen phosphate R*, 7.6 g of *sodium chloride R* and 10 g of *bovine albumin R* in *water R* and dilute to 1000.0 ml with the same solvent. Immediately before use adjust the pH (*2.2.3*) using *dilute sodium hydroxide solution R* or *dilute phosphoric acid R*.

Phosphate-albumin buffered saline pH 7.2 R1. *4009600.*
Dissolve 10.75 g of *disodium hydrogen phosphate R*, 7.6 g of *sodium chloride R* and 1 g of *bovine albumin R* in *water R* and dilute to 1000.0 ml with the same solvent. Immediately before use adjust the pH (*2.2.3*) using *dilute sodium hydroxide solution R* or *dilute phosphoric acid R*.

Phosphate buffer solution pH 7.2. *4004200.*
Mix 87.0 ml of a 71.5 g/l solution of *disodium hydrogen phosphate R* with 13.0 ml of a 21 g/l solution of *citric acid R*.

Imidazole buffer solution pH 7.3. *4004500.*
Dissolve 3.4 g of *imidazole R* and 5.8 g of *sodium chloride R* in *water R*, add 18.6 ml of *1 M hydrochloric acid* and dilute to 1000.0 ml with *water R*. Adjust the pH (*2.2.3*) if necessary.

Barbital buffer solution pH 7.4. *4004700.*
Mix 50 ml of a solution in *water R* containing 19.44 g/l of *sodium acetate R* and 29.46 g/l of *barbital sodium R* with 50.5 ml of *0.1 M hydrochloric acid*, add 20 ml of an 85 g/l of *sodium chloride R* and dilute to 250 ml with *water R*.

Buffer solution pH 7.4. *4004600.*
Dissolve 0.6 g of *potassium dihydrogen phosphate R*, 6.4 g of *disodium hydrogen phosphate R* and 5.85 g of *sodium chloride R* in *water R*, and dilute to 1000.0 ml with the same solvent. Adjust the pH (*2.2.3*) if necessary.

Phosphate buffered saline pH 7.4. *4005000.*
Dissolve 2.38 g of *disodium hydrogen phosphate R*, 0.19 g of *potassium dihydrogen phosphate R* and 8.0 g of *sodium chloride R* in water. Dilute to 1000.0 ml with the same solvent. Adjust the pH (*2.2.3*) if necessary.

Phosphate buffer solution pH 7.4. *4004800.*
Add 250.0 ml of *0.2 M potassium dihydrogen phosphate R* to 393.4 ml of *0.1 M sodium hydroxide*.

Tris(hydroxymethyl)aminomethane sodium chloride buffer solution pH 7.4. *4004900.*
Dissolve 6.08 g of *tris(hydroxymethyl)aminomethane R*, 8.77 g of *sodium chloride R* in 500 ml of *distilled water R*. Add 10.0 g of *bovine albumin R*. Adjust the pH (*2.2.3*) using *hydrochloric acid R*. Dilute to 1000.0 ml with *distilled water R*.

Borate buffer solution pH 7.5. *4005200.*
Dissolve 2.5 g of *sodium chloride R*, 2.85 g of *disodium tetraborate R* and 10.5 g of *boric acid R* in *water R* and dilute to 1000.0 ml with the same solvent. Adjust the pH (*2.2.3*) if necessary.
Store at 2 °C to 8 °C.

Buffer (HEPES) solution pH 7.5. *4009700.*
Dissolve 2.38 g of *2-[4-(2-hydroxyethyl)piperazin-1-yl]ethanesulphonic acid R* in about 90 ml of *water R*. Adjust the pH to 7.5 with *sodium hydroxide solution R*. Dilute to 100 ml with *water R*.

0.2 M Phosphate buffer solution pH 7.5. *4005400.*
Dissolve 27.22 g of *potassium dihydrogen phosphate R* in 930 ml of *water R*, adjust to pH 7.5 (*2.2.3*) with a 300 g/l solution of *potassium hydroxide R* and dilute to 1000.0 ml with *water R*.

0.33 M Phosphate buffer solution pH 7.5. *4005300.*
Solution I. Dissolve 119.31 g of *disodium hydrogen phosphate R* in *water R* and dilute to 1000.0 ml with the same solvent.
Solution II. Dissolve 45.36 g of *potassium dihydrogen phosphate R* in *water R* and dilute to 1000.0 ml with the same solvent.
Mix 85 ml of solution I and 15 ml of solution II. Adjust the pH (*2.2.3*) if necessary.

0.05 M Tris-hydrochloride buffer solution pH 7.5. *4005600.*
Dissolve 6.057 g of *tris(hydroxymethyl)aminomethane R* in *water R* and adjust the pH (*2.2.3*) with *hydrochloric acid R*. Dilute to 1000.0 ml with *water R*.

Tris(hydroxymethyl)aminomethane buffer solution pH 7.5. *4005500.*
Dissolve 7.27 g of *tris(hydroxymethyl)aminomethane R* and 5.27 g of *sodium chloride R* in *water R*, and adjust the pH (*2.2.3*) if necessary. Dilute to 1000.0 ml with *water R*.

Sodium citrate buffer solution pH 7.8 (0.034 M sodium citrate, 0.101 M sodium chloride). *4009800.*
Dissolve 10.0 g of *sodium citrate R* and 5.90 g of *sodium chloride R* in 900 ml of *water R*. Adjust the pH (*2.2.3*) by addition of *hydrochloric acid R* and dilute to 1000 ml with *water R*.

0.0015 M Borate buffer solution pH 8.0. *4006000.*
Dissolve 0.572 g of *disodium tetraborate R* and 2.94 g of *calcium chloride R* in 800 ml of *water R*. Adjust the pH (*2.2.3*) with *1 M hydrochloric acid*. Dilute to 1000.0 ml with *water R*.

Buffer solution pH 8.0. *4005900.*
To 50.0 ml of *0.2 M potassium dihydrogen phosphate R* add 46.8 ml of *0.2 M sodium hydroxide*. Dilute to 200.0 ml with *water R*.

Buffer solution pH 8.0 R1. *4010400.*
Dissolve 20 g of *dipotassium hydrogen phosphate R* in 900 ml of *water R*. Adjust the pH (*2.2.3*) with *phosphoric acid R*. Dilute to 1000 ml with *water R*.

0.02 M Phosphate buffer solution pH 8.0. *4006100.*
To 50.0 ml of *0.2 M potassium dihydrogen phosphate R* add 46.8 ml of *0.2 M sodium hydroxide*. Dilute to 500 ml with *water R*.

0.1 M Phosphate buffer solution pH 8.0. *4008400.*
Dissolve 0.523 g of *potassium dihydrogen phosphate R* and 16.73 g of *dipotassium hydrogen phosphate R* in *water R* and dilute to 1000.0 ml with the same solvent.

1 M Phosphate buffer solution pH 8.0. *4007800.*
Dissolve 136.1 g of *potassium dihydrogen phosphate R* in *water R*, adjust the pH (*2.2.3*) with *1 M sodium hydroxide*. Dilute to 1000.0 ml with *water R*.

Tris(hydroxymethyl)aminomethane buffer solution pH 8.1. *4006200.*
Dissolve 0.294 g of *calcium chloride R* in 40 ml of *tris(hydroxymethyl)aminomethane solution R* and adjust the pH (*2.2.3*) with *1 M hydrochloric acid*. Dilute to 100.0 ml with *water R*.

Tris-glycine buffer solution pH 8.3. *4006300.*
Dissolve 6.0 g of *tris(hydroxymethyl)aminomethane R* and 28.8 g of *glycine R* in *water R* and dilute to 1000.0 ml with the same solvent. Dilute 1 volume to 10 volumes with *water R* immediately before use.

Tris-hydrochloride buffer solution pH 8.3. *4011800.*
Dissolve 9.0 g of *tris(hydroxymethyl)aminomethane R* in 2.9 litres of *water R*. Adjust the pH (*2.2.3*) with *1 M hydrochloric acid*. Adjust the volume to 3 litres with *water R*.

Barbital buffer solution pH 8.4. *4006400.*
Dissolve 8.25 g of *barbital sodium R* in *water R* and dilute to 1000.0 ml with the same solvent.

Tris-EDTA BSA buffer solution pH 8.4. *4006500.*
Dissolve 6.1 g of *tris(hydroxymethyl)aminomethane R*, 2.8 g of *sodium edetate R*, 10.2 g of *sodium chloride R* and 10 g of *bovine albumin R* in *water R*, adjust to pH 8.4 (*2.2.3*) using *1 M hydrochloric acid* and dilute to 1000.0 ml with *water R*.

Tris(hydroxymethyl)aminomethane EDTA buffer solution pH 8.4. *4006600.*
Dissolve 5.12 g of *sodium chloride R*, 3.03 g of *tris(hydroxymethyl)aminomethane R* and 1.40 g of *sodium edetate R* in 250 ml of *distilled water R*. Adjust the pH (*2.2.3*) to 8.4 using *hydrochloric acid R*. Dilute to 500.0 ml with *distilled water R*.

Tris acetate buffer solution pH 8.5. *4006700.*
Dissolve 0.294 g of *calcium chloride R* and 12.11 g of *tris(hydroxymethyl)aminomethane R* in *water R*. Adjust the pH (*2.2.3*) with *acetic acid R*. Dilute to 1000.0 ml with *water R*.

Barbital buffer solution pH 8.6 R1. *4006900.*
Dissolve in *water R* 1.38 g of *barbital R*, 8.76 g of *barbital sodium R* and 0.38 g of *calcium lactate R* and dilute to 1000.0 ml with the same solvent.

1.5 M tris-hydrochloride buffer solution pH 8.8. *4009900.*
Dissolve 90.8 g of *tris(hydroxymethyl)aminomethane R* in 400 ml of *water R*. Adjust the pH (*2.2.3*) with *hydrochloric acid R* and dilute to 500.0 ml with *water R*.

Buffer (phosphate) solution pH 9.0. *4008300.*
Dissolve 1.74 g of *potassium dihydrogen phosphate R* in 80 ml of *water R*, adjust the pH (*2.2.3*) with *1 M potassium hydroxide* and dilute to 100.0 ml with *water R*.

Buffer solution pH 9.0. *4007000.*
Solution I. Dissolve 6.18 g of *boric acid R* in *0.1 M potassium chloride R* and dilute to 1000.0 ml with the same solvent.

Solution II. 0.1 M sodium hydroxide.

Mix 1000.0 ml of solution I and 420.0 ml of solution II.

Buffer solution pH 9.0 R1. *4007100.*
Dissolve 6.20 g of *boric acid R* in 500 ml of *water R* and adjust the pH (*2.2.3*) with *1 M sodium hydroxide* (about 41.5 ml). Dilute to 1000.0 ml with *water R*.

Ammonium chloride buffer solution pH 9.5. *4007200.*
Dissolve 33.5 g of *ammonium chloride R* in 150 ml of *water R*, add 42.0 ml of *concentrated ammonia R* and dilute to 250.0 ml with *water R*.

Store in a polyethylene container.

Ammonium chloride buffer solution pH 10.0. *4007300.*
Dissolve 5.4 g of *ammonium chloride R* in 20 ml of *water R*, add 35.0 ml of *ammonia R* and dilute to 100.0 ml with *water R*.

Diethanolamine buffer solution pH 10.0. *4007500.*
Dissolve 96.4 g of *diethanolamine R* in *water R* and dilute to 400 ml with the same solvent. Add 0.5 ml of an 186 g/l solution of *magnesium chloride R* and adjust the pH (*2.2.3*) with *1 M hydrochloric acid*. Dilute to 500.0 ml with *water R*.

0.1 M Ammonium carbonate buffer solution pH 10.3. *4011900.*
Dissolve 7.91 g of *ammonium carbonate R* in 800 ml of *water R*. Adjust the pH (*2.2.3*) with *dilute sodium hydroxide solution R*. Dilute to 1000.0 ml with *water R*.

Ammonium chloride buffer solution pH 10.4. *4011000.*
Dissolve 70 g of *ammonium chloride R* in 200 ml of *water R*, add 330 ml of *concentrated ammonia R* and dilute to 1000.0 ml with *water R*. If necessary, adjust to pH 10.4 with *ammonia R*.

Borate buffer solution pH 10.4. *4011100.*
Dissolve 24.64 g of *boric acid R* in 900 ml of *distilled water R*. Adjust the pH (*2.2.3*) using a 400 g/l solution of *sodium hydroxide R*. Dilute to 1000 ml with *distilled water R*.

Buffer solution pH 10.9. *4007600.*
Dissolve 6.75 g of *ammonium chloride R* in *ammonia R* and dilute to 100.0 ml with the same solvent.

Total-ionic-strength-adjustment buffer. *4007700.*
Dissolve 58.5 g of *sodium chloride R*, 57.0 ml of *glacial acetic acid R*, 61.5 g of *sodium acetate R* and 5.0 g of *cyclohexylene-dinitrilotetra-acetic acid R* in *water R* and dilute to 500.0 ml with the same solvent. Adjust to pH 5.0 to 5.5 with a 335 g/l solution of *sodium hydroxide R* and dilute to 1000.0 ml with *distilled water R*.

Total-ionic-strength-adjustment buffer R1. *4008800.*
Solution (a). Dissolve 210 g of *citric acid R* in 400 ml of *distilled water R*. Adjust to pH 7.0 (*2.2.3*) with *concentrated ammonia R*. Dilute to 1000.0 ml with *distilled water R*.

Solution (b). Dissolve 132 g of *ammonium phosphate R* in *distilled water R* and dilute to 1000.0 ml with the same solvent.

Solution (c). To a suspension of 292 g of (ethylenedinitrilo)tetra-*acetic acid R* in about 500 ml of *distilled water R*, add about 200 ml of *concentrated ammonia R* to dissolve. Adjust the pH to 6 to 7 (*2.2.3*) with *concentrated ammonia R*. Dilute to 1000.0 ml with *distilled water R*.

Mix equal volumes of solution (a), (b), and (c) and adjust to pH 7.5 with *concentrated ammonia R*.

4.2. VOLUMETRIC ANALYSIS

4.2.1. PRIMARY STANDARDS FOR VOLUMETRIC SOLUTIONS

Primary standards for volumetric solutions are indicated by the suffix RV. Primary standards of suitable quality may be obtained from commercial sources or prepared by the following methods.

Benzoic acid. $C_7H_6O_2$. (M_r 122.1). *2000200.* [65-85-0].
Sublime *benzoic acid R* in a suitable apparatus.

Potassium bromate. $KBrO_3$. (M_r 167.0). *2000300.* [7758-01-2].
Crystallise *potassium bromate R* from boiling *water R*. Collect the crystals and dry to constant mass at 180 °C.

Potassium hydrogen phthalate. $C_8H_5KO_4$. (M_r 204.2). *2000400.* [877-24-7].
Recrystallise *potassium hydrogen phthalate R* from boiling *water R*, collect the crystals at a temperature above 35 °C and dry to constant mass at 110 °C.

Sodium carbonate. Na_2CO_3 . (M_r 106.0). *2000500.* [497-19-8].
Filter at room temperature a saturated solution of *sodium carbonate R*. Introduce slowly into the filtrate a stream of *carbon dioxide R* with constant cooling and stirring. After about 2 h, collect the precipitate on a sintered-glass filter. Wash the filter with iced *water R* containing carbon dioxide. After drying at 100 °C to 105 °C, heat to constant mass at 270 °C to 300 °C, stirring from time to time.

Sodium chloride. NaCl. (M_r 58.44). *2000600.* [7647-14-5].
To 1 volume of a saturated solution of *sodium chloride R* add 2 volumes of *hydrochloric acid R*. Collect the crystals formed and wash with *hydrochloric acid R1*. Remove the hydrochloric acid by heating on a water-bath and dry the crystals to constant mass at 300 °C.

Sulphanilic acid. $C_6H_7NO_3S$. (M_r 173.2). *2000700.* [121-57-3].
Recrystallise *sulphanilic acid R* from boiling *water R*. Filter and dry to constant mass at 100 °C to 105 °C.

Zinc. Zn. (M_r 65.4). *2000800.* [7440-66-6].
Use a quality containing not less than 99.9 per cent of Zn.

4.2.2. VOLUMETRIC SOLUTIONS

Volumetric solutions are prepared according to the usual chemical analytical methods. The accuracy of the apparatus used is verified to ensure that it is appropriate for the intended use.

The concentration of volumetric solutions is indicated in terms of molarity. Molarity expresses, as the number of moles, the amount of substance dissolved in 1 litre of solution. A solution which contains x moles of substance per litre is said to be x M.

Volumetric solutions do not differ from the prescribed strength by more than 10 per cent. The molarity of the volumetric solutions is determined by an appropriate number of titrations. The repeatability does not exceed 0.2 per cent (relative standard deviation).

Volumetric solutions are standardised by the methods described below. When a volumetric solution is to be used in an assay in which the end-point is determined by an electrochemical process (for example, amperometry or potentiometry) the solution is standardised by the same method. The composition of the medium in which a volumetric solution is standardised should be the same as that in which it is to be used.

Solutions more dilute than those described are obtained by diluting the latter with *carbon dioxide-free water R*. The correction factors of these solutions are the same as those from which the dilutions were prepared.

0.1 M Acetic acid. *3008900.*
Dilute 6.0 g of *glacial acetic acid R* to 1000.0 ml with *water R*.

Standardisation. To 25.0 ml of acetic acid add 0.5 ml of *phenolphthalein solution R* and titrate with *0.1 M sodium hydroxide*.

0.1 M Ammonium and cerium nitrate. *3000100.*
Shake for 2 min a solution containing 56 ml of sulphuric acid R and 54.82 g of *ammonium and cerium nitrate R*, add five successive quantities, each of 100 ml, of *water R*, shaking after each addition. Dilute the clear solution to 1000.0 ml with *water R*. Standardise the solution after 10 days.

Standardisation. To 25.0 ml of the ammonium and cerium nitrate solution add 2.0 g of *potassium iodide R* and 150 ml of *water R*. Titrate immediately with *0.1 M sodium thiosulphate*, using 1 ml of *starch solution R* as indicator.

Store protected from light.

0.01 M Ammonium and cerium nitrate. *3000200.*
To 100.0 ml of *0.1 M ammonium and cerium nitrate* add, with cooling, 30 ml of sulphuric acid R and dilute to 1000.0 ml with *water R*.

0.1 M Ammonium and cerium sulphate. *3000300.*
Dissolve 65.0 g of *ammonium and cerium sulphate R* in a mixture of 500 ml of *water R* and 30 ml of sulphuric acid R. Allow to cool and dilute to 1000.0 ml with *water R*.

Standardisation. To 25.0 ml of the ammonium and cerium sulphate solution add 2.0 g of *potassium iodide R* and 150 ml of *water R*. Titrate immediately with *0.1 M sodium thiosulphate*, using 1 ml of *starch solution R* as indicator.

0.01 M Ammonium and cerium sulphate. *3000400.*
To 100.0 ml of *0.1 M ammonium and cerium sulphate* add, with cooling, 30 ml of sulphuric acid R and dilute to 1000.0 ml with *water R*.

0.1 M Ammonium thiocyanate. *3000500.*
Dissolve 7.612 g of *ammonium thiocyanate R* in *water R* and dilute to 1000.0 ml with the same solvent.

Standardisation. To 20.0 ml of *0.1 M silver nitrate* add 25 ml of *water R*, 2 ml of *dilute nitric acid R* and 2 ml of *ferric ammonium sulphate solution R2*. Titrate with the ammonium thiocyanate solution until a reddish-yellow colour is obtained.

0.1 M Barium chloride. *3000600.*
Dissolve 24.4 g of *barium chloride R* in *water R* and dilute to 1000.0 ml with the same solvent.

Standardisation. To 10.0 ml of the barium chloride solution add 60 ml of *water R*, 3 ml of *concentrated ammonia R* and 0.5 mg to 1 mg of *phthalein purple R*. Titrate with *0.1 M sodium edetate*. When the solution begins to decolorise, add 50 ml of *alcohol R* and continue the titration until the blue-violet colour disappears.

0.05 M Barium perchlorate. *3000700.*
Dissolve 15.8 g of *barium hydroxide R* in a mixture of 7.5 ml of *perchloric acid R* and 75 ml of *water R* , adjust the solution to pH 3 by adding *perchloric acid R* and filter if necessary. Add 150 ml of *alcohol R* and dilute to 250 ml with *water R*. Dilute to 1000.0 ml with *buffer solution pH 3.7 R*.

Standardisation. To 5.0 ml of *0.05 M sulphuric acid* add 5 ml of *water R*, 50 ml of *buffer solution pH 3.7 R* and 0.5 ml of *alizarin s solution R*. Titrate with the barium perchlorate solution until an orange-red colour appears. Standardise immediately before use.

0.025 M Barium perchlorate. *3009600.*
Dilute 500.0 ml of *0.05 M barium perchlorate* to 1000.0 ml with *buffer solution pH 3.7 R*.

0.004 M Benzethonium chloride. *3000900.*
Dissolve in *water R* 1.792 g of *benzethonium chloride R*, previously dried to constant mass at 100 °C to 105 °C, and dilute to 1000.0 ml with the same solvent.

Standardisation. Calculate the molarity of the solution from the content of $C_{27}H_{42}ClNO_2$ in the dried benzethonium chloride determined as follows. Dissolve 0.350 g of the dried substance in 30 ml of *anhydrous acetic acid R* and add 6 ml of *mercuric acetate solution R*. Titrate with *0.1 M perchloric acid*, using 0.05 ml of *crystal violet solution R* as indicator. Carry out a blank titration.

1 ml of *0.1 M perchloric acid* is equivalent to 44.81 mg of $C_{27}H_{42}ClNO_2$.

0.0167 M Bromide-bromate. *3001000.*
Dissolve 2.7835 g of *potassium bromate RV* and 13 g of *potassium bromide R* in *water R* and dilute to 1000.0 ml with the same solvent.

0.1 M Cerium sulphate. *3001100.*
Dissolve 40.4 g of *cerium sulphate R* in a mixture of 500 ml of *water R* and 50 ml of sulphuric acid R. Allow to cool and dilute to 1000.0 ml with *water R*.

Standardisation. To 25.0 ml of the cerium sulphate solution, add 2.0 g of *potassium iodide R* and 150 ml of *water R*. Titrate immediately with *0.1 M sodium thiosulphate* using 1 ml of *starch solution R* as indicator.

0.02 M Copper sulphate. *3001200.*
Dissolve 5.0 g of *copper sulphate R* in *water R* and dilute to 1000.0 ml with the same solvent.

Standardisation. To 20.0 ml of the copper sulphate solution add 2 g of *sodium acetate R* and 0.1 ml of *pyridylazonaphthol solution R*. Titrate with *0.02 M sodium edetate* until the colour changes from violet-blue to bright green. Titrate slowly towards the end of the titration.

1 M Cupriethylenediamine hydroxide solution. *3008700.*
The molar ratio of ethylenediamine to copper is 2.00 ± 0.04.

This solution is commercially available.

0.1 M Ferric ammonium sulphate. *3001300.*
Dissolve 50.0 g of *ferric ammonium sulphate R* in a mixture of 6 ml of sulphuric acid R and 300 ml of *water R* and dilute to 1000.0 ml with *water R*.

Standardisation. To 25.0 ml of the ferric ammonium sulphate solution, add 3 ml of *hydrochloric acid R* and 2 g of *potassium iodide R*. Allow to stand for 10 min. Titrate with *0.1 M sodium thiosulphate*, using 1 ml of *starch solution R* as indicator.

1 ml of *0.1 M sodium thiosulphate* is equivalent to 48.22 mg of $FeNH_4(SO_4)_2,12H_2O$.

0.1 M Ferrous sulphate. *3001400.*
Dissolve 27.80 g of *ferrous sulphate R* in 500 ml of *dilute sulphuric acid R* and dilute to 1000.0 ml with *water R*.

Standardisation. To 25.0 ml of the ferrous sulphate solution add 3 ml of *phosphoric acid R* and titrate immediately with *0.02 M potassium permanganate*. Standardise immediately before use.

6 M Hydrochloric acid. *3001500.*
Dilute 618.0 g of *hydrochloric acid R* to 1000.0 ml with *water R*.

3 M Hydrochloric acid. *3001600.*
Dilute 309.0 g of *hydrochloric acid R* to 1000.0 ml with *water R*.

2 M Hydrochloric acid. *3001700.*
Dilute 206.0 g of *hydrochloric acid R* to 1000.0 ml with *water R*.

1 M Hydrochloric acid. *3001800.*
Dilute 103.0 g of *hydrochloric acid R* to 1000.0 ml with *water R*.

Standardisation. Dissolve 1.000 g of *sodium carbonate RV* in 50 ml of *water R*, add 0.1 ml of *methyl orange solution R* and titrate with the hydrochloric acid until the solution just becomes yellowish-red. Boil for 2 min. The solution reverts to yellow. Cool and continue the titration until a yellowish-red colour is obtained.

1 ml of *1 M hydrochloric acid* is equivalent to 53.00 mg of Na_2CO_3.

0.1 M Hydrochloric acid. *3002100.*
Dilute 100.0 ml of *1 M hydrochloric acid* to 1000.0 ml with *water R*.

Standardisation. Carry out the titration described for *1 M hydrochloric acid* using 0.100 g of *sodium carbonate RV* dissolved in 20 ml of *water R*.

1 ml of *0.1 M hydrochloric acid* is equivalent to 5.30 mg of Na_2CO_3.

0.1 M Hydrochloric acid, alcoholic. *3008800.*
Dilute 9.0 ml of *hydrochloric acid R* to 1000.0 ml with *aldehyde-free alcohol R*.

0.5 M Iodine. *3009400.*
Dissolve 127 g of *iodine R* and 200 g of *potassium iodide R* in *water R* and dilute to 1000.0 ml with the same solvent.

Standardisation. To 2.0 ml of the iodine solution add 1 ml of *dilute acetic acid R* and 50 ml of *water R*. Titrate with *0.1 M sodium thiosulphate*, using *starch solution R* as indicator.

Store protected from light.

0.05 M Iodine. *3002700.*
Dissolve 12.7 g of *iodine R* and 20 g of *potassium iodide R* in *water R* and dilute to 1000.0 ml with the same solvent.

Standardisation. To 20.0 ml of the iodine solution add 1 ml of *dilute acetic acid R* and 30 ml of *water R*. Titrate with *0.1 M sodium thiosulphate*, using *starch solution R* as indicator.

Store protected from light.

0.01 M Iodine. *3002900.*
Add 0.3 g of *potassium iodide R* to 20.0 ml of *0.05 M iodine* and dilute to 100.0 ml with *water R*.

0.1 M Lead nitrate. *3003100.*
Dissolve 33 g of *lead nitrate R* in *water R* and dilute to 1000.0 ml with the same solvent.

Standardisation. To 20.0 ml of the lead nitrate solution add 300 ml of *water R* and carry out the determination of lead by complexometry (*2.5.11*).

0.05 M Lead nitrate. *3009700.*
Dilute 50.0 ml of *0.1 M Lead nitrate* to 100.0 ml with *water R*.

0.1 M Lithium methoxide. *3003300.*
Dissolve 0.694 g of *lithium R* in 150 ml of *anhydrous methanol R* and dilute to 1000.0 ml with *toluene R*.

Standardisation. To 10 ml of *dimethylformamide R* add 0.05 ml of a 3 g/l solution of *thymol blue R* in *methanol R* and titrate with the lithium methoxide solution until a pure blue colour is obtained. Immediately add 0.200 g of *benzoic acid RV*. Stir to effect solution and titrate with the lithium methoxide solution until the pure blue colour is again obtained. Protect the solution from atmospheric carbon dioxide throughout the titration. From the volume of titrant used in the second titration ascertain the exact strength of the lithium methoxide solution. Standardise immediately before use.

1 ml of *0.1 M lithium methoxide* is equivalent to 12.21 mg of $C_7H_6O_2$.

0.1 M Magnesium chloride. *3003400.*
Dissolve 20.33 g of *magnesium chloride R* in *water R* and dilute to 1000.0 ml with the same solvent.

Standardisation. Carry out the determination of magnesium by complexometry (*2.5.11*).

1 M Nitric acid. *3003600.*
Dilute 96.6 g of *nitric acid R* to 1000.0 ml with *water R*.

Standardisation. Dissolve 1.000 g of *sodium carbonate RV* in 50 ml of *water R*, add 0.1 ml of *methyl orange solution R* and titrate with the nitric acid until the solution just becomes reddish-yellow; boil for 2 min. The solution reverts to yellow. Cool and continue the titration until a reddish-yellow colour is obtained.

1 ml of *1 M nitric acid* is equivalent to 53.00 mg of Na_2CO_3.

0.1 M Perchloric acid. *3003900.*
Place 8.5 ml of *perchloric acid R* in a volumetric flask containing about 900 ml of *glacial acetic acid R* and mix. Add 30 ml of *acetic anhydride R*, dilute to 1000.0 ml with *glacial acetic acid R*, mix and allow to stand for 24 h. Determine the water content (*2.5.12*) without addition of methanol and, if necessary, adjust the water content to between 0.1 per cent and 0.2 per cent by adding either *acetic anhydride R* or *water R*. Allow to stand for 24 h.

Standardisation. Dissolve 0.350 g of *potassium hydrogen phthalate RV* in 50 ml of *anhydrous acetic acid R*, warming gently if necessary. Allow to cool protected from the air, and titrate with the perchloric acid solution, using 0.05 ml of *crystal violet solution R* as indicator. Note the temperature of the perchloric acid solution at the time of the titration. If the temperature at which an assay is carried out is different from that at which the *perchloric acid R* has been standardised the volume used in the assay becomes:

$$V_c = V\left[1 + (t_1 - t_2)\,0.0011\right]$$

where t_1 is the temperature during standardisation, and t_2 is the temperature during the assay, V_c is the corrected volume and V the observed volume.

1 ml of *0.1 M perchloric acid* is equivalent to 20.42 mg of $C_8H_5KO_4$.

0.05 M Perchloric acid. *3004000.*
Dilute 50.0 ml of *0.1 M perchloric acid* to 100.0 ml with *anhydrous acetic acid R*.

0.033 M Potassium bromate. *3004200.*
Dissolve 5.5670 g of *potassium bromate RV* in *water R* and dilute to 1000.0 ml with the same solvent.

0.02 M Potassium bromate. *3004300.*
Dissolve 3.340 g of *potassium bromate RV* in *water R* and dilute to 1000.0 ml with the same solvent.

0.0167 M Potassium bromate. *3004400.*
Prepare by diluting *0.033 M Potassium bromate*.

0.0083 M Potassium bromate. *3004500.*
Prepare by diluting *0.033 M Potassium bromate*.

0.0167 M Potassium dichromate. *3004600.*
Dissolve 4.90 g of *potassium dichromate R* in *water R* and dilute to 1000.0 ml with the same solvent.

Standardisation. To 20.0 ml of the potassium dichromate solution add 1 g of *potassium iodide R* and 7 ml of *dilute hydrochloric acid R*. Add 250 ml of *water R* and titrate with *0.1 M sodium thiosulphate*, using 3 ml of *starch solution R* as indicator, until the colour changes from blue to light green.

0.1 M Potassium hydrogen phthalate. *3004700.*
In a conical flask containing about 800 ml of *anhydrous acetic acid R*, dissolve 20.42 g of *potassium hydrogen phthalate RV*. Heat on a water-bath until completely dissolved, protected from humidity. Cool to 20 °C and dilute to 1000.0 ml with *anhydrous acetic acid R*.

1 M Potassium hydroxide. *3009100.*
Dissolve 60 g of *potassium hydroxide R* in *carbon dioxide-free water R* and dilute to 1000.0 ml with the same solvent.

Standardisation. Titrate 20.0 ml of the potassium hydroxide solution with *1 M hydrochloric acid*, using 0.5 ml of *phenolphthalein solution R* as indicator.

0.1 M Potassium hydroxide. *3004800.*
Dissolve 6 g of *potassium hydroxide R* in *carbon dioxide-free water R* and dilute to 1000.0 ml with the same solvent.

Standardisation. Titrate 20.0 ml of the potassium hydroxide solution with *0.1 M hydrochloric acid*, using 0.5 ml of *phenolphthalein solution R* as indicator.

0.5 M Potassium hydroxide in alcohol (60 per cent *V/V*). *3004900.*
Dissolve 3 g of *potassium hydroxide R* in *aldehyde-free alcohol R* (60 per cent *V/V*) and dilute to 100.0 ml with the same solvent.

Standardisation. Titrate 20.0 ml of the alcoholic potassium hydroxide solution (60 per cent *V/V*) with *0.5 M hydrochloric acid*, using 0.5 ml of *phenolphthalein solution R* as indicator.

0.5 M Potassium hydroxide, alcoholic. *3005000.*
Dissolve 3 g of *potassium hydroxide R* in 5 ml of *water R* and dilute to 100.0 ml with *aldehyde-free alcohol R*.

Standardisation. Titrate 20.0 ml of the alcoholic potassium hydroxide solution with *0.5 M hydrochloric acid*, using 0.5 ml of *phenolphthalein solution R* as indicator.

0.1 M Potassium hydroxide, alcoholic. *3005100.*
Dilute 20 ml of *0.5 M alcoholic potassium hydroxide* to 100.0 ml with *aldehyde-free alcohol R*.

0.01 M Potassium hydroxide, alcoholic. *3009000.*
Dilute 2.0 ml of *0.5 M alcoholic potassium hydroxide* to 100.0 ml with *aldehyde-free alcohol R*.

0.05 M Potassium iodate. *3005200.*
Dissolve 10.70 g of *potassium iodate R* in *water R* and dilute to 1000.0 ml with the same solvent.

Standardisation. Dilute 25.0 ml of the potassium iodate solution to 100.0 ml with *water R*. To 20.0 ml of this solution add 2 g of *potassium iodide R* and 10 ml of *dilute sulphuric acid R*. Titrate with *0.1 M sodium thiosulphate*, using 1 ml of *starch solution R*, added towards the end of the titration, as indicator.

0.001 M Potassium iodide. *3009200.*
Dilute 10.0 ml of *potassium iodide solution R* (166 g/l) to 100.0 ml with *water R*. Dilute 5.0 ml of this solution to 500.0 ml with *water R*.

0.02 M Potassium permanganate. *3005300.*
Dissolve 3.2 g of *potassium permanganate R* in *water R* and dilute to 1000.0 ml with the same solvent. Heat the solution for 1 h on a water-bath, allow to cool and filter through a sintered-glass filter.

Standardisation. To 20.0 ml of the potassium permanganate solution, add 2 g of *potassium iodide R* and 10 ml of *dilute sulphuric acid R*. Titrate with *0.1 M sodium thiosulphate*, using 1 ml of *starch solution R*, added towards the end of the titration, as indicator. Standardise immediately before use.

Store protected from light.

0.1 M Silver nitrate. *3005600.*
Dissolve 17.0 g of *silver nitrate R* in *water R* and dilute to 1000.0 ml with the same solvent.

Standardisation. Dissolve 0.100 g of *sodium chloride RV* in 30 ml of *water R*. Titrate with the silver nitrate solution, determining the end-point potentiometrically (*2.2.20*).

1 ml of *0.1 M silver nitrate* is equivalent to 5.844 mg of NaCl.

Store protected from light.

0.001 M Silver nitrate. *3009300.*
Dilute 5.0 ml of silver nitrate 0.1 M to 500.0 ml with *water R*.

0.1 M Sodium arsenite. *3005800.*
Dissolve *arsenious trioxide RV* equivalent to 4.946 g of As_2O_3 in a mixture of 20 ml of *strong sodium hydroxide solution R* and 20 ml of *water R*, dilute to 400 ml with *water R* and add *dilute hydrochloric acid R* until the solution is neutral to *litmus paper R*. Dissolve 2 g of *sodium hydrogen carbonate R* in the solution and dilute to 500.0 ml with *water R*.

0.1 M Sodium edetate. *3005900.*
Dissolve 37.5 g of *sodium edetate R* in 500 ml of *water R*, add 100 ml of *1 M sodium hydroxide* and dilute to 1000.0 ml with *water R*.

Standardisation. Dissolve 0.120 g of *zinc RV* in 4 ml of *hydrochloric acid R1* and add 0.1 ml of *bromine water R*. Drive off the excess of bromine by boiling, add *dilute sodium hydroxide solution R* until the solution is weakly acid or neutral and carry out the assay of zinc by complexometry *(2.5.11)*.

1 ml of *0.1 M sodium edetate* is equivalent to 6.54 mg of Zn.

Store in a polyethylene container.

0.02 M Sodium edetate. *3006000.*
Dissolve 7.444 g of *sodium edetate R* in *water R* and dilute to 1000.0 ml with the same solvent.

Standardisation. Dissolve 0.100 g of *zinc RV* in 4 ml of *hydrochloric acid R1* and add 0.1 ml of *bromine water R*. Drive off the excess of bromine by boiling. Transfer the solution to a volumetric flask and dilute to 100.0 ml with *water R*. Transfer 25.0 ml of the solution to a 500 ml conical flask and dilute to 200 ml with *water R*. Add about 50 mg of *xylenol orange triturate R* and *hexamethylenetetramine R* until the solution becomes violet-pink. Add 2 g of *hexamethylenetetramine R* in excess. Titrate with the sodium edetate solution until the violet-pink colour changes to yellow.

1 ml of *0.02 M sodium edetate* is equivalent to 1.308 mg of Zn.

1 M Sodium hydroxide. *3006300.*
Dissolve 42 g of *sodium hydroxide R* in *carbon dioxide-free water R* and dilute to 1000.0 ml with the same solvent.

Standardisation. Titrate 20.0 ml of the sodium hydroxide solution with *1 M hydrochloric acid* using the indicator prescribed in the assay in which *1 M sodium hydroxide* is used.

If sodium hydroxide free from carbonate is prescribed, prepare it as follows. Dissolve *sodium hydroxide R* in *water R* to give a concentration of 400 g/l to 600 g/l and allow to stand. Decant the clear supernatant liquid, taking precautions to avoid the introduction of carbon dioxide, and dilute with *carbon dioxide-free water R* to the required molarity. The solution complies with the following test. Titrate 20.0 ml of hydrochloric acid of the same molarity with the solution of sodium hydroxide, using 0.5 ml of *phenolphthalein solution R* as indicator. At the end-point add just sufficient of the acid to discharge the pink colour and concentrate the solution to 20 ml by boiling. During boiling add just sufficient acid to discharge the pink colour, which should not reappear after prolonged boiling. The volume of acid used does not exceed 0.1 ml.

0.1 M Sodium hydroxide. *3006600.*
Dilute 100.0 ml of *1 M sodium hydroxide* to 1000.0 ml with *carbon dioxide-free water R*.

Standardisation. Titrate 20.0 ml of the sodium hydroxide solution with *0.1 M hydrochloric acid*, using the end-point detection prescribed for the assay in which the *0.1 M sodium hydroxide* is used.

Standardisation (for use in the assay of halide salts of organic bases). Dissolve 0.100 g of *benzoic acid RV* in a mixture of 5 ml of *0.01 M hydrochloric acid* and 50 ml of *alcohol R*. Carry out the titration *(2.2.20)*, using the sodium hydroxide solution. Note the volume added between the 2 points of inflexion.

2 M Sodium hydroxide. *3009800.*
Dissolve 84 g of *sodium hydroxide R* in *carbon dioxide-free water R* and dilute to 1000.0 ml with the same solvent.

0.1 M Sodium hydroxide, ethanolic. *3007000.*
To 250 ml of *ethanol R* add 3.3 g of *strong sodium hydroxide solution R*.

Standardisation. Dissolve 0.100 g of *benzoic acid RV* in 2 ml of *water R* and 10 ml of *alcohol R*. Titrate with the ethanolic sodium hydroxide solution, using 0.2 ml of *thymolphthalein solution R* as indicator. Standardise immediately before use.

1 ml of *0.1 M ethanolic sodium hydroxide* is equivalent to 12.21 mg of $C_7H_6O_2$.

0.1 M Sodium methoxide. *3007100.*
Cool 175 ml of *anhydrous methanol R* in iced *water R* and add, in small portions, about 2.5 g of freshly cut *sodium R*. When the metal has dissolved, dilute to 1000.0 ml with *toluene R*.

Standardisation. To 10 ml of *dimethylformamide R* add 0.05 ml of a 3 g/l solution of *thymol blue R* in *methanol R*, and titrate with the sodium methoxide solution until a pure blue colour is obtained. Immediately add 0.200 g of *benzoic acid RV*. Stir to effect solution and titrate with the sodium methoxide solution until the pure blue colour is again obtained. Protect the solution from atmospheric carbon dioxide throughout the titration. From the volume of titrant used in the second titration ascertain the exact strength of the sodium methoxide solution. Standardise immediately before use.

1 ml of *0.1 M sodium methoxide* is equivalent to 12.21 mg of $C_7H_6O_2$.

0.1 M Sodium nitrite. *3007200.*
Dissolve 7.5 g of *sodium nitrite R* in *water R* and dilute to 1000.0 ml with the same solvent.

Standardisation. Dissolve 0.300 g of *sulphanilic acid RV* in 50 ml of *dilute hydrochloric acid R* and carry out the determination of primary aromatic amino-nitrogen *(2.5.8)*, using the sodium nitrite solution and determining the end-point electrometrically. Standardise immediately before use.

1 ml of *0.1 M sodium nitrite* is equivalent to 17.32 mg of $C_6H_7NO_3S$.

0.1 M Sodium periodate. *3009500.*
Dissolve 21.4 g of *sodium periodate R* in about 500 ml of *water R* and dilute to 1000.0 ml with the same solvent.

Standardisation. In a stoppered flask, introduce 20.0 ml of the sodium periodate solution and add 5 ml of *perchloric acid R*. Close the flask and shake. Adjust the solution to pH 6.4 *(2.2.3)* using a saturated solution of *sodium hydrogen carbonate R*. Add 10 ml of *potassium iodide solution R*, close, shake and allow to stand for 2 min. Titrate with *0.025 M sodium arsenite* until the yellow colour almost disappears. Add 2 ml of *starch solution R* and titrate slowly until the colour is completely discharged.

0.1 M Sodium thiosulphate. *3007300.*
Dissolve 25 g of *sodium thiosulphate R* and 0.2 g of *sodium carbonate R* in *carbon dioxide-free water R* and dilute to 1000.0 ml with the same solvent.

Standardisation. To 10.0 ml of *0.033 M potassium bromate*, add 40 ml of *water R*, 10 ml of *potassium iodide solution R* and 5 ml of *hydrochloric acid R1*. Titrate with the sodium thiosulphate solution, using 1 ml of *starch solution R*, added towards the end of the titration, as indicator.

0.5 M Sulphuric acid. *3007800.*
Dissolve 28 ml of sulphuric acid R in *water R* and dilute to 1000.0 ml with the same solvent.

Standardisation. Dissolve 1.000 g of *sodium carbonate RV* in 50 ml of *water R*, add 0.1 ml of *methyl orange solution R*, and titrate with the sulphuric acid until the solution begins to turn reddish-yellow. Boil for about 2 min. The colour of the solutions reverts to yellow. Cool and titrate again until the reddish-yellow colour reappears.

1 ml of *0.5 M sulphuric acid* is equivalent to 53.00 mg of Na_2CO_3.

0.05 M Sulphuric acid. *3008000.*
Dilute 100.0 ml of *0.5 M sulphuric acid* to 1000.0 ml with *water R*.

Standardisation. Carry out the titration described for *0.5 M sulphuric acid*, using 0.100 g of *sodium carbonate RV*, dissolved in 20 ml of *water R*.

1 ml of *0.05 M sulphuric acid* is equivalent to 5.30 mg of Na_2CO_3.

0.1 M Tetrabutylammonium hydroxide. *3008300.*
Dissolve 40 g of *tetrabutylammonium iodide R* in 90 ml of *anhydrous methanol R*, add 20 g of finely powdered *silver oxide R* and shake vigorously for 1 h. Centrifuge a few millilitres of the mixture and test the supernatant liquid for iodides. If a positive reaction is obtained, add an additional 2 g of *silver oxide R* and shake for a further 30 min. Repeat this procedure until the liquid is free from iodides, filter the mixture through a fine sintered-glass filter and rinse the reaction vessel and filter with three quantities, each of 50 ml, of *toluene R*. Add the washings to the filtrate and dilute to 1000.0 ml with *toluene R*. Pass dry carbon dioxide-free nitrogen through the solution for 5 min.

Standardisation. To 10 ml of *dimethylformamide R* add 0.05 ml of a 3 g/l solution of *thymol blue R* in *methanol R* and titrate with the tetrabutylammonium hydroxide solution until a pure blue colour is obtained. Immediately add 0.200 g of *benzoic acid RV*. Stir to effect solution, and titrate with the tetrabutylammonium hydroxide solution until the pure blue colour is again obtained. Protect the solution from atmospheric carbon dioxide throughout the titration. From the volume of titrant used in the second titration ascertain the exact strength of the tetrabutylammonium hydroxide solution. Standardise immediately before use.

1 ml of *0.1 M tetrabutylammonium hydroxide* is equivalent to 12.21 mg of $C_7H_6O_2$.

0.1 M Tetrabutylammonium hydroxide in 2-propanol. *3008400.*
Prepare as described for *0.1 M tetrabutylammonium hydroxide* using *2-propanol R* instead of *toluene R* and standardise as described.

0.05 M Zinc chloride. *3008500.*
Dissolve 6.82 g of *zinc chloride R*, weighed with appropriate precautions, in *water R*. If necessary, add dropwise *dilute hydrochloric acid R* until the opalescence disappears. Dilute to 1000.0 ml with *water R*.

Standardisation. To 20.0 ml of the zinc chloride solution add 5 ml of *dilute acetic acid R* and carry out the determination of zinc by complexometry (*2.5.11*).

0.1 M Zinc sulphate. *3008600.*
Dissolve 29 g of *zinc sulphate R* in *water R* and dilute to 1000.0 ml with the same solvent.

Standardisation. To 20.0 ml of the zinc sulphate solution add 5 ml of *dilute acetic acid R* and carry out the determination of zinc by complexometry (*2.5.11*).

5.1. GENERAL TEXTS ON STERILITY

5.1.3. EFFICACY OF ANTIMICROBIAL PRESERVATION

If a pharmaceutical preparation does not itself have adequate antimicrobial activity, antimicrobial preservatives may be added, particularly to aqueous preparations, to prevent proliferation or to limit microbial contamination which, during normal conditions of storage and use, particularly for multidose containers, could occur in a product and present a hazard to the patient from infection and spoilage of the preparation. Antimicrobial preservatives must not be used as a substitute for good manufacturing practice.

The efficacy of an antimicrobial preservative may be enhanced or diminished by the active constituent of the preparation or by the formulation in which it is incorporated or by the container and closure used. The antimicrobial activity of the preparation in its final container is investigated over the period of validity to ensure that such activity has not been impaired by storage. Such investigations may be carried out on samples removed from the final container immediately prior to testing.

During development of a pharmaceutical preparation, it shall be demonstrated that the antimicrobial activity of the preparation as such or, if necessary, with the addition of a suitable preservative or preservatives provides adequate protection from adverse effects that may arise from microbial contamination or proliferation during storage and use of the preparation.

The efficacy of the antimicrobial activity may be demonstrated by the test described below. The test is not intended to be used for routine control purposes.

TEST FOR EFFICACY OF ANTIMICROBIAL PRESERVATION

The test consists of challenging the preparation, wherever possible in its final container, with a prescribed inoculum of suitable micro-organisms, storing the inoculated preparation at a prescribed temperature, withdrawing samples from the container at specified intervals of time and counting the organisms in the samples so removed.

The preservative properties of the preparation are adequate if, in the conditions of the test, there is a significant fall or no increase, as appropriate, in the number of micro-organisms in the inoculated preparation after the times and at the temperatures prescribed. The criteria of acceptance, in terms of decrease in the number of micro-organisms with time, vary for different types of preparations according to the degree of protection intended (see Tables 5.1.3.-1/2/3).

Test micro-organisms

Pseudomonas aeruginosa	ATCC 9027; NCIMB 8626; CIP 82.118.
Staphylococcus aureus	ATCC 6538; NCTC 10788; NCIMB 9518; CIP 4.83.
Candida albicans	ATCC 10231; NCPF 3179; IP 48.72.
Aspergillus niger	ATCC 16404; IMI 149007; IP 1431.83.

Single-strain challenges are used and the designated micro-organisms are supplemented, where appropriate, by other strains or species that may represent likely contaminants to the preparation. It is recommended, for example, that *Escherichia coli* (ATCC 8739; NCIMB 8545; CIP 53.126) is used for all oral preparations and *Zygosaccharomyces rouxii* (NCYC 381; IP 2021.92) for oral preparations containing a high concentration of sugar.

Preparation of inoculum

Preparatory to the test, inoculate the surface of agar medium B (*2.6.12*) for bacteria or agar medium C without the addition of antibiotics (*2.6.12*) for fungi, with the recently grown stock culture of each of the specified micro-organisms. Incubate the bacterial cultures at 30-35 °C for 18-24 h, the culture of *C. albicans* at 20-25 °C for 48 h, and the culture of *A. niger* at 20-25 °C for 1 week or until good sporulation is obtained. Subcultures may be needed after revival before the micro-organism is in its optimal state, but it is recommended that their number be kept to a minimum.

To harvest the bacterial and *C. albicans* cultures, use a sterile suspending fluid, containing 9 g/l of *sodium chloride R*, for dispersal and transfer of the surface growth into a suitable vessel. Add sufficient suspending fluid to reduce the microbial count to about 10^8 micro-organisms per millilitre. To harvest the *A. niger* culture, use a sterile suspending fluid containing 9 g/l of *sodium chloride R* and 0.5 g/l of *polysorbate 80 R* and adjust the spore count to about 10^8 per millilitre by adding the same solution.

Remove immediately a suitable sample from each suspension and determine the number of colony-forming units per millilitre in each suspension by plate count or membrane filtration (*2.6.12*). This value serves to determine the inoculum and the baseline to use in the test. The suspensions shall be used immediately.

METHOD

To count the viable micro-organisms in the inoculated products, use the agar medium used for the initial cultivation of the respective micro-organisms.

Inoculate a series of containers of the product to be examined, each with a suspension of one of the test organisms to give an inoculum of 10^5 to 10^6 micro-organisms per millilitre or per gram of the preparation. The volume of the suspension of inoculum does not exceed 1 per cent of the volume of the product. Mix thoroughly to ensure homogeneous distribution.

Maintain the inoculated product at 20-25 °C, protected from light. Remove a suitable sample from each container, typically 1 ml or 1 g, at zero hour and at appropriate intervals according to the type of the product and determine the number of viable micro-organisms by plate count or membrane filtration (*2.6.12*). Ensure that any residual antimicrobial activity of the product is eliminated by dilution, by filtration or by the use of a specific inactivator. When dilution procedures are used, due allowance is made for the reduced sensitivity in the recovery of small numbers of viable micro-organisms. When a specific inactivator is used, the ability of the system to support the growth of the test organisms is confirmed by the use of appropriate controls.

The procedure is validated to verify its ability to demonstrate the required reduction in count of viable micro-organisms.

CRITERIA OF ACCEPTANCE

The criteria for evaluation of antimicrobial activity are given in Tables 5.1.3.-1/2/3 in terms of the log reduction in the number of viable micro-organisms against the value obtained for the inoculum.

5. General texts

Table 5.1.3.-1. - *Parenteral and ophthalmic preparations*

		Log reduction				
		6 h	24 h	7 d	14 d	28 d
Bacteria	A	2	3	-	-	NR*
	B	-	1	3	-	NI**
Fungi	A	-	-	2	-	NI
	B	-	-	-	1	NI

*NR: no recover

**NI: no increase

The A criteria express the recommended efficacy to be achieved. In justified cases where the A criteria cannot be attained, for example for reasons of an increased risk of adverse reactions, the B criteria must be satisfied.

Table 5.1.3.-2. - *Topical preparations*

		Log reduction			
		2 d	7 d	14 d	28 d
Bacteria	A	2	3	-	NI
	B	-	-	3	NI
Fungi	A	-	-	2	NI
	B	-	-	1	NI

The A criteria express the recommended efficacy to be achieved. In justified cases where the A criteria cannot be attained, for example for reasons of an increased risk of adverse reactions, the B criteria must be satisfied.

Table 5.1.3.-3. - *Oral preparations*

	Log reduction	
	14 d	28 d
Bacteria	3	NI
Fungi	1	NI

The above criteria express the recommended efficacy to be achieved.

DOSAGE FORMS

04/2003:1163

EYE PREPARATIONS

Ophthalmica

DEFINITION

Eye preparations are sterile liquid, semi-solid or solid preparations intended for administration upon the eyeball and/or to the conjunctiva or for insertion in the conjunctival sac.

Where applicable, containers for eye preparations comply with the requirements of *Materials used for the manufacture of containers* (*3.1* and subsections) and *Containers* (*3.2* and subsections).

Several categories of eye preparations may be distinguished:

— eye drops,

— eye lotions,

— powders for eye drops and eye lotions,

— semi-solid eye preparations,

— ophthalmic inserts.

PRODUCTION

During the development of an eye preparation, the formulation for which contains an antimicrobial preservative, the effectiveness of the chosen preservative shall be demonstrated to the satisfaction of the competent authority. A suitable test method together with criteria for judging the preservative properties of the formulation are provided in the text on *Efficacy of antimicrobial preservation* (*5.1.3*).

Eye preparations are prepared using materials and methods designed to ensure sterility and to avoid the introduction of contaminants and the growth of micro-organisms; recommendations on this aspect are provided in the text on *Methods of preparation of sterile products* (*5.1.1*).

In the manufacture of eye preparations containing dispersed particles, measures are taken to ensure a suitable and controlled particle size with regard to the intended use.

TESTS

Sterility (*2.6.1*). Eye preparations comply with the test for sterility. Applicators supplied separately also comply with the test for sterility. Remove the applicator with aseptic precautions from its package and transfer it to a tube of culture medium so that it is completely immersed. Incubate and interpret the results as described in the test for sterility.

Deliverable mass or volume (*2.9.28*). Liquid and semi-solid eye preparations supplied in single-dose containers comply with the test.

STORAGE

Unless otherwise prescribed, store in a sterile, airtight, tamper-proof container.

LABELLING

The label states the name of any added antimicrobial preservative.

Eye-drops

DEFINITION

Eye-drops are sterile aqueous or oily solutions or suspensions of one or more active substances intended for instillation into the eye.

Eye-drops may contain excipients, for example, to adjust the tonicity or the viscosity of the preparation, to adjust or stabilise the pH, to increase the solubility of the active substance, or to stabilise the preparation. These substances do not adversely affect the intended medicinal action or, at the concentrations used, cause undue local irritation.

Aqueous preparations supplied in multidose containers contain a suitable antimicrobial preservative in appropriate concentration except when the preparation itself has adequate antimicrobial properties. The antimicrobial preservative chosen must be compatible with the other ingredients of the preparation and must remain effective throughout the period of time during which eye-drops are in use.

If eye-drops are prescribed without antimicrobial preservatives they are supplied wherever possible in single-dose containers. Eye-drops intended for use in surgical procedures do not contain antimicrobial preservatives and are supplied in single-dose containers.

Eye-drops that are solutions, examined under suitable conditions of visibility, are practically clear and practically free from particles.

Eye-drops that are suspensions may show a sediment that is readily redispersed on shaking to give a suspension which remains sufficiently stable to enable the correct dose to be delivered.

Multidose preparations are supplied in containers that allow successive drops of the preparation to be administered. The containers contain at most 10 ml of the preparation, unless otherwise justified and authorised.

TESTS

Particle size. Unless otherwise justified and authorised, eye-drops in the form of a suspension comply with the following test: introduce a suitable quantity of the suspension into a counting cell or with a micropipette onto a slide, as appropriate, and scan under a microscope an area corresponding to 10 μg of the solid phase. For practical reasons, it is recommended that the whole sample is first scanned at low magnification (e.g. × 50) and particles greater than 25 μm are identified. These larger particles can then be measured at a larger magnification (e.g. × 200 to × 500). For each 10 μg of solid active substance, not more than 20 particles have a maximum dimension greater than 25 μm, and not more than 2 of these particles have a maximum dimension greater than 50 μm. None of the particles has a maximum dimension greater than 90 μm.

LABELLING

The label states:

— for multidose containers, the period after opening the container after which the contents must not be used. This period does not exceed 4 weeks, unless otherwise justified and authorised.

Eye lotions

DEFINITION

Eye lotions are sterile aqueous solutions intended for use in washing or bathing the eye or for impregnating eye dressings.

Eye lotions may contain excipients, for example to adjust the tonicity or the viscosity of the preparation or to adjust or stabilise the pH. These substances do not adversely affect the intended action or, at the concentrations used, cause undue local irritation.

Eye lotions supplied in multidose containers contain a suitable antimicrobial preservative in appropriate concentration except when the preparation itself has adequate antimicrobial properties. The antimicrobial preservative chosen is compatible with the other ingredients of the preparation and remains effective throughout the period of time during which the eye lotions are in use.

If eye lotions are prescribed without an antimicrobial preservative, they are supplied in single-dose containers. Eye lotions intended for use in surgical procedures or in first-aid treatment do not contain an antimicrobial preservative and are supplied in single-dose containers.

Eye lotions examined under suitable conditions of visibility, are practically clear and practically free from particles.

The containers for multidose preparations do not contain more than 200 ml of eye lotion, unless otherwise justified and authorised.

LABELLING

The label states:

— where applicable, that the contents are to be used on one occasion only,

— for multidose preparations, the period after opening the container after which the contents must not be used. This period does not exceed 4 weeks, unless otherwise justified and authorised.

Powders for eye-drops and powders for eye lotions

DEFINITION

Powders for the preparation of eye-drops and eye lotions are supplied in a dry, sterile form to be dissolved or suspended in an appropriate liquid vehicle at the time of administration. They may contain excipients to facilitate dissolution or dispersion, to prevent caking, to adjust the tonicity, to adjust or stabilise the pH or to stabilise the preparation.

After dissolution or suspension in the prescribed liquid, they comply with the requirements for eye-drops or eye lotions, as appropriate.

TESTS

Uniformity of content (*2.9.6*). Unless otherwise prescribed or justified and authorised, single-dose powders for eye-drops and eye lotions with a content of active substance less then 2 mg or less than 2 per cent of the total mass comply with test B for uniformity of content of single-dose preparations. If the preparation has more than one active substance, the requirement applies only to those substances which correspond to the above condition.

Uniformity of mass (*2.9.5*). Single-dose powders for eye-drops and eye lotions comply with the test for uniformity of mass of single-dose preparations. If the test for uniformity of content is prescribed for all the active substances, the test for uniformity of mass is not required.

Semi-solid eye preparations

DEFINITION

Semi-solid eye preparations are sterile ointments, creams or gels intended for application to the conjunctiva. They contain one or more active substances dissolved or dispersed in a suitable basis. They have a homogeneous appearance.

Semi-solid eye preparations comply with the requirements of the monograph on *Semi-solid preparations for cutaneous application (0132)*. The basis is non-irritant to the conjunctiva.

Semi-solid eye preparations are packed in small, sterilised collapsible tubes fitted or provided with a cannula and having a content of not more than 5 g of the preparation. The tubes must be well-closed to prevent microbial contamination. Semi-solid eye preparations may also be packed in suitably designed single-dose containers. The containers, or the nozzles of tubes, are of such a shape as to facilitate administration without contamination. Tubes are tamper-proof.

TESTS

Particle size. Semi-solid eye preparations containing dispersed solid particles comply with the following test: spread gently a quantity of the preparation corresponding to at least 10 µg of solid active substance as a thin layer. Scan under a microscope the whole area of the sample. For practical reasons, it is recommended that the whole sample is first scanned at a small magnification (e.g. × 50) and particles greater than 25 µm are identified. These larger particles can then be measured at a larger magnification (e.g. × 200 to × 500). For each 10 µg of solid active substance, not more than 20 particles have a maximum dimension greater than 25 µm, and not more than 2 of these particles have a maximum dimension greater than 50 µm. None of the particles has a maximum dimension greater than 90 µm.

Ophthalmic inserts

DEFINITION

Ophthalmic inserts are sterile, solid or semi-solid preparations of suitable size and shape, designed to be inserted in the conjunctival sac, to produce an ocular effect. They generally consist of a reservoir of active substance embedded in a matrix or bounded by a rate-controlling membrane. The active substance, which is more or less soluble in physiological fluids, is released over a determined period of time.

Ophthalmic inserts are individually distributed into sterile containers.

PRODUCTION

In the manufacture of ophthalmic inserts, means must be taken to ensure a suitable dissolution behaviour.

TESTS

Uniformity of content (*2.9.6*). Ophthalmic inserts comply, where applicable, with test A for uniformity of content.

LABELLING

The label states:

— where applicable, the total quantity of active substance per insert,

— where applicable, the dose released per unit time.

04/2003:0499

GRANULES

Granulata

Requirements for granules to be used for the preparation of oral solutions or suspensions are given in the monograph on Liquid preparations for oral use (0672). Where justified and authorised, the requirements of this monograph do not apply to granules for veterinary use.

DEFINITION

Granules are preparations consisting of solid, dry aggregates of powder particles sufficiently resistant to withstand handling. They are intended for oral administration. Some are swallowed as such, some are chewed and some are dissolved or dispersed in water or another suitable liquid before being administered.

Granules contain one or more active substances with or without excipients and, if necessary, colouring matter authorised by the competent authority and flavouring substances.

Granules are presented as single-dose or multidose preparations. Each dose of a multidose preparation is administered by means of a device suitable for measuring the quantity prescribed. For single-dose granules, each dose is enclosed in an individual container, for example a sachet or a vial.

Where applicable, containers for granules comply with the requirements of *Materials used for the manufacture of containers* (*3.1* and subsections) and *Containers* (*3.2* and subsections).

Several categories of granules may be distinguished:

— effervescent granules,
— coated granules,
— gastro-resistant granules,
— modified-release granules.

PRODUCTION

In the manufacture, packaging, storage and distribution of granules, suitable means are taken to ensure their microbial quality; recommendations on this aspect are provided in the text on *Microbiological quality of pharmaceutical preparations* (*5.1.4*).

TESTS

Uniformity of content (*2.9.6*). Unless otherwise prescribed or justified and authorised, single-dose granules with a content of active substance less than 2 mg or less than 2 per cent of the total mass comply with test B for uniformity of content of single-dose preparations. If the preparation has more than one active substance, the requirement applies only to those substances which correspond to the above conditions.

Uniformity of mass (*2.9.5*). Single-dose granules except for coated granules comply with the test for uniformity of mass of single-dose preparations. If the test for uniformity of content is prescribed for all the active substances, the test for uniformity of mass is not required.

Uniformity of mass of delivered doses from multidose containers (*2.9.27*). Granules supplied in multidose containers comply with the test.

STORAGE

If the preparation contains volatile ingredients or the contents have to be protected, store in an airtight container.

Effervescent granules

DEFINITION

Effervescent granules are uncoated granules generally containing acid substances and carbonates or hydrogen carbonates which react rapidly in the presence of water to release carbon dioxide. They are intended to be dissolved or dispersed in water before administration.

TESTS

Disintegration. Place one dose of the effervescent granules in a beaker containing 200 ml of *water R* at 15-25 °C; numerous bubbles of gas are evolved. When the evolution of gas around the individual grains ceases, the granules have disintegrated, being either dissolved or dispersed in the water. Repeat the operation on 5 other doses. The preparation complies with the test if each of the 6 doses used disintegrates within 5 min.

STORAGE

In an airtight container.

Coated granules

DEFINITION

Coated granules are usually multidose preparations and consist of granules coated with one or more layers of mixtures of various excipients.

PRODUCTION

The substances used as coatings are usually applied as a solution or suspension in conditions in which evaporation of the vehicle occurs.

TESTS

Dissolution. A suitable test may be carried out to demonstrate the appropriate release of the active substance(s), for example one of the tests described in *Dissolution test for solid dosage forms* (*2.9.3*).

Modified-release granules

DEFINITION

Modified-release granules are coated or uncoated granules which contain special excipients or which are prepared by special procedures, or both, designed to modify the rate, the place or the time at which the active substance or substances are released.

Modified-release granules include prolonged-release granules and delayed-release granules.

PRODUCTION

A suitable test is carried out to demonstrate the appropriate release of the active substance(s).

TESTS

Dissolution. Carry out a suitable test to demonstrate the appropriate release of the active substance(s), for example the test described in *Dissolution test for solid dosage forms* (*2.9.3*).

Gastro-resistant granules

DEFINITION

Gastro-resistant granules are delayed-release granules that are intended to resist the gastric fluid and to release the active substance(s) in the intestinal fluid. These properties are achieved by covering the granules with a gastro-resistant material (enteric-coated granules) or by other suitable means.

General Notices (1) apply to all monographs and other texts

PRODUCTION

A suitable test is carried out to demonstrate the appropriate release of the active substance(s).

TESTS

Dissolution. Carry out a suitable test to demonstrate the appropriate release of the active substance(s), for example the test described in *Dissolution test for solid dosage forms (2.9.3)*.

04/2003:0927

LIQUID PREPARATIONS FOR CUTANEOUS APPLICATION

Praeparationes liquidae ad usum dermicum

Where justified and authorised, the requirements of this monograph do not apply to preparations intended for systemic and veterinary use.

DEFINITION

Liquid preparations for cutaneous application are preparations of a variety of viscosities intended for local or transdermal delivery of active ingredients. They are solutions, emulsions or suspensions which may contain one or more active substances in a suitable vehicle. They may contain suitable antimicrobial preservatives, antioxidants and other excipients such as stabilisers, emulsifiers and thickeners.

Emulsions may show evidence of phase separation but are readily redispersed on shaking. Suspensions may show a sediment which is readily dispersed on shaking to give a suspension which is sufficiently stable to enable a homogeneous preparation to be delivered.

Where applicable, containers for liquid preparations for cutaneous application comply with the requirements of *Materials used for the manufacture of containers (3.1* and subsections) and *Containers (3.2* and subsections).

When liquid preparations for cutaneous application are dispensed in pressurised containers, the containers comply with the requirements of the monograph on *Pressurised pharmaceutical preparations (0523)*.

Preparations specifically intended for use on severely injured skin are sterile.

Several categories of liquid preparations for cutaneous application may be distinguished, for example:

— shampoos,

— cutaneous foams.

PRODUCTION

During the development of a liquid preparation for cutaneous application, the formulation for which contains an antimicrobial preservative, the effectiveness of the chosen preservative shall be demonstrated to the satisfaction of the competent authority. A suitable test method together with criteria for judging the preservative properties of the formulation are provided in the text on *Efficacy of antimicrobial preservation (5.1.3)*.

In the manufacture, packaging, storage and distribution of liquid preparations for cutaneous application, suitable means are taken to ensure their microbial quality; recommendations on this aspect are provided in the text on *Microbiological quality of pharmaceutical preparations (5.1.4)*.

Sterile liquid preparations for cutaneous application are prepared using materials and methods designed to ensure sterility and to avoid the introduction of contaminants and the growth of micro-organisms; recommendations on this aspect are provided in the text on *Methods of preparation of sterile products (5.1.1)*.

In the manufacture of liquid preparations for cutaneous application containing dispersed particles, measures are taken to ensure a suitable and controlled particle size with regard to the intended use.

TESTS

Deliverable mass or volume (*2.9.28*). Liquid preparations for cutaneous application supplied in single-dose containers comply with the test.

Sterility (*2.6.1*). Where the label indicates that the preparation is sterile, it complies with the test for sterility.

STORAGE

If the preparation is sterile, store in a sterile, airtight, tamper-proof container.

LABELLING

The label states:

— the name of any added antimicrobial preservative,

— where applicable, that the preparation is sterile.

Shampoos

DEFINITION

Shampoos are liquid or, occasionally semi-solid preparations intended for application to the scalp and subsequent washing away with water. Upon rubbing with water they usually form a foam.

They are emulsions, suspensions or solutions. Shampoos normally contain surface active agents.

Cutaneous foams

DEFINITION

Cutaneous foams comply with the requirements of the monograph on *Medicated foams (1105)*.

04/2003:0672

LIQUID PREPARATIONS FOR ORAL USE

Praeparationes liquidae peroraliae

Where justified and authorised, the requirements of this monograph do not apply to liquid preparations for oral use intended for veterinary use.

DEFINITION

Liquid preparations for oral use are usually solutions, emulsions or suspensions containing one or more active substances in a suitable vehicle; they may, however, consist of liquid active substances used as such (oral liquids).

Some preparations for oral use are prepared by dilution of concentrated liquid preparations, or from powders or granules for the preparation of oral solutions or suspensions, for oral drops or for syrups, using a suitable vehicle.

The vehicle for any preparations for oral use is chosen having regard to the nature of the active substance(s) and to provide organoleptic characteristics appropriate to the intended use of the preparation.

Liquid preparations for oral use may contain suitable antimicrobial preservatives, antioxidants and other excipients such as dispersing, suspending, thickening, emulsifying, buffering, wetting, solubilising, stabilising, flavouring and sweetening agents and colouring matter, authorised by the competent authority.

Emulsions may show evidence of phase separation but are readily redispersed on shaking. Suspensions may show a sediment which is readily dispersed on shaking to give a suspension which remains sufficiently stable to enable the correct dose to be delivered.

Where applicable, containers for liquid preparations for oral use comply with the requirements of *Materials used for the manufacture of containers* (*3.1* and subsections) and *Containers* (*3.2* and subsections).

Several categories of preparations may be distinguished:
— oral solutions, emulsions and suspensions,
— powders and granules for oral solutions and suspensions,
— oral drops,
— powders for oral drops,
— syrups,
— powders and granules for syrups.

PRODUCTION

During the development of a preparation for oral use, the formulation for which contains an antimicrobial preservative, the effectiveness of the chosen preservative shall be demonstrated to the satisfaction of the competent authority. A suitable test method together with criteria for judging the preservative properties of the formulation are provided in the text on *Efficacy of antimicrobial preservation* (*5.1.3*).

In the manufacturing, packaging, storage and distribution of liquid preparations for oral use, suitable means are taken to ensure their microbial quality; recommendations on this aspect are provided in the text on *Microbiological quality of pharmaceutical preparations* (*5.1.4*).

In the manufacture of liquid preparations for oral use containing dispersed particles, measures are taken to ensure a suitable and controlled particle size with regard to the intended use.

TESTS

Uniformity of content (*2.9.6*). Unless otherwise prescribed or justified and authorised, single-dose preparations that are suspensions comply with the following test. After shaking, empty each container as completely as possible and carry out the test on the individual contents. They comply with test B for uniformity of content of single-dose preparations.

Uniformity of mass. Single-dose preparations that are solutions or emulsions comply with the following test: weigh individually the contents of 20 containers, emptied as completely as possible, and determine the average mass. Not more than 2 of the individual masses deviate by more than 10 per cent from the average mass and none deviates by more than 20 per cent.

Dose and uniformity of dose of oral drops. Into a suitable, graduated cylinder, introduce by means of the dropping device the number of drops usually prescribed for one dose or introduce by means of the measuring device, the usually prescribed quantity. The dropping speed does not exceed 2 drops per second. Weigh the liquid, repeat the addition, weigh again and carry on repeating the addition and weighing until a total of 10 masses are obtained. No single mass deviates by more than 10 per cent from the average mass. The total of 10 masses does not differ by more than 15 per cent from the nominal mass of 10 doses. If necessary, measure the total volume of 10 doses. The volume does not differ by more than 15 per cent from the nominal volume of 10 doses.

Deliverable mass or volume (*2.9.28*). Liquid preparations for oral use supplied in single-dose containers comply with the test.

Uniformity of mass of delivered doses from multidose containers (*2.9.27*). Liquid preparations for oral use supplied in multidose containers comply with the test.

LABELLING

The label states the name of any added antimicrobial preservative.

Oral solutions, emulsions and suspensions

DEFINITION

Oral solutions, emulsions and suspensions are supplied in single-dose or multi-dose containers. Each dose from a multi-dose container is administered by means of a device suitable for measuring the prescribed volume. The device is usually a spoon or a cup for volumes of 5 ml or multiples thereof or an oral syringe for other volumes.

Powders and granules for oral solutions and suspensions

DEFINITION

Powders and granules for the preparation of oral solutions or suspensions generally conform to the definitions in the monographs on *Oral powders (1165)* or *Granules (0499)* as appropriate. They may contain excipients in particular to facilitate dispersion or dissolution and to prevent caking.

After dissolution or suspension, they comply with the requirements for oral solutions or oral suspensions, as appropriate.

TESTS

Uniformity of content (*2.9.6*). Unless otherwise prescribed or justified and authorised, single-dose powders and single-dose granules with a content of active substance less than 2 mg or less than 2 per cent of the total mass comply with test B for uniformity of content of single-dose preparations. If the preparation has more than one active substance, the requirement applies only to those substances that correspond to the above conditions.

Uniformity of mass (*2.9.5*). Single-dose powders and single-dose granules comply with the test for uniformity of mass of single-dose preparations. If the test for uniformity of content is prescribed for all the active substances, the test for uniformity of mass is not required.

LABELLING

The label states:
— the method of preparation of the solution or suspension,
— the conditions and the duration of storage after constitution.

Oral drops

DEFINITION

Oral drops are solutions, emulsions or suspensions which are administered in small volumes such as drops by the means of a suitable device.

LABELLING

The label states the number of drops per millilitre of preparation or per gram of preparation if the dose is measured in drops.

Powders for oral drops

DEFINITION

Powders for the preparation of oral drops generally conform to the definition of *Oral powders (1165)*. They may contain excipients to facilitate dissolution or suspension in the prescribed liquid or to prevent caking.

After dissolution or suspension, they comply with the requirements for oral drops.

TESTS

Uniformity of content (*2.9.6*). Unless otherwise prescribed or justified and authorised, single-dose powders for oral drops with a content of active substance less than 2 mg or less than 2 per cent of the total mass comply with test B for uniformity of content of single-dose preparations. If the preparation has more than one active substance, the requirement applies only to those substances that correspond to the above conditions.

Uniformity of mass (*2.9.5*). Single-dose powders for oral drops comply with the test for uniformity of mass of single-dose preparations. If the test for uniformity of content is prescribed for all the active substances, the test for uniformity of mass is not required.

Syrups

DEFINITION

Syrups are aqueous preparations characterised by sweet taste and a viscous consistency. They may contain sucrose at a concentration of at least 45 per cent *m/m*. The sweet taste can also be obtained by using other polyols or sweetening agents. Syrups usually contain aromatic or other flavouring agents. Each dose from a multi-dose container is administered by means of a device suitable for measuring the prescribed volume. The device is usually a spoon or a cup for volumes of 5 ml or multiples thereof.

LABELLING

The label states the name and concentration of the polyol or sweetening agent.

Powders and granules for syrups

DEFINITION

Powders and granules for syrups generally conform to the definitions in the monograph on *Oral powders (1165)* or *Granules (0499)*. They may contain excipients to facilitate dissolution.

After dissolution, they comply with the requirements for syrups.

TESTS

Uniformity of content (*2.9.6*). Unless otherwise prescribed or justified and authorised, single-dose powders and granules for syrups with a content of active substance less than 2 mg or less than 2 per cent of the total mass comply with test B for uniformity of content of single-dose preparations. If the preparation has more than one active substance, the requirement applies only to those substances that correspond to the above conditions.

Uniformity of mass (*2.9.5*). Single-dose powders and granules for syrups comply with the test for uniformity of mass of single-dose preparations. If the test for uniformity of content is prescribed for all the active substances, the test for uniformity of mass is not required.

04/2003:1165

POWDERS, ORAL

Pulveres perorales

Requirements for powders to be used for the preparation of oral solutions or suspensions are given in the monograph for Liquid preparations for oral use (0672). Where justified and authorised, the requirements of this monograph do not apply to oral powders intended for veterinary use.

DEFINITION

Oral powders are preparations consisting of solid, loose, dry particles of varying degrees of fineness. They contain one or more active substances, with or without excipients and, if necessary, colouring matter authorised by the competent authority and flavouring substances. They are generally administered in or with water or another suitable liquid. They may also be swallowed directly. They are presented as single-dose or multidose preparations.

Where applicable, containers for oral powders comply with the requirements of *Materials used for the manufacture of containers (3.1 and subsections)* and *Containers (3.2 and subsections)*.

Multidose oral powders require the provision of a measuring device capable of delivering the quantity prescribed. Each dose of a single-dose powder is enclosed in an individual container, for example a sachet or a vial.

PRODUCTION

In the manufacture of oral powders, means are taken to ensure a suitable particle size with regard to the intended use.

In the manufacture, packaging, storage and distribution of oral powders, suitable means are taken to ensure their microbial quality; recommendations on this aspect are provided in the text on *Microbiological quality of pharmaceutical preparations (5.1.4)*.

TESTS

Uniformity of content (*2.9.6*). Unless otherwise prescribed or justified and authorised, single-dose oral powders with a content of active substance less than 2 mg or less than 2 per cent of the total mass comply with test B for uniformity of content of single-dose preparations. If the preparation has more than one active substance, the requirement applies only to those substances which correspond to the above conditions.

Uniformity of mass (*2.9.5*). Single-dose oral powders comply with the test for uniformity of mass of single-dose preparations. If the test for uniformity of content is prescribed for all the active substances, the test for uniformity of mass is not required.

Uniformity of mass of delivered doses from multidose containers (*2.9.27*). Oral powders supplied in multidose containers comply with the test.

STORAGE

If the preparation contains volatile ingredients, or the contents have to be protected, store in an airtight container.

Effervescent powders

Effervescent powders are presented as single-dose or multidose preparations and generally contain acid substances and carbonates or hydrogen carbonates which react rapidly in the presence of water to release carbon dioxide. They are intended to be dissolved or dispersed in water before administration.

STORAGE

In an airtight container.

04/2003:0671

PREPARATIONS FOR INHALATION

Inhalanda

DEFINITION

Preparations for inhalation are liquid or solid preparations intended for administration as vapours or aerosols to the lung in order to obtain a local or systemic effect. They contain one or more active substances which may be dissolved or dispersed in a suitable vehicle.

Preparations for inhalation may, depending on the type of preparation, contain propellants, co-solvents, diluents, antimicrobial preservatives, solubilising and stabilising agents, etc. These excipients do not adversely affect the functions of the mucosa of the respiratory tract or its cilia.

Preparations for inhalation are supplied in multidose or single-dose containers. When supplied in pressurised containers, they comply with the requirements of the monograph on *Pressurised pharmaceutical preparations (0523)*.

Preparations intended to be administered as aerosols (dispersions of solid or liquid particles in a gas) are administered by one of the following devices:

– nebuliser,

– pressurised metered-dose inhaler,

– dry-powder inhaler.

PRODUCTION

During the development of a preparation for inhalation which contains an antimicrobial preservative, the effectiveness of the chosen preservative shall be demonstrated to the satisfaction of the competent authority. A suitable test method together with the criteria for judging the preservative properties of the formulation are described in the text on *Efficacy of antimicrobial preservation (5.1.3)*.

The size of aerosol particles to be inhaled is controlled so that a significant fraction is deposited in the lung. The fine-particle characteristics of preparations for inhalation are determined by the method for *Aerodynamic assessment of fine particles (2.9.18)*.

In assessing the uniformity of delivered dose of a multidose inhaler, it is not sufficient to test a single inhaler. Manufacturers must substitute procedures which take both inter- and intra-inhaler dose uniformity into account. A suitable procedure based on the intra-inhaler test would be to collect each of the specified doses at the beginning, middle and end of the number of doses stated on the label from separate inhalers.

Pressurised metered-dose inhalers are tested for leakage. All inhalers are tested for extraneous particulate contamination.

LABELLING

For metered-dose preparations the label states:

– the delivered dose, except for preparations for which the dose has been established as a metered-dose or as a predispensed-dose,

– where applicable, the number of deliveries from the inhaler to provide the minimum recommended dose,

– the number of deliveries per inhaler.

The label states, where applicable, the name of any added antimicrobial preservative.

Liquid preparations for inhalation

Three categories of liquid preparations for inhalation may be distinguished:

A. preparations intended to be converted into vapour,

B. liquid preparations for nebulisation,

C. pressurised metered-dose preparations for inhalation.

Liquid preparations for inhalation are solutions or dispersions.

Dispersions are readily dispersible on shaking and they remain sufficiently stable to enable the correct dose to be delivered. Suitable excipients may be used.

A. PREPARATIONS INTENDED TO BE CONVERTED INTO VAPOUR

DEFINITION

Preparations intended to be converted into vapour are solutions, dispersions or solid preparations. They are usually added to hot water and the vapour generated is inhaled.

B. LIQUID PREPARATIONS FOR NEBULISATION

DEFINITION

Liquid preparations for inhalation intended to be converted into aerosols by continuously operating nebulisers or metered-dose nebulisers are solutions, suspensions or emulsions. Suitable co-solvents or solubilisers may be used to increase the solubility of the active substances.

Liquid preparations for nebulisation in concentrated form for use in continuously operating nebulisers are diluted to the prescribed volume with the prescribed liquid before use. Liquids for nebulisation may also be prepared from powders. The pH of the liquid preparations for use in continuously operating nebulisers is not lower than 3 and not higher than 8.5.

Suspensions and emulsions are readily dispersible on shaking and they remain sufficiently stable to enable the correct dose to be delivered.

Aqueous preparations for nebulisation supplied in multidose containers may contain a suitable antimicrobial preservative at a suitable concentration except where the preparation itself has adequate antimicrobial properties.

Continuously operating nebulisers are devices that convert liquids into aerosols by high-pressure gases, ultrasonic vibration or other methods. They allow the dose to be inhaled at an appropriate rate and particle size which ensures deposition of the preparation in the lungs.

Metered-dose nebulisers are devices that convert liquids into aerosols by high-pressure gases, ultrasonic vibration or other methods. The volume of liquid to be nebulised is metered so that the aerosol dose can be inhaled with one breath.

C. PRESSURISED METERED-DOSE PREPARATIONS FOR INHALATION

DEFINITION

Pressurised metered-dose preparations for inhalation are solutions, suspensions or emulsions supplied in special containers equipped with a metering valve and which are held under pressure with suitable propellants or suitable mixtures of liquefied propellants, which can act also as solvents. Suitable co-solvents, solubilisers and stabilisers may be added.

Dosage forms

The delivered dose is the dose delivered from the inhaler to the patient. For some preparations, the dose has been established as a metered-dose. The metered-dose is determined by adding the amount deposited within the device to the delivered dose. It may also be determined directly.

TESTS

Uniformity of delivered dose. Containers usually operate in an inverted position. For containers that operate in an upright position, an equivalent test is applied using methods that ensure the complete collection of the delivered dose. In all cases, prepare the inhaler as directed in the instructions to the patient.

The dose collection apparatus must be capable of quantitatively capturing the delivered dose.

The following apparatus and procedure may be used.

The apparatus (Figure 0671.-1) consists of a filter-support base with an open-mesh filter-support, such as a stainless steel screen, a collection tube that is clamped or screwed to the filter-support base, and a mouthpiece adapter to ensure an airtight seal between the collection tube and the mouthpiece. Use a mouthpiece adapter which ensures that the front face of the inhaler mouthpiece is flush with the front face of the sample collection tube. The vacuum connector is connected to a system comprising a vacuum source and a flow regulator. The source should be adjusted to draw air through the complete assembly, including the filter and the inhaler to be tested, at 28.3 ± 1.5 litres/min. Air should be drawn continuously through the apparatus to avoid loss of the active substance into the atmosphere. The filter support base is designed to accommodate 25 mm

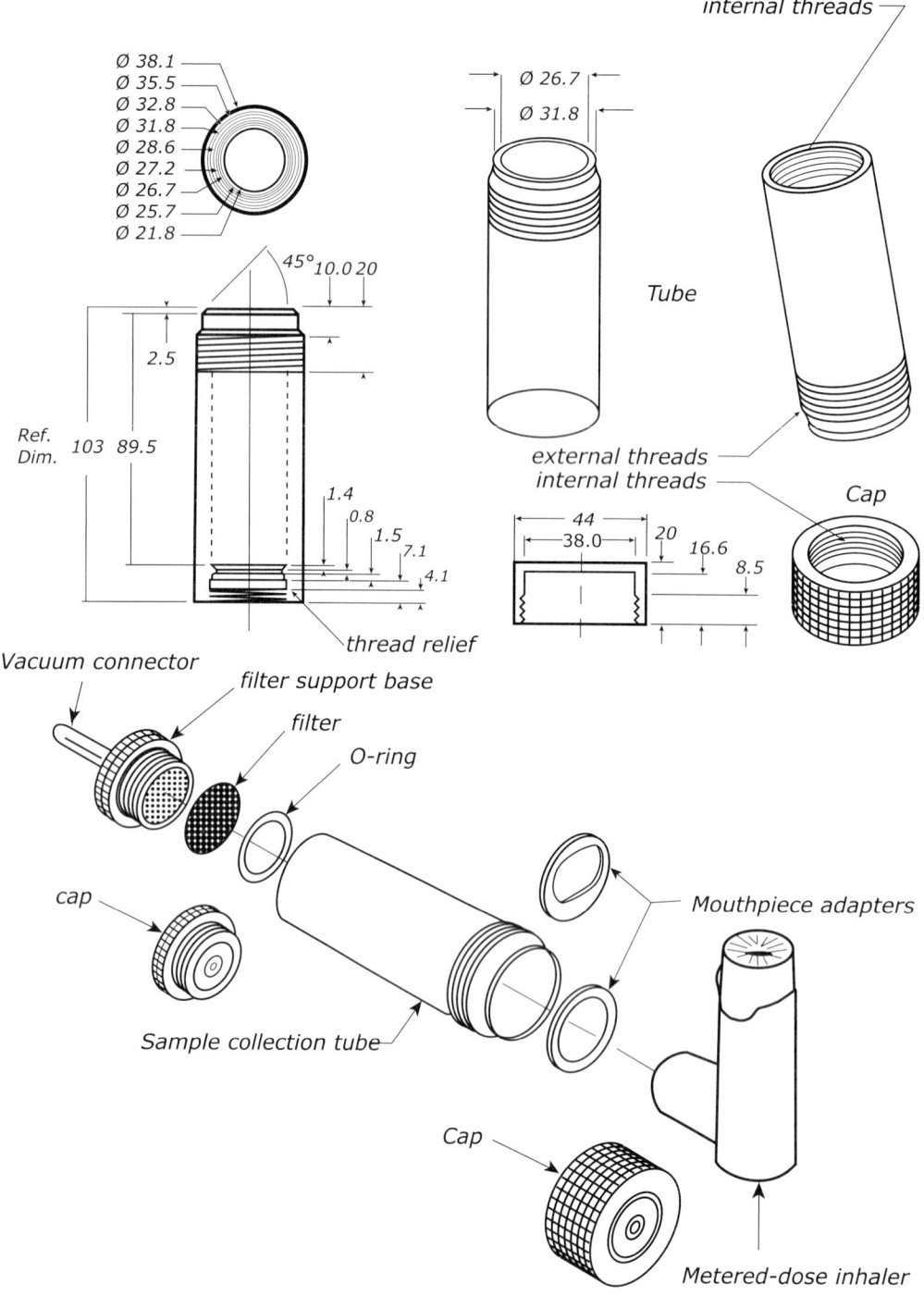

Figure 0671.-1. – *Dose collection apparatus for pressurised metered-dose preparations*
Dimensions in millimetres

diameter filter disks. The filter disk and other materials used in the construction of the apparatus must be compatible with the active substance and solvents that are used to extract the active substance from the filter. One end of the collection tube is designed to hold the filter disk tightly against the filter-support base. When assembled, the joints between the components of the apparatus are airtight so that when a vacuum is applied to the base of the filter, all of the air drawn through the collection tube passes through the inhaler.

Unless otherwise prescribed in the instructions to the patient, shake the inhaler for 5 s and discharge one delivery to waste. Fire the inverted inhaler into the apparatus, depressing the valve for a sufficient time to ensure complete discharge. Repeat the procedure until the number of deliveries that constitute the minimum recommended dose have been sampled. Quantitatively collect the contents of the apparatus and determine the amount of active substance.

Repeat the procedure for a further 2 doses.

Discharge the device to waste, waiting not less than 5 s between actuations until $(n/2)+1$ deliveries remain, where n is the number of deliveries stated on the label. Collect 4 doses using the procedure described above.

Discharge the device to waste, waiting not less than 5 s between actuations until 3 doses remain. Collect these 3 doses using the procedure described above.

For preparations containing more than one active substance, carry out the test for uniformity of delivered dose for each active substance.

Unless otherwise justified and authorised, the preparation complies with the test if 9 out of 10 results lie between 75 per cent and 125 per cent of the average value and all lie between 65 per cent and 135 per cent. If 2 or 3 values lie outside the range of 75 per cent to 125 per cent, repeat the test for 2 more inhalers. Not more than 3 of the 30 values lie outside the range 75 per cent to 125 per cent and no value lies outside the range 65 per cent to 135 per cent.

Fine particle dose. Using an apparatus and procedure described in *Aerodynamic assessment of fine particles* (*2.9.18 - apparatus C or D*), calculate the fine particle dose.

Number of deliveries per inhaler. Take one inhaler and discharge the contents to waste, actuating the valve at intervals of not less than 5 s. The total number of deliveries so discharged from the inhaler is not less than the number stated on the label (this test may be combined with the test for uniformity of delivered dose).

Powders for inhalation

DEFINITION

Powders for inhalation are presented as single-dose powders or multidose powders. To facilitate their use, active substances may be combined with a suitable carrier. They are generally administered by dry-powder inhalers. In pre-metered systems, the inhaler is loaded with powders pre-dispensed in capsules or other suitable pharmaceutical forms. For devices using a powder reservoir, the dose is created by a metering mechanism within the inhaler.

The delivered dose is the dose delivered from the inhaler. For some preparations, the dose has been established as a metered dose or as a predispensed dose. The metered dose is determined by adding the amount deposited within the device to the delivered dose. It may also be determined directly.

TESTS

Uniformity of delivered dose. In all cases, prepare the inhaler as directed in the instructions to the patient. The dose collection apparatus must be capable of quantitatively capturing the delivered dose. A dose collection apparatus similar to that described for the evaluation of pressurised metered-dose inhalers may be used provided that the dimensions of the tube and the filter can accommodate the measured flow rate. A suitable tube is defined in Figure 0671.-1. Connect the tube to a flow system according to the scheme specified in Figure 0671.-2 and Table 0671.-1.

Unless otherwise stated, determine the test flow rate and duration using the dose collection tube, the associated flow system, a suitable differential pressure meter and a suitable volumetric flow meter, calibrated for the flow leaving the meter, according to the following procedure.

Prepare the inhaler for use and connect it to the inlet of the apparatus using a mouthpiece adapter to ensure an airtight seal. Use a mouthpiece adapter which ensures that the front face of the inhaler mouthpiece is flush with the front face of the sample collection tube. Connect one port of a differential pressure meter to the pressure reading point, P1, in Figure 0671.-2 and let the other be open to the atmosphere. Switch on the pump, open the two way valve and adjust the flow control valve until the pressure drop across the inhaler is 4.0 kPa (40.8 cm H_2O) as indicated by the differential pressure meter. Remove the inhaler from the mouthpiece adapter and without touching the flow control valve, connect a flow meter to the inlet of the sampling apparatus. If the flow rate is above 100 litres/min adjust the flow control valve to obtain a flow rate of 100 ± 5 litres/min. Note the volumetric airflow rate and define this as the test flow rate, Q, in litres per minute. Define the test flow duration, T, in seconds so that a volume of 4 litres of air is drawn through the inhaler.

Ensure that critical flow occurs in the flow control valve by the following procedure. With the inhaler in place and the test flow rate Q, measure the absolute pressure on both sides of the control valve (pressure reading points P2 and P3 in Figure 0671.-2). A ratio P3/P2 $\leq$ 0.5 indicates critical flow. Switch to a more powerful pump and re-measure the test flow rate if critical flow is not indicated.

Predispensed systems. Prepare the inhaler as directed in the instructions to the patient and connect it to the apparatus using an adapter which ensures a good seal. Draw air through the inhaler using the predetermined conditions. Repeat the procedure until the number of deliveries which constitute the minimum recommended dose have been sampled. Quantitatively collect the contents of the apparatus and determine the amount of active substance.

Repeat the procedure for a further 9 doses.

Reservoir systems. Prepare the inhaler as directed in the instructions to the patient and connect it to the apparatus using an adapter which ensures a good seal. Draw air through the inhaler under the predetermined conditions. Repeat the procedure until the number of deliveries which constitute the minimum recommended dose have been sampled. Quantitatively collect the contents of the apparatus and determine the amount of active substance.

Repeat the procedure for a further 2 doses.

Discharge the device to waste until $(n/2)+1$ deliveries remain, where n is the number of deliveries stated on the label. If necessary, store the inhaler to discharge electrostatic charges. Collect 4 doses using the procedure described above.

Discharge the device to waste until 3 doses remain. If necessary, store the inhaler to discharge electrostatic charges. Collect 3 doses using the procedure described above.

For preparations containing more than 1 active substance, carry out the test for uniformity of delivered dose for each active substance.

The preparation complies with the test if 9 out of 10 results lie between 75 per cent and 125 per cent of the average value and all lie between 65 per cent and 135 per cent. If 2 or 3 values lie outside the range of 75 per cent to 125 per cent, repeat the test for 2 more inhalers. Not more than 3 of the 30 values lie outside the range 75 per cent to 125 per cent and no value lies outside the range 65 per cent to 135 per cent.

In justified and authorised cases, these ranges may be extended but no value should be greater than 150 per cent or less than 50 per cent of the average value.

Table 0671.-1. – *Specifications of the apparatus described in figure 0671.-2*

Code	Item	Description
A	Sample collection tube	Capable of quantitatively capturing the delivered dose, e.g. Dose collection tube similar to that described in Fig. 0671.-1 with dimensions of 34.85 mm ID × 12 cm length (e.g. product number XX40 047 00, Millipore Corporation, Bedford, MA 01732 with modified exit tube, ID ≥ 8 mm, fitted with Gelman product number 61631), or equivalent.
B	Filter	47 mm filter, e.g. A/E glass fibre filter (Gelman Sciences, Ann Arbor, MI 48106), or equivalent.
C	Connector	ID ≥ 8 mm, e.g., short metal coupling, with low-diameter branch to P3.
D	Vacuum tubing	8 ± 0.5 mm ID × 50 ± 10 cm length, e.g., silicone tubing with an OD of 14 mm and an ID of 8 mm.

Code	Item	Description
E	Two-way solenoid valve	Minimum airflow resistance orifice having an ID of ≥ 8 mm and a maximum response time of 100 ms (e.g. type 256-A08, Bürkert GmbH, D-74653 Ingelfingen), or equivalent.
F	Vacuum pump	Pump must be capable of drawing the required flow rate through the assembled apparatus with the dry powder inhaler in the mouthpiece adapter (e.g. product type 1023, 1423 or 2565, Gast Manufacturing Inc., Benton Harbor, MI 49022), or equivalent. Connect the pump to the solenoid valve using short and/or wide (≥ 10 mm ID) vacuum tubing and connectors to minimise pump capacity requirements.
G	Timer	Timer capable of driving the solenoid valve for the required time period (e.g. type G814, RS Components International, Corby, NN17 9RS, UK), or equivalent.
P1	Pressure tap	2.2 mm ID, 3.1 mm OD, flush with internal surface of the sample collection tube, centred and burr-free, 59 mm from its inlet.
P1 P2 P3	Pressure measurements	Differential pressure to atmosphere (P1) or absolute pressure (P2 and P3).
H	Flow control valve	Adjustable regulating valve with maximum $Cv \geq 1$, (e.g. type 8FV12LNSS, Parker Hannifin plc., Barnstaple, EX31 1NP, UK), or equivalent.

Fine particle dose. Using the apparatus and procedure described in *Aerodynamic assessment of fine particles (2.9.18 - apparatus C or D)*, calculate the fine particle dose.

Number of deliveries per inhaler for multidose inhalers. Discharge doses from the inhaler until empty, at the predetermined flow rate. Record the deliveries discharged. The total number of doses delivered is not less than the number stated on the label (this test may be combined with the test for uniformity of delivered dose).

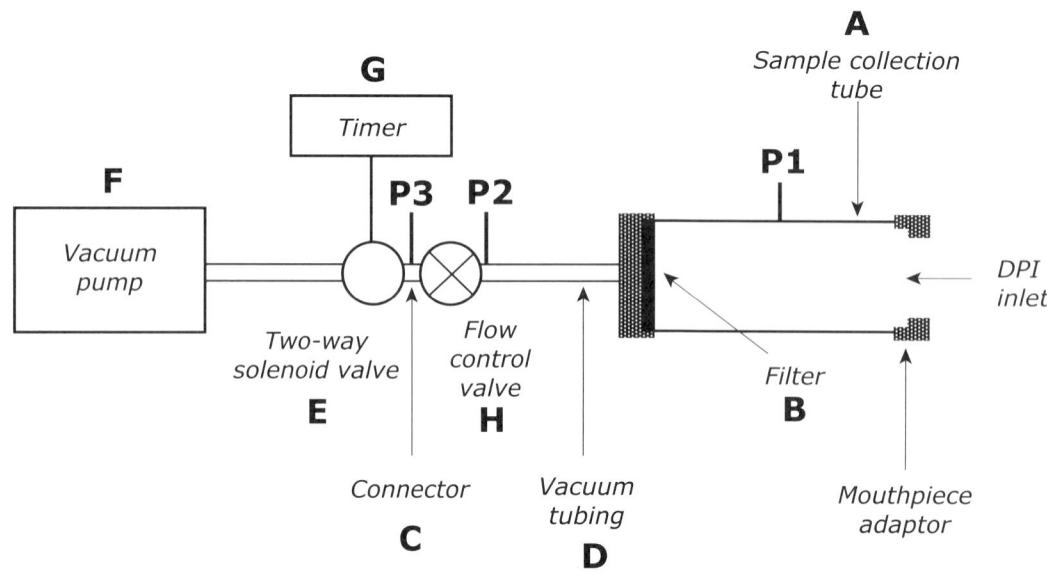

Figure 0671.-2. – *Apparatus suitable for measuring the uniformity of delivered dose for powder inhalers*

A

Monographs
A - C

01/2002:0580
corrected

APROTININ

Aprotininum

DEFINITION

Aprotinin is a polypeptide consisting of a chain of 58 amino acids. It inhibits stoichiometrically the activity of several proteolytic enzymes such as chymotrypsin, kallikrein, plasmin and trypsin. It contains not less than 3.0 Ph. Eur. U. of aprotinin activity per milligram, calculated with reference to the dried substance.

PRODUCTION

The animals from which aprotinin is derived must fulfil the requirements for the health of animals suitable for human consumption to the satisfaction of the competent authority.

The manufacturing process is validated to demonstrate suitable inactivation or removal of any contamination by viruses or other infectious agents.

The method of manufacture is validated to demonstrate that the product, if tested, would comply with the following tests:

Abnormal toxicity (*2.6.9*). Inject into each mouse a quantity of the substance to be examined containing 2 Ph. Eur. U. dissolved in a sufficient quantity of *water for injections R* to give a volume of 0.5 ml.

Histamine (*2.6.10*): maximum 0.2 μg of histamine base per 3 Ph. Eur. U.

CHARACTERS

Appearance: almost white powder, hygroscopic.

Solubility: soluble in water and in isotonic solutions, practically insoluble in organic solvents.

IDENTIFICATION

A. Thin-layer chromatography (*2.2.27*).

Test solution. Solution S (see Tests).

Reference solution. Aprotinin solution BRP.

Plate: *TLC silica gel G plate R.*

Mobile phase: *water R, glacial acetic acid R* (80:100 *V/V*) containing 100 g/l of *sodium acetate R.*

Application: 10 μl.

Development: over a path of 12 cm.

Drying: in air.

Detection: spray with a solution of 0.1 g of *ninhydrin R* in a mixture of 6 ml of a 10 g/l solution of *cupric chloride R*, 21 ml of *glacial acetic acid R* and 70 ml of *ethanol R*. Dry the plate at 60 °C.

Results: the principal spot in the chromatogram obtained with the test solution is similar in position, colour and size to the principal spot in the chromatogram obtained with the reference solution.

B. Determine the ability of the substance to be examined to inhibit trypsin activity using the method described below.

Test solution. Dilute 1 ml of solution S to 50 ml with *buffer solution pH 7.2 R.*

Trypsin solution. Dissolve 10 mg of *trypsin BRP* in *0.002 M hydrochloric acid* and dilute to 100 ml with the same acid.

Casein solution. Dissolve 0.2 g of *casein R* in *buffer solution pH 7.2 R* and dilute to 100 ml with the same buffer solution.

Precipitating solution. Mix 1 volume of *glacial acetic acid R*, 49 volumes of *water R* and 50 volumes of *ethanol R*.

Mix 1 ml of the test solution with 1 ml of the trypsin solution. Allow to stand for 10 min and add 1 ml of the casein solution. Incubate at 35 °C for 30 min. Cool in iced water and add 0.5 ml of the precipitating solution. Shake and allow to stand at room temperature for 15 min. The solution is cloudy. Carry out a blank test under the same conditions using *buffer solution pH 7.2 R* instead of the test solution. The solution is not cloudy.

TESTS

Solution S. Prepare a solution of the substance to be examined containing 15 Ph. Eur. U./ml, calculated from the activity stated on the label.

Appearance of solution. Solution S is clear (*2.2.1*).

Absorbance (*2.2.25*): maximum 0.80 by measuring at the absorption maximum at 277 nm.

Prepare a solution of the substance to be examined containing 3.0 Ph. Eur. U./ml.

Protein impurities of higher molecular mass. Size-exclusion chromatography (*2.2.30*).

Use *cross-linked dextran for chromatography R2*. Use a 180 g/l solution of *anhydrous acetic acid R* to swell the gel and as the eluent. Prepare a column of gel 0.8 m to 1.0 m long and 25 mm in diameter, taking care to avoid the introduction of air bubbles. Place at the top of the column a quantity of the substance to be examined containing 300 Ph. Eur. U. dissolved in 1 ml of a 180 g/l solution of *anhydrous acetic acid R* and allow to elute. Collect the eluate in fractions of 2 ml. Measure the absorbance (*2.2.25*) of each fraction at the absorption maximum at 277 nm and plot the values on a graph. The chromatogram obtained does not present an absorption maximum before the elution of the aprotinin.

Loss on drying (*2.2.32*): maximum 6.0 per cent, determined on 0.100 g by drying *in vacuo*.

Sterility (*2.6.1*). If intended for use in the manufacture of parenteral dosage forms without a further appropriate sterilisation procedure, it complies with the test for sterility.

Bacterial endotoxins (*2.6.14*): less than 0.14 IU per European Pharmacopoeia Unit of aprotinin, if intended for use in the manufacture of parenteral dosage forms without a further appropriate procedure for the removal of bacterial endotoxins.

ASSAY

The activity of aprotinin is determined by measuring its inhibitory action on a solution of trypsin of known activity. The inhibiting activity of the aprotinin is calculated from the difference between the initial activity and the residual activity of the trypsin.

The inhibiting activity of aprotinin is expressed in European Pharmacopoeia Units. 1 Ph. Eur. U. inhibits 50 per cent of the enzymatic activity of 2 microkatals of trypsin.

Use a reaction vessel with a capacity of about 30 ml and provided with:

— a device that will maintain a temperature of 25 ± 0.1 °C;

— a stirring device, such as a magnetic stirrer;

— a lid with 5 holes for accommodating the electrodes, the tip of a burette, a tube for the admission of nitrogen and the introduction of the reagents.

An automatic or manual titration apparatus may be used. In the latter case the burette is graduated in 0.05 ml and the pH-meter is provided with a wide reading scale and glass and calomel electrodes.

Test solution. Prepare a solution of the substance to be examined in *0.0015 M borate buffer solution pH 8.0 R* expected to contain 1.67 Ph. Eur. U./ml (about 0.6 mg (*m* mg) per millilitre).

Trypsin solution. Prepare a solution of *trypsin BRP* containing about 0.8 microkatals per millilitre (about 1 mg/ml), using *0.001 M hydrochloric acid* as the solvent. Use a freshly prepared solution and keep in iced water.

Trypsin and aprotinin solution. To 4.0 ml of the trypsin solution add 1.0 ml of the test solution. Dilute immediately to 40.0 ml with *0.0015 M borate buffer solution pH 8.0 R.* Allow to stand at room temperature for 10 min and then keep in iced water. Use within 6 h of preparation.

Dilute trypsin solution. Dilute 0.5 ml of the trypsin solution to 10.0 ml with *0.0015 M borate buffer solution pH 8.0 R.* Allow to stand at room temperature for 10 min and then keep in iced water.

Maintain an atmosphere of nitrogen in the reaction flask and stir continuously; introduce 9.0 ml of *0.0015 M borate buffer solution pH 8.0 R* and 1.0 ml of a freshly prepared 6.9 g/l solution of *benzoylarginine ethyl ester hydrochloride R.* Adjust to pH 8.0 with *0.1 M sodium hydroxide.* When the temperature has reached equilibrium at 25 ± 0.1 °C, add 1.0 ml of the trypsin and aprotinin solution and start a timer. Maintain at pH 8.0 by the addition of *0.1 M sodium hydroxide* and note the volume added every 30 s. Continue the reaction for 6 min. Determine the number of millilitres of *0.1 M sodium hydroxide* used per second (n_1 ml). Carry out, under the same conditions, a titration using 1.0 ml of the dilute trypsin solution. Determine the number of millilitres of *0.1 M sodium hydroxide* used per second (n_2 ml).

Calculate the aprotinin activity in European Pharmacopoeia Units per milligram from the expression:

$$\frac{4000\,(2n_2 - n_1)}{m}$$

The estimated activity is not less than 90 per cent and not more than 110 per cent of the activity stated on the label.

STORAGE

In an airtight, tamper-proof container, protected from light.

LABELLING

The label states:

— the number of European Pharmacopoeia Units of aprotinin activity per milligram,

— where applicable, that the substance is sterile,

— where applicable, that the substance is free from bacterial endotoxins.

01/2002:0579
corrected

APROTININ CONCENTRATED SOLUTION

Aprotinini solutio concentrata

DEFINITION

Aprotinin concentrated solution is a solution of aprotinin, a polypeptide consisting of a chain of 58 amino acids, which inhibits stoichiometrically the activity of several proteolytic enzymes such as chymotrypsin, kallikrein, plasmin and trypsin. It contains not less than 15.0 Ph. Eur. U. of aprotinin activity per millilitre.

PRODUCTION

The animals from which aprotinin is derived must fulfil the requirements for the health of animals suitable for human consumption to the satisfaction of the competent authority.

The manufacturing process is validated to demonstrate suitable inactivation or removal of any contamination by viruses or other infectious agents.

The method of manufacture is validated to demonstrate that the product, if tested, would comply with the following tests:

Abnormal toxicity (*2.6.9*). Inject into each mouse a quantity of the preparation to be examined containing 2 Ph. Eur. U. diluted with a sufficient quantity of *water for injections R* to give a volume of 0.5 ml.

Histamine (*2.6.10*): maximum 0.2 μg of histamine base per 3 Ph. Eur. U.

CHARACTERS

Appearance: clear and colourless liquid.

IDENTIFICATION

A. Thin-layer chromatography (*2.2.27*).

Test solution. Solution S (see Tests).

Reference solution. Aprotinin solution BRP.

Plate: TLC silica gel G plate R.

Mobile phase: water R, glacial acetic acid R (80:100 V/V) containing 100 g/l of *sodium acetate R*).

Application: 10 μl.

Development: over a path of 12 cm.

Drying: in air.

Detection: spray with a solution of 0.1 g of *ninhydrin R* in a mixture of 6 ml of a 10 g/l solution of *cupric chloride R*, 21 ml of *glacial acetic acid R* and 70 ml of *ethanol R.* Dry the plate at 60 °C.

Results: the principal spot in the chromatogram obtained with the test solution is similar in position, colour and size to the principal spot in the chromatogram obtained with the reference solution.

B. Determine the ability of the preparation to be examined to inhibit trypsin activity using the method described below.

Test solution. Dilute 1 ml of solution S to 50 ml with *buffer solution pH 7.2 R.*

Trypsin solution. Dissolve 10 mg of *trypsin BRP* in *0.002 M hydrochloric acid* and dilute to 100 ml with the same acid.

Casein solution. Dissolve 0.2 g of *casein R* in *buffer solution pH 7.2 R* and dilute to 100 ml with the same buffer solution.

Precipitating solution. Mix 1 volume of *glacial acetic acid R*, 49 volumes of *water R* and 50 volumes of *ethanol R.*

Mix 1 ml of the test solution with 1 ml of the trypsin solution. Allow to stand for 10 min and add 1 ml of the casein solution. Incubate at 35 °C for 30 min. Cool in iced water and add 0.5 ml of the precipitating solution. Shake and allow to stand at room temperature for 15 min. The solution is cloudy. Carry out a blank test under the same conditions using *buffer solution pH 7.2 R* instead of the test solution. The solution is not cloudy.

TESTS

Solution S. Prepare a solution containing 15 Ph. Eur. U./ml, if necessary by dilution on the basis of the activity stated on the label.

Appearance of solution. Solution S is clear (*2.2.1*).

Absorbance (*2.2.25*): maximum 0.80 by measuring at the absorption maximum at 277 nm.

Prepare from the concentrated solution a dilution containing 3.0 Ph. Eur. U./ml.

Protein impurities of higher molecular mass. Size-exclusion chromatography (*2.2.30*).

Freeze-dry the preparation to be examined using a pressure of 2.7 Pa and a temperature of -30 °C; the operation, including freeze-drying and a period of drying at 15-25 °C, takes 6-12 h.

Use *cross-linked dextran for chromatography R2*. Use a 180 g/l solution of *anhydrous acetic acid R* to swell the gel and as the eluent. Prepare a column of gel 0.8 m to 1.0 m long and 25 mm in diameter, taking care to avoid the introduction of air bubbles. Place at the top of the column a quantity of the preparation to be examined containing 300 Ph. Eur. U. dissolved in 1 ml of a 180 g/l solution of *anhydrous acetic acid R* and allow to elute. Collect the eluate in fractions of 2 ml. Measure the absorbance (*2.2.25*) of each fraction at the absorption maximum at 277 nm and plot the values on a graph. The chromatogram obtained does not present an absorption maximum before the elution of the aprotinin.

Specific activity of the dry residue: minimum 3.0 Ph. Eur. U. of aprotinin activity per milligram of dry residue.

Evaporate 25.0 ml to dryness in a water-bath, dry the residue at 110 °C for 15 h and weigh. From the mass of the residue and the activity determined as described below, calculate the number of European Pharmacopoeia Units per milligram of dry residue.

Sterility (*2.6.1*). If intended for use in the manufacture of parenteral dosage forms without a further appropriate sterilisation procedure, it complies with the test for sterility.

Bacterial endotoxins (*2.6.14*): less than 0.14 IU per European Pharmacopoeia Unit of aprotinin, if intended for use in the manufacture of parenteral dosage forms without a further appropriate procedure for the removal of bacterial endotoxins.

ASSAY

The activity of aprotinin is determined by measuring its inhibitory action on a solution of trypsin of known activity. The inhibiting activity of the aprotinin is calculated from the difference between the initial activity and the residual activity of the trypsin.

The inhibiting activity of aprotinin is expressed in European Pharmacopoeia Units. 1 Ph. Eur. U. inhibits 50 per cent of the enzymatic activity of 2 microkatals of trypsin.

Use a reaction vessel with a capacity of about 30 ml and provided with:

— a device that will maintain a temperature of 25 ± 0.1 °C;

— a stirring device, such as a magnetic stirrer;

— a lid with 5 holes for accommodating the electrodes, the tip of a burette, a tube for the admission of nitrogen and the introduction of the reagents.

An automatic or manual titration apparatus may be used. In the latter case the burette is graduated in 0.05 ml and the pH-meter is provided with a wide reading scale and glass and calomel electrodes.

Test solution. With *0.0015 M borate buffer solution pH 8.0 R* prepare an appropriate dilution (*D*) of the concentrated solution expected on the basis of the stated potency to contain 1.67 Ph. Eur. U./ml.

Trypsin solution. Prepare a solution of *trypsin BRP* containing about 0.8 microkatals per millilitre (about 1 mg/ml), using *0.001 M hydrochloric acid* as the solvent. Use a freshly prepared solution and keep in iced water.

Trypsin and aprotinin solution. To 4.0 ml of the trypsin solution add 1.0 ml of the test solution. Dilute immediately to 40.0 ml with *0.0015 M borate buffer solution pH 8.0 R*. Allow to stand at room temperature for 10 min and then keep in iced water. Use within 6 h of preparation.

Dilute trypsin solution. Dilute 0.5 ml of the trypsin solution to 10.0 ml with *0.0015 M borate buffer solution pH 8.0 R*. Allow to stand at room temperature for 10 min and then keep in iced water.

Maintain an atmosphere of nitrogen in the reaction flask and stir continuously; introduce 9.0 ml of *0.0015 M borate buffer solution pH 8.0 R* and 1.0 ml of a freshly prepared 6.9 g/l solution of *benzoylarginine ethyl ester hydrochloride R*. Adjust to pH 8.0 with *0.1 M sodium hydroxide*. When the temperature has reached equilibrium at 25 ± 0.1 °C, add 1.0 ml of the trypsin and aprotinin solution and start a timer. Maintain at pH 8.0 by the addition of *0.1 M sodium hydroxide* and note the volume added every 30 s. Continue the reaction for 6 min. Determine the number of millilitres of *0.1 M sodium hydroxide* used per second (n_1 ml). Carry out, under the same conditions, a titration using 1.0 ml of the dilute trypsin solution. Determine the number of millilitres of *0.1 M sodium hydroxide* used per second (n_2 ml).

Calculate the aprotinin activity in European Pharmacopoeia Units per millilitre from the expression:

$$4000\,(2n_2 - n_1) \times D$$

D =   dilution factor of the aprotinin concentrated solution to be examined in order to obtain a solution containing 1.67 Ph. Eur. U./ml.

The estimated activity is not less than 90 per cent and not more than 110 per cent of the activity stated on the label.

STORAGE

In an airtight, tamper-proof container, protected from light.

LABELLING

The label states:

— the number of European Pharmacopoeia Units of aprotinin activity per millilitre.

— where applicable, that the solution is sterile,

— where applicable, that the solution is free from bacterial endotoxins.

Monographs A - C

B

Monographs A - C

04/2003:1975

BASIC BUTYLATED METHACRYLATE COPOLYMER

Copolymerum methacrylatis butylati basicum

DEFINITION

Copolymer of 2-(dimethylamino)ethyl methacrylate, butyl methacrylate and methyl methacrylate having a mean relative molecular mass of about 150 000. The ratio of 2-dimethylaminoethyl methacrylate groups to butyl methacrylate and methyl methacrylate groups is about 2:1:1.

Content of dimethylaminoethyl groups: 20.8 per cent to 25.5 per cent (dried substance).

CHARACTERS

Appearance: colourless or yellowish granules or white powder, slightly hygroscopic.

Solubility: practically insoluble in water, freely soluble in methylene chloride. It dissolves slowly in alcohol.

IDENTIFICATION

A. Infrared absorption spectrophotometry (*2.2.24*).

> *Comparison*: *Ph. Eur. reference spectrum of basic butylated methacrylate copolymer*.

B. It complies with the limits of the assay.

TESTS

Solution S. Dissolve 12.5 g in a mixture of 35.0 g of *acetone R* and 52.5 g of *2-propanol R*.

Viscosity (*2.2.10*): 3 mPa·s to 6 mPa·s, determined on solution S.

Apparatus: rotating viscosimeter.

Dimensions:

— *spindle*: diameter = 25.15 mm, height = 90.74 mm, shaft diameter = 4 mm,

— *cylinder*: diameter = 27.62 mm, height = 0.135 m.

Stirring speed: 30 r/min.

Volume of solution: 16 ml of solution S.

Temperature: 20 °C.

Absorbance (*2.2.25*): maximum 0.30 at 420 nm, determined on solution S.

Appearance of film. Spread evenly 1.0 ml of solution S on a glass plate. Upon drying a clear film is formed.

Monomers: maximum 0.3 per cent, for the sum of contents of butyl methacrylate, methyl methacrylate and 2-dimethylaminoethyl methacrylate calculated by procedures A and B.

A. Butyl methacrylate and methyl methacrylate. Liquid chromatography (*2.2.29*).

> *Test solution*. Dissolve 1.00 g of the substance to be examined in *phosphate buffer solution pH 2.0 R* and dilute to 50.0 ml with the same buffer solution.

> *Reference solution*. Dissolve 10.0 mg of *butyl methacrylate R* and 10.0 mg of *methyl methacrylate R* in 10.0 ml of *acetonitrile R* and dilute to 50.0 ml with *water R*. Dilute 1.0 ml of the solution to 50.0 ml with *water R*.

> *Column*:

> — *size*: *l* = 0.125 m, Ø = 4.6 mm,

> — *stationary phase*: *octadecylsilyl silica gel for chromatography R* (7 µm).

> *Mobile phase*: *phosphate buffer solution pH 2.0 R*, *methanol R* (45:55 *V/V*).

> *Flow rate*: 2.0 ml/min.

> *Detection*: spectrophotometer at 205 nm.

> *Injection*: 50 µl.

B. 2-Dimethylaminoethyl methacrylate. Liquid chromatography (*2.2.29*).

> *Test solution*. Dissolve 1.00 g of the substance to be examined in *tetrahydrofuran R* and dilute to 50.0 ml with the same solvent.

> *Reference solution*. Dissolve 10.0 mg of 2-(dimethylamino)ethyl methacrylate R in *tetrahydrofuran R* and dilute to 50.0 ml with the same solvent. Dilute 2.0 ml of the solution to 50.0 ml with *tetrahydrofuran R*.

> *Column*:

> — *size*: *l* = 0.125 m, Ø = 4.6 mm,

> — *stationary phase*: *aminopropylsilyl silica gel for chromatography R* (10 µm).

> *Mobile phase*: mix 25 volumes of a 3.404 g/l solution of *potassium dihydrogen phosphate R* and 75 volumes of *tetrahydrofuran R*.

> *Flow rate*: 2.0 ml/min.

> *Detection*: spectrophotometer at 215 nm.

> *Injection*: 50 µl.

Heavy metals (*2.4.8*): maximum 20 ppm.

2.0 g complies with limit test C. Prepare the standard using 4.0 ml of *lead standard solution (10 ppm Pb) R*.

Loss on drying (*2.2.32*): maximum 2.0 per cent, determined on 1.000 g by drying in an oven at 110 °C for 3 h.

Sulphated ash (*2.4.14*): maximum 0.1 per cent, determined on 1.0 g.

ASSAY

Dissolve 0.200 g in a mixture of 4 ml of *water R* and 96 ml of *anhydrous acetic acid R*. Titrate with *0.1 M perchloric acid*, determining the end-point potentiometrically (*2.2.20*).

1 ml of *0.1 M perchloric acid* is equivalent to 7.21 mg of $C_4H_{10}N$.

STORAGE

In an airtight container.

IMPURITIES

A. R = $[CH_2]_3$-CH_3: butyl methacrylate,

B. R = CH_3: methyl methacrylate,

C. R = CH_2-CH_2-$N(CH_3)_2$: 2-(dimethylamino)ethyl methacrylate.

04/2003:0256

BENZYL ALCOHOL

Alcohol benzylicus

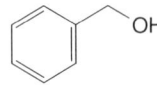

C₇H₈O M_r 108.1

DEFINITION

Phenylmethanol.

Content: 98.0 per cent to 100.5 per cent.

CHARACTERS

Appearance: clear, colourless, oily liquid.

Solubility: soluble in water, miscible with alcohol and with fatty and essential oils.

Relative density: 1.043 to 1.049.

IDENTIFICATION

Infrared absorption spectrophotometry (*2.2.24*).

Comparison: *Ph. Eur. reference spectrum of benzyl alcohol*.

TESTS

Appearance of solution. The solution is clear (*2.2.1*) and colourless (*2.2.2, Method II*).

Shake 2.0 ml with 60 ml of *water R*. It dissolves completely.

Acidity. To 10 ml add 10 ml of *alcohol R* and 1 ml of *phenolphthalein solution R*. Not more than 1 ml of *0.1 M sodium hydroxide* is required to change the colour of the indicator to pink.

Refractive index (*2.2.6*): 1.538 to 1.541.

Peroxide value (*2.5.5*): maximum 5.

Benzaldehyde and other related substances. Gas chromatography (*2.2.28*).

Test solution. The substance to be examined.

Standard solution (a). Dissolve 0.100 g of *ethylbenzene R* in 10.0 ml of the test solution. Dilute 2.0 ml of this solution to 20.0 ml with the test solution.

Standard solution (b). Dissolve 2.000 g of *dicyclohexyl R* in 10.0 ml of the test solution. Dilute 2.0 ml of this solution to 20.0 ml with the test solution.

Reference solution (a). Dissolve 0.750 g of *benzaldehyde R* and 0.500 g of *cyclohexylmethanol R* in the test solution and dilute to 25.0 ml with the test solution. Add 1.0 ml of this solution to a mixture of 2.0 ml of standard solution (a) and 3.0 ml of standard solution (b) and dilute to 20.0 ml with the test solution.

Reference solution (b). Dissolve 0.250 g of *benzaldehyde R* and 0.500 g of *cyclohexylmethanol R* in the test solution and dilute to 25.0 ml with the test solution. Add 1.0 ml of this solution to a mixture of 2.0 ml of standard solution (a) and 2.0 ml of standard solution (b) and dilute to 20.0 ml with the test solution.

Column:

— *material*: fused silica,

— *size*: l = 30 m, Ø = 0.32 mm,

— *stationary phase*: *macrogol 20 000 R* (film thickness 0.5 µm).

Carrier gas: *helium for chromatography R*.

Linear velocity: 25 cm/s.

Temperature:

	Time (min)	Temperature (°C)
Column	0 - 34	50 → 220
	34 - 69	220
Injection port		200
Detector		310

Detection: flame ionisation.

Benzyl alcohol not intended for parenteral use.

Injection: without air-plug, 0.1 µl of the test solution and 0.1 µl of reference solution (a).

Relative retention with reference to benzyl alcohol (retention time = about 26 min): ethylbenzene = about 0.28; dicyclohexyl = about 0.59; benzaldehyde = about 0.68; cyclohexylmethanol = about 0.71.

System suitability: reference solution (a):

— *resolution*: minimum 3.0 between the peaks corresponding to benzaldehyde and to cyclohexylmethanol.

In the chromatogram obtained with the test solution, verify that there are no peaks with the same retention time as the standards.

Limits:

— *benzaldehyde*: not more than the difference between the area of the peak due to benzaldehyde in the chromatogram obtained with reference solution (a) and the area of the peak due to benzaldehyde in the chromatogram obtained with the test solution (0.15 per cent).

— *cyclohexylmethanol*: not more than the difference between the area of the peak due to cyclohexylmethanol in the chromatogram obtained with reference solution (a) and the area of the peak due to cyclohexylmethanol in the chromatogram obtained with the test solution (0.10 per cent).

— *total of other peaks with a relative retention less than that of benzyl alcohol*: not more than 4 times the area of the peak due to ethylbenzene in the chromatogram obtained with reference solution (a) (0.04 per cent).

— *total of peaks with a relative retention greater than that of benzyl alcohol*: not more than the area of the peak due to dicyclohexyl in the chromatogram obtained with reference solution (a) (0.3 per cent).

— *disregard limit*: 0.01 times the area of the peak due to ethylbenzene in the chromatogram obtained with reference solution (a) (0.0001 per cent).

Benzyl alcohol intended for parenteral use.

Injection: without air-plug, 0.1 µl of the test solution and 0.1 µl of reference solution (b).

Relative retention with reference to benzyl alcohol (retention time = about 26 min): ethylbenzene = about 0.28; dicyclohexyl = about 0.59; benzaldehyde = about 0.68; cyclohexylmethanol = about 0.71.

System suitability: reference solution (b):

— *resolution*: minimum 3.0 between the peaks corresponding to benzaldehyde and to cyclohexylmethanol.

In the chromatogram obtained with the test solution, verify that there are no peaks with the same retention time as the standards.

Limits:

— *benzaldehyde*: not more than the difference between the area of the peak due to benzaldehyde in the chromatogram obtained with reference solution (b) and the area of the peak due to benzaldehyde in the chromatogram obtained with the test solution (0.05 per cent).

— *cyclohexylmethanol*: not more than the difference between the area of the peak due to cyclohexylmethanol in the chromatogram obtained with reference solution (b) and the area of the peak due to cyclohexylmethanol in the chromatogram obtained with the test solution (0.10 per cent).

— *total of other peaks with a relative retention less than that of benzyl alcohol*: not more than twice the area of the peak due to ethylbenzene in the chromatogram obtained with reference solution (b) (0.02 per cent).

— *total of peaks with a relative retention greater than that of benzyl alcohol*: not more than the area of the peak due to dicyclohexyl in the chromatogram obtained with reference solution (b) (0.2 per cent).

— *disregard limit*: 0.01 times the area of the peak due to ethylbenzene in the chromatogram obtained with reference solution (b) (0.0001 per cent).

Residue on evaporation: maximum 0.05 per cent.

After ensuring that the substance to be examined complies with the test for peroxide value, evaporate 10.0 g to dryness on a water-bath, dry at 100-105 °C for 1 h and allow to cool in a desiccator. The residue weighs a maximum of 5 mg.

ASSAY

To 0.900 g (*m* g) add 15.0 ml of a freshly prepared mixture of 1 volume of *acetic anhydride R* and 7 volumes of *pyridine R* and boil under a reflux condenser for 30 min. Cool and add 25 ml of *water R*. Using 0.25 ml of *phenolphthalein solution R* as indicator, titrate with *1 M sodium hydroxide* (n_1 ml). Carry out a blank titration (n_2 ml).

Calculate the percentage content of C_7H_8O from the expression:

$$\frac{10.81\left(n_2 - n_1\right)}{m}$$

STORAGE

In an airtight container, under nitrogen, protected from light at a temperature between 2 °C and 8 °C.

LABELLING

The label states, where applicable, that the substance is suitable for use in the manufacture of parenteral dosage forms.

04/2003:1826

BITTER-FENNEL FRUIT OIL

Foeniculi amari fructus aetheroleum

DEFINITION

Essential oil obtained by steam distillation from the ripe fruits of *Foeniculum vulgare* Miller, ssp. *vulgare* var. *vulgare*.

Content:

— fenchone: 12.0 per cent to 25.0 per cent,

— *trans*-anethole: 55.0 per cent to 75.0 per cent.

CHARACTERS

Appearance: clear, colourless or pale yellow liquid.

It has a characteristic odour.

IDENTIFICATION

First identification: B.

Second identification: A.

A. Thin-layer chromatography (*2.2.27*).

Test solution. Dissolve 0.1 ml of the oil to be examined in 5 ml of *toluene R*.

Reference solution. Dissolve 10 µl of *fenchone R* and 80 µl of *anethole R* in 5 ml of *toluene R*.

Plate: TLC silica gel plate R.

Mobile phase: ethyl acetate R, toluene R (5:95 V/V).

Application: 10 µl, as bands.

Development: over a path of 15 cm.

Drying: in air.

Detection: spray with a freshly prepared 200 g/l solution of *phosphomolybdic acid R* in *alcohol R* and heat at 150 °C for 15 min; examine in daylight.

Results: see below the sequence of the zones present in the chromatograms obtained with the reference solution and the test solution. Furthermore, other zones may be present in the chromatogram obtained with the test solution.

Top of the plate	
Anethole: a dark blue to dark violet zone	A dark blue to dark violet zone (anethole)
———	———
Fenchone: a blue or bluish-grey zone	A blue or bluish-grey zone (fenchone)
———	———
Reference solution	**Test solution**

B. Examine the chromatograms obtained in the test for chromatographic profile.

Results: the characteristic peaks in the chromatogram obtained with the test solution are similar in retention time to those in the chromatogram obtained with the reference solution.

TESTS

Relative density (*2.2.5*): 0.961 to 0.975.

Refractive index (*2.2.6*): 1.528 to 1.539.

Optical rotation (*2.2.7*): + 10.0° to + 24.0°.

Chromatographic profile. Gas chromatography (*2.2.28*): use the normalisation procedure.

Test solution. Dissolve 0.20 ml of the oil to be examined in *heptane R* and dilute to 10.0 ml with the same solvent.

Reference solution. Dissolve 20 µl of *α-pinene R*, 20 µl of *limonene R*, 50 µl of *fenchone R*, 20 µl of *estragole R*, 10 µl of *cis-anethole R*, 100 µl of *anethole R* and 20 µl of *anisaldehyde R* in *heptane R* and dilute to 10.0 ml with the same solvent.

Column:

— *material*: fused silica,

— *size*: *l* = 30 m (a film thickness of 1 µm may be used) to 60 m (a film thickness of 0.2 µm may be used), Ø = 0.25-0.53 mm; when using a column longer than 30 m, an adjustment of the temperature programme may be necessary,

— *stationary phase*: macrogol 20 000 R.

The following chromatogram is published for information.

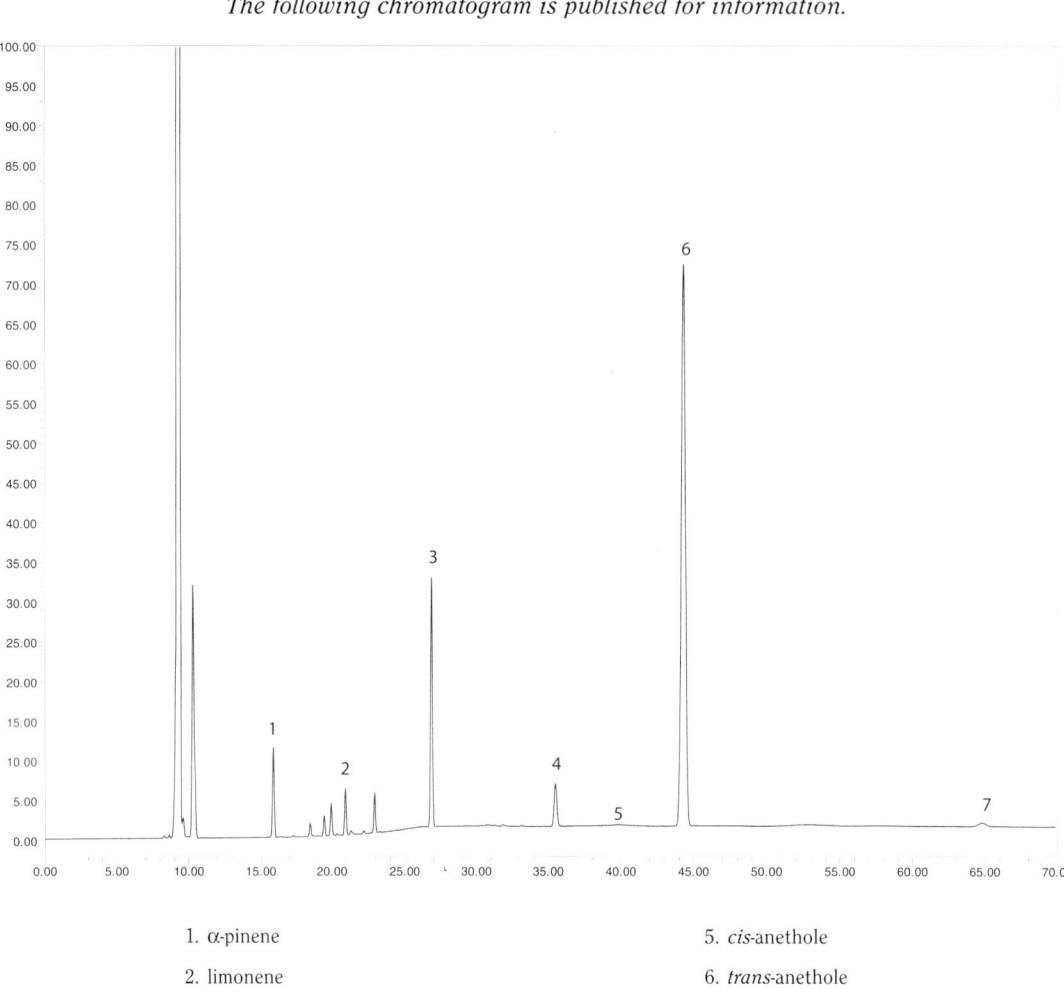

1. α-pinene
2. limonene
3. fenchone
4. estragole

5. *cis*-anethole
6. *trans*-anethole
7. anisaldehyde

Figure 1826.-1. – *Chromatogram of bitter-fennel fruit oil for the test for chromatographic profile*

Carrier gas: *helium for chromatography R.*

Flow rate: 1 ml/min.

Split ratio: 1:200.

Temperature:

	Time (min)	Temperature (°C)
Column	0 – 4	60
	4 – 26	60 → 170
	26 – 41	170
Injection port		220
Detector		270

Detection: flame ionisation.

Injection: 1.0 µl.

Elution order: order indicated in the composition of the reference solution. Record the retention times of these substances.

System suitability: reference solution:

— *resolution*: minimum of 1.5 between the peaks due to *cis*-anethole and *trans*-anethole.

Using the retention times determined from the chromatogram obtained with the reference solution, locate the components of the reference solution on the chromatogram obtained with the test solution (disregard the peak due to heptane). Determine the percentage content of these components. The limits are within the following ranges:

— *α-pinene*: 1.0 per cent to 10.0 per cent,
— *limonene*: 0.9 per cent to 5.0 per cent,
— *fenchone*: 12.0 per cent to 25.0 per cent,
— *estragole*: maximum 6.0 per cent,
— *cis-anethole*: maximum 0.5 per cent,
— *trans-anethole*: 55.0 per cent to 75.0 per cent,
— *anisaldehyde*: maximum 2.0 per cent.

The ratio of α-pinene content to limonene content is greater than 1.

STORAGE

In an airtight, well-filled container, protected from light at a temperature not exceeding 25 °C.

04/2003:0706

BROMHEXINE HYDROCHLORIDE

Bromhexini hydrochloridum

$C_{14}H_{21}Br_2ClN_2$ M_r 412.6

DEFINITION

N-(2-Amino-3,5-dibromobenzyl)-N-methylcyclohexanamine hydrochloride.

Content: 98.5 per cent to 101.5 per cent (dried substance).

CHARACTERS

Appearance: white or almost white, crystalline powder.

Solubility: very slightly soluble in water, slightly soluble in alcohol and in methylene chloride.

It shows polymorphism.

IDENTIFICATION

First identification: A, E.

Second identification: B, C, D, E.

A. Infrared absorption spectrophotometry (*2.2.24*).

   Comparison: bromhexine hydrochloride CRS.

   If the spectra obtained in the solid state show differences, dissolve the substance to be examined and the reference substance separately in *methanol R*, evaporate to dryness and record new spectra using the residues.

B. Thin-layer chromatography (*2.2.27*).

   Test solution. Dissolve 20 mg of the substance to be examined in *methanol R* and dilute to 10 ml with the same solvent.

   Reference solution. Dissolve 20 mg of *bromhexine hydrochloride CRS* in *methanol R* and dilute to 10 ml with the same solvent.

   Plate: TLC silica gel F$_{254}$ plate R.

   Mobile phase: glacial acetic acid R, water R, butanol R (17:17:66 *V/V/V*).

   Application: 20 µl.

   Development: over 3/4 of the plate.

   Drying: in air.

   Detection: examine in ultraviolet light at 254 nm.

   Results: the principal spot in the chromatogram obtained with the test solution is similar in position and size to the principal spot in the chromatogram obtained with the reference solution.

C. Dissolve about 25 mg in a mixture of 1 ml of *dilute sulphuric acid R* and 50 ml of *water R*. Add 2 ml of *methylene chloride R* and 5 ml of *chloramine solution R* and shake. A brownish-yellow colour develops in the lower layer.

D. Dissolve about 1 mg in 3 ml of *0.1 M hydrochloric acid*. The solution gives the reaction of primary aromatic amines (*2.3.1*).

E. Dissolve about 20 mg in 1 ml of *methanol R* and add 1 ml of *water R*. The solution gives reaction (a) of chlorides (*2.3.1*).

TESTS

Related substances. Liquid chromatography (*2.2.29*).

Test solution. Dissolve 50 mg of the substance to be examined in *methanol R* and dilute to 10.0 ml with the same solvent.

Reference solution (a). Dissolve 5 mg of *bromhexine impurity C CRS* in *methanol R*, add 1.0 ml of the test solution and dilute to 10.0 ml with the same solvent.

Reference solution (b). Dilute 1.0 ml of the test solution to 100.0 ml with *methanol R*. Dilute 1.0 ml to 10.0 ml with *methanol R*.

Column:

- *size*: l = 0.12 m, Ø = 4.6 mm,
- *stationary phase*: octadecylsilyl silica gel for chromatography R (3 µm),

Mobile phase: mix 0.50 ml of *phosphoric acid R* in 950 ml of *water R*, adjust to pH 7.0 with *triethylamine R* (about 1.5 ml) and dilute to 1000 ml with *water R*; mix 20 volumes of this solution with 80 volumes of *acetonitrile R*.

Flow rate: 1.0 ml/min.

Detection: spectrophotometer at 248 nm.

Injection: 10 µl.

Run time: 2.5 times the retention time of bromhexine.

Relative retention with reference to bromhexine (retention time = about 11 min): impurity A = about 0.1; impurity B = about 0.2; impurity C = about 0.4; impurity D = about 0.5.

System suitability: reference solution (a):

- *resolution*: minimum 12.0 between the peaks due to impurity C and bromhexine.

Limits:

- *any impurity*: not more than twice the area of the principal peak in the chromatogram obtained with reference solution (b) (0.2 per cent), and not more than 1 such peak has an area greater than the area of the principal peak in the chromatogram obtained with reference solution (b) (0.1 per cent),
- *total*: not more than 3 times the area of the principal peak in the chromatogram obtained with reference solution (b) (0.3 per cent),
- *disregard limit*: 0.5 times the area of the principal peak in the chromatogram obtained with reference solution (b) (0.05 per cent).

Loss on drying (*2.2.32*): maximum 1.0 per cent, determined on 1.000 g by drying in an oven at 100-105 °C.

Sulphated ash (*2.4.14*): maximum 0.1 per cent, determined on 1.0 g.

ASSAY

Dissolve 0.300 g in 70 ml of *alcohol R* and add 1 ml of *0.1 M hydrochloric acid*. Carry out a potentiometric titration (*2.2.20*), using *0.1 M sodium hydroxide*. Read the volume between the 2 points of inflexion.

1 ml of *0.1 M sodium hydroxide* is equivalent to 41.26 mg of $C_{14}H_{21}Br_2ClN_2$.

STORAGE

Protected from light.

IMPURITIES

Qualified impurities: A, B, C, D.

Other detectable impurities: E.

A. R = CH₂OH: (2-amino-3,5-dibromophenyl)methanol,

B. R = CHO: 2-amino-3,5-dibromobenzaldehyde,

C. R = H: *N*-(2-aminobenzyl)-*N*-methylcyclohexanamine,

D. R = Br: *N*-(2-amino-5-bromobenzyl)-*N*-methylcyclohexan-amine,

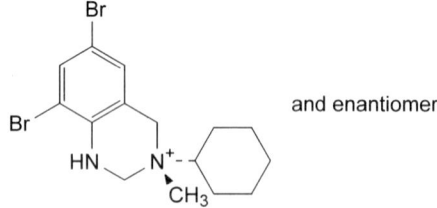

and enantiomer

E. (3*RS*)-6,8-dibromo-3-cyclohexyl-3-methyl-1,2,3,4-tetrahydroquinazolin-3-ium.

C

Monographs A - C

04/2003:0597

CARNAUBA WAX

Cera carnauba

DEFINITION

Purified wax obtained from the leaves of *Copernicia cerifera* Mart.

CHARACTERS

Appearance: pale yellow or yellow powder, flakes or hard masses.

Solubility: practically insoluble in water, soluble on heating in ethyl acetate and in xylene, practically insoluble in alcohol.

Relative density: about 0.97.

IDENTIFICATION

Thin-layer chromatography (*2.2.27*).

Test solution. Dissolve 0.10 g of the substance to be examined with heating in 5 ml of *chloroform R*. Use the warm solution.

Reference solution. Dissolve 5 mg of *menthol R*, 5 µl of *menthyl acetate R* and 5 mg of *thymol R* in 10 ml of *toluene R*.

Plate: TLC silica gel plate R.

Mobile phase: ethyl acetate R, chloroform R (2:98 V/V).

Application: 30 µl of the test solution and 10 µl of the reference solution as bands 20 mm by 3 mm.

Development: over half of the plate.

Drying: in air.

Detection: spray with a freshly prepared 200 g/l solution of *phosphomolybdic acid R* in *alcohol R* (about 10 ml for a 20 cm plate). Heat at 100-105 °C for 10-15 min.

Results: the chromatogram obtained with the reference solution shows in the lower part a dark blue zone (menthol), above this zone a reddish zone (thymol) and in the upper part a dark blue zone (menthyl acetate). The chromatogram obtained with the test solution shows a large blue zone (triacontanol = melissyl alcohol) at a level between the thymol and menthol zones in the chromatogram obtained with the reference solution. Further blue zones are visible in the upper part of the chromatogram obtained with the test solution, at levels between those of the menthyl acetate and thymol zones in the chromatogram obtained with the reference solution; above these zones further zones are visible in the chromatogram obtained with the test solution; the zone with the highest R_f value is very pronounced. A number of faint zones are visible below the triacontanol zone and the starting point is coloured blue.

TESTS

Appearance of solution. The solution is clear (*2.2.1*) and not more intensely coloured than a 50 mg/l solution of *potassium dichromate R* (*2.2.2, Method II*).

Dissolve 0.10 g with heating in *chloroform R* and dilute to 10 ml with the same solvent.

Melting point (*2.2.15*): 80 °C to 88 °C.

Melt the substance to be examined carefully on a water-bath before introduction into the capillary tubes. Allow the tubes to stand in the refrigerator for 24 h or at 0 °C for 2 h.

Acid value: 2 to 7.

To 2.000 g (*m* g) in a 250 ml conical flask fitted with a reflux condenser add 40 ml of *xylene R* and a few glass beads. Heat with stirring until the substance is completely dissolved.

Add 20 ml of *alcohol R* and 1 ml of *bromothymol blue solution R3* and titrate the hot solution with *0.5 M alcoholic potassium hydroxide* until a green colour persisting for at least 10 s is obtained (n_1 ml). Carry out a blank test (n_2 ml). Calculate the acid value from the expression:

$$\frac{28.05\,(n_1 - n_2)}{m}$$

Saponification value: 78 to 95.

To 2.000 g (*m* g) in a 250 ml conical flask fitted with a reflux condenser add 40 ml of *xylene R* and a few glass beads. Heat with stirring until the substance is completely dissolved. Add 20 ml of *alcohol R* and 20.0 ml of *0.5 M alcoholic potassium hydroxide*. Boil under a reflux condenser for 3 h. Add 1 ml of *phenolphthalein solution R1* and titrate the hot solution immediately with *0.5 M hydrochloric acid* until the red colour disappears. Repeat the heating and titration until the colour no longer reappears on heating (n_3 ml). Carry out a blank test (n_4 ml). Calculate the saponification value from the expression:

$$\frac{28.05\,(n_4 - n_3)}{m}$$

Total ash (*2.4.16*): maximum 0.25 per cent, determined on 2.0 g.

STORAGE

Protected from light.

01/2002:1497
corrected

CASTOR OIL, HYDROGENATED

Ricini oleum hydrogenatum

DEFINITION

Hydrogenated castor oil is the oil obtained by hydrogenation of *Virgin Castor oil (0051)*. It consists mainly of the triglyceride of 12-hydroxystearic acid.

CHARACTERS

A fine, almost white or pale yellow powder or almost white or pale yellow masses or flakes, practically insoluble in water, freely soluble in methylene chloride, slightly soluble in light petroleum, very slightly soluble in ethanol.

IDENTIFICATION

A. Melting point (*2.2.14*): 83 °C to 88 °C.

B. It complies with the test for hydroxyl value (see Tests).

C. It complies with the test for composition of fatty acids (see Tests).

TESTS

Acid value (*2.5.1*). Not more than 4.0, determined on 10.0 g dissolved in 75 ml of hot *alcohol R*.

Hydroxyl value (*2.5.3, Method A*): 145 to 165, determined on a warm solution.

Iodine value (*2.5.4*). Not more than 5.0.

Alkaline impurities. Dissolve 1.0 g by gentle heating in a mixture of 1.5 ml of *alcohol R* and 3 ml of *toluene R*. Add 0.05 ml of a 0.4 g/l solution of *bromophenol blue R* in *alcohol R*. Not more than 0.2 ml of *0.01 M hydrochloric acid* is required to change the colour of the indicator to yellow.

Composition of fatty acids. Examine by gas chromatography (*2.4.22, Method A*) with the following modifications.

Test solution. Introduce 75 mg of the substance to be examined in a 10 ml centrifuge tube with a screw cap. Dissolve in 2 ml of *1,1-dimethylethyl methyl ether R1* by shaking and heat gently (50-60 °C). Add, when still warm, 1 ml of a 12 g/l solution of *sodium R* in *anhydrous methanol R*, prepared with the necessary precautions, and mix vigorously for at least 5 min. Add 5 ml of *distilled water R* and mix vigorously for about 30 s. Centrifuge for 15 min at 1500 *g*. Use the upper layer.

Reference solution. Dissolve 50 mg of *methyl 12-hydroxystearate CRS* and 50 mg of *methyl stearate CRS* in 10.0 ml of *1,1-dimethylethyl methyl ether R1*.

The chromatographic procedure may be carried out using:

– a fused-silica column 30 m long and 0.25 mm in internal diameter coated with *macrogol 20 000 R* (film thickness 0.25 μm),
– *helium for chromatography R* as the carrier gas at a flow rate of 0.9 ml/min,
– a flame-ionisation detector,
– a split injector (1:100),

maintaining the temperature of the column at 215 °C for 55 min and maintaining the temperature of the injection port and that of the detector at 250 °C.

Inject 1 μl of each solution.

Calculate the fraction of each fatty acid using the following expression:

$$A_{x,s,c}/\sum A_{x,s,c} \times 100 \text{ per cent } m/m$$

$A_{x,s,c}$ = corrected peak area of the fatty acid in the test solution:

$$A_{x,s,c} = A_{x,s} \times R_c$$

R_c = relative correction factor for the peak corresponding to methyl 12-hydroxystearate:

$$R_c = \frac{m_{1,r} \times A_{2,r}}{A_{1,r} \times m_{2,r}}$$

R_c = 1 for peaks corresponding to each of the other specified fatty acids or any unspecified fatty acid,

$m_{1,r}$ = mass of methyl 12-hydroxystearate in the reference solution,

$m_{2,r}$ = mass of methyl stearate in the reference solution,

$A_{1,r}$ = area of any peak corresponding to methyl 12-hydroxystearate in the chromatogram obtained with the reference solution,

$A_{2,r}$ = area of any peak corresponding to methyl stearate in the chromatogram obtained with the reference solution,

$A_{x,s}$ = area of the peaks corresponding to any specified or unspecified fatty acid methyl esters.

The fatty acid fraction of the oil has the following composition:

– *palmitic acid*: not more than 2.0 per cent,
– *stearic acid*: 7.0 per cent to 14.0 per cent,
– *arachidic acid*: not more than 1.0 per cent,
– *12-oxostearic acid* (equivalent chain length on macrogol 20 000: 22.7): not more than 5.0 per cent,
– *12-hydroxystearic acid* (equivalent chain length on macrogol 20 000: 23.9): 78.0 per cent to 91.0 per cent,
– *any other fatty acid*: not more than 3.0 per cent.

Nickel (*2.4.27*). Not more than 1 ppm of Ni.

STORAGE

Store in a well-filled container.

IMPURITIES

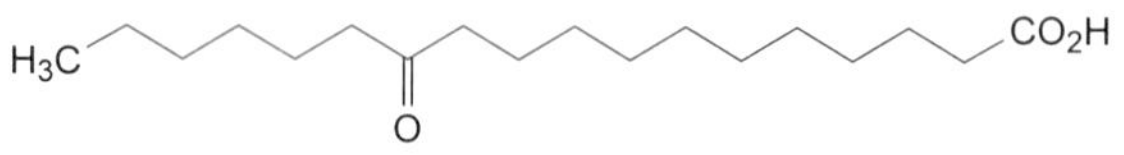

A. 12-oxostearic acid.

01/2002:0051
corrected

CASTOR OIL, VIRGIN

Ricini oleum virginale

DEFINITION

Virgin castor oil is the fatty oil obtained by cold expression from the seeds of *Ricinus communis* L. A suitable antioxidant may be added.

CHARACTERS

A clear, almost colourless or slightly yellow, viscous, hygroscopic liquid, slightly soluble in light petroleum, miscible with alcohol and with glacial acetic acid.

It has a refractive index of about 1.479 and a relative density of about 0.958.

IDENTIFICATION

First identification: D.

Second identification: A, B, C.

A. It complies with the test for optical rotation (see Tests).

B. It complies with the test for hydroxyl value (see Tests).

C. It complies with the test for iodine value (see Tests).

D. It complies with the test for composition of fatty acids (see Tests).

TESTS

Optical rotation (*2.2.7*): + 3.5° to + 6.0°.

Absorbance (*2.2.25*). To 1.0 g add *alcohol R* and dilute to 100.0 ml with the same solvent. The solution shows an absorption maximum at 269 nm. The specific absorbance measured at this maximum is not greater than 1.5.

Acid value (*2.5.1*). Dissolve 5.0 g in 25 ml of the prescribed mixture of solvents. The acid value is not greater than 2.0.

Hydroxyl value (*2.5.3, Method A*). Not less than 150.

Iodine value (*2.5.4*): 82 to 90.

Peroxide value (*2.5.5*). Not greater than 10.0.

Unsaponifiable matter (*2.5.7*). Not more than 0.8 per cent, determined on 5.0 g.

Composition of fatty acids. Examine by gas chromatography (*2.4.22, Method A*) with the following modifications.

Test solution. Introduce 75 mg of the substance to be examined in a 10 ml centrifuge tube with a screw cap. Dissolve in 2 ml of *1,1-dimethylethyl methyl ether R1* with shaking and heat gently (50-60 °C). Add, when still warm, 1 ml of a 12 g/l solution of *sodium R* in *anhydrous methanol R*, prepared with the necessary precautions, and mix vigorously for at least 5 min. Add 5 ml of *distilled water R* and mix vigorously for about 30 s. Centrifuge for 15 min at 1500 *g*. Use the upper layer.

Reference solution. Dissolve 50 mg of *methyl ricinoleate CRS* and 50 mg of *methyl stearate CRS* in 10.0 ml of *1,1-dimethylethyl methyl ether R1*.

The chromatographic procedure may be carried out using:
- a fused-silica column 30 m long and 0.25 mm in internal diameter coated with *macrogol 20 000 R* (film thickness 0.25 µm),
- *helium for chromatography R* as the carrier gas at a flow rate of 0.9 ml/min,
- a flame-ionisation detector,
- a split injector (1:100),

maintaining the temperature of the column at 215 °C for 55 min and maintaining the temperature of the injection port and that of the detector at 250 °C.

Inject 1 µl of each solution.

Calculate the fraction of each fatty acid using the following expression:

$$A_{x,s,c} / \sum A_{x,s,c} \times 100 \text{ per cent } m/m$$

$A_{x,s,c}$ = corrected peak area of the fatty acid in the test solution:

$$A_{x,s,c} = A_{x,s} \times R_c$$

R_c = relative correction factor:

$$R_c = \frac{m_{1,r} \times A_{2,r}}{A_{1,r} \times m_{2,r}}$$

for the peak corresponding to methyl ricinoleate.

R_c = 1 for peaks corresponding to each of the other specified fatty acids or any unspecified fatty acid,

$m_{1,r}$ = mass of methyl ricinoleate in the reference solution,

$m_{2,r}$ = mass of methyl stearate in the reference solution,

$A_{1,r}$ = area of any peak corresponding to methyl ricinoleate in the chromatogram obtained with the reference solution,

$A_{2,r}$ = area of any peak corresponding to methyl stearate in the chromatogram obtained with the reference solution,

$A_{x,s}$ = area of the peaks corresponding to any specified or unspecified fatty acid methyl esters.

The fatty acid fraction of the oil has the following composition:
- *palmitic acid*: not more than 2.0 per cent,

- *stearic acid*: not more than 2.5 per cent,
- *oleic acid and isomers* (C18:1 equivalent chain length on macrogol 20 000: 18.3): 2.5 per cent to 6.0 per cent,
- *linoleic acid* (C18:2 equivalent chain length on macrogol 20 000: 18.8): 2.5 per cent to 7.0 per cent,
- *linolenic acid* (C18:3 equivalent chain length on macrogol 20 000: 19.2): not more than 1.0 per cent,
- *eicosenoic acid* (C20:1 equivalent chain length on macrogol 20 000: 20.2): not more than 1.0 per cent,
- *ricinoleic acid* (equivalent chain length on macrogol 20 000: 23.9): 85.0 per cent to 92.0 per cent,
- *any other fatty acid*: not more than 1.0 per cent.

Water (*2.5.12*). Not more than 0.3 per cent, determined on 5.0 g by the semi-micro determination of water.

STORAGE

Store in a well-filled container, protected from light, at a temperature not exceeding 25 °C.

LABELLING

The label states the name and concentration of any added antioxidant.

07/2002:0813
corrected

CEFADROXIL MONOHYDRATE

Cefadroxilum monohydricum

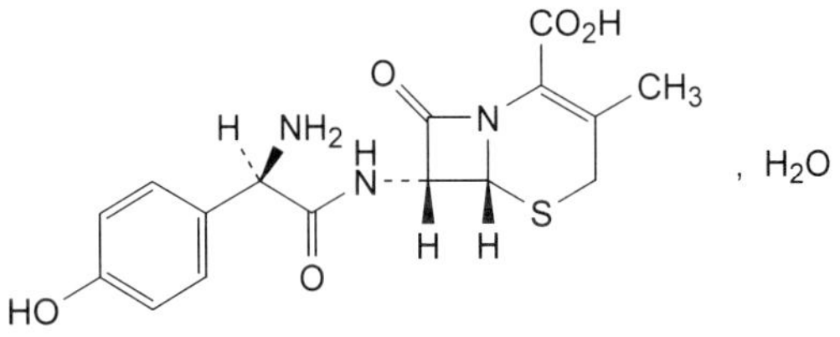

$C_{16}H_{17}N_3O_5S,H_2O$ M_r 381.4

DEFINITION

(6R,7R)-7-[[(2R)-2-Amino-2-(4-hydroxyphenyl)acetyl]amino]-3-methyl-8-oxo-5-thia-1-azabicyclo[4.2.0]oct-2-ene-2-carboxylic acid monohydrate.

Content: 95.0 per cent to 102.0 per cent (anhydrous substance).

CHARACTERS

Appearance: white or almost white powder.

Solubility: slightly soluble in water, very slightly soluble in alcohol.

IDENTIFICATION

First identification: A.

Second identification: B, C.

A. Infrared absorption spectrophotometry (*2.2.24*).

   Comparison: *cefadroxil CRS*.

B. Thin-layer chromatography (*2.2.27*).

   Test solution. Dissolve 20 mg of the substance to be examined in 5 ml of a mixture of equal volumes of *methanol R* and *0.067 M phosphate buffer solution pH 7.0 R*.

   Reference solution (a). Dissolve 20 mg of *cefadroxil CRS* in 5 ml of a mixture of equal volumes of *methanol R* and *0.067 M phosphate buffer solution pH 7.0 R*.

Reference solution (b). Dissolve 20 mg of *cefadroxil CRS* and 20 mg of *cefalexin CRS* in 5 ml of a mixture of equal volumes of *methanol R* and *0.067 M phosphate buffer solution pH 7.0 R.*

Plate: TLC silanised silica gel F$_{254}$ plate R.

Mobile phase: mix 10 volumes of *tetrahydrofuran R* and 90 volumes of a 154 g/l solution of *ammonium acetate R* adjusted to pH 6.2 with *acetic acid R.*

Application: 1 µl.

Development: over a path of 15 cm.

Drying: in air.

Detection: examine in ultraviolet light at 254 nm.

System suitability: the chromatogram obtained with reference solution (b) shows 2 clearly separated spots.

Results: the principal spot in the chromatogram obtained with the test solution is similar in position and size to the principal spot in the chromatogram obtained with reference solution (a).

C. Place about 2 mg in a test-tube about 150 mm long and 15 mm in diameter. Moisten with 0.05 ml of *water R* and add 2 ml of *sulphuric acid-formaldehyde reagent R.* Mix the contents of the tube by swirling; the solution is yellow. Place the test-tube in a water-bath for 1 min; an orange colour develops.

TESTS

pH (*2.2.3*): 4.0 to 6.0.

Suspend 1.0 g in *carbon dioxide-free water R* and dilute to 20 ml with the same solvent.

Specific optical rotation (*2.2.7*): + 165 to + 178 (anhydrous substance).

Dissolve 0.500 g in *water R* and dilute to 50.0 ml with the same solvent.

Absorbance (*2.2.25*). Dissolve 20.0 mg in *phosphate buffer solution pH 6.0 R* and dilute to 100.0 ml with the same solvent. The absorbance of the solution determined at 330 nm is not greater than 0.05. Dilute 10.0 ml of the solution to 100.0 ml with *phosphate buffer solution pH 6.0 R.* Examined between 235 nm and 340 nm, the diluted solution shows an absorption maximum at 264 nm. The specific absorbance at this maximum is 225 to 250 (anhydrous substance).

Related substances. Liquid chromatography (*2.2.29*).

Test solution. Dissolve 50.0 mg of the substance to be examined in mobile phase A and dilute to 50.0 ml with mobile phase A.

Reference solution (a). Dissolve 10.0 mg of D-α-(4-hydroxyphenyl)glycine CRS (impurity A) in mobile phase A and dilute to 10.0 ml with mobile phase A.

Reference solution (b). Dissolve 10.0 mg of 7-aminodesacetoxycephalosporanic acid CRS (impurity B) in *phosphate buffer solution pH 7.0 R5* and dilute to 10.0 ml with the same buffer solution.

Reference solution (c). Dilute 1.0 ml of reference solution (a) and 1.0 ml of reference solution (b) to 100.0 ml with mobile phase A.

Reference solution (d). Dissolve 10 mg of *dimethylformamide R* and 10 mg of *dimethylacetamide R* in mobile phase A and dilute to 10.0 ml with mobile phase A. Dilute 1.0 ml to 100.0 ml with mobile phase A.

Reference solution (e). Dilute 1.0 ml of reference solution (c) to 25.0 ml with mobile phase A.

Column:
- *size:* l = 0.10 m, Ø = 4.6 mm,

- *stationary phase:* spherical *octadecylsilyl silica gel for chromatography R* (5 µm).

Mobile phase:
- *mobile phase A: phosphate buffer solution pH 5.0 R,*
- *mobile phase B: methanol R2,*

Time (min)	Mobile phase A (per cent V/V)	Mobile phase B (per cent V/V)
0 - 1	98	2
1 - 20	98 → 70	2 → 30
20 - 23	70 → 98	30 → 2
23 - 30	98	2

Flow rate: 1.5 ml/min.

Detection: spectrophotometer at 220 nm.

Injection: 20 µl; inject the test solution and reference solutions (c), (d) and (e).

Relative retention with reference to cefadroxil (retention time = about 6 min): dimethylformamide = about 0.4; dimethylacetamide = about 0.75.

System suitability:

- *resolution:* minimum 5.0 between the peaks due to impurity A and to impurity B in the chromatogram obtained with reference solution (c),

- *signal-to-noise ratio:* minimum 10 for the second peak in the chromatogram obtained with reference solution (e).

Limits:

- *impurity A:* not more than the area of the first peak in the chromatogram obtained with reference solution (c) (1.0 per cent),

- *any other impurity:* not more than the area of the second peak in the chromatogram obtained with reference solution (c) (1.0 per cent),

- *total:* not more than 3 times the area of the second peak in the chromatogram obtained with reference solution (c) (3.0 per cent),

- *disregard limit:* 0.05 times the area of the second peak in the chromatogram obtained with reference solution (c) (0.05 per cent); disregard the peaks due to dimethylformamide and dimethylacetamide.

N,N-Dimethylaniline (*2.4.26, Method B*): maximum 20 ppm.

Water (*2.5.12*): 4.0 per cent to 6.0 per cent, determined on 0.200 g.

Sulphated ash (*2.4.14*): maximum 0.5 per cent, determined on 1.0 g.

ASSAY

Liquid chromatography (*2.2.29*).

Test solution. Dissolve 50.0 mg of the substance to be examined in the mobile phase and dilute to 100.0 ml with the mobile phase.

Reference solution (a). Dissolve 50.0 mg of *cefadroxil CRS* in the mobile phase and dilute to 100.0 ml with the mobile phase.

Reference solution (b). Dissolve 5 mg of *cefadroxil CRS* and 50 mg of *amoxicillin trihydrate CRS* in the mobile phase and dilute to 100 ml with the mobile phase.

Column:
- *size:* l = 0.25 m, Ø = 4.6 mm,

- *stationary phase: octadecylsilyl silica gel for chromatography R* (5 µm).

Mobile phase: acetonitrile R, a 2.72 g/l solution of *potassium dihydrogen phosphate R* (4:96 V/V).

Flow rate: 1 ml/min.

Detection: spectrophotometer at 254 nm.

Injection: 20 µl.

System suitability: reference solution (b):

— *resolution*: minimum 5.0 between the peaks due to cefadroxil and to amoxicillin.

Calculate the percentage content of cefadroxil.

STORAGE

Protected from light.

IMPURITIES

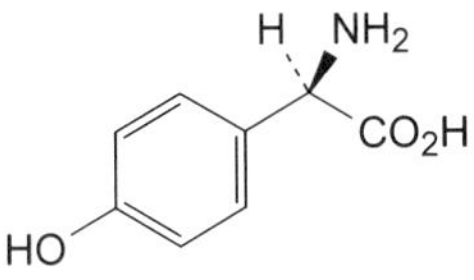

A. (2R)-2-amino-2-(4-hydroxyphenyl)acetic acid,

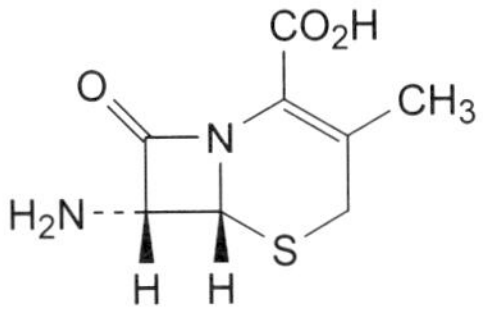

B. (6R,7R)-7-amino-3-methyl-8-oxo-5-thia-1-azabicyclo[4.2.0]oct-2-ene-2-carboxylic acid (7-ADCA),

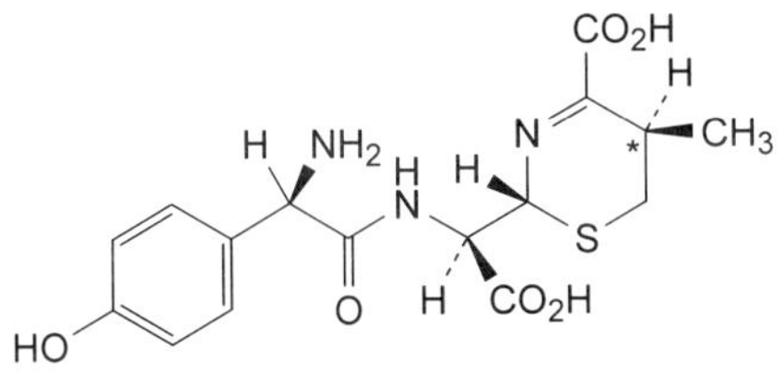

and epimer at C*

C. (2R,5RS)-2-[(R)-[[(2R)-2-amino-2-(4-hydroxyphenyl)acetyl]amino]carboxymethyl]-5-methyl-5,6-dihydro-2H-1,3-thiazine-4-carboxylic acid,

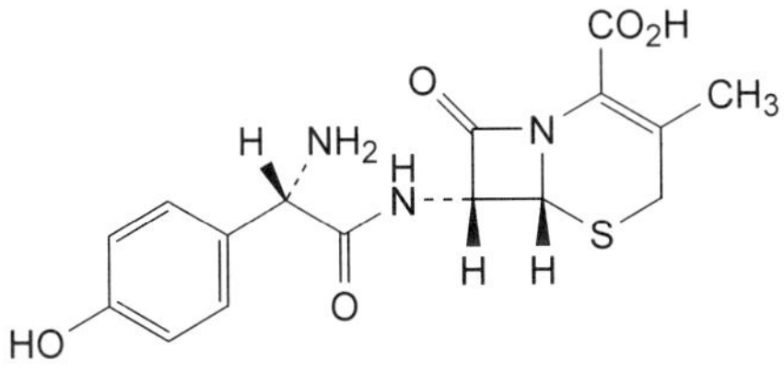

D. (6R,7R)-7-[[(2S)-2-amino-2-(4-hydroxyphenyl)acetyl]amino]-3-methyl-8-oxo-5-thia-1-azabicyclo[4.2.0]oct-2-ene-2-carboxylic acid (L-cefadroxil),

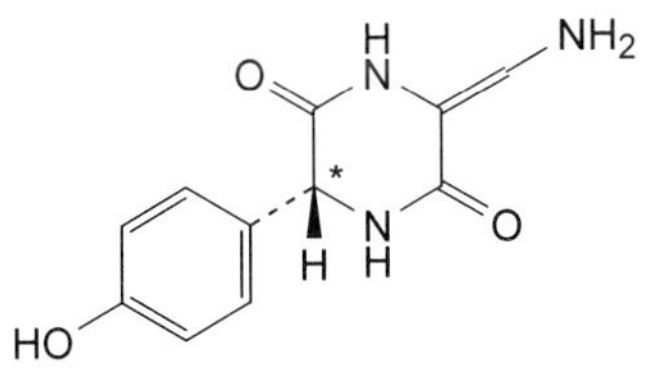

and epimer at C*

E. (6RS)-3-(aminomethylene)-6-(4-hydroxyphenyl)piperazine-2,5-dione,

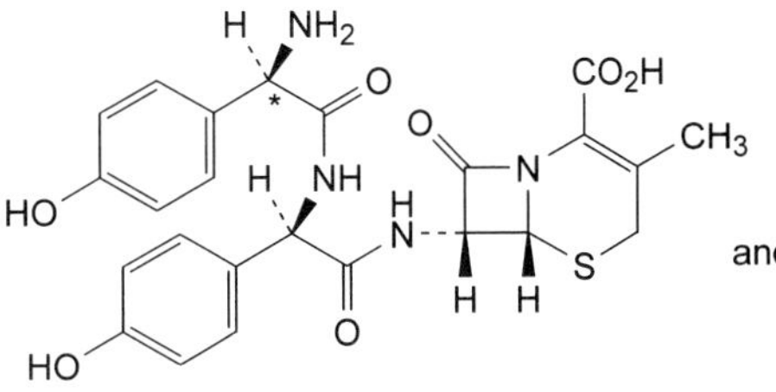

and epimer at C*

F. (6R,7R)-7-[[(2R)-2-[[(2RS)-2-amino-2-(4-hydroxyphenyl)acetyl]amino]-2-(4-hydroxyphenyl)acetyl]amino]-3-methyl-8-oxo-5-thia-1-azabicyclo[4.2.0]oct-2-ene-2-carboxylic acid,

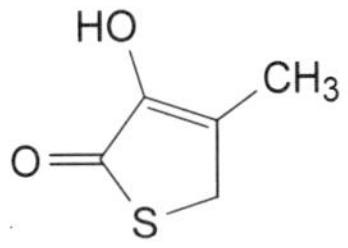

G. 3-hydroxy-4-methylthiophen-2(5H)-one,

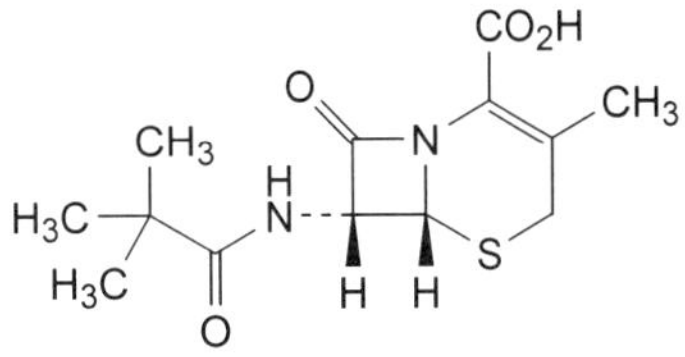

H. (6R,7R)-7-[(2,2-dimethylpropanoyl)amino]-3-methyl-8-oxo-5-thia-1-azabicyclo[4.2.0]oct-2-ene-2-carboxylic acid (7-ADCA pivalamide).

04/2003:1650

CEFAPIRIN SODIUM

Cefapirinum natricum

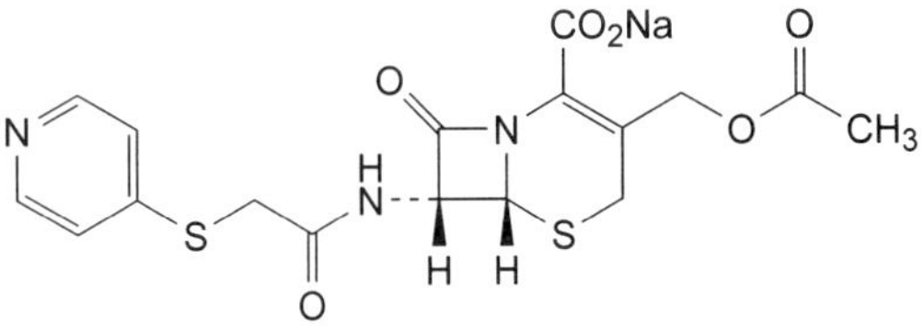

$C_{17}H_{16}N_3NaO_6S_2$ M_r 445.5

DEFINITION

Sodium (6R,7R)-3-[(acetyloxy)methyl]-8-oxo-7-[[[(pyridin-4-yl)sulphanyl]acetyl]amino]-5-thia-1-azabicyclo[4.2.0]oct-2-ene-2-carboxylate.

Content: 96.0 per cent to 102.0 per cent (anhydrous substance).

CHARACTERS

Appearance: white or pale yellow powder.

Solubility: soluble in water, practically insoluble in methylene chloride.

IDENTIFICATION

A. Infrared absorption spectrophotometry (*2.2.24*).
   Comparison: cefapirin sodium CRS.

B. It gives reaction (a) of sodium (*2.3.1*).

TESTS

Appearance of solution. The solution is not more opalescent than reference suspension I (*2.2.1*).

Dissolve 2.0 g in *water R* and dilute to 10 ml with the same solvent.

pH (*2.2.3*): 6.5 to 8.5.

Dissolve 0.100 g in *carbon dioxide-free water R* and dilute to 10.0 ml with the same solvent.

Specific optical rotation (*2.2.7*): + 150 to + 165 (anhydrous substance).

Dissolve 0.500 g in *water R* and dilute to 25.0 ml with the same solvent.

Related substances. Liquid chromatography (*2.2.29*). *Prepare the solutions immediately before use.*

Test solution. Dissolve 42 mg of the substance to be examined in the mobile phase and dilute to 200.0 ml with the mobile phase.

Reference solution (a). Dissolve 42 mg of *cefapirin sodium CRS* in the mobile phase and dilute to 200.0 ml with the mobile phase.

Reference solution (b). Dilute 1.0 ml of the test solution to 100.0 ml with the mobile phase.

Reference solution (c). Dilute 1.0 ml of reference solution (b) to 20.0 ml with the mobile phase.

Reference solution (d). Mix 1 ml of the test solution, 8 ml of the mobile phase and 1 ml of *hydrochloric acid R1*. Heat at 60 °C for 10 min.

Column:
- *size*: $l = 0.30$ m, $\emptyset = 4$ mm,
- *stationary phase*: *octadecylsilyl silica gel for chromatography R* (10 μm).

Mobile phase: mix 80 ml of *dimethylformamide R*, 4.0 ml of *glacial acetic acid R* and 20 ml of a 4.5 per cent (*m/m*) solution of *potassium hydroxide R* and dilute to 2 litres with *water R*.

Flow rate: 2.0 ml/min.

Detection: spectrophotometer at 254 nm.

Injection: 20 μl; inject the test solution and reference solutions (b), (c) and (d).

Run time: twice the retention time of cefapirin.

System suitability: reference solution (d):
- *resolution*: minimum 2.0 between the peaks due to cefapirin and to impurity A.

Limits:
- *any impurity*: not more than the area of the principal peak in the chromatogram obtained with reference solution (b) (1.0 per cent), and not more than 1 such peak has an area greater than 0.3 times the area of the principal peak in the chromatogram obtained with reference solution (b) (0.3 per cent),
- *total*: not more than twice the area of the principal peak in the chromatogram obtained with reference solution (b) (2.0 per cent),
- *disregard limit*: the area of the principal peak in the chromatogram obtained with reference solution (c) (0.05 per cent).

N,N-Dimethylaniline (*2.4.26, Method B*): maximum 20 ppm.

2-Ethylhexanoic acid (*2.4.28*): maximum 0.5 per cent.

Water (*2.5.12*): maximum 2.0 per cent, determined on 0.300 g.

Sterility (*2.6.1*). If intended for use in the manufacture of parenteral dosage forms without a further appropriate sterilisation procedure, it complies with the test for sterility.

Bacterial endotoxins (*2.6.14*): less than 0.17 IU/mg, if intended for use in the manufacture of parenteral dosage forms without a further appropriate procedure for the removal of bacterial endotoxins.

ASSAY

Liquid chromatography (*2.2.29*) as described in the test for related substances with the following modifications.

Injection: 20 μl; inject the test solution and reference solution (a).

Calculate the percentage content of $C_{17}H_{16}N_3NaO_6S_2$.

STORAGE

Protected from light. If the substance is sterile, store in a sterile, tamper-proof container.

LABELLING

The label states:
- where applicable, that the substance is sterile,
- where applicable, that the substance is free from bacterial endotoxins.

IMPURITIES

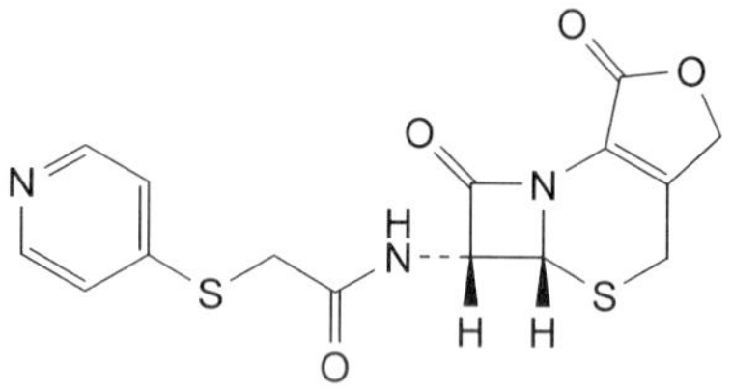

A. (5a*R*,6*R*)-6-[[[(pyridin-4-yl)sulphanyl]acetyl]amino]-5a,6-dihydro-3*H*,7*H*-azeto[2,1-*b*]furo[3,4-*d*][1,3]thiazine-1,7(4*H*)-dione (deacetylcefapirin lactone),

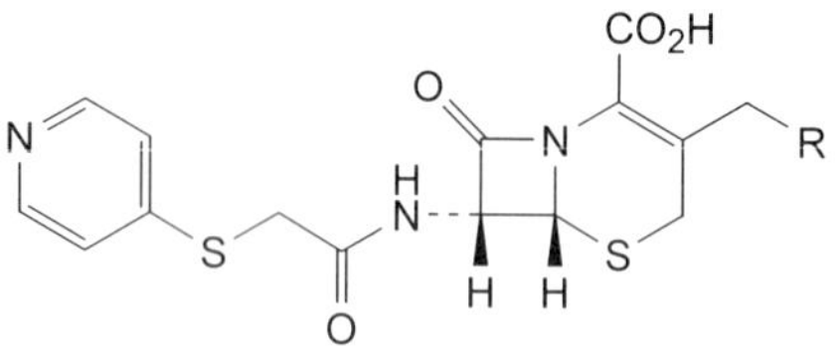

B. R = OH: (6*R*,7*R*)-3-(hydroxymethyl)-8-oxo-7-[[[(pyridin-4-yl)sulphanyl]acetyl]amino]-5-thia-1-azabicyclo[4.2.0]oct-2-ene-2-carboxylic acid (deacetylcefapirin),

C. R = H: (6*R*,7*R*)-3-methyl-8-oxo-7-[[[(pyridin-4-yl)sulphanyl]acetyl]amino]-5-thia-1-azabicyclo[4.2.0]oct-2-ene-2-carboxylic acid (deacetoxycefapirin).

07/2002:0988
corrected

CEFAZOLIN SODIUM

Cefazolinum natricum

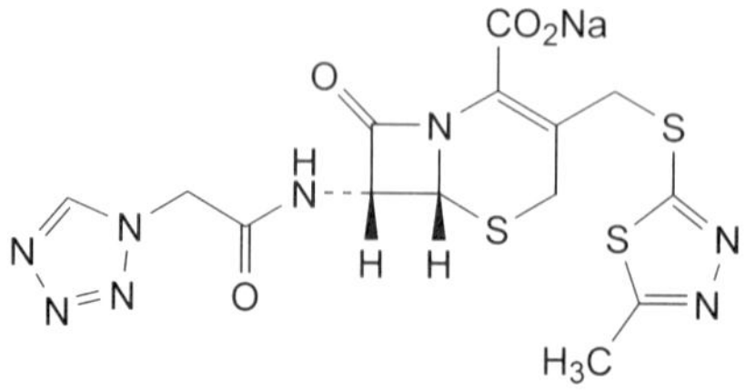

$C_{14}H_{13}N_8NaO_4S_3$ M_r 476.5

DEFINITION

Sodium (6*R*,7*R*)-3-[[(5-methyl-1,3,4-thiadiazol-2-yl)sulphanyl]methyl]-8-oxo-7-[(1*H*-tetrazol-1-ylacetyl)amino]-5-thia-1-azabicyclo[4.2.0]oct-2-ene-2-carboxylate.

Content: 95.0 per cent to 102.0 per cent (anhydrous substance).

CHARACTERS

Appearance: white or almost white powder, very hygroscopic.

Solubility: freely soluble in water, very slightly soluble in alcohol.

It shows polymorphism.

IDENTIFICATION

A. Infrared absorption spectrophotometry (*2.2.24*).

Preparation: dissolve 0.150 g in 5 ml of *water R*, add 0.5 ml of *dilute acetic acid R*, swirl and allow to stand for 10 min in iced water. Filter the precipitate and rinse with 1-2 ml of *water R*. Dissolve in a mixture of 1 volume of *water R* and 9 volumes of *acetone R*. Evaporate the solvent almost to dryness, then dry in an oven at 60 °C for 30 min.

Comparison: cefazolin CRS.

B. It gives reaction (a) of sodium (*2.3.1*).

TESTS

Solution S. Dissolve 2.50 g in *carbon dioxide-free water R* and dilute to 25.0 ml with the same solvent.

Appearance of solution. Solution S is clear (*2.2.1*) and its absorbance (*2.2.25*) at 430 nm has a maximum of 0.15.

pH (*2.2.3*): 4.0 to 6.0 for solution S.

Specific optical rotation (*2.2.7*): −15 to −24 (anhydrous substance).

Dissolve 1.25 g in *water R* and dilute to 25.0 ml with the same solvent.

Absorbance (*2.2.25*). Dissolve 0.100 g in *water R* and dilute to 100.0 ml with the same solvent. Dilute 2.0 ml of the solution to 100.0 ml with *sodium hydrogen carbonate solution R*. Examined between 220 nm and 350 nm, the solution shows an absorption maximum at 272 nm. The specific absorbance at the maximum is 260 to 300 (anhydrous substance).

Related substances. Liquid chromatography (*2.2.29*).

Test solution. Dissolve 50.0 mg of the substance to be examined in mobile phase A and dilute to 20.0 ml with the same mobile phase.

Reference solution (a). Dilute 1.0 ml of the test solution to 100.0 ml with mobile phase A.

Reference solution (b). Dissolve 20 mg of the substance to be examined in 10 ml of a 2 g/l solution of *sodium hydroxide R*. Allow to stand for 15-30 min. Dilute 1.0 ml of the solution to 20 ml with mobile phase A.

Column:

— *size*: l = 0.125 m, Ø = 4.0 mm,

— *stationary phase*: *octadecylsilyl silica gel for chromatography R* (3 µm),

— *temperature*: 45 °C.

Mobile phase:

— *mobile phase A*: solution containing 14.54 g/l of *disodium hydrogen phosphate R* and 3.53 g/l of *potassium dihydrogen phosphate R*,

— *mobile phase B*: *acetonitrile for chromatography R*,

The following chromatogram is published for information.

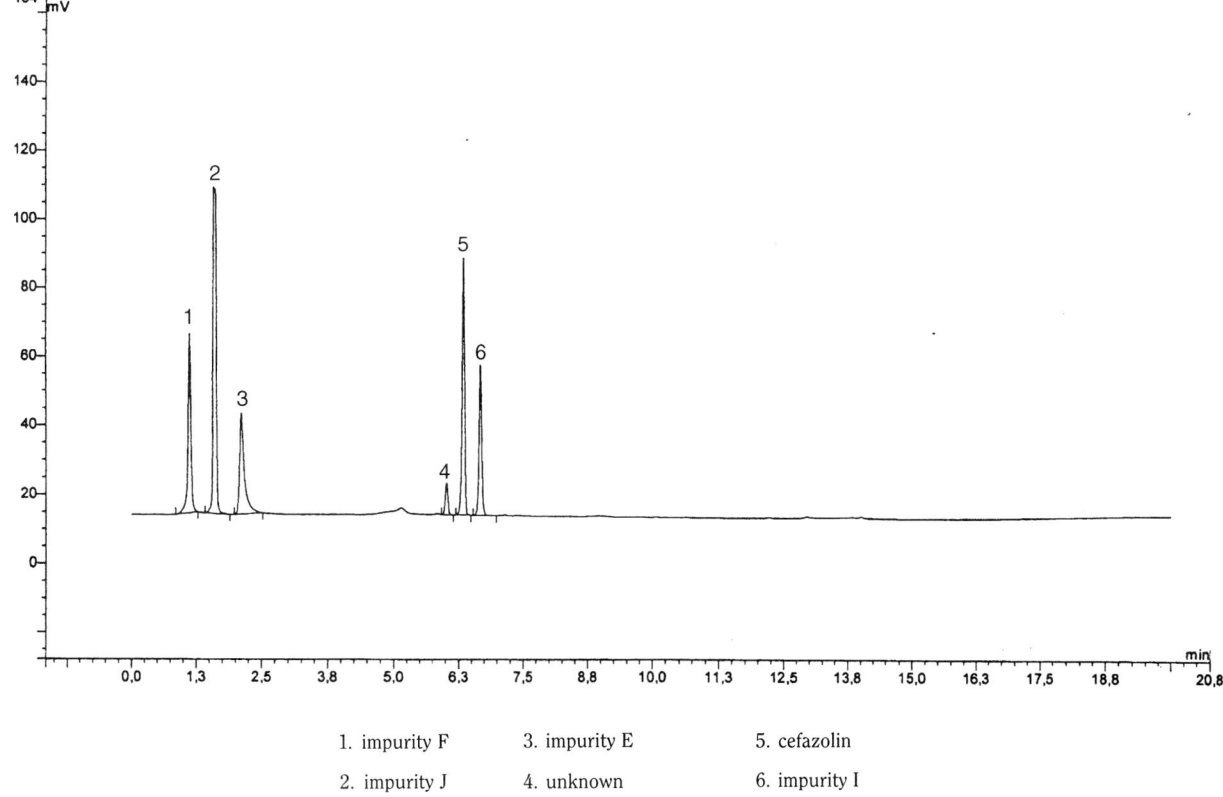

1. impurity F   3. impurity E   5. cefazolin

2. impurity J   4. unknown   6. impurity I

Figure 0988.-1. − *Chromatogram of reference solution (b) (in situ degradation) for the test for related substances of cefazolin sodium*

Time (min)	Mobile phase A (per cent V/V)	Mobile phase B (per cent V/V)	λ (nm)
0 - 1	98	2	210
1 - 2	98	2	254
2 - 4	98 → 85	2 → 15	254
4 - 10	85 → 60	15 → 40	254
10 - 11.5	60 → 35	40 → 65	254
11.5 - 12	35	65	254
12 - 15	35 → 98	65 → 2	254
15 - 16	98	2	254
16 - 21	98	2	210

Flow rate: 1.2 ml/min.

Detection: spectrophotometer at 210 nm and at 254 nm (see table above).

Injection: 5 μl.

System suitability: reference solution (b):

— *resolution*: minimum 2.0 between the peaks due to cefazolin and to impurity I.

Limits:

— *any impurity* (seen at 210 nm or 254 nm): not more than the area of the principal peak in the chromatogram obtained with reference solution (a) (1.0 per cent),

— *total*: not more than 3.5 times the area of the principal peak in the chromatogram obtained with reference solution (a) (3.5 per cent),

— *disregard limit*: 0.05 times the area of the principal peak in the chromatogram obtained with reference solution (a) (0.05 per cent).

N,N-Dimethylaniline (*2.4.26, Method B*): maximum 20 ppm.

Water (*2.5.12*): maximum 6.0 per cent, determined on 0.300 g.

Sterility (*2.6.1*). If intended for use in the manufacture of parenteral dosage forms without a further appropriate sterilisation procedure, it complies with the test for sterility.

Bacterial endotoxins (*2.6.14*): less than 0.15 IU/mg, if intended for use in the manufacture of parenteral dosage forms without a further appropriate procedure for the removal of bacterial endotoxins.

ASSAY

Liquid chromatography (*2.2.29*).

Test solution. Dissolve 50.0 mg of the substance to be examined in the mobile phase and dilute to 50.0 ml with the mobile phase.

Reference solution (a). Dissolve 50.0 mg of *cefazolin CRS* in the mobile phase and dilute to 50.0 ml with the mobile phase.

Reference solution (b). Dissolve 5.0 mg of *cefuroxime sodium CRS* in 10.0 ml of reference solution (a) and dilute to 100.0 ml with the mobile phase.

Column:

— *size*: *l* = 0.25 m, Ø = 4.6 mm,

— *stationary phase*: *octadecylsilyl silica gel for chromatography R* (5 μm).

Mobile phase: mix 10 volumes of *acetonitrile R* and 90 volumes of a solution containing 2.77 g/l of *disodium hydrogen phosphate R* and 1.86 g/l of *citric acid R*.

Flow rate: 1.0 ml/min.

Detection: spectrophotometer at 270 nm.

Injection: 20 μl.

System suitability: reference solution (b):

— *resolution*: minimum 2.0 between the peaks due to cefazolin and cefuroxime.

Calculate the percentage content of cefazolin sodium by multiplying the percentage content of cefazolin by 1.048.

STORAGE

In an airtight container, protected from light. If the substance is sterile, store in a sterile, airtight, tamper-proof container.

LABELLING

The label states:

— where applicable, that the substance is sterile,

— where applicable, that the substance is free from bacterial endotoxins.

IMPURITIES

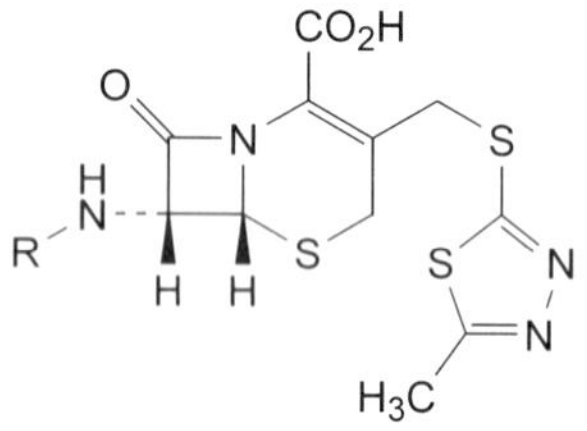

A. R = H: (6R,7R)-7-amino-3-[[(5-methyl-1,3,4-thiadiazol-2-yl)sulphanyl]methyl]-8-oxo-5-thia-1-azabicyclo[4.2.0]oct-2-ene-2-carboxylic acid,

B. R = CO-C(CH₃)₃: (6R,7R)-7-[(2,2-dimethylpropanoyl)amino]-3-[[(5-methyl-1,3,4-thiadiazol-2-yl)sulphanyl]methyl]-8-oxo-5-thia-1-azabicyclo[4.2.0]oct-2-ene-2-carboxylic acid,

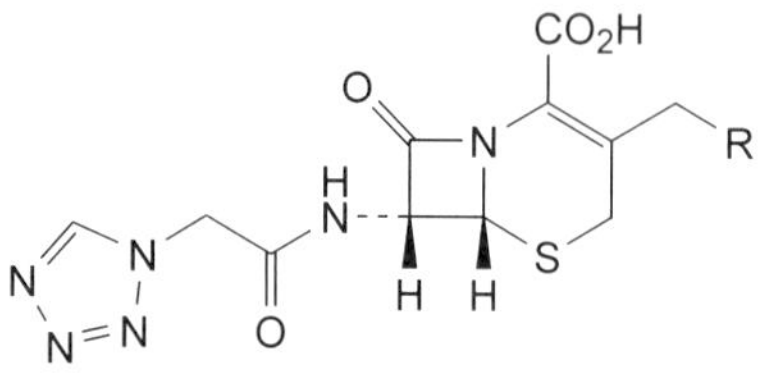

C. R = H: (6R,7R)-3-methyl-8-oxo-7-[(1H-tetrazol-1-ylacetyl)amino]-5-thia-1-azabicyclo[4.2.0]oct-2-ene-2-carboxylic acid,

D. R = O-CO-CH₃: (6R,7R)-3-[(acetyloxy)methyl]-8-oxo-7-[(1H-tetrazol-1-ylacetyl)amino]-5-thia-1-azabicyclo[4.2.0]oct-2-ene-2-carboxylic acid,

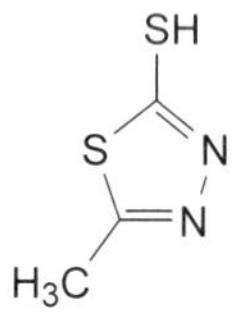

E. 5-methyl-1,3,4-thiadiazol-2-thiol (MMTD),

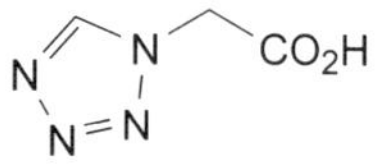

F. (1H-tetrazol-1-yl)acetic acid,

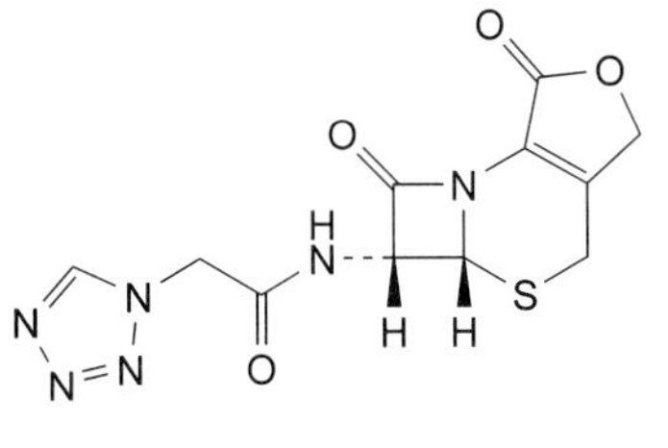

G. (5a*R*,6*R*)-6-[(1*H*-tetrazol-1-ylacetyl)amino]-5a,6-dihydro-3*H*,7*H*-azeto[2,1-*b*]furo[3,4-*d*][1,3]thiazine-1,7(4*H*)-dione,

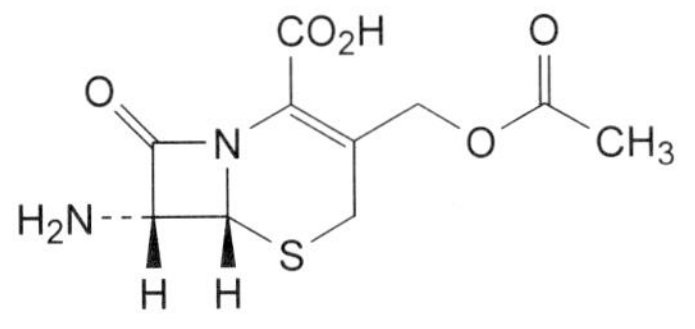

H. (6*R*,7*R*)-3-[(acetyloxy)methyl]-7-amino-8-oxo-5-thia-1-azabicyclo[4.2.0]oct-2-ene-2-carboxylic acid (7-ACA),

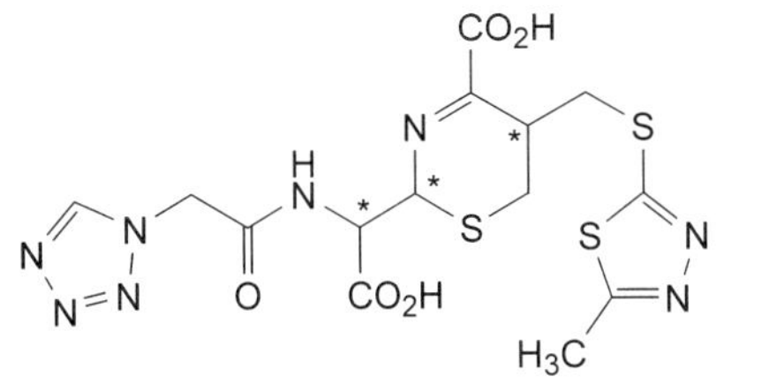

I. 2-[carboxy[(1*H*-tetrazol-1-ylacetyl)amino]methyl]-5-[[(5-methyl-1,3,4-thiadiazol-2-yl)sulphanyl]methyl]-5,6-dihydro-2*H*-1,3-thiazine-4-carboxylic acid (cefazoloic acid),

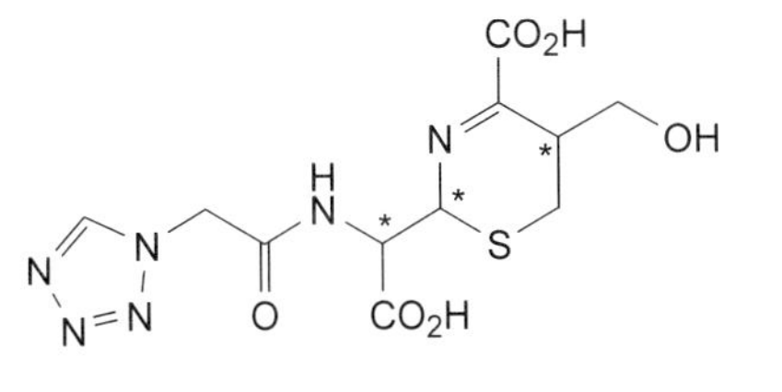

J. 2-[carboxy[(1*H*-tetrazol-1-ylacetyl)amino]methyl]-5-(hydroxymethyl)-5,6-dihydro-2*H*-1,3-thiazine-4-carboxylic acid (hydrolysed cefazoloic acid),

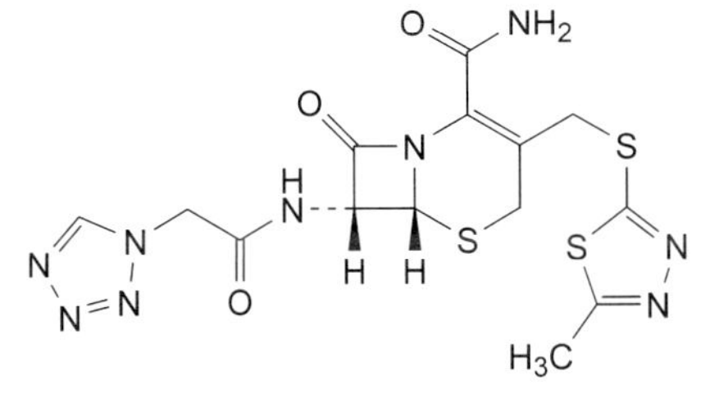

K. (6*R*,7*R*)-3-[[(5-methyl-1,3,4-thiadiazol-2-yl)sulphanyl]methyl]-8-oxo-7-[(1*H*-tetrazol-1-ylacetyl)amino]-5-thia-1-azabicyclo[4.2.0]oct-2-ene-2-carboxamide (cefazolinamide).

04/2003:0173

CHLORTETRACYCLINE HYDROCHLORIDE

Chlortetracyclini hydrochloridum

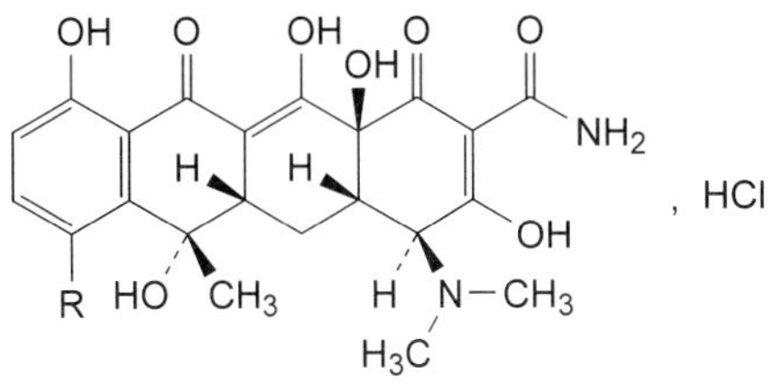

Compound	R	Molecular formula	Mr
Chlortetracycline hydrochloride	Cl	$C_{22}H_{24}Cl_2N_2O_8$	515.3
Tetracycline hydrochloride	H	$C_{22}H_{25}ClN_2O_8$	480.9

DEFINITION

Mixture of antibiotics, the main component being the hydrochloride of (4*S*,4a*S*,5a*S*,6*S*,12a*S*)-7-chloro-4-(dimethylamino)-3,6,10,12,12a-pentahydroxy-6-methyl-1,11-dioxo-1,4,4a,5,5a,6,11,12a-octahydrotetracene-2-carboxamide (chlortetracycline hydrochloride), a substance produced by the growth of certain strains of *Streptomyces aureofaciens* or obtained by any other means.

Content:

- $C_{22}H_{24}Cl_2N_2O_8$: minimum 89.5 per cent (anhydrous substance),
- $C_{22}H_{25}ClN_2O_8$: maximum 8.0 per cent (anhydrous substance),
- 94.5 per cent to 102.0 per cent for the sum of the contents of chlortetracycline hydrochloride and tetracycline hydrochloride (anhydrous substance).

CHARACTERS

Appearance: yellow powder.

Solubility: slightly soluble in water and in alcohol. It dissolves in solutions of alkali hydroxides and carbonates.

IDENTIFICATION

A. Thin-layer chromatography (*2.2.27*).

Test solution. Dissolve 5 mg of the substance to be examined in *methanol R* and dilute to 10 ml with the same solvent.

Reference solution (a). Dissolve 5 mg of *chlortetracycline hydrochloride CRS* in *methanol R* and dilute to 10 ml with the same solvent.

Reference solution (b). Dissolve 5 mg of *chlortetracycline hydrochloride CRS*, 5 mg of *doxycycline R* and 5 mg of *demeclocycline hydrochloride R* in *methanol R* and dilute to 10 ml with the same solvent.

Plate: *TLC octadecylsilyl silica gel F$_{254}$ plate R*.

Mobile phase: mix 20 volumes of *acetonitrile R*, 20 volumes of *methanol R* and 60 volumes of a 63 g/l solution of *oxalic acid R* previously adjusted to pH 2 with *concentrated ammonia R*.

Application: 1 µl.

Development: over 3/4 of the plate.

Drying: in air.

Detection: examine in ultraviolet light at 254 nm.

System suitability: the chromatogram obtained with reference solution (b) shows 3 clearly separated spots.

Results: the principal spot in the chromatogram obtained with the test solution is similar in position and size to the principal spot in the chromatogram obtained with reference solution (a).

B. To about 2 mg add 5 ml of *sulphuric acid R*. A deep blue colour develops which becomes bluish-green. Add the solution to 2.5 ml of *water R*. The colour becomes brownish.

C. It gives reaction (a) of chlorides (*2.3.1*).

TESTS

pH (*2.2.3*): 2.3 to 3.3.

Dissolve 0.1 g in 10 ml of *carbon dioxide-free water R*, heating slightly.

Specific optical rotation (*2.2.7*): −235 to −250 (anhydrous substance).

Dissolve 0.125 g in *water R* and dilute to 50.0 ml with the same solvent.

Absorbance (*2.2.25*): maximum 0.40 at 460 nm.

Dissolve 0.125 g in *water R* and dilute to 25.0 ml with the same solvent.

Related substances. Liquid chromatography (*2.2.29*). *Prepare the solutions immediately before use.*

Test solution. Dissolve 25.0 mg of the substance to be examined in *0.01 M hydrochloric acid* and dilute to 25.0 ml with the same acid.

Reference solution (a). Dissolve 25.0 mg of *chlortetracycline hydrochloride CRS* in *0.01 M hydrochloric acid* and dilute to 25.0 ml with the same acid.

Reference solution (b). Dissolve 10.0 mg of *4-epichlortetracycline hydrochloride CRS* in *0.01 M hydrochloric acid* and dilute to 25.0 ml with the same acid.

Reference solution (c). Dissolve 20.0 mg of *tetracycline hydrochloride CRS* in *0.01 M hydrochloric acid* and dilute to 25.0 ml with the same acid.

Reference solution (d). Mix 5.0 ml of reference solution (a) and 10.0 ml of reference solution (b) and dilute to 25.0 ml with *0.01 M hydrochloric acid.*

Reference solution (e). Mix 5.0 ml of reference solution (b) and 5.0 ml of reference solution (c) and dilute to 50.0 ml with *0.01 M hydrochloric acid.*

Reference solution (f). Dilute 1.0 ml of reference solution (c) to 20.0 ml with *0.01 M hydrochloric acid.* Dilute 5.0 ml of this solution to 200.0 ml with *0.01 M hydrochloric acid.*

Column:
- *size*: l = 0.25 m, Ø = 4.6 mm,
- *stationary phase*: *octylsilyl silica gel for chromatography R* (5 μm),
- *temperature*: 35 °C.

Mobile phase: to 500 ml of *water R*, add 50 ml of *perchloric acid solution R*, shake and add 450 ml of *dimethyl sulphoxide R*,

Flow rate: 1 ml/min.

Detection: spectrophotometer at 280 nm.

Injection: 20 μl; inject the test solution and reference solutions (d), (e) and (f).

System suitability: reference solution (d):
- *resolution*: minimum 2.0 between the peaks due to impurity A and to chlortetracycline; if necessary, adjust the dimethyl sulphoxide content in the mobile phase,
- *symmetry factor*: maximum 1.3 for the peak due to chlortetracycline.

Limits:
- *impurity A*: not more than the area of the corresponding peak in the chromatogram obtained with reference solution (e) (4.0 per cent),
- *total of other impurities eluting between the solvent peak and the peak corresponding to chlortetracycline*: not more than 0.25 times the area of the peak due to impurity A in the chromatogram obtained with reference solution (e) (1.0 per cent),
- *disregard limit*: area of the principal peak in the chromatogram obtained with reference solution (f) (0.1 per cent).

Heavy metals (*2.4.8*): maximum 50 ppm.

0.5 g complies with limit test C. Prepare the standard using 2.5 ml of *lead standard solution (10 ppm Pb) R.*

Water (*2.5.12*): maximum 2.0 per cent, determined on 0.300 g.

Sulphated ash (*2.4.14*): maximum 0.5 per cent, determined on 1.0 g.

Sterility (*2.6.1*). If intended for use in the manufacture of parenteral dosage forms without a further appropriate sterilisation procedure, it complies with the test for sterility.

Bacterial endotoxins (*2.6.14*): less than 1 IU/mg, if intended for use in the manufacture of parenteral dosage forms without a further appropriate procedure for the removal of bacterial endotoxins.

ASSAY

Liquid chromatography (*2.2.29*) as described in the test for related substances with the following modification.

Injection: test solution and reference solutions (a) and (e).

Calculate the percentage content of $C_{22}H_{24}Cl_2N_2O_8$ using the chromatogram obtained with reference solution (a). Calculate the percentage content of $C_{22}H_{25}ClN_2O_8$ using the chromatogram obtained with reference solution (e).

STORAGE

Protected from light. If the substance is sterile, store in a sterile, airtight, tamper-proof container.

LABELLING

The label states:
- where applicable, that the substance is sterile,
- where applicable, that the substance is free from bacterial endotoxins.

IMPURITIES

A. (4R,4aS,5aS,6S,12aS)-7-chloro-4-(dimethylamino)-3,6,10,12,12a-pentahydroxy-6-methyl-1,11-dioxo-1,4,4a,5,5a,6,11,12a-octahydrotetracene-2-carboxamide (4-epichlortetracycline),

B. demeclocycline.

04/2003:0993

CHOLESTEROL

Cholesterolum

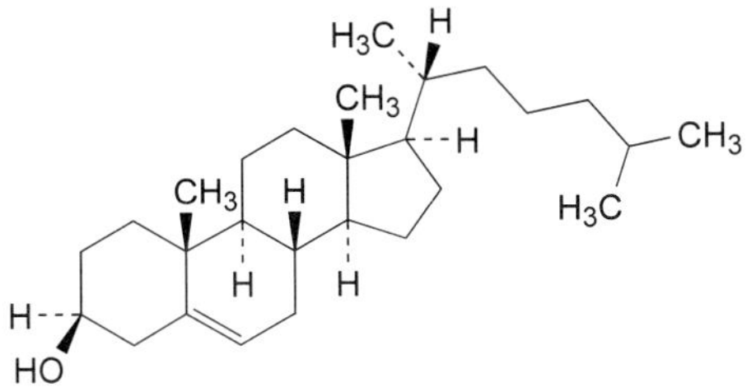

$C_{27}H_{46}O$ M_r 386.7

DEFINITION

Cholesterol contains not less than 95.0 per cent of cholest-5-en-3β-ol and not less than 97.0 per cent and not more than 103.0 per cent of total sterols, calculated with reference to the dried substance.

CHARACTERS

A white or almost white, crystalline powder, practically insoluble in water, sparingly soluble in acetone and in alcohol. It is sensitive to light.

IDENTIFICATION

A. Melting point (2.2.14): 147 °C to 150 °C.

B. Examine by thin-layer chromatography (2.2.27), using a *TLC silica gel G plate R*. Prepare the solutions immediately before use.

    Test solution. Dissolve 10 mg of the substance to be examined in *ethylene chloride R* and dilute to 5 ml with the same solvent.

    Reference solution. Dissolve 10 mg of *cholesterol CRS* in *ethylene chloride R* and dilute to 5 ml with the same solvent.

    Apply to the plate 20 µl of each solution. Develop immediately, protected from light, over a path of 15 cm using a mixture of 33 volumes of *ethyl acetate R* and 66 volumes of *toluene R*. Allow the plate to dry in air and spray 3 times with *antimony trichloride solution R*. Examine the chromatograms 3-4 min after spraying. The principal spot in the chromatogram obtained with the test solution is similar in position, colour and size to the principal spot in the chromatogram obtained with the reference solution.

C. Dissolve about 5 mg in 2 ml of *methylene chloride R*. Add 1 ml of *acetic anhydride R*, 0.01 ml of *sulphuric acid R* and shake. A pink colour is produced which rapidly changes to red, then to blue and finally to brilliant green.

TESTS

Solubility in alcohol. In a stoppered flask, dissolve 0.5 g in 50 ml of *alcohol R* at 50 °C. Allow to stand for 2 h. No deposit or turbidity is formed.

Acidity. Dissolve 1.0 g in 10 ml of *ether R*, add 10.0 ml of *0.1 M sodium hydroxide* and shake for about 1 min. Heat gently to eliminate ether and then boil for 5 min. Cool, add 10 ml of *water R* and 0.1 ml of *phenolphthalein solution R* as indicator and titrate with *0.1 M hydrochloric acid* until the pink colour just disappears, stirring the solution vigorously

throughout the titration. Carry out a blank titration. The difference between the volumes of *0.1 M hydrochloric acid* required to change the colour of the indicator in the blank and in the test is not more than 0.3 ml.

Loss on drying (2.2.32). Not more than 0.3 per cent, determined on 1.000 g by drying *in vacuo* at 60 °C for 4 h.

Sulphated ash (2.4.14). Not more than 0.1 per cent, determined on 1.0 g.

ASSAY

Examine by gas chromatography (2.2.28), using *pregnenolone isobutyrate CRS* as the internal standard.

Internal standard solution. Dissolve 0.100 g of *pregnenolone isobutyrate CRS* in *heptane R* and dilute to 100.0 ml with the same solvent.

Test solution. Dissolve 25.0 mg of the substance to be examined in the internal standard solution and dilute to 25.0 ml with the same solution.

Reference solution. Dissolve 25.0 mg of *cholesterol CRS* in the internal standard solution and dilute to 25.0 ml with the same solution.

The chromatographic procedure may be carried out using:

– a fused-silica column 30 m long and 0.25 mm in internal diameter coated with *poly(dimethyl)siloxane R* (film thickness 0.25 µm),

– *helium for chromatography R* as the carrier gas with a split ratio of 1:25 at a flow rate of 2 ml/min,

– a flame-ionisation detector,

maintaining the temperature of the column at 275 °C, that of the injection port at 285 °C and that of the detector at 300 °C.

Inject 1.0 µl of each solution. The assay is not valid unless the resolution between the peaks due to pregnenolone isobutyrate and cholest-5-en-3β-ol in the chromatogram obtained with the reference solution is at least 10.0.

Calculate the percentage content of cholest-5-en-3β-ol, using the declared content of cholest-5-en-3β-ol in *cholesterol CRS*. Calculate the percentage content of total sterols by adding together the contents of cholest-5-en-3β-ol and other substances with a retention time less than or equal to 1.5 times the retention time of cholest-5-en-3β-ol. Disregard the peaks due to the internal standard and the solvent.

STORAGE

Store protected from light.

LABELLING

The label states the source material for the production of cholesterol (for example bovine brain and spinal cord, wool fat or chicken eggs).

IMPURITIES

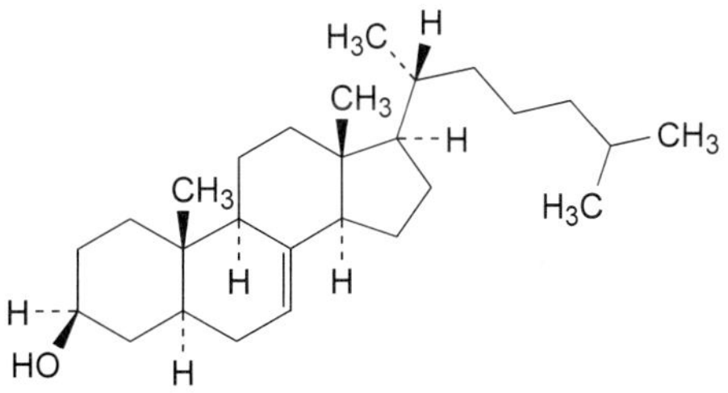

A. 5α-cholest-7-en-3β-ol (lathosterol),

B. cholesta-5,24-dien-3β-ol (desmosterol),

C. 5α-cholesta-7,24-dien-3β-ol.

04/2003:1192

COD-LIVER OIL (TYPE A)

Iecoris aselli oleum A

DEFINITION

Purified fatty oil obtained from the fresh livers of *Gadus morhua* L. and other species of *Gadidae*, solid substances being removed by cooling and filtering. A suitable antioxidant may be added.

Content: 600 IU (180 µg) to 2500 IU (750 µg) of vitamin A per gram and 60 IU (1.5 µg) to 250 IU (6.25 µg) of vitamin D_3 per gram.

CHARACTERS

Appearance: clear, yellowish, viscous liquid.

Solubility: practically insoluble in water, slightly soluble in alcohol, miscible with light petroleum.

IDENTIFICATION

First identification: A, B, C.

Second identification: C, D.

A. In the assay for vitamin A using method A, the test solution shows an absorption maximum (2.2.25) at 325 ± 2 nm. In the assay for vitamin A using method B, the chromatogram obtained with the test solution shows a peak corresponding to the peak of all-*trans*-retinol in the chromatogram obtained with the reference solution.

B. In the assay for vitamin D_3, the chromatogram obtained with test solution (a) shows a peak corresponding to the peak of cholecalciferol in the chromatogram obtained with reference solution (b).

C. It complies with the test for composition of fatty acids (see Tests).

D. To 0.1 g add 0.5 ml of *methylene chloride R* and 1 ml of *antimony trichloride solution R*. Mix. A deep blue colour develops in about 10 s.

TESTS

Colour: not more intensely coloured than a reference solution prepared as follows: to 3.0 ml of red primary solution add 25.0 ml of yellow primary solution and dilute to 50.0 ml with a 10 g/l solution of *hydrochloric acid R* (2.2.2, Method II).

Relative density (2.2.5): 0.917 to 0.930.

Refractive index (2.2.6): 1.477 to 1.484.

Acid value (2.5.1): maximum 2.0.

Anisidine value (2.5.36): maximum 30.0.

Iodine value (2.5.4, *Method B*): 150 to 180. Use *starch solution R2*.

Peroxide value (2.5.5, *Method B*): maximum 10.0.

Unsaponifiable matter (2.5.7): maximum 1.5 per cent, determined on 2.0 g, and extracting with 3 quantities, each of 50 ml, of *peroxide-free ether R*.

Stearin. 10 ml remains clear after cooling in iced water for 3 h.

Composition of fatty acids. Gas chromatography (2.2.28).

Trivial name of fatty acid	Nomenclature	Lower limit area (per cent)	Upper limit area (per cent)
Saturated fatty acids:			
Myristic acid	14:0	2.0	6.0
Palmitic acid	16:0	7.0	14.0
Stearic acid	18:0	1.0	4.0
Mono-unsaturated fatty acids:			
Palmitoleic acid	16:1 n-7	4.5	11.5
cis-Vaccenic acid	18:1 n-7	2.0	7.0
Oleic acid	18:1 n-9	12.0	21.0
Gadoleic acid	20:1 n-11	1.0	5.5
Gondoic acid	20:1 n-9	5.0	17.0
Erucic acid	22:1 n-9	0	1.5
Cetoleic acid (22:1 n-11)	22:1 n-11+13	5.0	12.0
Poly-unsaturated fatty acids:			
Linoleic acid	18:2 n-6	0.5	3.0
α-Linolenic acid	18:3 n-3	0	2.0
Moroctic acid	18:4 n-3	0.5	4.5
Timnodonic (eicosapentaenoic) acid (EPA)	20:5 n-3	7.0	16.0
Cervonic (docosahexaenoic) acid (DHA)	22:6 n-3	6.0	18.0

Test solution. Introduce about 0.45 g of the substance to be examined into a 10 ml volumetric flask, dissolve in *hexane R* containing 50 mg of *butylhydroxytoluene R* per litre and dilute to 10.0 ml with the same solvent. Transfer 2.0 ml of the solution into a quartz tube and evaporate the solvent with a gentle current of *nitrogen R*. Add 1.5 ml of a 20 g/l solution of *sodium hydroxide R* in *methanol R*, cover with *nitrogen R*, cap tightly with a polytetrafluoroethylene lined cap, mix and heat in a water-bath for 7 min. Cool, add 2 ml of *boron trichloride-methanol solution R*, cover with *nitrogen R*, cap tightly, mix and heat in a water-bath for 30 min. Cool to 40-50 °C, add 1 ml of *trimethylpentane R*, cap and vortex or shake vigorously for at least 30 s. Immediately add 5 ml of *saturated sodium chloride solution R*, cover with *nitrogen R*, cap and vortex or shake thoroughly for at least 15 s. Allow the upper layer to become clear and transfer to a separate tube. Shake the methanol layer once more with 1 ml of *trimethylpentane R* and combine the trimethylpentane extracts. Wash the combined extracts with 2 quantities, each of 1 ml, of *water R* and dry over *anhydrous sodium sulphate R*. Prepare 2 solutions for each sample.

Column:

— *material*: fused silica,

— *size*: l = 30 m, Ø = 0.25 mm,

— *stationary phase*: *macrogol 20 000 R* (film thickness 0.25 µm).

Carrier gas: *hydrogen for chromatography R* or *helium for chromatography R*, where oxygen scrubber is applied.

Split ratio: 1:200.

Temperature:

	Time (min)	Temperature (°C)
Column	0 - 55	170 → 225
	55 - 75	225
Injection port		250
Detection		280

Detection: flame ionisation.

Injection: 1 µl, twice.

System suitability:

— the 15 fatty acids to be tested are satisfactorily identified from the chromatogram shown in Figure 1192.-1,

— injection of a mixture of equal amounts of *methyl palmitate R*, *methyl stearate R*, *methyl arachidate R* and *methyl behenate R* give area percentages of 24.4, 24.8, 25.2 and 25.6 (± 0.5 per cent), respectively,

— *resolution*: minimum of 1.3 between the peaks due to methyl oleate and methyl *cis*-vaccenate; the resolution between the pair due to methyl gadoleate and methyl gondoate is sufficient for purposes of identification and area measurement.

Calculate the area per cent for each fatty acid methyl ester from the expression:

$$\frac{A_x}{A_t} \times 100$$

A_x = peak area of fatty acid x,

A_t = sum of the peak areas (up to C22:6 n-3).

The calculation is not valid unless:

— the total area is based only on peaks due to solely fatty acids methyl esters,

— the number of fatty acid methyl ester peaks exceeding 0.05 per cent of the total area is at least 24,

— the 24 largest peaks of the methyl esters account for more than 90 per cent of the total area. (These correspond to, in common elution order: 14:0, 15:0, 16:0, 16:1 n-7, 16:4 n-1, 18:0, 18:1 n-9, 18:1 n-7, 18:2 n-6, 18:3 n-3, 18:4 n-3, 20:1 n-11, 20:1 n-9, 20:1 n-7, 20:2 n-6, 20:4 n-6, 20:3 n-3, 20:4 n-3, 20:5 n-3, 22:1 n-11, 22:1 n-9, 21:5 n-3, 22:5 n-3, 22:6 n-3).

ASSAY

Vitamin A. *Carry out the test as rapidly as possible, avoiding exposure to actinic light and air, oxidising agents, oxidation catalysts (for example, copper and iron) and acids.*

Use method A. If method A is found not to be valid, use method B.

METHOD A

Ultraviolet absorption spectrophotometry (*2.2.25*).

Test solution. To 1.00 g in a round-bottomed flask, add 3 ml of a freshly prepared 50 per cent *m/m* solution of *potassium hydroxide R* and 30 ml of *ethanol R*. Boil under reflux in a current of *nitrogen R* for 30 min. Cool rapidly and add 30 ml of *water R*. Extract with 50 ml of *ether R*. Repeat the extraction 3 times and discard the lower layer after complete separation. Wash the combined upper layers with 4 quantities, each of 50 ml, of *water R* and evaporate to dryness under a gentle current of *nitrogen R* at a temperature not exceeding 30 °C or in a rotary evaporator at a temperature not exceeding 30 °C under reduced pressure (water ejector). Dissolve the residue in sufficient *2-propanol R1* to give an expected concentration of vitamin A equivalent to 10-15 IU/ml.

Measure the absorbances of the solution at 300 nm, 310 nm, 325 nm and 334 nm and at the wavelength of maximum absorption with a suitable spectrophotometer in 1 cm specially matched cells, using *2-propanol R1* as the compensation liquid.

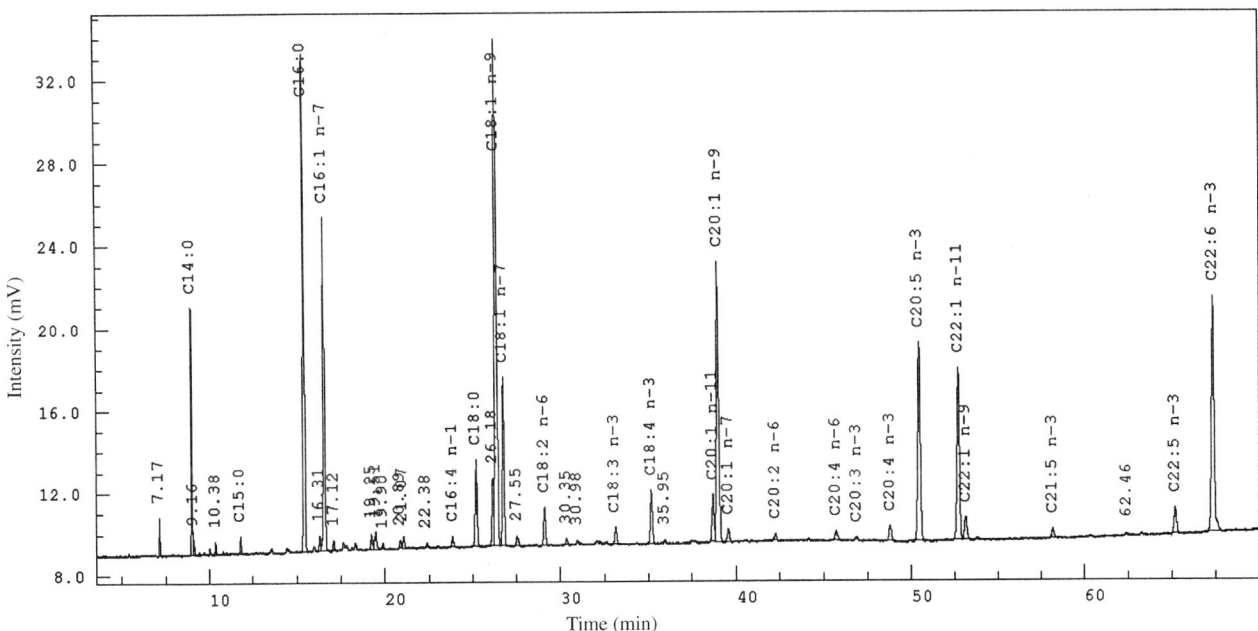

Figure 1192.-1. – *Chromatogram of cod-liver oil (type A) for the test for composition of fatty acids*

Calculate the content of vitamin A, as all-*trans*-retinol, in International Units per gram from the expression:

$$A_{325} \times \frac{1830}{100m} \times V$$

A_{325} = absorbance at 325 nm,

m = mass of the substance to be examined, in grams,

V = total volume of solution containing 10-15 IU of vitamin A per millilitre,

1830 = conversion factor for the specific absorbance of all-*trans*-retinol, in International Units.

The above expression can be used only if A_{325} has a value of not greater than $A_{325,\text{corr}}/0.970$ where $A_{325,\text{corr}}$ is the corrected absorbance at 325 nm and is given by the equation:

$$A_{325,\,\text{corr}} = 6.815A_{325} - 2.555A_{310} - 4.260A_{334}$$

A designates the absorbance at the wavelength indicated by the subscript.

If A_{325} has a value greater than $A_{325,\text{corr}}/0.970$, calculate the content of vitamin A from the following expression:

$$A_{325,\,\text{corr}} \times \frac{1830}{100m} \times V$$

The assay is not valid unless:

— the wavelength of maximum absorption lies between 323 nm and 327 nm,

— the absorbance at 300 nm relative to that at 325 nm is at most 0.73.

METHOD B

Liquid chromatography (*2.2.29*).

Test solution. To 2.00 g in a round-bottomed flask, add 5 ml of a freshly prepared 100 g/l solution of *ascorbic acid R* and 10 ml of a freshly prepared 800 g/l solution of *potassium hydroxide R* and 100 ml of *ethanol R*. Boil under a reflux condenser on a water-bath for 15 min. Add 100 ml of a 10 g/l solution of *sodium chloride R* and cool. Transfer the solution to a 500 ml separating funnel rinsing the round-bottomed flask with about 75 ml of a 10 g/l solution of *sodium chloride R* and then with 150 ml of a mixture of equal volumes of *light petroleum R3* and *ether R*. Shake for 1 min. When the layers have separated completely, discard the lower layer and wash the upper layer, first with 50 ml of a 30 g/l solution of *potassium hydroxide R* in a 10 per cent V/V solution of *ethanol R* and then with 3 quantities, each of 50 ml, of a 10 g/l solution of *sodium chloride R*. Filter the upper layer through 5 g of *anhydrous sodium sulphate R* on a fast filter paper into a 250 ml flask suitable for a rotary evaporator. Wash the funnel with 10 ml of fresh extraction mixture, filter and combine the upper layers. Distil them at a temperature not exceeding 30 °C under reduced pressure (water ejector) and fill with *nitrogen R* when evaporation is completed. Alternatively evaporate the solvent under a gentle current of *nitrogen R* at a temperature not exceeding 30 °C. Dissolve the residue in *2-propanol R*, transfer to a 25 ml volumetric flask and dilute to 25 ml with *2-propanol R*. Gentle heating in an ultrasonic bath may be required. (A large fraction of the white residue is cholesterol, constituting approximately 50 per cent of the unsaponifiable matter of cod-liver oil).

Reference solution (a). Prepare a solution of *retinyl acetate CRS* in *2-propanol R1* so that 1 ml contains about 1000 IU of all-*trans*-retinol.

The exact concentration of reference solution (a) is assessed by ultraviolet absorption spectrophotometry (*2.2.25*). Dilute reference solution (a) with *2-propanol R1* to a presumed concentration of 10-15 IU/ml and measure the absorbance at 326 nm in matched 1 cm cells using *2-propanol R1* as the compensation liquid.

Calculate the content of vitamin A in International Units per millilitre of reference solution (a) from the following expression, taking into account the assigned content of *retinyl acetate CRS*:

$$A_{326} \times \frac{1900 \times V_2}{100 \times V_1}$$

A_{326} = absorbance at 326 nm,

V_1 = volume of reference solution (a) used,

V_2 = volume of the diluted solution,

1900 = conversion factor for the specific absorbance of *retinyl acetate CRS*, in International Units.

Reference solution (b). Proceed as described for the test solution but using 2.00 ml of reference solution (a) in place of the substance to be examined.

The exact concentration of reference solution (b) is assessed by ultraviolet absorption spectrophotometry (*2.2.25*). Dilute reference solution (b) with *2-propanol R1* to a presumed concentration of 10-15 IU/ml of all-*trans*-retinol and measure the absorbance at 325 nm in matched 1 cm cells using *2-propanol R1* as the compensation liquid.

Calculate the content of all-*trans*-retinol in International Units per millilitre of reference solution (b) from the expression:

$$A_{325} \times \frac{1830 \times V_3}{100 \times V_4}$$

A_{325} = absorbance at 325 nm,

V_3 = volume of the diluted solution,

V_4 = volume of reference solution (b) used,

1830 = conversion factor for the specific absorbance of all-*trans*-retinol, in International Units.

Column:

— *size*: l = 0.25 m, Ø = 4.6 mm,

— *stationary phase*: *octadecylsilyl silica gel for chromatography R* (film thickness 5-10 μm).

Mobile phase: *water R*, *methanol R* (3:97 V/V).

Flow rate: 1 ml/min.

Detection: spectrophotometer at 325 nm.

Injection: 10 μl; inject in triplicate the test solution and reference solution (b).

Retention time: all-*trans*-retinol = 5 ± 1 min.

System suitability:

— the chromatogram obtained with the test solution shows a peak due to that of all-*trans*-retinol in the chromatogram obtained with reference solution (b),

— when using the method of standard additions to the test solution there is greater than 95 per cent recovery of the added *retinyl acetate CRS*,

— the recovery of all-*trans*-retinol in reference solution (b) as assessed by direct absorption spectrophotometry is greater than 95 per cent.

Calculate the content of vitamin A using the following expression:

$$A_1 \times \frac{C \times V}{A_2} \times \frac{1}{m}$$

A_1 = area of the peak due to all-*trans*-retinol in the chromatogram obtained with the test solution,

A_2 = area of the peak due to all-*trans*-retinol in the chromatogram obtained with reference solution (b),

C = concentration of *retinyl acetate CRS* in reference solution (a) as assessed prior to the saponification, in International Units per millilitre (= 1000 IU/ml),

V = volume of reference solution (a) treated (2.00 ml),

m = mass of the substance to be examined in the test solution (2.00 g).

Vitamin D$_3$. Liquid chromatography (*2.2.29*). *Carry out the assay as rapidly as possible, avoiding exposure to actinic light and air.*

Internal standard solution. Dissolve 0.50 mg of *ergocalciferol CRS* in 100 ml of *ethanol R*.

Test solution (a). To 4.00 g in a round-bottomed flask, add 5 ml of a freshly prepared 100 g/l solution of *ascorbic acid R*, 10 ml of a freshly prepared 800 g/l solution of *potassium hydroxide R* and 100 ml of *ethanol R*. Boil under a reflux condenser on a water-bath for 30 min. Add 100 ml of a 10 g/l solution of *sodium chloride R* and cool the solution to room temperature. Transfer the solution to a 500 ml separating funnel rinsing the round-bottomed flask with about 75 ml of a 10 g/l solution of *sodium chloride R* and then with 150 ml of a mixture of equal volumes of *light petroleum R3* and *ether R*. Shake for 1 min. When the layers have separated completely, discard the lower layer and wash the upper layer, first with 50 ml of a 30 g/l solution of *potassium hydroxide R* in a 10 per cent *V/V* solution of *ethanol R*, and then with 3 quantities, each of 50 ml, of a 10 g/l solution of *sodium chloride R*. Filter the upper layer through 5 g of *anhydrous sodium sulphate R* on a fast filter paper into a 250 ml flask suitable for a rotary evaporator. Wash the funnel with 10 ml of fresh extraction mixture, filter and combine the upper layers. Distil them at a temperature not exceeding 30 °C under reduced pressure (water ejector) and fill with *nitrogen R* when evaporation is completed. Alternatively evaporate the solvent under a gentle current of *nitrogen R* at a temperature not exceeding 30 °C. Dissolve the residue in 1.5 ml of the mobile phase described under Purification. Gentle heating in an ultrasonic bath may be required. (A large fraction of the white residue is cholesterol, constituting approximately 50 per cent *m/m* of the unsaponifiable matter of cod-liver oil).

Test solution (b). To 4.00 g add 2.0 ml of the internal standard solution and proceed as described for test solution (a).

Reference solution (a). Dissolve 0.50 mg of *cholecalciferol CRS* in 100.0 ml of *ethanol R*.

Reference solution (b). In a round-bottomed flask, add 2.0 ml of reference solution (a) and 2.0 ml of the internal standard solution and proceed as described for test solution (a).

PURIFICATION

Column:

– *size*: $l = 0.25$ m, Ø = 4.6 mm,

– *stationary phase*: *nitrile silica gel for chromatography R* (film thickness 10 µm).

Mobile phase: *isoamyl alcohol R*, *hexane R* (1.6:98.4 *V/V*).

Flow rate: 1.1 ml/min.

Detection: spectrophotometer at 265 nm.

Inject 350 µl of reference solution (b). Collect the eluate from 2 min before until 2 min after the retention time of cholecalciferol, in a ground-glass-stoppered tube containing 1 ml of a 1 g/l solution of *butylhydroxytoluene R* in *hexane R*. Repeat the procedure with test solutions (a) and (b). Evaporate the eluates obtained from reference solution (b) and from test solutions (a) and (b), separately, to dryness at a temperature not exceeding 30 °C under a gentle current of *nitrogen R*. Dissolve each residue in 1.5 ml of *acetonitrile R*.

DETERMINATION

Column:

– *size*: $l = 0.15$ m, Ø = 4.6 mm,

– *stationary phase*: *octadecylsilyl silica gel for chromatography R* (film thickness 5 µm).

Mobile phase: *phosphoric acid R*, 96 per cent *V/V* solution of *acetonitrile R* (0.2:99.8 *V/V*).

Flow rate: 1.0 ml/min.

Detection: spectrophotometer at 265 nm.

Injection: 2 quantities not exceeding 200 µl of each of the 3 solutions obtained under Purification.

System suitability:

– *resolution*: minimum 1.4 between the peaks corresponding to ergocalciferol and cholecalciferol in the chromatogram obtained with reference solution (b),

– when using the method of standard additions to test solution (a) there is greater than 95 per cent recovery of the added *cholecalciferol CRS* when due consideration has been given to correction by the internal standard.

Calculate the content of vitamin D$_3$ in International Units per gram using the following expression, taking into account the assigned content of *cholecalciferol CRS*:

$$\frac{A_2}{A_6} \times \frac{A_3}{A_4 - \left[\frac{A_5}{A_1}\right] \times A_2} \times \frac{m_2}{m_1} \times \frac{V_2}{V_1} \times 40$$

m_1 = mass of the sample in test solution (b) in grams,

m_2 = total mass of *cholecalciferol CRS* used for the preparation of reference solution (a) in micrograms (500 µg),

A_1 = area (or height) of the peak due to cholecalciferol in the chromatogram obtained with test solution (a),

A_2 = area (or height) of the peak due to cholecalciferol in the chromatogram obtained with test solution (b),

A_3 = area (or height) of the peak due to ergocalciferol in the chromatogram obtained with reference solution (b),

A_4 = area (or height) of the peak due to ergocalciferol in the chromatogram obtained with test solution (b),

A_5 = area (or height) of a possible peak in the chromatogram obtained with test solution (a) with the same retention time as the peak co-eluting with ergocalciferol in test solution (b),

A_6 = area (or height) of the peak due to cholecalciferol in the chromatogram obtained with reference solution (b),

V_1 = total volume of reference solution (a) (100 ml),

V_2 = volume of reference solution (a) used for preparing reference solution (b) (2.0 ml).

STORAGE

In an airtight and well-filled container, protected from light. If no antioxidant is added, store under an inert gas.

Once the container has been opened, its contents are used as soon as possible and any part of the contents not used at once is protected by an atmosphere of inert gas.

LABELLING

The label states:

- the number of International Units of vitamin A,
- the number of International Units of vitamin D_3,
- the name and concentration of any added antioxidant.

04/2003:1193

COD-LIVER OIL (TYPE B)

Iecoris aselli oleum B

DEFINITION

Purified fatty oil obtained from the fresh livers of *Gadus morhua* L. and other species of *Gadidae*, solid substances being removed by cooling and filtering. A suitable antioxidant may be added.

Content: 600 IU (180 µg) to 2500 IU (750 µg) of vitamin A per gram and 60 IU (1.5 µg) to 250 IU (6.25 µg) of vitamin D_3 per gram.

CHARACTERS

Appearance: clear, yellowish, viscous liquid.

Solubility: practically insoluble in water, slightly soluble in alcohol, miscible with light petroleum.

IDENTIFICATION

First identification: A, B, C.

Second identification: C, D.

A. In the assay for vitamin A using method A, the test solution shows an absorption maximum (*2.2.25*) at 325 ± 2 nm. In the assay for vitamin A using method B, the chromatogram obtained with the test solution shows a peak corresponding to the peak of all-*trans*-retinol in the chromatogram obtained with the reference solution.

B. In the assay for vitamin D_3, the chromatogram obtained with test solution (a) shows a peak corresponding to the peak of cholecalciferol in the chromatogram obtained with reference solution (b).

C. It complies with the test for composition of fatty acids (see Tests).

D. To 0.1 g add 0.5 ml of *methylene chloride R* and 1 ml of *antimony trichloride solution R*. Mix. A deep blue colour develops in about 10 s.

TESTS

Colour: not more intensely coloured than a reference solution prepared as follows: to 3.0 ml of red primary solution add 25.0 ml of yellow primary solution and dilute to 50.0 ml with a 10 g/l solution of *hydrochloric acid R* (*2.2.2, Method II*).

Relative density (*2.2.5*): 0.917 to 0.930.

Refractive index (*2.2.6*): 1.477 to 1.484.

Acid value (*2.5.1*): maximum 2.0.

Iodine value (*2.5.4, Method B*): 150 to 180. Use *starch solution R2*.

Peroxide value (*2.5.5, Method B*): maximum 10.0.

Unsaponifiable matter (*2.5.7*): maximum 1.5 per cent, determined on 2.0 g and extracting with 3 quantities, each of 50 ml, of *peroxide-free ether R*.

Stearin. 10 ml remains clear after cooling in iced water for 3 h.

Composition of fatty acids. Gas chromatography (*2.2.28*).

Trivial name of fatty acid	Nomenclature	Lower limit area (per cent)	Upper limit area (per cent)
Saturated fatty acids:			
Myristic acid	14:0	2.0	6.0
Palmitic acid	16:0	7.0	14.0
Stearic acid	18:0	1.0	4.0
Mono-unsaturated fatty acids:			
Palmitoleic acid	16:1 n-7	4.5	11.5
cis-Vaccenic acid	18:1 n-7	2.0	7.0
Oleic acid	18:1 n-9	12.0	21.0
Gadoleic acid	20:1 n-11	1.0	5.5
Gondoic acid	20:1 n-9	5.0	17.0
Erucic acid	22:1 n-9	0	1.5
Cetoleic acid (22:1 n-11)	22:1 n-11+13	5.0	12.0
Poly-unsaturated fatty acids:			
Linoleic acid	18:2 n-6	0.5	3.0
α-Linolenic acid	18:3 n-3	0	2.0
Moroctic acid	18:4 n-3	0.5	4.5
Timnodonic (eicosapentaenoic) acid (EPA)	20:5 n-3	7.0	16.0
Cervonic (docosahexaenoic) acid (DHA)	22:6 n-3	6.0	18.0

Test solution. Introduce about 0.45 g of the substance to be examined into a 10 ml volumetric flask, dissolve in *hexane R* containing 50 mg of *butylhydroxytoluene R* per litre and dilute to 10.0 ml with the same solvent. Transfer 2.0 ml of the solution into a quartz tube and evaporate the solvent with a gentle current of *nitrogen R*. Add 1.5 ml of a 20 g/l solution of *sodium hydroxide R* in *methanol R*, cover with *nitrogen R*, cap tightly with a polytetrafluoroethylene lined cap, mix and heat in a water-bath for 7 min. Cool, add 2 ml of *boron trichloride-methanol solution R*, cover with *nitrogen R*, cap tightly, mix and heat in a water-bath for 30 min. Cool to 40-50 °C, add 1 ml of *trimethylpentane R*, cap and vortex or shake vigorously for at least 30 s. Immediately add 5 ml of *saturated sodium chloride solution R*, cover with *nitrogen R*, cap and vortex or shake thoroughly for at least 15 s. Allow the upper layer to become clear and transfer to a separate tube. Shake the methanol layer once more with 1 ml of *trimethylpentane R* and combine the trimethylpentane extracts. Wash the combined extracts with 2 quantities, each of 1 ml, of *water R* and dry over *anhydrous sodium sulphate R*. Prepare 2 solutions for each sample.

Column:

- *material*: fused silica,
- *size*: $l = 30$ m, $\emptyset = 0.25$ mm,
- *stationary phase*: *macrogol 20 000 R* (film thickness 0.25 µm).

Carrier gas: *hydrogen for chromatography R* or *helium for chromatography R*, where oxygen scrubber is applied.

Split ratio: 1:200.

Temperature:

	Time (min)	Temperature (°C)
Column	0 - 55	170 → 225
	55 - 75	225
Injection port		250
Detector		280

Detection: flame ionisation.

Injection: 1 μl, twice.

System suitability:

– the 15 fatty acids to be tested are satisfactorily identified from the chromatogram shown in Figure 1193.-1.

– injection of a mixture of equal amounts of *methyl palmitate R*, *methyl stearate R*, *methyl arachidate R*, and *methyl behenate R* give area percentages of 24.4, 24.8, 25.2 and 25.6 (± 0.5 per cent), respectively,

– *resolution*: minimum of 1.3 between the peaks due to methyl oleate and methyl *cis*-vaccenate; the resolution between the pair due to methyl gadoleate and methyl gondoate is sufficient for purposes of identification and area measurement.

Calculate the area per cent for each fatty acid methyl ester from the expression:

$$\frac{A_x}{A_t} \times 100$$

A_x = peak area of fatty acid x,

A_t = sum of the peak areas (up to C22:6 n-3).

The calculation is not valid unless:

– the total area is based only on peaks due to solely fatty acids methyl esters,

– the number of fatty acid methyl ester peaks exceeding 0.05 per cent of the total area is at least 24,

– the 24 largest peaks of the methyl esters account for more than 90 per cent of the total area. (These correspond to, in common elution order: 14:0, 15:0, 16:0, 16:1 n-7, 16:4 n-1, 18:0, 18:1 n-9, 18:1 n-7, 18:2 n-6, 18:3 n-3, 18:4 n-3, 20:1 n-11, 20:1 n-9, 20:1 n-7, 20:2 n-6, 20:4 n-6, 20:3 n-3, 20:4 n-3, 20:5 n-3, 22:1 n-11, 22:1 n-9, 21:5 n-3, 22:5 n-3, 22:6 n-3).

ASSAY

Vitamin A. *Carry out the test as rapidly as possible, avoiding exposure to actinic light and air, oxidising agents, oxidation catalysts (for example, copper and iron) and acids.*

Use method A. If method A is found not to be valid, use method B.

METHOD A

Ultraviolet absorption spectrophotometry (*2.2.25*).

Test solution. To 1.00 g in a round-bottomed flask, add 3 ml of a freshly prepared 50 per cent *m/m* solution of *potassium hydroxide R* and 30 ml of *ethanol R*. Boil under reflux in a current of *nitrogen R* for 30 min. Cool rapidly and add 30 ml of *water R*. Extract with 50 ml of *ether R*. Repeat the extraction 3 times and discard the lower layer after complete separation. Wash the combined upper layers with 4 quantities, each of 50 ml, of *water R* and evaporate to dryness under a gentle current of *nitrogen R* at a temperature not exceeding 30 °C or in a rotary evaporator at a temperature not exceeding 30 °C under reduced pressure (water ejector). Dissolve the residue in sufficient *2-propanol R1* to give an expected concentration of vitamin A equivalent to 10-15 IU/ml.

Measure the absorbances of the solution at 300 nm, 310 nm, 325 nm and 334 nm and at the wavelength of maximum absorption with a suitable spectrophotometer in 1 cm specially matched cells, using *2-propanol R1* as the compensation liquid.

Calculate the content of vitamin A, as all-*trans*-retinol, in International Units per gram from the expression:

$$A_{325} \times \frac{1830}{100m} \times V$$

A_{325} = absorbance at 325 nm,

m = mass of the substance to be examined, in grams,

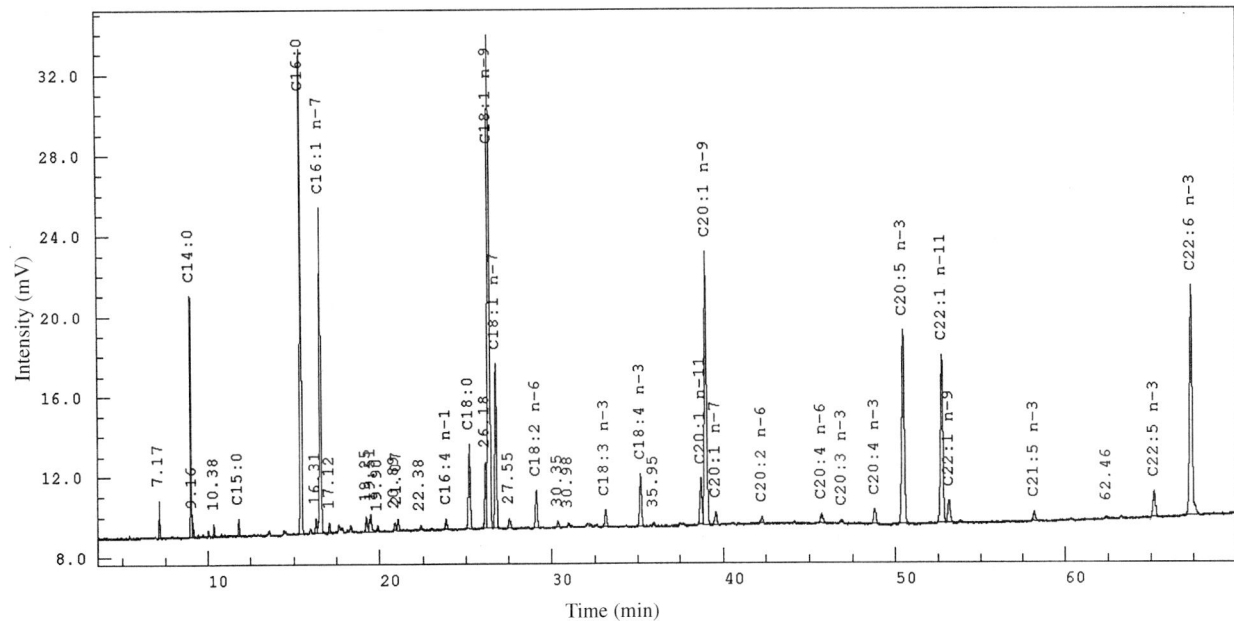

Figure 1193.-1. – *Chromatogram of cod-liver oil (type B) for the test for composition of fatty acids*

V = total volume of solution containing 10-15 IU of vitamin A per millilitre,

1830 = conversion factor for the specific absorbance of all-*trans*-retinol, in International Units.

The above expression can be used only if A_{325} has a value of not greater than $A_{325,corr}/0.970$ where $A_{325,corr}$ is the corrected absorbance at 325 nm and is given by the equation:

$$A_{325,\,corr} = 6.815A_{325} - 2.555A_{310} - 4.260A_{334}$$

A designates the absorbance at the wavelength indicated by the subscript.

If A_{325} has a value greater than $A_{325,corr}/0.970$, calculate the content of vitamin A from the expression:

$$A_{325,\,corr} \times \frac{1830}{100m} \times V$$

The assay is not valid unless:

— the wavelength of maximum absorption lies between 323 nm and 327 nm,

— the absorbance at 300 nm relative to that at 325 nm is at most 0.73.

METHOD B

Liquid chromatography (*2.2.29*).

Test solution. To 2.00 g in a round-bottomed flask, add 5 ml of a freshly prepared 100 g/l solution of *ascorbic acid R* and 10 ml of a freshly prepared 800 g/l solution of *potassium hydroxide R* and 100 ml of *ethanol R*. Boil under a reflux condenser on a water-bath for 15 min. Add 100 ml of a 10 g/l solution of *sodium chloride R* and cool. Transfer the solution to a 500 ml separating funnel rinsing the round-bottomed flask with about 75 ml of a 10 g/l solution of *sodium chloride R* and then with 150 ml of a mixture of equal volumes of *light petroleum R3* and *ether R*. Shake for 1 min. When the layers have separated completely, discard the lower layer and wash the upper layer, first with 50 ml of a 30 g/l solution of *potassium hydroxide R* in a 10 per cent *V/V* solution of *ethanol R* and then with 3 quantities, each of 50 ml, of a 10 g/l solution of *sodium chloride R*. Filter the upper layer through 5 g of *anhydrous sodium sulphate R* on a fast filter paper into a 250 ml flask suitable for a rotary evaporator. Wash the funnel with 10 ml of fresh extraction mixture, filter and combine the upper layers. Distil them at a temperature not exceeding 30 °C under reduced pressure (water ejector) and fill with *nitrogen R* when evaporation is completed. Alternatively evaporate the solvent under a gentle current of *nitrogen R* at a temperature not exceeding 30 °C. Dissolve the residue in *2-propanol R*, transfer to a 25 ml volumetric flask and dilute to 25 ml with *2-propanol R*. Gentle heating in an ultrasonic bath may be required. (A large fraction of the white residue is cholesterol, constituting approximately 50 per cent of the unsaponifiable matter of cod-liver oil).

Reference solution (a). Prepare a solution of *retinyl acetate CRS* in *2-propanol R1* so that 1 ml contains about 1000 IU of all-*trans*-retinol.

The exact concentration of reference solution (a) is assessed by ultraviolet absorption spectrophotometry (*2.2.25*). Dilute reference solution (a) with *2-propanol R1* to a presumed concentration of 10-15 IU/ml and measure the absorbance at 326 nm in matched 1 cm cells using *2-propanol R1* as the compensation liquid.

Calculate the content of vitamin A in International Units per millilitre of reference solution (a) using the following expression, taking into account the assigned content of *retinyl acetate CRS*:

$$A_{326} \times \frac{1900 \times V_2}{100 \times V_1}$$

A_{326} = absorbance at 326 nm,

V_1 = volume of reference solution (a) used,

V_2 = volume of the diluted solution,

1900 = conversion factor for the specific absorbance of *retinyl acetate CRS*, in International Units.

Reference solution (b). Proceed as described for the test solution but using 2.00 ml of reference solution (a) in place of the substance to be examined.

The exact concentration of reference solution (b) is assessed by ultraviolet absorption spectrophotometry (*2.2.25*). Dilute reference solution (b) with *2-propanol R1* to a presumed concentration of 10-15 IU/ml of all-*trans*-retinol and measure the absorbance at 325 nm in matched 1 cm cells using *2-propanol R1* as the compensation liquid.

Calculate the content of all-*trans*-retinol in International Units per millilitre of reference solution (b) from the expression:

$$A_{325} \times \frac{1830 \times V_3}{100 \times V_4}$$

A_{325} = absorbance at 325 nm,

V_3 = volume of the diluted solution,

V_4 = volume of reference solution (b) used,

1830 = conversion factor for the specific absorbance of all-*trans*-retinol, in International Units.

Column:

— *size*: l = 0.25 m, $\varnothing$ = 4.6 mm,

— *stationary phase*: *octadecylsilyl silica gel for chromatography R* (film thickness 5-10 µm).

Mobile phase: *water R, methanol R* (3:97 *V/V*).

Flow rate: 1 ml/min.

Detection: spectrophotometer at 325 nm.

Injection: 10 µl; inject in triplicate the test solution and reference solution (b).

Retention time: all-*trans*-retinol = 5 ± 1 min.

System suitability:

— the chromatogram obtained with the test solution shows a peak due to that of all-*trans*-retinol in the chromatogram obtained with reference solution (b),

— when using the method of standard additions to the test solution there is greater than 95 per cent recovery of the added *retinyl acetate CRS*,

— the recovery of all-*trans*-retinol in reference solution (b) as assessed by direct absorption spectrophotometry is greater than 95 per cent.

Calculate the content of vitamin A using the following expression:

$$A_1 \times \frac{C \times V}{A_2} \times \frac{1}{m}$$

A_1 = area of the peak due to all-*trans*-retinol in the chromatogram obtained with the test solution,

A_2 = area of the peak due to all-*trans*-retinol in the chromatogram obtained with reference solution (b),

C = concentration of *retinyl acetate CRS* in reference solution (a) as assessed prior to the saponification, in International Units per millilitre (= 1000 IU/ml),

V = volume of reference solution (a) treated (2.00 ml),

m = mass of the substance to be examined in the test solution (2.00 g).

Vitamin D$_3$. Liquid chromatography (*2.2.29*). *Carry out the assay as rapidly as possible, avoiding exposure to actinic light and air.*

Internal standard solution. Dissolve 0.50 mg of *ergocalciferol CRS* in 100 ml of *ethanol R*.

Test solution (a). To 4.00 g in a round-bottomed flask, add 5 ml of a freshly prepared 100 g/l solution of *ascorbic acid R*, 10 ml of a freshly prepared 800 g/l solution of *potassium hydroxide R* and 100 ml of *ethanol R*. Boil under a reflux condenser on a water-bath for 30 min. Add 100 ml of a 10 g/l solution of *sodium chloride R* and cool the solution to room temperature. Transfer the solution to a 500 ml separating funnel rinsing the round-bottomed flask with about 75 ml of a 10 g/l solution of *sodium chloride R* and then with 150 ml of a mixture of equal volumes of *light petroleum R3* and *ether R*. Shake for 1 min. When the layers have separated completely, discard the lower layer and wash the upper layer, first with 50 ml of a 30 g/l solution of *potassium hydroxide R* in a 10 per cent *V/V* solution of *ethanol R*, and then with 3 quantities, each of 50 ml, of a 10 g/l solution of *sodium chloride R*. Filter the upper layer through 5 g of *anhydrous sodium sulphate R* on a fast filter paper into a 250 ml flask suitable for a rotary evaporator. Wash the funnel with 10 ml of fresh extraction mixture, filter and combine the upper layers. Distil them at a temperature not exceeding 30 °C under reduced pressure (water ejector) and fill with *nitrogen R* when evaporation is completed. Alternatively evaporate the solvent under a gentle current of *nitrogen R* at a temperature not exceeding 30 °C. Dissolve the residue in 1.5 ml of the mobile phase described under Purification. Gentle heating in an ultrasonic bath may be required. (A large fraction of the white residue is cholesterol, constituting approximately 50 per cent *m/m* of the unsaponifiable matter of cod-liver oil).

Test solution (b). To 4.00 g add 2.0 ml of the internal standard solution and proceed as described for test solution (a).

Reference solution (a). Dissolve 0.50 mg of *cholecalciferol CRS* in 100.0 ml of *ethanol R*.

Reference solution (b). In a round-bottomed flask, add 2.0 ml of reference solution (a) and 2.0 ml of the internal standard solution and proceed as described for test solution (a).

PURIFICATION

Column:

- *size*: $l = 0.25$ m, Ø = 4.6 mm,
- *stationary phase*: *nitrile silica gel for chromatography R* (film thickness 10 µm).

Mobile phase: *isoamyl alcohol R, hexane R* (1.6:98.4 *V/V*).

Flow rate: 1.1 ml/min.

Detection: spectrophotometer at 265 nm.

Inject 350 µl of reference solution (b). Collect the eluate from 2 min before until 2 min after the retention time of cholecalciferol, in a ground-glass-stoppered tube containing 1 ml of a 1 g/l solution of *butylhydroxytoluene R* in *hexane R*. Repeat the procedure with test solutions (a) and (b). Evaporate the eluates obtained from reference solution (b) and from test solutions (a) and (b), separately, to dryness at a temperature not exceeding 30 °C under a gentle current of *nitrogen R*. Dissolve each residue in 1.5 ml of *acetonitrile R*.

DETERMINATION

Column:

- *size*: $l = 0.15$ m, Ø = 4.6 mm,
- *stationary phase*: *octadecylsilyl silica gel for chromatography R* (film thickness 5 µm).

Mobile phase: *phosphoric acid R*, a 96 per cent *V/V* solution of *acetonitrile R* (0.2:99.8 *V/V*).

Flow rate: 1.0 ml/min.

Detection: spectrophotometer at 265 nm.

Injection: 2 quantities not exceeding 200 µl of each of the 3 solutions obtained under Purification.

System suitability:

- *resolution*: minimum 1.4 between the peaks due to ergocalciferol and cholecalciferol in the chromatogram obtained with reference solution (b),
- when using the method of standard additions to test solution (a) there is greater than 95 per cent recovery of the added *cholecalciferol CRS* when due consideration has been given to correction by the internal standard.

Calculate the content of vitamin D$_3$ in International Units per gram using the following expression, taking into account the assigned content of *cholecalciferol CRS*:

$$\frac{A_2}{A_6} \times \frac{A_3}{A_4 - \left[\frac{A_5}{A_1}\right] \times A_2} \times \frac{m_2}{m_1} \times \frac{V_2}{V_1} \times 40$$

m_1 = mass of the sample in test solution (b) in grams,

m_2 = total mass of *cholecalciferol CRS* used for the preparation of reference solution (a) in micrograms (500 µg),

A_1 = area (or height) of the peak due to cholecalciferol in the chromatogram obtained with test solution (a),

A_2 = area (or height) of the peak due to cholecalciferol in the chromatogram obtained with test solution (b),

A_3 = area (or height) of the peak due to ergocalciferol in the chromatogram obtained with reference solution (b),

A_4 = area (or height) of the peak due to ergocalciferol in the chromatogram obtained with test solution (b),

A_5 = area (or height) of a possible peak in the chromatogram obtained with test solution (a) with the same retention time as the peak co-eluting with ergocalciferol in test solution (b),

A_6 = area (or height) of the peak due to cholecalciferol in the chromatogram obtained with reference solution (b),

V_1 = total volume of reference solution (a) (100 ml),

V_2 = volume of reference solution (a) used for preparing reference solution (b) (2.0 ml).

STORAGE

In an airtight and well-filled container, protected from light. If no antioxidant is added, store under an inert gas.

Once the container has been opened, its contents are used as soon as possible and any part of the contents not used at once is protected by an atmosphere of inert gas.

LABELLING

The label states:

- the number of International Units of vitamin A,
- the number of International Units of vitamin D_3,
- the name and concentration of any added antioxidant.

04/2003:0758

COLCHICINE

Colchicinum

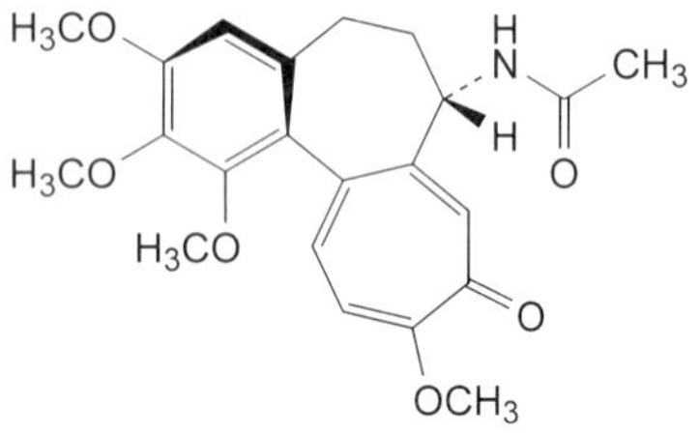

$C_{22}H_{25}NO_6$ M_r 399.4

DEFINITION

(-)-N-[(7S,12aS)-1,2,3,10-Tetramethoxy-9-oxo-5,6,7,9-tetrahydrobenzo[a]heptalen-7-yl]acetamide.

Content: 97.0 per cent to 102.0 per cent (anhydrous and ethyl acetate-free substance).

CHARACTERS

Appearance: yellowish-white, amorphous or crystalline powder.

Solubility: very soluble in water, rapidly recrystallising from concentrated solutions as the sesquihydrate, freely soluble in alcohol, practically insoluble in cyclohexane.

IDENTIFICATION

First identification: B.

Second identification: A, C, D.

A. Dissolve 5 mg in alcohol R and dilute to 100.0 ml with the same solvent. Dilute 5.0 ml of the solution to 25.0 ml with alcohol R. Examined between 230 nm and 400 nm (2.2.25), the solution shows 2 absorption maxima, at 243 nm and 350 nm. The ratio of the absorbance measured at 243 nm to that measured at 350 nm is 1.7 to 1.9.

B. Infrared absorption spectrophotometry (2.2.24).

Preparation: discs of potassium bromide R.

Comparison: colchicine CRS.

C. To 0.5 ml of solution S (see Tests) add 0.5 ml of dilute hydrochloric acid R and 0.15 ml of ferric chloride solution R1. The solution is yellow and becomes dark green on boiling for 30 s. Cool, add 2 ml of methylene chloride R and shake. The organic layer is greenish-yellow.

D. Dissolve about 30 mg in 1 ml of alcohol R and add 0.15 ml of ferric chloride solution R1. A brownish-red colour develops.

TESTS

Solution S. Dissolve 0.10 g in water R and dilute to 20 ml with the same solvent.

Appearance of solution. Solution S is clear (2.2.1) and not more intensely coloured than reference solution GY_3 (2.2.2, Method II).

Acidity or alkalinity. To 10 ml of solution S add 0.1 ml of bromothymol blue solution R1. Either the solution does not change colour or it becomes green. Not more than 0.1 ml of 0.01 M sodium hydroxide is required to change the colour of the indicator to blue.

Specific optical rotation (2.2.7): −235 to −250 (anhydrous and ethyl acetate-free substance).

Dissolve 50.0 mg in alcohol R and dilute to 10.0 ml with the same solvent.

Related substances. Liquid chromatography (2.2.29).

Test solution. Dissolve 20.0 mg of the substance to be examined in a mixture of equal volumes of methanol R and water R and dilute to 20.0 ml with the same mixture of solvents.

Reference solution (a). Dissolve 20.0 mg of colchicine for system suitability CRS in a mixture of equal volumes of methanol R and water R and dilute to 20.0 ml with the same mixture of solvents.

Reference solution (b). Dilute 1.0 ml of the test solution to 100.0 ml with a mixture of equal volumes of methanol R and water R.

Reference solution (c). Dilute 1 ml of reference solution (b) to 20.0 ml with a mixture of equal volumes of methanol R and water R.

Column:

- size: l = 0.25 m, Ø = 4.6 mm,
- stationary phase: octylsilyl silica gel for chromatography R1 (5 µm).

Mobile phase: mix 450 volumes of a 6.8 g/l solution of potassium dihydrogen phosphate R and 530 volumes of methanol R. After cooling to room temperature, adjust the volume to 1000 ml with methanol R. Adjust the apparent pH to 5.5 with dilute phosphoric acid R.

Flow rate: 1 ml/min.

Detection: spectrophotometer at 254 nm.

Injection: 20 µl.

Run time: 3 times the retention time of colchicine.

Relative retention with reference to colchicine (retention time = about 7 min): impurity D = about 0.4; impurity E = about 0.7; impurity B = about 0.8; impurity A = about 0.94; impurity C = about 1.2.

System suitability: reference solution (a):

Peak-to-valley ratio: minimum 2, where H_P = height above the baseline of the peak due to impurity A and H_V = height above the baseline of the lowest point of the curve separating this peak from the peak due to colchicine.

Limits:

- impurity A: not more than 3.5 times the area of the principal peak in the chromatogram obtained with reference solution (b) (3.5 per cent),
- any other impurity: not more than the area of the principal peak in the chromatogram obtained with reference solution (b) (1 per cent),

— *total*: not more than 5 times the area of the principal peak in the chromatogram obtained with reference solution (b) (5 per cent),

— *disregard limit*: area of the principal peak in the chromatogram obtained with reference solution (c) (0.05 per cent).

Colchiceine: maximum 0.2 per cent.

Dissolve 50 mg in *water R* and dilute to 5 ml with the same solvent. Add 0.1 ml of *ferric chloride solution R1*. The solution is not more intensely coloured than a mixture of 1 ml of red primary solution, 2 ml of yellow primary solution and 2 ml of blue primary solution (*2.2.2, Method II*).

Chloroform (*2.4.24*): maximum 500 ppm.

Ethyl acetate (*2.4.24*): maximum 6.0 per cent *m/m*.

Water (*2.5.12*): maximum 2.0 per cent, determined on 0.500 g.

Sulphated ash (*2.4.14*): maximum 0.1 per cent, determined on 0.5 g.

ASSAY

Dissolve 0.250 g with gentle heating in a mixture of 10 ml of *acetic anhydride R* and 20 ml of *toluene R*. Titrate with *0.1 M perchloric acid*, determining the end-point potentiometrically (*2.2.20*).

1 ml of *0.1 M perchloric acid* is equivalent to 39.94 mg of $C_{22}H_{25}NO_6$.

STORAGE

Protected from light.

IMPURITIES

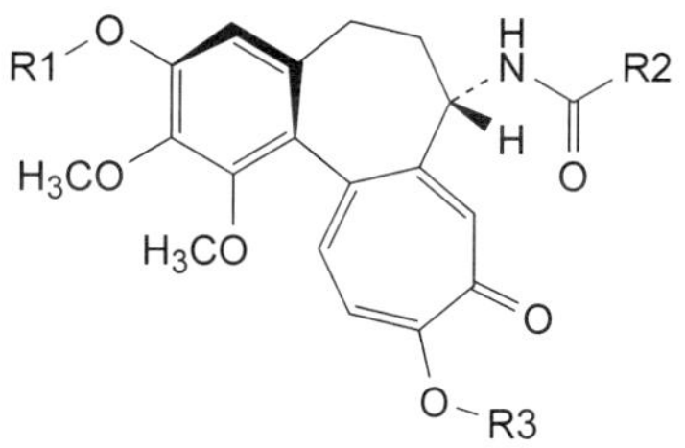

A. R1 = R3 = CH_3, R2 = H: *N*-[(7*S*,12a*S*)-1,2,3,10-tetramethoxy-9-oxo-5,6,7,9-tetrahydrobenzo[*a*]heptalen-7-yl]formamide (*N*-deacetyl-*N*-formylcolchicine),

E. R1 = H, R2 = R3 = CH_3: *N*-[(7*S*,12a*S*)-3-hydroxy-1,2,10-trimethoxy-9-oxo-5,6,7,9-tetrahydrobenzo[*a*]heptalen-7-yl]acetamide (3-*O*-demethylcolchicine),

F. R1 = R2 = CH_3, R3 = H: *N*-[(7*S*,12a*S*)-10-hydroxy-1,2,3-trimethoxy-9-oxo-5,6,7,9-tetrahydrobenzo[*a*]heptalen-7-yl]acetamide (colchiceine),

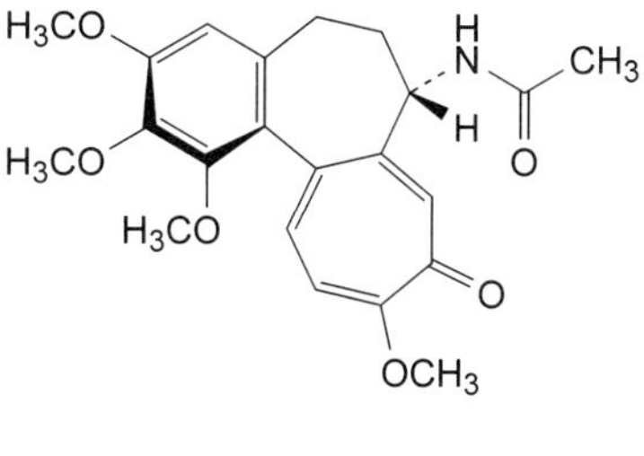

B. (-)-*N*-[(7*S*,12a*R*)-1,2,3,10-tetramethoxy-9-oxo-5,6,7,9-tetrahydrobenzo[*a*]heptalen-7-yl]acetamide (conformationnal isomer),

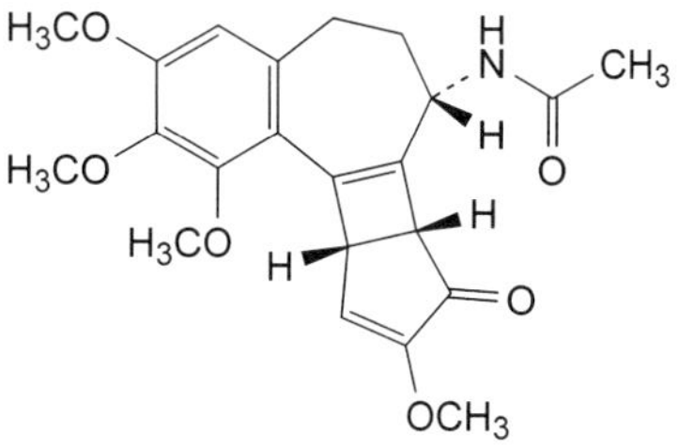

C. *N*-[(7*S*,7b*R*,10a*S*)-1,2,3,9-tetramethoxy-8-oxo-5,6,7,7b,8,10a-hexahydrobenzo[*a*]cyclopenta[3,4]-cyclobuta[1,2-*c*]cyclohepten-7-yl]acetamide (β-lumicolchicine),

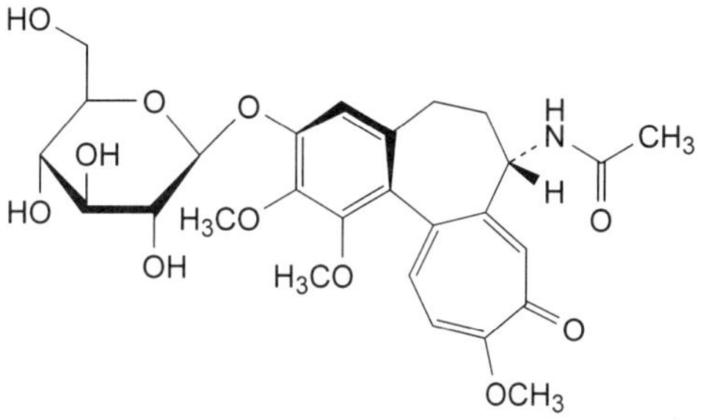

D. *N*-[(7*S*,12a*S*)-3-(β-D-glucopyranosyloxy)-1,2,10-trimethoxy-9-oxo-5,6,7,9-tetrahydrobenzo[*a*]heptalen-7-yl]acetamide (colchicoside).

04/2003:1862

COLOPHONY

Colophonium

DEFINITION

Residue remaining after distillation of the volatile oil from the oleoresin obtained from various species of *Pinus*.

CHARACTERS

Macroscopic characters described under identification A.

IDENTIFICATION

A. Translucent, pale yellow to brownish-yellow, angular, irregularly-shaped, brittle, glassy pieces of different sizes the surfaces of which bear conchoidal markings.

B. Thin-layer chromatography (*2.2.27*).

Test solution. Dissolve 1 g in 10 ml of *methanol R* by gently warming.

Reference solution. Dissolve 10 mg of *thymol R* and 10 mg of *linalol R* in 10 ml of *methanol R*.

Plate: TLC silica gel plate R.

Mobile phase: methylene chloride R.

Application: 10 µl, as bands.

Development: over a path of 15 cm.

Drying: in air.

Detection: spray with *anisaldehyde solution R* and heat at 100-105 °C for 10 min; examine in daylight.

Results: see below the sequence of the zones present in the chromatograms obtained with the reference solution and the test solution. Furthermore, other coloured zones are present in the chromatogram obtained with the test solution.

Top of the plate	
	A purple band
	A purple band
———	———
	2 purple bands
Thymol: an orange band	
———	———
Linalol: a purple band	Sequence of narrow purple bands
	Purple extended baseline band
Reference solution	**Test solution**

TESTS

Acid value (*2.5.1*): 145 to 180, determined on 1.0 g.

Foreign matter (*2.8.2*): maximum 2 per cent.

Total ash (*2.4.16*): maximum 0.2 per cent.

STORAGE

Do not reduce to a powder.

01/2002:0891
corrected

COPOVIDONE

Copovidonum

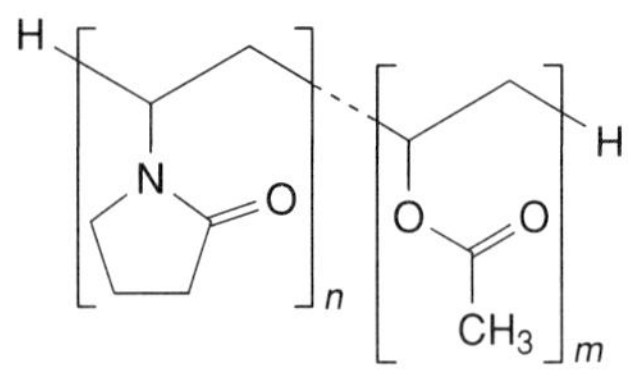

$n = 1.2m$

$(C_6H_9NO)_n$, $(C_4H_6O_2)_m$ M_r $(111.1)_n + (86.1)_m$

DEFINITION

Copovidone is a copolymer of 1-ethenylpyrrolidin-2-one and ethenyl acetate in the mass proportion 3:2.

Content:
- nitrogen (N; A_r 14.01): 7.0 per cent to 8.0 per cent (dried substance),
- ethenyl acetate $C_4H_6O_2$; M_r 86.10): 35.3 per cent to 42.0 per cent (dried substance).

K-value: 90.0 per cent to 110.0 per cent of the value stated on the label.

CHARACTERS

Aspect: white or yellowish-white powder or flakes, hygroscopic.

Solubility: freely soluble in water, in alcohol and in methylene chloride.

IDENTIFICATION

First identification: A.

Second identification: B, C.

A. Infrared absorption spectrophotometry (*2.2.24*).
   Comparison: Ph. Eur. reference spectrum of copovidone.

B. To 1 ml of solution S (see Tests) add 5 ml of *water R* and 0.2 ml of *0.05 M iodine*. A red colour appears.

C. Dissolve 0.7 g of *hydroxylamine hydrochloride R* in 10 ml of *methanol R*, add 20 ml of a 40 g/l solution of *sodium hydroxide R* and filter if necessary. To 5 ml of the solution add 0.1 g of the substance to be examined and boil for 2 min. Transfer 50 µl to a filter paper and add 0.1 ml of a mixture of equal volumes of *ferric chloride solution R1* and *hydrochloric acid R*. A violet colour appears.

TESTS

Solution S. Dissolve 10 g in *water R* and dilute to 100 ml with the same solvent. Add the substance to be examined to the *water R* in small portions with constant stirring.

Appearance of solution. Solution S is not more opalescent than reference suspension III (*2.2.1*) and not more intensely coloured than reference solution B_5, R_5 or BY_5 (*2.2.2, Method II*).

Aldehydes: maximum 500 ppm, expressed as acetaldehyde.

Test solution. Dissolve 1.0 g of the substance to be examined in *phosphate buffer solution pH 9.0 R* and dilute to 100.0 ml with the same solvent. Stopper the flask and heat at 60 °C for 1 h. Allow to cool.

Reference solution. Dissolve 0.140 g of *acetaldehyde ammonia trimer trihydrate R* in *water R* and dilute to 200.0 ml with the same solvent. Dilute 1.0 ml of this solution to 100.0 ml with *phosphate buffer solution pH 9.0 R*.

Into 3 identical spectrophotometric cells with a path length of 1 cm, introduce separately 0.5 ml of the test solution, 0.5 ml of the reference solution and 0.5 ml of *water R* (blank). To each cell, add 2.5 ml of *phosphate buffer solution pH 9.0 R* and 0.2 ml of *nicotinamide-adenine dinucleotide solution R*. Mix and stopper tightly. Allow to stand at 22 ± 2 °C for 2-3 min and measure the absorbance (*2.2.25*) of each solution at 340 nm, using *water R* as the compensation liquid. To each cell, add 0.05 ml of *aldehyde dehydrogenase solution R*, mix and stopper tightly. Allow to stand at 22 ± 2 °C for 5 min. Measure the absorbance of each solution at 340 nm using *water R* as compensation liquid. Determine the content of aldehydes using the expression:

$$\frac{(A_{t2} - A_{t1}) - (A_{b2} - A_{b1})}{(A_{s2} - A_{s1}) - (A_{b2} - A_{b1})} \times \frac{100\,000 \times C}{m}$$

A_{t1} = absorbance of the test solution before the addition of aldehyde dehydrogenase,

A_{t2} = absorbance of the test solution after the addition of aldehyde dehydrogenase,

A_{s1} = absorbance of the reference solution before the addition of aldehyde dehydrogenase,

A_{s2} = absorbance of the reference solution after the addition of aldehyde dehydrogenase,

A_{b1} = absorbance of the blank before the addition of aldehyde dehydrogenase,

A_{b2} = absorbance of the blank after the addition of aldehyde dehydrogenase,

m = mass of povidone, in grams, calculated with reference to the dried substance,

C = concentration (mg/ml), of acetaldehyde in the reference solution, calculated from the weight of the acetaldehyde ammonia trimer trihydrate with the factor 0.72.

Peroxides: maximum 400 ppm, expressed as H_2O_2.

Dilute 10 ml of solution S to 25 ml with *water R*. Add 2 ml of *titanium trichloride-sulphuric acid reagent R* and allow to stand for 30 min. The absorbance (*2.2.25*) of the solution, measured at 405 nm using a mixture of 25 ml of a 40 g/l solution of the substance to be examined and 2 ml of a 13 per cent *V/V* solution of *sulphuric acid R* as the compensation liquid, is not greater than 0.35.

Hydrazine. Thin-layer chromatography (*2.2.27*). *Use freshly prepared solutions.*

Test solution. To 25 ml of solution S add 0.5 ml of a 50 g/l solution of *salicylaldehyde R* in *methanol R*, mix and heat in a water-bath at 60 °C for 15 min. Allow to cool, add 2.0 ml of *xylene R*, shake for 2 min and centrifuge. Use the clear supernatant layer.

Reference solution. Dissolve 9 mg of *salicylaldehyde azine R* in *xylene R* and dilute to 100 ml with the same solvent. Dilute 1 ml of this solution to 10 ml with *xylene R*.

Plate: *TLC silica gel silanised plate R*.

Mobile phase: *water R, methanol R* (20:80 *V/V*).

Application: 10 µl.

Development: over a path of 15 cm.

Drying: in air.

Detection: examine in ultraviolet light at 365 nm.

Limits:

— *hydrazine*: any spot corresponding to salicylaldehyde azine in the chromatogram obtained with the test solution is not more intense than the spot in the chromatogram obtained with the reference solution (1 ppm).

Monomers: maximum 0.1 per cent.

Dissolve 10.0 g in 30 ml of *methanol R* and add slowly 20.0 ml of *iodine bromide solution R*. Allow to stand for 30 min protected from light with repeated shaking. Add 10 ml of a 100 g/l solution of *potassium iodide R* and titrate with *0.1 M sodium thiosulphate* until a yellow colour is obtained. Continue titration dropwise until the solution becomes colourless. Carry out a blank titration. Not more than 1.8 ml of *0.1 M sodium thiosulphate* is used.

Impurity A. Liquid chromatography (*2.2.29*).

Test solution. Dissolve 100 mg of the substance to be examined in *water R* and dilute to 50.0 ml with the same solvent.

Reference solution. Dissolve 100 mg of *2-pyrrolidone R* in *water R* and dilute to 100 ml with the same solvent. Dilute 1.0 ml to 100.0 ml with *water R*.

Precolumn:

— *size*: *l* = 0.025 m, Ø = 4 mm,

— *stationary phase*: *end-capped octadecylsilyl silica gel for chromatography R* (5 µm).

Column:

— *size*: *l* = 0.25 m, Ø = 4 mm,

— *stationary phase*: spherical *aminohexadecylsilyl silica gel for chromatography R* (5 µm),

— *temperature*: 30 °C.

Mobile phase: *water R*, adjusted to pH 2.4 with *phosphoric acid R*.

Flow rate: 1 ml/min.

Detection: spectrophotometer at 205 nm. A detector is placed between the precolumn and the analytical column. A second detector is placed after the analytical column.

Injection: 10 µl. When impurity A has left the precolumn (after about 1.2 min) switch the flow directly from the pump to the analytical column. Before the next chromatogram is run, wash the precolumn by reversed flow.

Limits:

— *impurity A*: not more than the area of the principal peak obtained with the reference solution (0.5 per cent).

Heavy metals (*2.4.8*): maximum 20 ppm.

12 ml of solution S complies with limit test A. Prepare the standard using *lead standard solution (2 ppm Pb) R*.

Loss on drying (*2.2.32*): maximum 5.0 per cent, determined on 0.500 g by drying in an oven at 100-105 °C.

Sulphated ash (*2.4.14*): maximum 0.1 per cent, determined on 1.0 g.

Viscosity, expressed as *K*-value. Dilute 5.0 ml of solution S to 50.0 ml with *water R*. Allow to stand for 1 h and determine the viscosity (*2.2.9*) of the solution at 25 ± 0.1 °C using viscometer No. 1 with a minimum flow time of 100 s. Calculate the *K*-value from the expression:

$$\frac{1.5 log\eta - 1}{0.15 + 0.003c} + \frac{\sqrt{300c\,log\eta + (c + 1.5c\,log\eta)^2}}{0.15c + 0.003c^2}$$

c = percentage concentration (g/100 ml) of the substance to be examined, calculated with reference to the dried substance,

η = viscosity of the solution relative to that of water.

ASSAY

Ethenyl acetate. Determine the saponification value (*2.5.6*) on 2.00 g of the substance to be examined. Multiply the result obtained by 0.1534 to obtain the percentage content of the ethenyl acetate component.

Nitrogen. Carry out the determination of nitrogen (*2.5.9*) using 30.0 mg of the substance to be examined and 1 g of a mixture of 3 parts of *copper sulphate R* and 997 parts of *dipotassium sulphate R*, heating until a clear, light green solution is obtained and then for a further 45 min.

STORAGE

In an airtight container.

LABELLING

The label states the *K*-value.

IMPURITIES

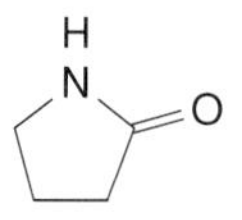

A. pyrrolidin-2-one (2-pyrrolidone).

04/2003:0892

CROSPOVIDONE

Crospovidonum

$(C_6H_9NO)_n$ M_r $(111.1)_n$

DEFINITION

Crospovidone is a cross-linked homopolymer of 1-ethenylpyrrolidin-2-one. It is available in different degrees of powder fineness (type A and type B).

Content: 11.0 per cent to 12.8 per cent of nitrogen (N; A_r 14.01) (dried substance).

CHARACTERS

Appearance: white or yellowish-white powder or flakes, hygroscopic.

Solubility: practically insoluble in water, in alcohol and in methylene chloride.

IDENTIFICATION

A. Infrared absorption spectrophotometry (*2.2.24*).

Comparison: Ph. Eur. reference spectrum of crospovidone.

B. Suspend 1 g in 10 ml of *water R*, add 0.1 ml of *0.05 M iodine* and shake for 30 s. Add 1 ml of *starch solution R* and shake. No blue colour develops within 30 s.

C. To 10 ml of *water R*, add 0.1 g and shake. A suspension is formed and no clear solution is obtained within 15 min.

D. Weigh a suitable quantity of the substance to be examined (for example 10 mg to 100 mg) and suspend it in 10.0 ml of *water R*, adding a wetting agent. Observe under a microscope at a suitable magnification using a calibrated ocular micrometer. If the majority of particles are in the range 50 μm to 300 μm, the product is classified as type A. If almost all the particles are below 50 μm, the product is classified as type B.

TESTS

Peroxides. Type A: maximum 400 ppm expressed as H_2O_2; type B: maximum 1000 ppm expressed as H_2O_2.

Suspend 2.0 g in 50 ml of *water R*. To 25 ml of this suspension add 2 ml of *titanium trichloride-sulphuric acid reagent R*. Allow to stand for 30 min and filter. The absorbance (*2.2.25*) of the filtrate, measured at 405 nm using a mixture of 25 ml of a filtered 40 g/l suspension of the substance to be examined and 2 ml of a 13 per cent *V/V* solution of *sulphuric acid R* as the compensation liquid has a maximum of 0.35.

For type B use 10 ml of the suspension diluted to 25 ml with *water R* for the test.

Water-soluble substances: maximum 1.0 per cent.

Transfer 25.0 g to a 400 ml beaker, add 200 ml of *water R* and stir for 1 h using a magnetic stirrer. Transfer the suspension to a 250.0 ml volumetric flask, rinsing with *water R*, and dilute to volume with the same solvent. Allow the bulk of the solids to settle. Filter about 100 ml of the almost clear supernatant liquid through a 0.45 μm membrane filter, protected by superimposing a 3 μm membrane filter. While filtering, stir the liquid above the filter manually or by means

of a mechanical stirrer, taking care not to damage the filter. Transfer 50.0 ml of the clear filtrate to a tared 100 ml beaker, evaporate to dryness and dry at 105-110 °C for 3 h. The residue weighs a maximum of 50 mg.

Impurity A. Liquid chromatography (*2.2.29*).

Test solution. Suspend 1.250 g in 50.0 ml of *methanol R* and shake for 60 min. Leave the bulk to settle and filter through a 0.2 μm filter.

Reference solution (a). Dissolve 50 mg of *1-vinylpyrrolidin-2-one R* in *methanol R* and dilute to 100.0 ml with the same solvent. Dilute 1.0 ml of the solution to 100.0 ml with *methanol R*. Dilute 5.0 ml of this solution to 100.0 ml with the mobile phase.

Reference solution (b). Dissolve 10 mg of *1-vinylpyrrolidin-2-one R* and 0.50 g of *vinyl acetate R* in *methanol R* and dilute to 100 ml with the same solvent. Dilute 1.0 ml of the solution to 100.0 ml with the mobile phase.

Precolumn:

— *size*: $l = 0.025$ m, Ø = 4 mm,

— *stationary phase*: *octadecylsilyl silica gel for chromatography R* (5 μm).

Column:

— *size*: $l = 0.25$ m, Ø = 4 mm,

— *stationary phase*: *octadecylsilyl silica gel for chromatography R* (5 μm),

— *temperature*: 40 °C.

Mobile phase: acetonitrile R, water R (10:90 *V/V*).

Flow rate: adjusted so that the retention time of the peak corresponding to impurity A is about 10 min.

Detection: spectrophotometer at 235 nm.

Injection: 50 μl. After each injection of the test solution, wash the precolumn by passing the mobile phase backward, at the same flow rate as applied in the test, for 30 min.

System suitability:

— *resolution*: minimum of 2.0 between the peaks corresponding to impurity A and to vinyl acetate in the chromatogram obtained with reference solution (b),

— *repeatability*: maximum relative standard deviation of 2.0 per cent after 5 injections of reference solution (a).

Limits:

— *impurity A*: not more than the area of the principal peak in the chromatogram obtained with reference solution (a) (10 ppm).

Heavy metals (*2.4.8*): maximum 10 ppm.

2.0 g complies with limit test D. Prepare the standard using 2 ml of *lead standard solution (10 ppm Pb) R*.

Loss on drying (*2.2.32*): maximum 5.0 per cent, determined on 0.500 g by drying in an oven at 100-105 °C.

Sulphated ash (*2.4.14*): maximum 0.1 per cent, determined on 1.0 g.

ASSAY

Place 100.0 mg of the substance to be examined (*m* mg) in a combustion flask, add 5 g of a mixture of 1 g of *copper sulphate R*, 1 g of *titanium dioxide R* and 33 g of *dipotassium sulphate R*, and 3 glass beads. Wash any adhering particles from the neck into the flask with a small quantity of *water R*. Add 7 ml of *sulphuric acid R*, allowing it to run down the sides of the flask, and mix the contents by rotation. Close the mouth of the flask loosely, for example by means of a glass bulb with a short stem, to avoid excessive loss of sulphuric acid. Heat gradually at first, then increase the temperature until there is vigorous boiling with condensation of sulphuric acid in the neck of the flask; precautions are to be taken to prevent the upper part of the flask from becoming overheated. Continue the heating for 45 min. Cool, dissolve the solid material by cautiously adding to the mixture 20 ml of *water R*, cool again and place in a steam-distillation apparatus. Add 30 ml of *strong sodium hydroxide solution R* through the funnel, rinse the funnel cautiously with 10 ml of *water R* and distil immediately by passing steam through the mixture. Collect 80-100 ml of distillate in a mixture of 30 ml of a 40 g/l solution of *boric acid R* and 0.05 ml of *bromocresol green-methyl red solution R* and enough *water R* to cover the tip of the condenser. Towards the end of the distillation lower the receiver so that the tip of the condenser is above the surface of the acid solution and rinse the end part of the condenser with a small quantity of *water R*. Titrate the distillate with *0.025 M sulphuric acid* until the colour of the solution changes from green through pale greyish-blue to pale greyish-red-purple (n_1 ml of *0.025 M sulphuric acid*).

Repeat the test using about 100 mg of *glucose R* in place of the substance to be examined (n_2 ml of *0.025 M sulphuric acid*).

$$\text{Percentage content of nitrogen} = \frac{0.7004\,(n_1 - n_2)}{m} \times 100$$

STORAGE

In an airtight container.

LABELLING

The label states the type (type A or type B).

IMPURITIES

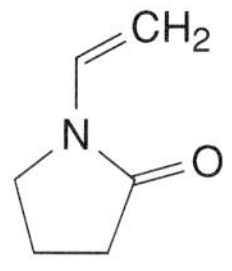

A. 1-ethenylpyrrolidin-2-one (1-vinylpyrrolidin-2-one).

D

Monographs
D - K

04/2003:0176

DEMECLOCYCLINE HYDROCHLORIDE

Demeclocyclini hydrochloridum

$C_{21}H_{22}Cl_2N_2O_8$ M_r 501.3

DEFINITION

(4S,4aS,5aS,6S,12aS)-7-Chloro-4-(dimethylamino)-3,6,10,12,12a-pentahydroxy-1,11-dioxo-1,4,4a,5,5a,6,11,12a-octahydrotetracene-2-carboxamide hydrochloride.

Substance produced by certain strains of *Streptomyces aureofaciens* or obtained by any other means.

Content: 89.5 per cent to 102.0 per cent (anhydrous substance).

CHARACTERS

Appearance: yellow powder.

Solubility: soluble or sparingly soluble in water, slightly soluble in alcohol, very slightly soluble in acetone. It dissolves in solutions of alkali hydroxides and carbonates.

IDENTIFICATION

A. Thin-layer chromatography (*2.2.27*).

Test solution. Dissolve 5 mg of the substance to be examined in *methanol R* and dilute to 10 ml with the same solvent.

Reference solution (a). Dissolve 5 mg of *demeclocycline hydrochloride CRS* in *methanol R* and dilute to 10 ml with the same solvent.

Reference solution (b). Dissolve 5 mg of *demeclocycline hydrochloride CRS*, 5 mg of *chlortetracycline hydrochloride R* and 5 mg of *tetracycline hydrochloride R* in *methanol R* and dilute to 10 ml with the same solvent.

Plate: TLC octadecylsilyl silica gel F_{254} plate R.

Mobile phase: mix 20 volumes of *acetonitrile R*, 20 volumes of *methanol R* and 60 volumes of a 63 g/l solution of *oxalic acid R* previously adjusted to pH 2 with *concentrated ammonia R*.

Application: 1 µl.

Development: over 3/4 of the plate.

Drying: in air.

Detection: examine in ultraviolet light at 254 nm.

System suitability: the chromatogram obtained with reference solution (b) shows 3 clearly separated spots.

Results: the principal spot in the chromatogram obtained with the test solution is similar in position and size to the principal spot in the chromatogram obtained with reference solution (a).

B. To about 2 mg add 5 ml of *sulphuric acid R*. A violet colour develops. Add the solution to 2.5 ml of *water R*. The colour becomes yellow.

C. It gives reaction (a) of chlorides (*2.3.1*).

TESTS

pH (*2.2.3*): 2.0 to 3.0.
Dissolve 0.1 g in *carbon dioxide-free water R* and dilute to 10 ml with the same solvent.

Specific optical rotation (*2.2.7*): −248 to −263 (anhydrous substance).
Dissolve 0.250 g in *0.1 M hydrochloric acid* and dilute to 25.0 ml with the same acid.

Specific absorbance (*2.2.25*): 340 to 370 determined at the maximum at 385 nm (anhydrous substance).
Dissolve 10.0 mg in *0.01 M hydrochloric acid* and dilute to 100.0 ml with the same acid. To 10.0 ml of the solution add 12 ml of *dilute sodium hydroxide solution R* and dilute to 100.0 ml with *water R*.

Related substances. Liquid chromatography (*2.2.29*).
Prepare the solutions immediately before use.

Test solution. Dissolve 25.0 mg of the substance to be examined in *0.01 M hydrochloric acid* and dilute to 25.0 ml with the same acid.

Reference solution (a). Dissolve 25.0 mg of *demeclocycline hydrochloride CRS* in *0.01 M hydrochloric acid* and dilute to 25.0 ml with the same acid.

Reference solution (b). Dissolve 5.0 mg of *4-epidemeclocycline hydrochloride CRS* in *0.01 M hydrochloric acid* and dilute to 25.0 ml with the same acid.

Reference solution (c). Mix 1.0 ml of reference solution (a) and 5.0 ml of reference solution (b) and dilute to 25.0 ml with *0.01 M hydrochloric acid*.

Reference solution (d). Dilute 5.0 ml of reference solution (a) to 100.0 ml with *0.01 M hydrochloric acid*.

Column:
– *size*: l = 0.25 m, Ø = 4.6 mm,
– *stationary phase*: *styrene-divinylbenzene copolymer R* (8 µm),
– *temperature*: 60 °C,

Mobile phase: weigh 80.0 g of *2-methyl-2-propanol R* and transfer to a 1000 ml volumetric flask with the aid of 200 ml of *water R*; add 100 ml of a 35 g/l solution of *dipotassium hydrogen phosphate R* adjusted to pH 9.0 with *dilute phosphoric acid R*, 150 ml of a 10 g/l solution of *tetrabutylammonium hydrogen sulphate R* adjusted to pH 9.0 with *dilute sodium hydroxide solution R* and 10 ml of a 40 g/l solution of *sodium edetate R* adjusted to pH 9.0 with *dilute sodium hydroxide solution R*; dilute to 1000 ml with *water R*.

Flow rate: 1 ml/min.

Detection: spectrophotometer at 254 nm.

Injection: 20 µl; inject the test solution and reference solutions (c) and (d).

System suitability: reference solution (c):
– *resolution*: minimum of 2.8 between the peaks due to impurity B (1st peak) and demeclocycline (2nd peak); if necessary, adjust the 2-methyl-2-propanol content of the mobile phase or lower the pH of the mobile phase,
– *symmetry factor*: maximum 1.25 for the peak due to demeclocycline.

Limits:
– *any impurity*: not more than the area of the principal peak in the chromatogram obtained with reference solution (d) (5.0 per cent), and not more than 1 such peak has an area greater than 0.8 times the area of the principal peak in the chromatogram obtained with reference solution (d) (4.0 per cent),

— *total*: not more than twice the area of the principal peak in the chromatogram obtained with reference solution (d) (10.0 per cent),

— *disregard limit*: 0.02 times the area of the principal peak in the chromatogram obtained with reference solution (d) (0.1 per cent).

Heavy metals (*2.4.8*): maximum 50 ppm.

0.5 g complies with limit test C. Prepare the standard using 2.5 ml of *lead standard solution (10 ppm Pb) R*.

Water (*2.5.12*): maximum 3.0 per cent, determined on 1.000 g.

Sulphated ash (*2.4.14*): maximum 0.5 per cent, determined on 1.0 g.

ASSAY

Liquid chromatography (*2.2.29*) as described in the test for related substances with the following modification.

Injection: test solution and reference solution (a).

Calculate the percentage content of $C_{21}H_{22}Cl_2N_2O_8$.

STORAGE

Protected from light.

IMPURITIES

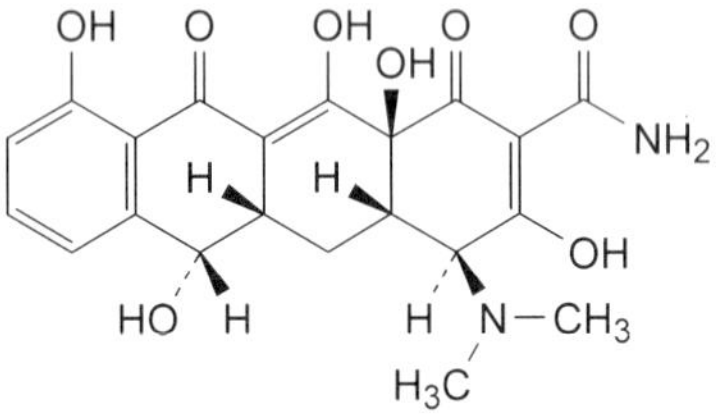

A. (4S,4aS,5aS,6S,12aS)-4-(dimethylamino)-3,6,10,12,12a-pentahydroxy-1,11-dioxo-1,4,4a,5,5a,6,11,12a-octahydrotetracene-2-carboxamide (demethyltetracycline),

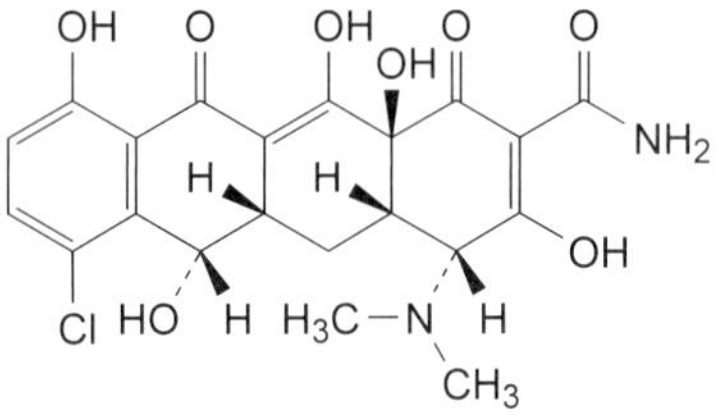

B. (4R,4aS,5aS,6S,12aS)-7-chloro-4-(dimethyl-amino)-3,6,10,12,12a-pentahydroxy-1,11-di-oxo-1,4,4a,5,5a,6,11,12a-octahydrotetracene-2-car-boxamide (4-epidemeclocycline).

01/2003:0388
corrected

DEXAMETHASONE

Dexamethasonum

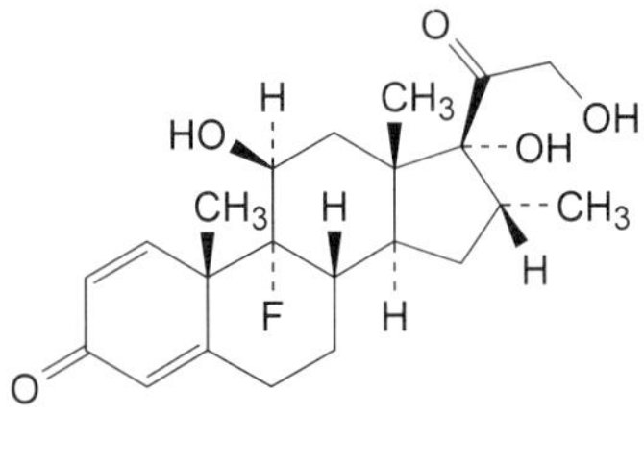

$C_{22}H_{29}FO_5$ M_r 392.5

DEFINITION

Dexamethasone contains not less than 97.0 per cent and not more than the equivalent of 103.0 per cent of 9-fluoro-11β,17,21-trihydroxy-16α-methylpregna-1,4-diene-3,20-dione, calculated with reference to the dried substance.

CHARACTERS

A white or almost white, crystalline powder, practically insoluble in water, sparingly soluble in ethanol, slightly soluble in methylene chloride.

IDENTIFICATION

First identification: B, C.

Second identification: A, C, D, E.

A. Dissolve 10.0 mg in *ethanol R* and dilute to 100.0 ml with the same solvent. Place 2.0 ml of the solution in a stoppered test tube, add 10.0 ml of *phenylhydrazine-sulphuric acid solution R*, mix and heat in a water-bath at 60 °C for 20 min. Cool immediately. The absorbance (*2.2.25*) of the solution at the maximum at 419 nm is not less than 0.4.

B. Examine by infrared absorption spectrophotometry (*2.2.24*), comparing with the spectrum obtained with *dexamethasone CRS*.

C. Examine by thin-layer chromatography (*2.2.27*), using as the coating substance a suitable silica gel with a fluorescent indicator having an optimal intensity at 254 nm.

Test solution. Dissolve 10 mg of the substance to be examined in a mixture of 1 volume of *methanol R* and 9 volumes of *methylene chloride R* and dilute to 10 ml with the same mixture of solvents.

Reference solution (a). Dissolve 20 mg of *dexamethasone CRS* in a mixture of 1 volume of *methanol R* and 9 volumes of *methylene chloride R* and dilute to 20 ml with the same mixture of solvents.

Reference solution (b). Dissolve 10 mg of *betamethasone CRS* in reference solution (a) and dilute to 10 ml with the same solution.

Apply to the plate 5 μl of each solution. Develop over a path of 15 cm, using a mixture of 5 volumes of *butanol R* saturated with *water R*, 10 volumes of *toluene R* and 85 volumes of *ether R*. Allow the plate to dry in air and examine in ultraviolet light at 254 nm. The principal spot in the chromatogram obtained with the test solution is similar in position and size to the principal spot in the chromatogram obtained with reference solution (a). Spray with *alcoholic solution of sulphuric acid R*. Heat at 120 °C for 10 min or until the spots appear. Allow to cool. Examine the chromatograms in daylight and in ultraviolet light at 365 nm. The principal spot in the chromatogram obtained with the test solution is similar in position, colour in daylight, fluorescence in ultraviolet light at 365 nm and size to the principal spot in the chromatogram obtained with reference solution (a). The test is not valid unless the chromatogram obtained with reference solution (b) shows 2 spots which may, however, not be completely separated.

D. Add about 2 mg to 2 ml of *sulphuric acid R* and shake to dissolve. Within 5 min, a faint reddish-brown colour develops. Add the solution to 10 ml of *water R* and mix. The colour is discharged.

E. Mix about 5 mg with 45 mg of *heavy magnesium oxide R* and ignite in a crucible until an almost white residue is obtained (usually less than 5 min). Allow to cool, add 1 ml of *water R*, 0.05 ml of *phenolphthalein solution R1* and about 1 ml of *dilute hydrochloric acid R* to render the solution colourless. Filter. To a freshly prepared mixture of 0.1 ml of *alizarin S solution R* and 0.1 ml of *zirconyl nitrate solution R*, add 1.0 ml of the filtrate. Mix, allow to stand for 5 min and compare the colour of the solution with that of a blank prepared in the same manner. The test solution is yellow and the blank is red.

TESTS

Specific optical rotation (*2.2.7*). Dissolve 0.250 g in *dioxan R* and dilute to 25.0 ml with the same solvent. The specific optical rotation is + 75 to + 80, calculated with reference to the dried substance.

Related substances. Examine by liquid chromatography (*2.2.29*).

Test solution. Place 25.0 mg of the substance to be examined in a 10.0 ml volumetric flask, add 1.5 ml of *acetonitrile R* and then 5 ml of mobile phase A. Mix with the aid of an ultrasonic bath until complete dissolution and dilute to 10.0 ml with mobile phase A.

Reference solution (a). Dissolve 2 mg of *dexamethasone CRS* and 2 mg of *methylprednisolone CRS* in mobile phase A and dilute to 100.0 ml with the same mobile phase.

Reference solution (b). Dilute 1.0 ml of the test solution to 100.0 ml with mobile phase A.

The chromatographic procedure may be carried out using:

— a stainless steel column 0.25 m long and 4.6 mm in internal diameter packed with *octadecylsilyl silica gel for chromatography R* (5 µm),

— as mobile phase at a flow rate of 2.5 ml/min a linear gradient programme using the following conditions:

Mobile phase A. In a 1000 ml volumetric flask, mix 250 ml of *acetonitrile R* with 700 ml of *water R* and allow to equilibrate; adjust the volume to 1000 ml with *water R* and mix again,

Mobile phase B. Acetonitrile R,

Time (min)	Mobile phase A (per cent *V/V*)	Mobile phase B (per cent *V/V*)	Comment
0	100	0	isocratic
15	100 → 0	0 → 100	begin linear gradient
40	0	100	end chromatogram, return to 100 A
41	100	0	begin equilibration with A
46 = 0	100	0	end equilibration, begin next chromatogram

— as detector a spectrophotometer set at 254 nm,

maintaining the temperature of the column at 45 °C.

Equilibrate the column for at least 30 min with mobile phase B at a flow rate of 2.5 ml/min and then with mobile phase A for 5 min. For subsequent chromatograms, use the conditions described from 40.0 min to 46.0 min.

Adjust the sensitivity of the system so that the height of the principal peak in the chromatogram obtained with 20 µl of reference solution (b) is at least 50 per cent of the full scale of the recorder.

Inject 20 µl of reference solution (a). When the chromatograms are recorded in the prescribed conditions, the retention times are: methylprednisolone about 11.5 min and dexamethasone about 13 min. The test is not valid unless the resolution between the peaks corresponding to

methylprednisolone and dexamethasone is at least 2.8; if necessary, adjust the concentration of acetonitrile in mobile phase A.

Inject 20 µl of mobile phase A as a blank, 20 µl of the test solution and 20 µl of reference solution (b). Record the chromatogram of the test solution for twice the retention time of the principal peak. In the chromatogram obtained with the test solution: the area of any peak, apart from the principal peak, is not greater than 0.5 times the area of the principal peak in the chromatogram obtained with reference solution (b) (0.5 per cent); the sum of the areas of all the peaks, apart from the principal peak, is not greater than the area of the principal peak in the chromatogram obtained with reference solution (b) (1 per cent). Disregard any peak due to the blank and any peak with an area less than 0.05 times the area of the principal peak in the chromatogram obtained with reference solution (b).

Loss on drying (*2.2.32*). Not more than 0.5 per cent, determined on 0.500 g by drying in an oven at 100-105 °C.

ASSAY

Dissolve 0.100 g in *alcohol R* and dilute to 100.0 ml with the same solvent. Dilute 2.0 ml of the solution to 100.0 ml with *alcohol R*. Measure the absorbance (*2.2.25*) at the maximum at 238.5 nm.

Calculate the content of $C_{22}H_{29}FO_5$ taking the specific absorbance to be 394.

STORAGE

Protected from light.

04/2003:1507

DEXTRIN

Dextrinum

DEFINITION

Dextrin is maize, potato or cassava starch partly hydrolysed and modified by heating with or without the presence of acids, alkalis or pH control agents.

CHARACTERS

White or almost white, free-flowing powder, very soluble in boiling water forming a mucilaginous solution, slowly soluble in cold water, practically insoluble in alcohol.

IDENTIFICATION

A. Suspend 1 g in 50 ml of *water R*, boil for 1 min and cool. To 1 ml of the solution add 0.05 ml of *iodine solution R1*. A dark blue to reddish-brown colour is produced which disappears on heating.

B. Centrifuge 5 ml of the mucilage obtained in identification test A. To the upper layer add 2 ml of *dilute sodium hydroxide solution R* and, dropwise with shaking, 0.5 ml of *copper sulphate solution R* and boil. A red precipitate is produced.

C. It is very soluble in boiling *water R*, forming a mucilaginous solution.

TESTS

pH (*2.2.3*). Disperse 5.0 g in 100 ml of *carbon dioxide-free water R*. The pH is 2.0 to 8.0.

Chlorides. Dissolve 2.5 g in 50 ml of boiling *water R*, dilute to 100 ml with *water R* and filter. Dilute 1 ml of the filtrate to 15 ml, add 1 ml of *dilute nitric acid R*, pour the mixture as a single addition into 1 ml of *silver nitrate solution R2* and allow to stand for 5 min protected from light. When viewed transversely against a black background any opalescence produced is not more intense than that obtained by treating a mixture of 10 ml of *chloride standard solution (5 ppm Cl) R* and 5 ml of *water R*, prepared in the same manner (0.2 per cent).

Reducing sugars. To a quantity of dextrin equivalent to 2.0 g (dried substance) add 100 ml of *water R*, shake for 30 min, dilute with *water R* to 200.0 ml and filter. To 10.0 ml of alkaline *cupri-tartaric solution R* add 20.0 ml of the filtrate, mix, and heat on a hot plate adjusted to bring the solution to boil within 3 min. Boil for 2 min, and cool immediately. Add 5 ml of a 300 g/l solution of *potassium iodide R* and 10 ml of *1 M sulphuric acid*, mix, and titrate immediately with *0.1 M sodium thiosulphate*, using *starch solution R*, added towards the end of the titration, as indicator. Repeat the procedure beginning with "To 10.0 ml of...", using, in place of the filtrate, 20.0 ml of a 1 g/l solution of *glucose R*, accurately prepared. Perform a blank titration. $(V_B - V_U)$ is not greater than $(V_B - V_S)$, in which V_B, V_U and V_S are the number of millilitres of *0.1 M sodium thiosulphate* consumed in the titrations of the blank, the dextrin and the glucose, respectively (10 per cent, calculated as glucose $C_6H_{12}O_6$).

Heavy metals (*2.4.8*). 1.0 g complies with limit test C for heavy metals (20 ppm). Prepare the standard using 2 ml of *lead standard solution (10 ppm Pb) R*.

Loss on drying (*2.2.32*). Not more than 13.0 per cent, determined on 1.000 g by drying at 130 °C to 135 °C for 90 min.

Sulphated ash (*2.4.14*). Not more than 0.5 per cent, determined on 1.0 g.

04/2003:0023

DIPHENHYDRAMINE HYDROCHLORIDE

Diphenhydramini hydrochloridum

C$_{17}$H$_{22}$ClNO $\qquad$ M$_r$ 291.8

DEFINITION

2-(Diphenylmethoxy)-*N*,*N*-dimethylethanamine hydrochloride.

Content: 99.0 per cent to 101.0 per cent (dried substance).

CHARACTERS

Appearance: white or almost white, crystalline powder.

Solubility: very soluble in water, freely soluble in alcohol.

IDENTIFICATION

First identification: C, D.

Second identification: A, B, D.

A. Melting point (*2.2.14*): 168 °C to 172 °C.

B. Dissolve 50 mg in *alcohol R* and dilute to 100.0 ml with the same solvent. Examined between 230 nm and 350 nm, the solution shows 3 absorption maxima (*2.2.25*), at

253 nm, 258 nm and 264 nm. The ratio of the absorbance measured at the maximum at 258 nm to that measured at the maximum at 253 nm is 1.1 to 1.3. The ratio of the absorbance measured at the maximum at 258 nm to that measured at the maximum at 264 nm is 1.2 to 1.4.

C. Infrared absorption spectrophotometry (*2.2.24*).
Preparation: discs.
Comparison: *diphenhydramine hydrochloride CRS*.

D. It gives the reactions of chlorides (*2.3.1*).

TESTS

Solution S. Dissolve 1.0 g in *carbon dioxide-free water R* and dilute to 20 ml with the same solvent.

Appearance of solution. Solution S and a fivefold dilution of solution S are clear (*2.2.1*). Solution S is not more intensely coloured than reference solution BY$_6$ (*2.2.2, Method II*).

Acidity or alkalinity. To 10 ml of solution S add 0.15 ml of *methyl red solution R* and 0.25 ml of *0.01 M hydrochloric acid*. The solution is pink. Not more than 0.5 ml of *0.01 M sodium hydroxide* is required to change the colour of the indicator to yellow.

Related substances. Liquid chromatography (*2.2.29*).

Test solution. Dissolve 70 mg of the substance to be examined in the mobile phase and dilute to 20.0 ml with the mobile phase. Dilute 2.0 ml of the solution to 10.0 ml with the mobile phase.

Reference solution (a). Dilute 1.0 ml of the test solution to 10.0 ml with the mobile phase. Dilute 1.0 ml of this solution to 20.0 ml with the mobile phase.

Reference solution (b). Dissolve 5 mg of *diphenhydramine impurity A CRS* and 5 mg of *diphenylmethanol R* in the mobile phase and dilute to 10.0 ml with the mobile phase. To 2.0 ml of this solution add 1.5 ml of the test solution and dilute to 10.0 ml with the mobile phase.

Column:

— *size*: l = 0.25 m, Ø = 4.6 mm,

— *stationary phase*: *base-deactivated octylsilyl silica gel for chromatography R* (5 µm).

Mobile phase: mix 35 volumes of *acetonitrile R* and 65 volumes of a 5.4 g/l solution of *potassium dihydrogen phosphate R* adjusted to pH 3.0 using *phosphoric acid R*.

Flow rate: 1.2 ml/min.

Detection: spectrophotometer at 220 nm.

Injection: 10 µl.

Run time: 7 times the retention time of diphenhydramine.

Relative retention with reference to diphenhydramine (retention time = about 6 min): impurity A = about 0.9; impurity B = about 1.5; impurity C = about 1.8; impurity D = about 2.6; impurity E = about 5.1.

System suitability: reference solution (b):

— *resolution*: minimum 2.0 between the peaks due to diphenhydramine and to impurity A.

Limits:

— *correction factor*: for the calculation of content, multiply the peak area of impurity D by 1.4,

— *impurity A*: not more than the area of the principal peak in the chromatogram obtained with reference solution (a) (0.5 per cent),

— *any other impurity*: not more than 0.6 times the area of the principal peak in the chromatogram obtained with reference solution (a) (0.3 per cent),

– *total*: not more than twice the area of the principal peak in the chromatogram obtained with reference solution (a) (1.0 per cent),

– *disregard limit*: 0.1 times the area of the principal peak in the chromatogram obtained with reference solution (a) (0.05 per cent).

Loss on drying (*2.2.32*): maximum 0.5 per cent, determined on 1.000 g by drying in an oven at 100-105 °C.

Sulphated ash (*2.4.14*): maximum 0.1 per cent, determined on 1.0 g.

ASSAY

Dissolve 0.250 g in 50 ml of *alcohol R* and add 5.0 ml of *0.01 M hydrochloric acid*. Carry out a potentiometric titration (*2.2.20*), using *0.1 M sodium hydroxide*. Read the volume added between the 2 points of inflexion.

1 ml of *0.1 M sodium hydroxide* is equivalent to 29.18 mg of $C_{17}H_{22}ClNO$.

STORAGE

Protected from light.

IMPURITIES

Qualified impurities: A, B, C, D, E.

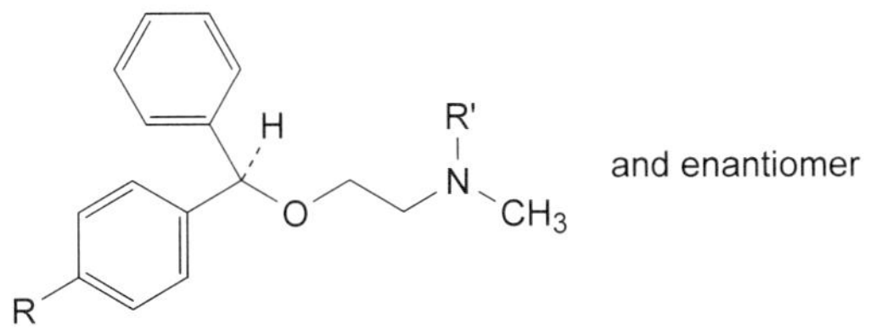

A. R = R′ = H: 2-(diphenylmethoxy)-*N*-methylethanamine,

B. R = R′ = CH₃: 2-[(*RS*)-(4-methylphenyl)phenylmethoxy]-*N*,*N*-dimethylethanamine,

C. R = Br, R′ = CH₃: 2-[(*RS*)-(4-bromophenyl)phenylmethoxy]-*N*,*N*-dimethylethanamine,

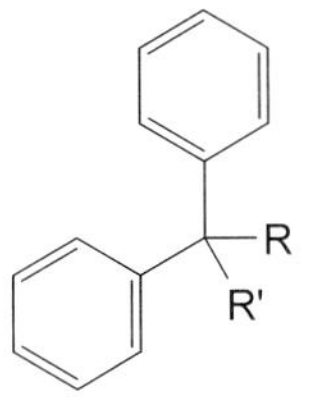

D. R = OH, R′ = H: diphenylmethanol (benzhydrol),

E. R + R′ = O: diphenylmethanone (benzophenone).

04/2003:1509

DISODIUM PHOSPHATE, ANHYDROUS

Dinatrii phosphas anhydricus

Na_2HPO_4 M_r 142.0

DEFINITION

Anhydrous disodium phosphate contains not less than 98.0 per cent and not more than the equivalent of 101.0 per cent of Na_2HPO_4, calculated with reference to the dried substance.

CHARACTERS

A white powder, hygroscopic, soluble in water, practically insoluble in alcohol.

IDENTIFICATION

A. Solution S (see Tests) is slightly alkaline (*2.2.4*).

B. It complies with the test for loss on drying (see Tests).

C. Solution S (see Tests) gives the reactions of phosphates (*2.3.1*).

D. Solution S (see Tests) gives reaction (a) of sodium (*2.3.1*).

TESTS

Solution S. Dissolve 5.0 g in *distilled water R* and dilute to 100.0 ml with the same solvent.

Appearance of solution. Solution S is clear (*2.2.1*) and colourless (*2.2.2, Method II*).

Reducing substances. To 10 ml of solution S add 5 ml of *dilute sulphuric acid R* and 0.25 ml of *0.02 M potassium permanganate* and heat on a water-bath for 5 min. The solution retains a slight red colour.

Monosodium phosphate. Calculated from the number of millilitres of *1 M hydrochloric acid* (25 ml) and of *1 M sodium hydroxide* (n_1 ml and n_2 ml) used in the assay, the ratio:

$$\frac{n_2 - 25}{25 - n_1}$$

does not exceed 0.025.

Chlorides (*2.4.4*). 5 ml of solution S diluted to 15 ml with *dilute nitric acid R* complies with the limit test for chlorides (200 ppm).

Sulphates (*2.4.13*). To 6 ml of solution S add 2 ml of *dilute hydrochloric acid R* and dilute to 15 ml with *distilled water R*. The solution complies with the limit test for sulphates (500 ppm).

Arsenic (*2.4.2*). 10 ml of solution S complies with limit test A for arsenic (2 ppm).

Iron (*2.4.9*). 10 ml of solution S complies with the limit test for iron (20 ppm).

Heavy metals (*2.4.8*). 12 ml of solution S complies with limit test A for heavy metals (10 ppm). Prepare the standard using 5 ml of *lead standard solution (1 ppm Pb) R* and 5 ml of *water R*.

Loss on drying (*2.2.32*). Not more than 1.0 per cent, determined on 1.000 g by drying in an oven at 100 °C to 105 °C for 4 h.

ASSAY

Dissolve 1.600 g (*m*) in 25.0 ml of *carbon dioxide-free water R* and add 25.0 ml of *1 M hydrochloric acid*. Using *1 M sodium hydroxide*, titrate potentiometrically (*2.2.20*) to the first inflexion point (n_1 ml). Continue the titration to the second inflexion point (total volume of *1 M sodium hydroxide* required, n_2 ml).

Calculate the percentage content of Na_2HPO_4 from the expression:

$$\frac{1420\,(25 - n_1)}{m\,(100 - d)}$$

d =   percentage loss on drying.

STORAGE

Store in an airtight container.

04/2003:0272

DOXYCYCLINE HYCLATE

Doxycyclini hyclas

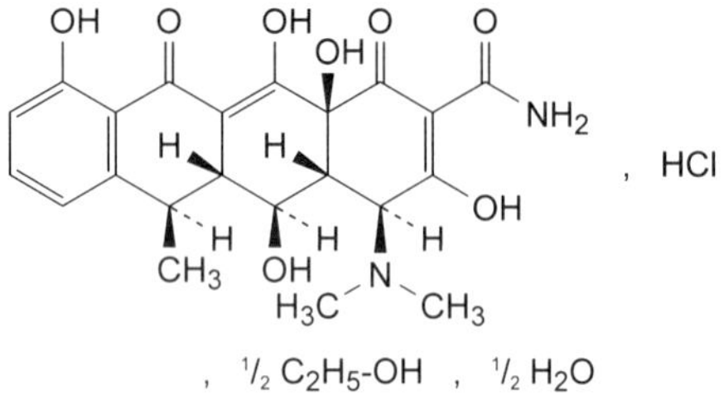

, HCl

, $^1/_2$ C$_2$H$_5$-OH , $^1/_2$ H$_2$O

$(C_{22}H_{25}ClN_2O_8),^1/_2\ C_2H_6O,^1/_2H_2O$ $\hspace{2cm}$ M_r 512.9

DEFINITION

Hydrochloride hemiethanol hemihydrate of
(4S,4aR,5S,5aR,6R,12aS)-4-(dimethylamino)-3,5,10,12,12a-
pentahydroxy-6-methyl-1,11-dioxo-1,4,4a,5,5a,6,11,12a-
octahydrotetracene-2-carboxamide.

Substance obtained from oxytetracycline or metacycline or
by any other means.

Content: 95.0 per cent to 102.0 per cent of C$_{22}$H$_{25}$ClN$_2$O$_8$
(anhydrous and ethanol-free substance).

CHARACTERS

Appearance: yellow, crystalline powder, hygroscopic.

Solubility: freely soluble in water and in methanol,
sparingly soluble in alcohol. It dissolves in solutions of alkali
hydroxides and carbonates.

IDENTIFICATION

A. Examine the chromatograms obtained in the assay.

$\quad$ *Results*: the principal peak in the chromatogram obtained
$\quad$ with the test solution is similar in retention time and size
$\quad$ to the principal peak in the chromatogram obtained with
$\quad$ reference solution (a).

B. To about 2 mg add 5 ml of *sulphuric acid R*. A yellow
$\quad$ colour develops.

C. It gives reaction (a) of chlorides (*2.3.1*).

TESTS

pH (*2.2.3*): 2.0 to 3.0.

Dissolve 0.1 g in *carbon dioxide-free water R* and dilute to
10 ml with the same solvent.

Specific optical rotation (*2.2.7*): − 105 to − 120 (anhydrous
and ethanol-free substance).

Dissolve 0.250 g in a mixture of 1 volume of *1 M hydrochloric
acid* and 99 volumes of *methanol R* and dilute to 25.0 ml with
the same mixture of solvents. Carry out the measurement
within 5 min of preparing the solution.

Specific absorbance (*2.2.25*): 300 to 335 determined at the
maximum at 349 nm (anhydrous and ethanol-free substance).

Dissolve 25.0 mg in a mixture of 1 volume of *1 M
hydrochloric acid* and 99 volumes of *methanol R* and dilute
to 25.0 ml with the same mixture of solvents. Dilute 1.0 ml
of the solution to 100.0 ml with a mixture of 1 volume of *1 M
hydrochloric acid* and 99 volumes of *methanol R*. Carry out
the measurement within 1 h of preparing the solution.

Light-absorbing impurities. The absorbance (*2.2.25*),
determined at 490 nm has a maximum of 0.07 (anhydrous
and ethanol-free substance).

Dissolve 0.10 g in a mixture of 1 volume of *1 M hydrochloric
acid* and 99 volumes of *methanol R* and dilute to 10.0 ml with
the same mixture of solvents. Carry out the measurement
within 1 h of preparing the solution.

Related substances. Liquid chromatography (*2.2.29*).
Prepare the solutions immediately before use.

Test solution. Dissolve 20.0 mg of the substance to be
examined in *0.01 M hydrochloric acid* and dilute to 25.0 ml
with the same acid.

Reference solution (a). Dissolve 20.0 mg of *doxycycline
hyclate CRS* in *0.01 M hydrochloric acid* and dilute to
25.0 ml with the same acid.

Reference solution (b). Dissolve 20.0 mg of *6-epidoxycycline
hydrochloride CRS* in *0.01 M hydrochloric acid* and dilute
to 25.0 ml with the same acid.

Reference solution (c). Dissolve 20.0 mg of *metacycline
hydrochloride CRS* in *0.01 M hydrochloric acid* and dilute
to 25.0 ml with the same acid.

Reference solution (d). Mix 4.0 ml of reference solution (a),
1.5 ml of reference solution (b) and 1.0 ml of reference
solution (c) and dilute to 25.0 ml with *0.01 M hydrochloric
acid*.

Reference solution (e). Mix 2.0 ml of reference solution (b)
and 2.0 ml of reference solution (c) and dilute to 100.0 ml
with *0.01 M hydrochloric acid*.

Column:

− *size*: l = 0.25 m, Ø = 4.6 mm,

− *stationary phase*: *styrene-divinylbenzene copolymer R*
$\quad$ (8 µm),

− *temperature*: 60 °C.

Mobile phase: weigh 60.0 g of *2-methyl-2-propanol R* and
transfer to a 1000 ml volumetric flask with the aid of 200 ml
of *water R*; add 400 ml of *buffer solution pH 8.0 R*, 50 ml
of a 10 g/l solution of *tetrabutylammonium hydrogen
sulphate R* adjusted to pH 8.0 with *dilute sodium hydroxide
solution R* and 10 ml of a 40 g/l solution of *sodium edetate R*
adjusted to pH 8.0 with *dilute sodium hydroxide solution R*;
dilute to 1000.0 ml with *water R*.

Flow rate: 1.0 ml/min.

Detection: spectrophotometer at 254 nm.

Injection: 20 µl; inject the test solution and reference
solutions (d) and (e).

Relative retention with reference to doxycycline:
impurity E = about 0.2; impurity D = about 0.3;
impurity C = about 0.5; impurity F = about 1.2.

System suitability: reference solution (d):

− *resolution*: minimum 1.25 between the peaks due to
$\quad$ impurity B (1st peak) and impurity A (2nd peak) and
$\quad$ minimum 2.0 between the peaks due to impurity A
$\quad$ and doxycycline (3rd peak); if necessary, adjust the
$\quad$ 2-methyl-2-propanol content in the mobile phase,

− *symmetry factor*: maximum 1.25 for the peak due to
$\quad$ doxycycline.

Limits:

− *impurity A*: not more than the area of the corresponding
$\quad$ peak in the chromatogram obtained with reference
$\quad$ solution (e) (2.0 per cent),

− *impurity B*: not more than the area of the corresponding
$\quad$ peak in the chromatogram obtained with reference
$\quad$ solution (e) (2.0 per cent),

− *any other impurity*: not more than 0.25 times the area of
$\quad$ the peak due to impurity A in the chromatogram obtained
$\quad$ with reference solution (e) (0.5 per cent),

- *disregard limit*: 0.05 times the area of the peak due to impurity A in the chromatogram obtained with reference solution (e) (0.1 per cent).

Ethanol (*2.4.24, System A*): 4.3 per cent to 6.0 per cent.

Heavy metals (*2.4.8*): maximum 50 ppm.

0.5 g complies with limit test C. Prepare the standard using 2.5 ml of *lead standard solution (10 ppm Pb) R*.

Water (*2.5.12*): 1.4 per cent to 2.8 per cent, determined on 1.20 g.

Sulphated ash (*2.4.14*): maximum 0.4 per cent, determined on 1.0 g.

Sterility (*2.6.1*). If intended for use in the manufacture of parenteral dosage forms without a further appropriate sterilisation procedure, it complies with the test for sterility.

Bacterial endotoxins (*2.6.14*): less than 1.14 IU/mg, if intended for use in the manufacture of parenteral dosage forms without a further appropriate procedure for the removal of bacterial endotoxins.

ASSAY

Liquid chromatography (*2.2.29*) as described in the test for related substances with the following modification.

Injection: test solution and reference solution (a).

Calculate the percentage content of $C_{22}H_{25}ClN_2O_8$ ($M_r = 480.9$).

STORAGE

In an airtight container, protected from light. If the substance is sterile, store in a sterile, airtight, tamper-proof container.

LABELLING

The label states:

— where applicable, that the substance is sterile,

— where applicable, that the substance is free from bacterial endotoxins.

IMPURITIES

A. R1 = NH$_2$, R2 = R5 = H, R3 = N(CH$_3$)$_2$, R4 = CH$_3$:
(4S,4aR,5S,5aR,6S,12aS)-4-(dimethylamino)-3,5,10,12,12a-pentahydroxy-6-methyl-1,11-dioxo-1,4,4a,5,5a,6,11,12-octahydrotetracene-2-carboxamide (6-epidoxycycline),

B. R1 = NH$_2$, R2 = H, R3 = N(CH$_3$)$_2$, R4 + R5 = CH$_2$:
(4S,4aR,5S,5aR,12aS)-4-(dimethylamino)-3,5,10,12,12a-pentahydroxy-6-methylene-1,11-dioxo-1,4,4a,5,5a,6,11,12a-octahydrotetracene-2-carboxamide (metacycline),

C. R1 = NH$_2$, R2 = N(CH$_3$)$_2$, R3 = R4 = H, R5 = CH$_3$:
(4R,4aR,5S,5aR,6R,12aS)-4-(dimethylamino)-3,5,10,12,12a-pentahydroxy-6-methyl-1,11-dioxo-1,4,4a,5,5a,6,11,12a-octahydrotetracene-2-carboxamide (4-epidoxycycline),

D. R1 = NH$_2$, R2 = N(CH$_3$)$_2$, R3 = R5 = H, R4 = CH$_3$:
(4R,4aR,5S,5aR,6S,12aS)-4-(dimethylamino)-3,5,10,12,12a-pentahydroxy-6-methyl-1,11-dioxo-1,4,4a,5,5a,6,11,12a-octahydrotetracene-2-carboxamide (4-epi-6-epidoxycycline),

E. R1 = NH$_2$, R2 = H, R3 = N(CH$_3$)$_2$, R4 = OH, R5 = CH$_3$:
oxytetracycline,

F. R1 = CH$_3$, R2 = R4 = H, R3 = N(CH$_3$)$_2$, R5 = CH$_3$:
(4S,4aR,5S,5aR,6R,12aS)-2-acetyl-4-(dimethylamino)-3,5,10,12,12a-pentahydroxy-6-methyl-4a,5a,6,12a-tetrahydrotetracene-1,11(4H,5H)-dione (2-acetyl-2-decarbamoyldoxycycline).

04/2003:0820

DOXYCYCLINE MONOHYDRATE

Doxycyclinum monohydricum

$C_{22}H_{24}N_2O_8,H_2O$ M_r 462.5

DEFINITION

(4S,4aR,5S,5aR,6R,12aS)-4-(Dimethylamino)-3,5,10,12,12a-pentahydroxy-6-methyl-1,11-dioxo-1,4,4a,5,5a,6,11,12a-octahydrotetracene-2-carboxamide monohydrate.

Substance obtained from oxytetracycline or metacycline or by any other means.

Content: 95.0 per cent to 102.0 per cent (anhydrous substance).

CHARACTERS

Appearance: yellow, crystalline powder.

Solubility: very slightly soluble in water and in alcohol. It dissolves in dilute solutions of mineral acids and in solutions of alkali hydroxides and carbonates.

IDENTIFICATION

A. Examine the chromatograms obtained in the assay.

Results: the principal peak in the chromatogram obtained with the test solution is similar in retention time and size to the principal peak in the chromatogram obtained with reference solution (a).

B. To about 2 mg add 5 ml of *sulphuric acid R*. A yellow colour develops.

C. Dissolve 25 mg in a mixture of 0.2 ml of *dilute nitric acid R* and 1.8 ml of *water R*. The solution does not give reaction (a) of chlorides (*2.3.1*).

TESTS

pH (*2.2.3*): 5.0 to 6.5.

Suspend 0.1 g in *carbon dioxide-free water R* and dilute to 10 ml with the same solvent.

Specific optical rotation (*2.2.7*): − 113 to − 130 (anhydrous substance).

Dissolve 0.250 g in a mixture of 0.5 volumes of *hydrochloric acid R* and 99.5 volumes of *methanol R* and dilute to 25.0 ml with the same mixture of solvents. Carry out the measurement within 5 min of preparing the solution.

Specific absorbance (*2.2.25*): 325 to 363 determined at the maximum at 349 nm (anhydrous substance).

Dissolve 25.0 mg in a mixture of 0.5 volumes of *hydrochloric acid R* and 99.5 volumes of *methanol R* and dilute to 50.0 ml with the same mixture of solvents. Dilute 2.0 ml of the solution to 100.0 ml with a mixture of 0.5 volumes of *1 M hydrochloric acid* and 99.5 volumes of *methanol R*. Carry out the measurement within 1 h of preparing the solution.

Light-absorbing impurities. The absorbance (*2.2.25*) determined at 490 nm has a maximum of 0.07 (anhydrous substance).

Dissolve 0.10 g in a mixture of 0.5 volumes of *hydrochloric acid R* and 99.5 volumes of *methanol R* and dilute to 10.0 ml with the same mixture of solvents. Carry out the measurement within 1 h of preparing the solution.

Related substances. Liquid chromatography (*2.2.29*). *Prepare the solutions immediately before use.*

Test solution. Dissolve 20.0 mg of the substance to be examined in *0.01 M hydrochloric acid* and dilute to 25.0 ml with the same acid.

Reference solution (a). Dissolve 20.0 mg of *doxycycline hyclate CRS* in *0.01 M hydrochloric acid* and dilute to 25.0 ml with the same acid.

Reference solution (b). Dissolve 20.0 mg of *6-epidoxycycline hydrochloride CRS* in *0.01 M hydrochloric acid* and dilute to 25.0 ml with the same acid.

Reference solution (c). Dissolve 20.0 mg of *metacycline hydrochloride CRS* in *0.01 M hydrochloric acid* and dilute to 25.0 ml with the same acid.

Reference solution (d). Mix 4.0 ml of reference solution (a), 1.5 ml of reference solution (b) and 1.0 ml of reference solution (c) and dilute to 25.0 ml with *0.01 M hydrochloric acid*.

Reference solution (e). Mix 2.0 ml of reference solution (b) and 2.0 ml of reference solution (c) and dilute to 100.0 ml with *0.01 M hydrochloric acid*.

Column:

– *size*: l = 0.25 m, Ø = 4.6 mm,

– *stationary phase*: *styrene-divinylbenzene copolymer R* (8 µm),

– *temperature*: 60 °C.

Mobile phase: weigh 60.0 g of *2-methyl-2-propanol R* and transfer into a 1000 ml volumetric flask with the aid of 200 ml of *water R*; add 400 ml of *buffer solution pH 8.0 R*, 50 ml of a 10 g/l solution of *tetrabutylammonium hydrogen sulphate R* adjusted to pH 8.0 with *dilute sodium hydroxide solution R* and 10 ml of a 40 g/l solution of *sodium edetate R* adjusted to pH 8.0 with *dilute sodium hydroxide solution R*; dilute to 1000.0 ml with *water R*.

Flow rate: 1.0 ml/min.

Detection: spectrophotometer at 254 nm.

Injection: 20 µl; inject the test solution and reference solutions (d) and (e).

Relative retention with reference to doxycycline: impurity E = about 0.2; impurity D = about 0.3; impurity C = about 0.5; impurity F = about 1.2.

System suitability: reference solution (d):

– *resolution*: minimum 1.25 between the peaks due to impurity B (1st peak) and impurity A (2nd peak) and minimum 2.0 between the peaks due to impurity A and doxycycline (3rd peak); if necessary, adjust the 2-methyl-2-propanol content in the mobile phase,

– *symmetry factor*: maximum 1.25 for the peak due to doxycycline.

Limits:

– *impurity A*: not more than the area of the corresponding peak in the chromatogram obtained with reference solution (e) (2.0 per cent),

– *impurity B*: not more than the area of the corresponding peak in the chromatogram obtained with reference solution (e) (2.0 per cent),

– *any other impurity*: not more than 0.25 times the area of the peak due to impurity A in the chromatogram obtained with reference solution (e) (0.5 per cent),

– *disregard limit*: 0.05 times the area of the peak due to impurity A in the chromatogram obtained with reference solution (e) (0.1 per cent).

Heavy metals (*2.4.8*): maximum 50 ppm.

0.5 g complies with limit test C. Prepare the standard using 2.5 ml of *lead standard solution (10 ppm Pb) R*.

Water (*2.5.12*): 3.6 per cent to 4.6 per cent, determined on 0.200 g.

Sulphated ash (*2.4.14*): maximum 0.4 per cent, determined on 1.0 g.

ASSAY

Liquid chromatography (*2.2.29*) as described in the test for related substances with the following modification.

Injection: test solution and reference solution (a).

Calculate the percentage content of $C_{22}H_{24}N_2O_8$.

STORAGE

Protected from light.

IMPURITIES

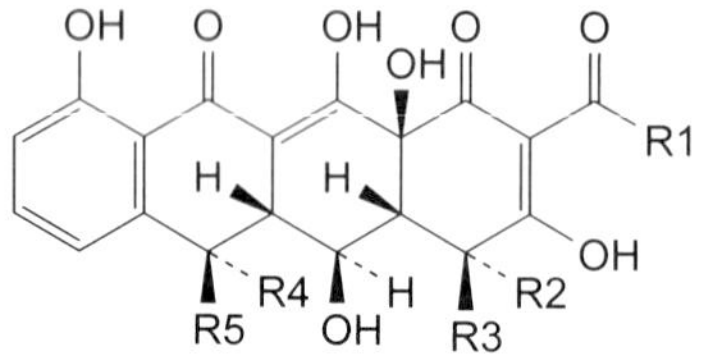

A. R1 = NH$_2$, R2 = R5 = H, R3 = N(CH$_3$)$_2$, R4 = CH$_3$: (4*S*,4a*R*,5*S*,5a*R*,6*S*,12a*S*)-4-(dimethylamino)-3,5,10,12,12a-pentahydroxy-6-methyl-1,11-dioxo-1,4,4a,5,5a,6,11,12a-octahydrotetracene-2-carboxamide (6-epidoxycycline),

B. R1 = NH$_2$, R2 = H, R3 = N(CH$_3$)$_2$, R4 + R5 = CH$_2$: (4*S*,4a*R*,5*S*,5a*R*,12a*S*)-4-(dimethylamino)-3,5,10,12,12a-pentahydroxy-6-methylene-1,11-dioxo-1,4,4a,5,5a,6,11,12a-octahydrotetracene-2-carboxamide (metacycline),

C. R1 = NH$_2$, R2 = N(CH$_3$)$_2$, R3 = R4 = H, R5 = CH$_3$: (4*R*,4a*R*,5*S*,5a*R*,6*R*,12a*S*)-4-(dimethylamino)-3,5,10,12,12a-pentahydroxy-6-methyl-1,11-dioxo-1,4,4a,5,5a,6,11,12a-octahydrotetracene-2-carboxamide (4-epidoxycycline),

D. R1 = NH$_2$, R2 = N(CH$_3$)$_2$, R3 = R5 = H, R4 = CH$_3$: (4*R*,4a*R*,5*S*,5a*R*,6*S*,12a*S*)-4-(dimethylamino)-3,5,10,12,12a-pentahydroxy-6-methyl-1,11-dioxo-1,4,4a,5,5a,6,11,12a-octahydrotetracene-2-carboxamide (4-epi-6-epidoxycycline),

E. R1 = NH$_2$, R2 = H, R3 = N(CH$_3$)$_2$, R4 = OH, R5 = CH$_3$: oxytetracycline,

F. R1 = CH$_3$, R2 = R4 = H, R3 = N(CH$_3$)$_2$, R5 = CH$_3$: (4*S*,4a*R*,5*S*,5a*R*,6*R*,12a*S*)-2-acetyl-4-(dimethylamino)-3,5,10,12,12a-pentahydroxy-6-methyl-4a,5a,6,12a-tetrahydrotetracene-1,11(4*H*,5*H*)-dione (2-acetyl-2-decarbamoyldoxycycline).

E

01/2003:1420
corrected

ENALAPRIL MALEATE

Enalaprili maleas

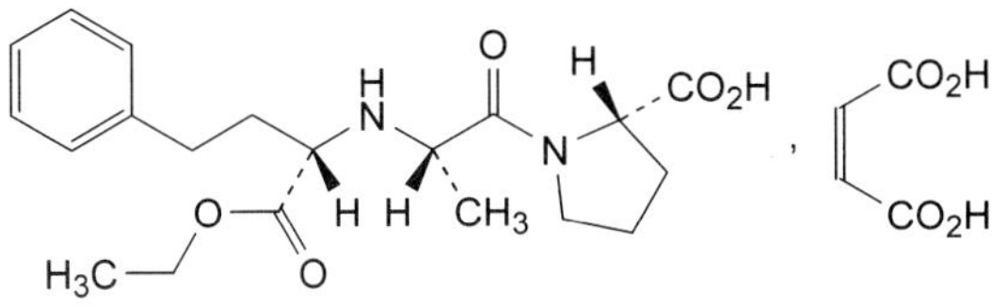

$C_{24}H_{32}N_2O_9$

M_r 492.5

DEFINITION

Enalapril maleate contains not less than 98.5 per cent and not more than the equivalent of 101.5 per cent of (2S)-1-[(2S)-2-[[(1S)-1-(ethoxycarbonyl)-3-phenylpropyl]amino]propanoyl]pyrrolidine-2-carboxylic acid (Z)-butenedioate, calculated with reference to the dried substance.

CHARACTERS

A white or almost white crystalline powder, sparingly soluble in water, freely soluble in methanol, practically insoluble in methylene chloride. It dissolves in dilute solutions of alkali hydroxides.

IDENTIFICATION

First identification: B.

Second identification: A, C, D.

A. Melting point (*2.2.14*): 143 °C to 145 °C.

B. Examine by infrared absorption spectrophotometry (*2.2.24*), comparing with the spectrum obtained with *enalapril maleate CRS*.

C. Dissolve about 30 mg in 3 ml of *water R*. Add 1 ml of *bromine water R* and heat on a water bath until bromine has disappeared completely and cool. To 0.2 ml of this solution, add 3 ml of a 3 g/l solution of *resorcinol R* in *sulphuric acid R* and heat on a water bath for 15 min. A reddish-brown colour develops.

D. To about 30 mg, add 0.5 ml of a 100 g/l solution of *hydroxylamine hydrochloride R* in *methanol R* and 1.0 ml of a 100 g/l solution of *potassium hydroxide R* in *alcohol R*. Heat to boiling, allow to cool and acidify with *dilute hydrochloric acid R*. Add 0.2 ml of *ferric chloride solution R1* diluted 1 to 10; a reddish-brown colour appears.

TESTS

Solution S. Dissolve 0.25 g in *carbon dioxide-free water R* and dilute to 25.0 ml with the same solvent.

Appearance of solution. Solution S is clear (*2.2.1*) and colourless (*2.2.2, Method II*).

pH (*2.2.3*). The pH of solution S is 2.4 to 2.9.

Specific optical rotation (*2.2.7*): −48 to −51, determined on solution S and calculated with reference to the dried substance.

Related substances. Examine by liquid chromatography (*2.2.29*).

Buffer solution A. Dissolve 2.8 g of *sodium dihydrogen phosphate monohydrate R* in 950 ml of *water R*. Adjust to pH 2.5 with *phosphoric acid R* and dilute to 1000 ml with *water R*.

Buffer solution B. Dissolve 2.8 g of *sodium dihydrogen phosphate monohydrate R* in 950 ml of *water R*. Adjust to pH 6.8 with *strong sodium hydroxide solution R* and dilute to 1000 ml with *water R*.

Dissolution mixture. Mix 50 ml of *acetonitrile R1* and 950 ml of buffer solution A.

Test solution. Dissolve 30.0 mg of the substance to be examined in the dissolution mixture and dilute to 100.0 ml with the same mixture.

Reference solution (a). Dilute 1.0 ml of the test solution to 100.0 ml with the dissolution mixture.

Reference solution (b). Dissolve 3.0 mg of *enalapril for system suitability CRS* in the dissolution mixture and dilute to 10.0 ml with the same mixture.

The chromatographic procedure may be carried out using:

— a stainless steel column 0.15 m long and 4.1 mm in internal diameter packed with *styrene-divinylbenzene copolymer R* (5 μm),

— as mobile phase at a flow rate of 1.4 ml/min,

   Mobile phase A. Mix 50 ml of *acetonitrile R1* and 950 ml of buffer solution B,

   Mobile phase B. Mix 340 ml of buffer solution B and 660 ml of *acetonitrile R1*,

Time (min)	Mobile phase A (per cent *V/V*)	Mobile phase B (per cent *V/V*)
0 - 20	95 → 40	5 → 60
20 - 25	40	60
25 - 26	40 → 95	60 → 5
26 - 30	95	5

— as detector a spectrophotometer set at 215 nm,

maintaining the temperature of the column at 70 °C.

Inject 50 μl of reference solution (b). When the chromatogram is recorded in the prescribed conditions, the retention times are: enalapril about 11 min and impurity A about 12 min. The test is not valid unless the resolution between the peaks corresponding to enalapril and impurity A is at least 1.5. Inject 50 μl of the test solution and 50 μl of reference solution (a). In the chromatogram obtained with the test solution: the area of any peak corresponding to impurity A is not greater than that of the principal peak in the chromatogram obtained with reference solution (a) (1.0 per cent); the area of any peak apart from the principal peak and any peak corresponding to impurity A, is not greater than 0.3 times the area of the principal peak in the chromatogram obtained with reference solution (a) (0.3 per cent) and the sum of the areas of any such peaks is not greater than the area of the principal peak in the chromatogram obtained with reference solution (a) (1.0 per cent). Disregard any peak with an area less than 0.05 times that of the principal peak in the chromatogram obtained with reference solution (a).

Heavy metals (*2.4.8*). 2.0 g complies with limit test C (10 ppm). Use 2 ml of *lead standard solution (10 ppm Pb) R*.

Loss on drying (*2.2.32*). Not more than 1.0 per cent determined on 1.000 g by heating in an oven at 100-105 °C for 3 h.

Sulphated ash (*2.4.14*). Not more than 0.1 per cent, determined on 1.0 g.

ASSAY

Dissolve 0.100 g in *carbon dioxide-free water R* and dilute to 30 ml with the same solvent. Titrate with *0.1 M sodium hydroxide* determining the end point potentiometrically (*2.2.20*). Titrate to the second point of inflexion.

1 ml of *0.1 M sodium hydroxide* is equivalent to 16.42 mg of $C_{24}H_{32}N_2O_9$.

STORAGE

Store protected from light.

IMPURITIES

Qualified impurities: A, B, C, D, E, H.

Other detectable impurities: F, G, I.

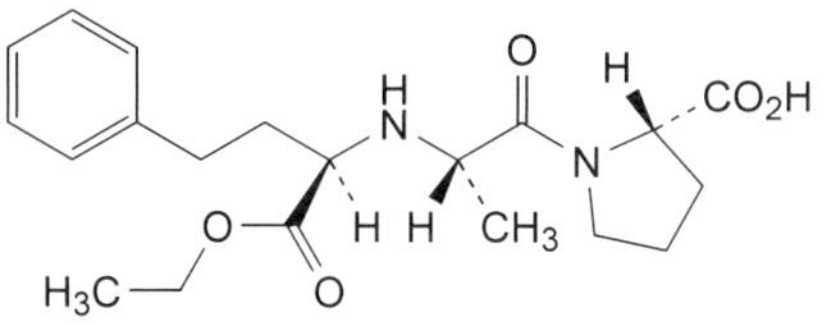

A. (2*S*)-1-[(2*S*)-2-[[(1*R*)-1-(ethoxycarbonyl)-3-phenylpropyl]amino]propanoyl]pyrrolidine-2-carboxylic acid,

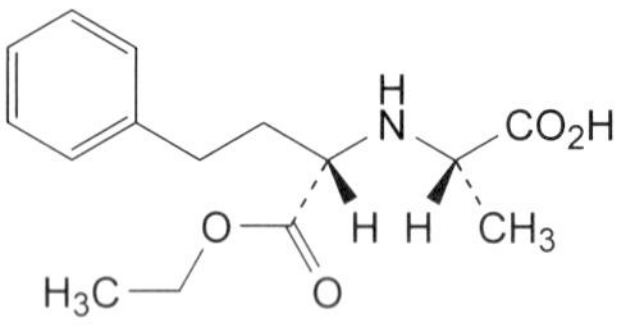

B. (2*S*)-2-[[(1*S*)-1-(ethoxycarbonyl)-3-phenylpropyl]amino]propanoic acid,

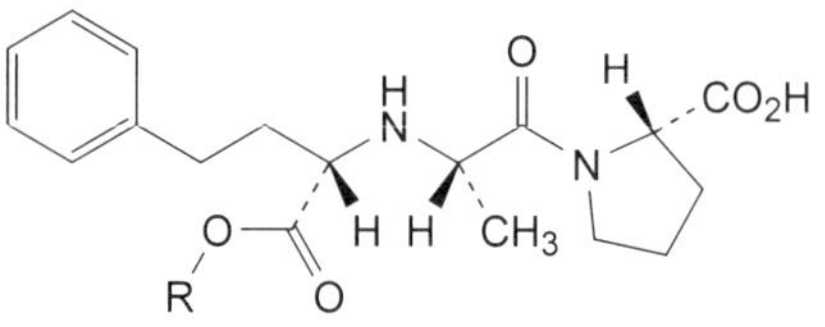

C. R = H: (2*S*)-1-[(2*S*)-2-[[(1*S*)-1-carboxy-3-phenylpropyl]amino]propanoyl]pyrrolidine-2-carboxylic acid,

E. R = CH$_2$-CH$_2$-C$_6$H$_5$: (2*S*)-1-[(2*S*)-2-[[(1*S*)-3-phenyl-1-[(2-phenylethoxy)carbonyl]propyl]amino]propanoyl]pyrrolidine-2-carboxylic acid,

F. R = C$_4$H$_9$: (2*S*)-1-[(2*S*)-2-[[(1*S*)-1-(butoxycarbonyl)-3-phenylpropyl]amino]propanoyl]pyrrolidine-2-carboxylic acid,

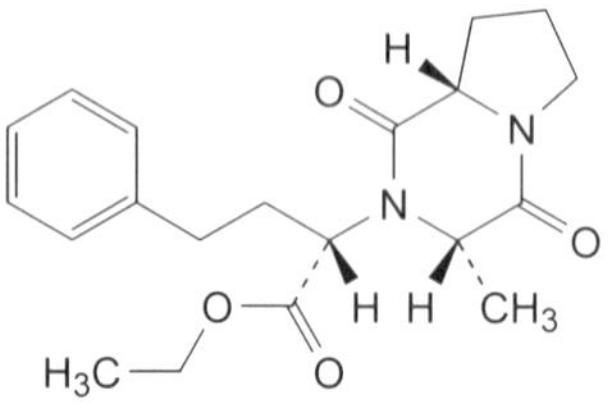

D. ethyl (2*S*)-2-[(3*S*,8a*S*)-3-methyl-1,4-dioxooctahydropyrrolo[1,2-*a*]pyrazin-2-yl]-4-phenylbutanoate,

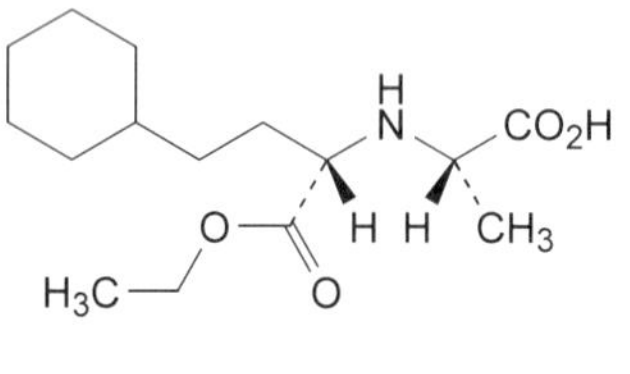

G. (2*S*)-2-[[(1*S*)-3-cyclohexyl-1-(ethoxycarbonyl)propyl]amino]propanoic acid,

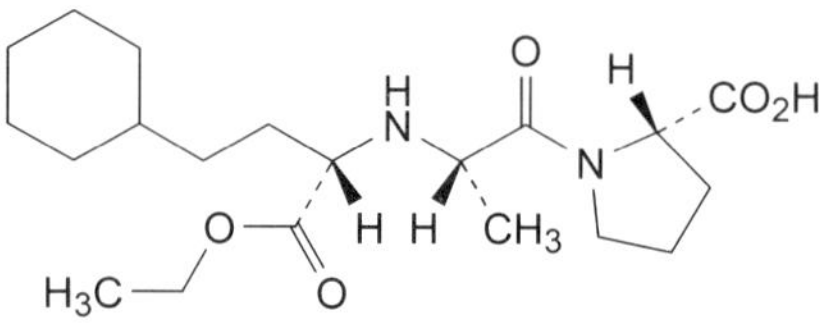

H. (2*S*)-1-[(2*S*)-2-[[(1*S*)-3-cyclohexyl-1-(ethoxycarbonyl)propyl]amino]propanoyl]pyrrolidine-2-carboxylic acid,

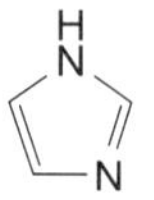

I. 1*H*-imidazole.

04/2003:0139

ESTRADIOL BENZOATE

Estradioli benzoas

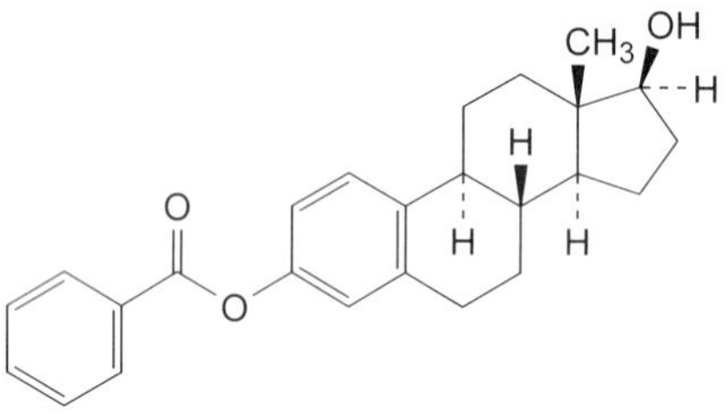

$C_{25}H_{28}O_3$ M_r 376.5

DEFINITION

17β-Hydroxyestra-1,3,5(10)-trien-3-yl benzoate.

Content: 97.0 per cent to 103.0 per cent (dried substance).

CHARACTERS

Appearance: almost white, crystalline powder or colourless crystals.

Solubility: practically insoluble in water, freely soluble in methylene chloride, sparingly soluble in acetone, slightly soluble in methanol.

It shows polymorphism.

IDENTIFICATION

Infrared absorption spectrophotometry (*2.2.24*).

Comparison: estradiol benzoate CRS.

If the spectra obtained show differences, dissolve the substance to be examined and the reference substance separately in *acetone R*, evaporate to dryness and record new spectra using the residues.

TESTS

Specific optical rotation (*2.2.7*): + 55.0 to + 59.0 (dried substance).

Dissolve 0.250 g in *acetone R* and dilute to 25.0 ml with the same solvent.

Related substances. Liquid chromatography (*2.2.29*).

Test solution. Dissolve 20 mg of the substance to be examined in *acetonitrile R* and dilute to 10.0 ml with the same solvent.

Reference solution (a). Dissolve 5 mg of *estradiol benzoate impurity E CRS* in 5 ml of *acetonitrile R*, add 2.5 ml of the test solution and dilute to 10 ml with *acetonitrile R*.

Reference solution (b). Dilute 1.0 ml of the test solution to 100.0 ml with *acetonitrile R.*

Column:

– *size: l* = 0.25 m, Ø = 4.6 mm,

– *stationary phase: octylsilyl silica gel for chromatography R* (5 µm).

Mobile phase:

– *mobile phase A: water R, acetonitrile R* (40:60 *V/V*),

– *mobile phase B: acetonitrile R,*

Time (min)	Mobile phase A (per cent *V/V*)	Mobile phase B (per cent *V/V*)
0 - t_R	100	0
t_R - (t_R + 1)	100 → 10	0 → 90
(t_R + 1) - (t_R + 10)	10	90

t_R = retention time of impurity E

Flow rate: 1.0 ml/min.

Detection: spectrophotometer at 230 nm.

Injection: 10 µl.

Elution order: impurity A, impurity F, estradiol benzoate, impurity E, impurity B, impurity D, impurity C.

System suitability: reference solution (a):

– *resolution:* minimum 2.0 between the peaks due to estradiol benzoate and to impurity E.

Limits:

– *any impurity:* not more than 0.5 times the area of the principal peak in the chromatogram obtained with reference solution (b) (0.5 per cent),

– *total:* not more than 1.5 times the area of the principal peak in the chromatogram obtained with reference solution (b) (1.5 per cent),

– *disregard limit:* 0.05 times the area of the principal peak in the chromatogram obtained with reference solution (b) (0.05 per cent).

Loss on drying *(2.2.32):* maximum 0.5 per cent, determined on 0.5 g by drying in an oven at 100-105 °C for 3 h.

ASSAY

Dissolve 25.0 mg in *ethanol R* and dilute to 250.0 ml with the same solvent. Dilute 10.0 ml of the solution to 100.0 ml with *ethanol R.* Measure the absorbance *(2.2.25)* at the maximum at 231 nm.

Calculate the content of $C_{25}H_{28}O_3$ taking the specific absorbance to be 500.

IMPURITIES

Qualified impurities: A, B, C, D, E, F.

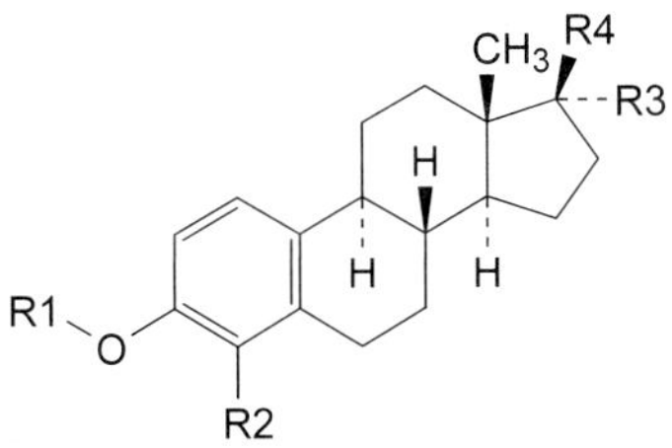

A. R1 = R2 = R3 = H, R4 = OH: estradiol,

B. R1 = CO-C$_6$H$_5$, R2 = CH$_3$, R3 = H, R4 = OH: 17β-hydroxy-4-methylestra-1,3,5(10)-trien-3-yl benzoate,

C. R1 = CO-C$_6$H$_5$, R2 = R3 = H, R4 = O-CO-C$_6$H$_5$: estra-1,3,5(10)-triene-3,17β-diyl dibenzoate,

D. R1 = R2 = R3 = H, R4 = O-CO-C$_6$H$_5$: 3-hydroxyestra-1,3,5(10)-trien-17β-yl benzoate,

E. R1 = CO-C$_6$H$_5$, R2 = R4 = H, R3 = OH: 17α-hydroxyestra-1,3,5(10)-trien-3-yl benzoate,

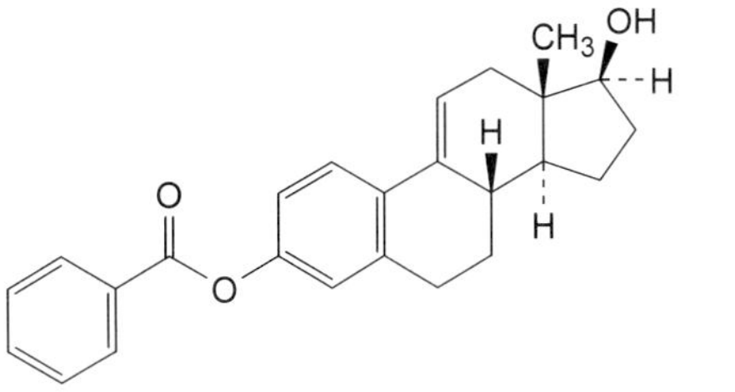

F. 17β-hydroxyestra-1,3,5(10),9(11)-tetraen-3-yl benzoate.

04/2003:1203

ESTRIOL

Estriolum

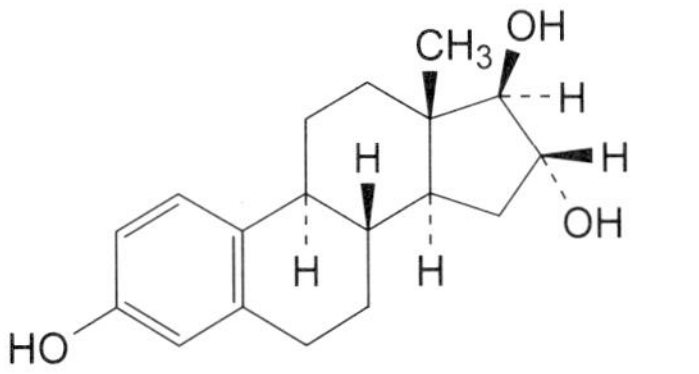

$C_{18}H_{24}O_3$ M_r 288.4

DEFINITION

Estriol contains not less than 97.0 per cent and not more than the equivalent of 103.0 per cent of estra-1,3,5(10)-triene-3,16α,17β-triol, calculated with reference to the dried substance.

CHARACTERS

A white or almost white, crystalline powder, practically insoluble in water, sparingly soluble in alcohol.

It melts about 282 °C.

IDENTIFICATION

A. Examine by infrared absorption spectrophotometry *(2.2.24),* comparing with the spectrum obtained with *estriol CRS.*

B. Examine by thin-layer chromatography *(2.2.27),* using a suitable silica gel as the coating substance.

Test solution. Dissolve 10 mg of the substance to be examined in *methanol R* and dilute to 10 ml with the same solvent.

Reference solution (a). Dissolve 10 mg of *estriol CRS* in *methanol R* and dilute to 10 ml with the same solvent.

Reference solution (b). Dissolve 5 mg of *estradiol hemihydrate CRS* in reference solution (a) and dilute to 5 ml with the same solvent.

Apply to the plate 5 µl of each solution. Develop over a path of 15 cm using a mixture of 20 volumes of *alcohol R* and 80 volumes of *toluene R.* Allow the plate to dry in air. Spray the plate with *alcoholic solution of sulphuric acid R.* Heat the plate at 100 °C for 10 min or until the spots appear. Allow to cool. Examine in daylight and ultraviolet light at 365 nm. The principal spot in the chromatogram obtained with the test solution is similar in position, colour in daylight, fluorescence in ultraviolet light at 365 nm and size to the principal spot in the chromatogram obtained with the reference solution (a). The test is not valid unless the chromatogram obtained with reference solution (b) shows 2 clearly separated spots.

TESTS

Specific optical rotation (2.2.7). Dissolve 80 mg in *ethanol R* and dilute to 10 ml with the same solvent. The specific optical rotation is + 60 to + 65, calculated with reference to the dried substance.

Related substances. Examine by liquid chromatography (2.2.29).

Solvent mixture. A mixture of 20 volumes of *2-propanol R1* and 80 volumes of *heptane R*.

Test solution. Dissolve 20.0 mg of the substance to be examined in 5 ml of *2-propanol R1* and dilute to 20.0 ml with the solvent mixture.

Reference solution (a). Dissolve 5 mg of *estriol CRS* and 2.0 mg of *estriol impurity A CRS* in 5 ml of *2-propanol R1* and dilute to 10.0 ml with the solvent mixture. Dilute 1.0 ml of the solution to 20.0 ml with the solvent mixture.

Reference solution (b). Dilute 1.0 ml of the test solution to 10.0 ml with the solvent mixture. Dilute 1.0 ml of the solution to 10.0 ml with the same solvent mixture.

The chromatographic procedure may be carried out using:

— a stainless steel column 0.15 m long and 4.0 mm in internal diameter packed with *diol silica gel for chromatography R* (5 μm),

— as mobile phase at a flow rate of 1.2 ml/min a linear gradient programme using the following conditions:

Mobile phase A. Heptane R,

Mobile phase B. 2-Propanol R1,

Time (min)	Mobile phase A (per cent V/V)	Mobile phase B (per cent V/V)	Comment
0 - 10	95 → 88	5 → 12	linear gradient
10 - 20	88	12	isocratic
20 - 30	88 → 95	12 → 5	switch to initial eluent composition
30 - 35	95	5	equilibration
35 = 0	95	5	restart gradient

— as detector a spectrophotometer set at 280 nm,

maintaining the temperature of the column at 40 °C.

Equilibrate the column with a mixture of 20 per cent *V/V* of *2-propanol R1* in *heptane R* until a stable baseline is obtained.

Adjust the sensitivity of the system so that the height of the principal peak in the chromatogram obtained with 20 μl of reference solution (b) is about 25 per cent of the full scale of the recorder.

Inject 20 μl of reference solution (a). When the chromatograms are recorded in the prescribed conditions, the retention times are: estriol about 19 min and estriol impurity A about 21 min. The test is not valid unless the resolution between the peaks corresponding to estriol and estriol impurity A is at least 2.2. If the retention times increase or the resolution decreases, wash the column first with *acetone R* and then with *heptane R*.

Inject separately 20 μl of the solvent mixture as a blank, 20 μl of the test solution and 20 μl of each of the reference solutions (a) and (b). In the chromatogram obtained with the test solution: the area of any peak corresponding to estriol impurity A is not greater than half the area of the peak corresponding to estriol impurity A in the chromatogram obtained with reference solution (a) (0.5 per cent) and any other peak, apart from the principal peak, is not greater than half the area of the principal peak in the chromatogram obtained with reference solution (b) (0.5 per cent); the sum of the areas of all the peaks, apart from the principal peak and the peak corresponding to estriol impurity A, is not greater than the area of the peak in the chromatogram obtained with reference solution (b) (1 per cent). Disregard any peak due to the blank and any peak with an area less than 0.05 times the area of the principal peak in the chromatogram obtained with reference solution (b).

Loss on drying (2.2.32). Not more than 0.5 per cent, determined on 1.000 g by drying in an oven at 100-105 °C for 3 h.

ASSAY

Dissolve 25.0 mg in *alcohol R* and dilute to 50.0 ml with the same solvent. Dilute 10.0 ml of this solution to 50.0 ml with the same solvent. Measure the absorbance (2.2.25) at the maximum at 281 nm.

Calculate the content of $C_{18}H_{24}O_3$ taking the specific absorbance to be 72.5.

IMPURITIES

Qualified impurities: A, B, C, D, E, F, G.

Other detectable impurities: H, I.

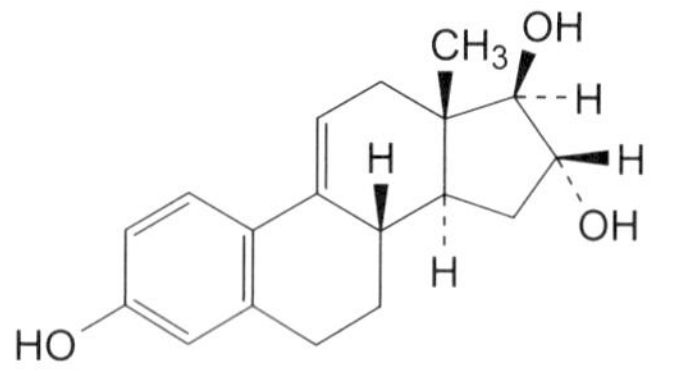

A. estra-1,3,5(10),9(11)-tetraene-3,16α,17β-triol (9,11-didehydroestriol),

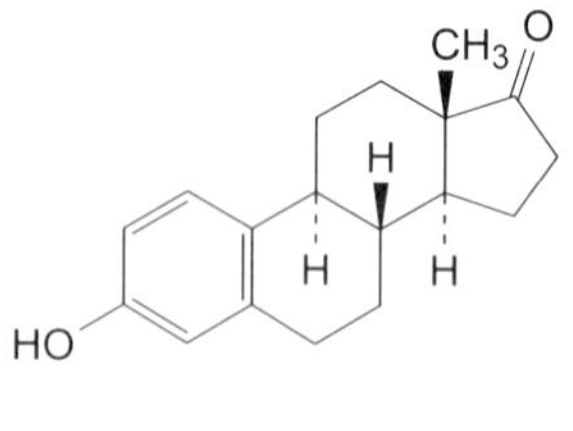

B. 3-hydroxyestra-1,3,5(10)-trien-17-one (estrone),

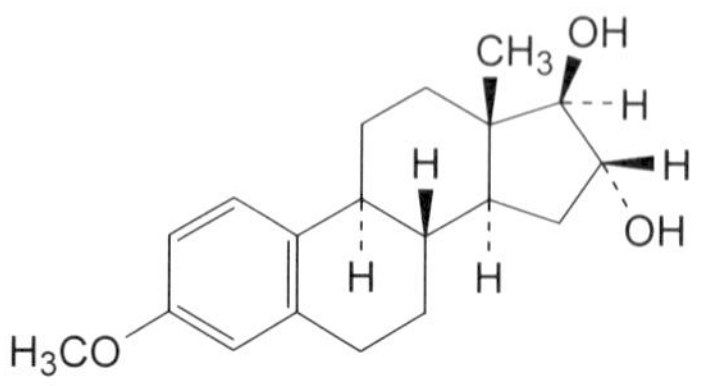

C. 3-methoxyestra-1,3,5(10)-triene-16α,17β-diol (estriol 3-methyl ether),

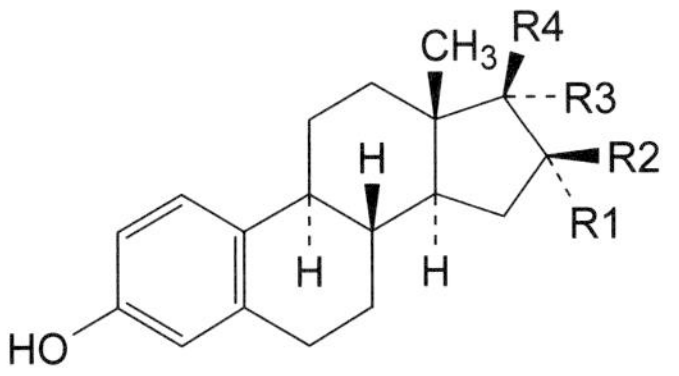

D. R1 = R2 = R3 = H, R4 = OH: estradiol,

E. R1 = R3 = OH, R2 = R4 = H: estra-1,3,5(10)-triene-3,16α,17α-triol (17-epi-estriol),

F. R1 = R3 = H, R2 = R4 = OH: estra-1,3,5(10)-triene-3,16β,17β-triol (16-epi-estriol),

G. R1 = R4 = H, R2 = R3 = OH: estra-1,3,5(10)-triene-3,16β,17α-triol (16,17-epi-estriol),

H. R1 = OH, R2 = H, R3 + R4 = O: 3,16α-dihydroxyestra-1,3,5(10)-trien-17-one,

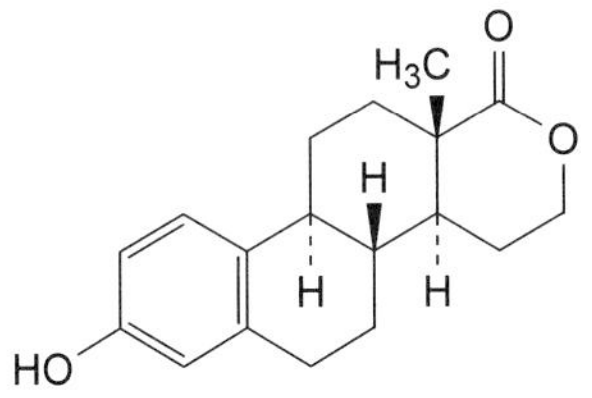

I. 3-hydroxy-17-oxa-D-homoestra-1,3,5(10)-trien-17a-one.

04/2003:0764

ETHOSUXIMIDE

Ethosuximidum

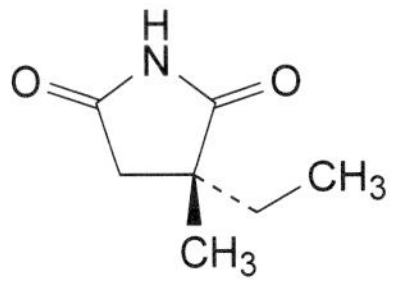

and enantiomer

C₇H₁₁NO₂ ... hold

$C_7H_{11}NO_2$　　　　　　　　　　　　　　　　　　M_r 141.2

DEFINITION

(RS)-3-Ethyl-3-methylpyrrolidine-2,5-dione.

Content: 99.0 per cent to 101.0 per cent (anhydrous substance).

CHARACTERS

Appearance: white or almost white powder or waxy solid.

Solubility: freely soluble in water, very soluble in alcohol and in methylene chloride.

It shows polymorphism.

IDENTIFICATION

First identification: A, C.

Second identification: A, B, D, E.

A. Melting point (2.2.14): 45 °C to 50 °C.

B. Dissolve 50.0 mg in alcohol R and dilute to 50.0 ml with the same solvent. Examined between 230 nm and 300 nm (2.2.25), the solution shows an absorption maximum at 248 nm. The specific absorbance at the maximum is 8 to 9.

C. Infrared absorption spectrophotometry (2.2.24).

Preparation: discs of potassium bromide R.

Comparison: ethosuximide CRS.

If the spectra obtained in the solid state show differences, dissolve the substance to be examined and the reference substance separately in methylene chloride R, evaporate to dryness and record new spectra using the residues.

D. Dissolve 0.1 g in 3 ml of methanol R. Add 0.05 ml of a 100 g/l solution of cobalt chloride R and 0.05 ml of a 100 g/l solution of calcium chloride R and add 0.1 ml of dilute sodium hydroxide solution R. A purple colour develops and no precipitate is formed.

E. To about 10 mg add 10 mg of resorcinol R and 0.2 ml of sulphuric acid R. Heat at 140 °C for 5 min and cool. Add 5 ml of water R and 2 ml of concentrated ammonia R1. A brown colour is produced. Add about 100 ml of water R. A green fluorescence is produced.

TESTS

Solution S. Dissolve 2.5 g in water R and dilute to 25 ml with the same solvent.

Appearance of solution. Solution S is clear (2.2.1) and colourless (2.2.2, Method II).

Cyanide. Liquid chromatography (2.2.29).

Test solution. Dissolve 0.50 g of the substance to be examined in water R and dilute to 10.0 ml with the same solvent.

Reference solution (a). Dissolve 0.125 g of potassium cyanide R in water R and dilute to 50.0 ml with the same solvent. Dilute 1.0 ml to 100.0 ml with water R. Dilute 0.5 ml of this solution to 10.0 ml with water R.

Reference solution (b). Dissolve 0.50 g of the substance to be examined in water R, add 0.5 ml of reference solution (a) and dilute to 10.0 ml with water R.

Column:
- size: l = 0.075 m, Ø = 7.5 mm,
- stationary phase: spherical weak anion exchange resin (10 μm).

Mobile phase: dissolve 2.1 g of lithium hydroxide R and 85 mg of sodium edetate R in water for chromatography R and dilute to 1000.0 ml with the same solvent.

Flow rate: 2.0 ml/min.

Detection: electrochemical detector (direct amperometry) with a silver working electrode, a silver-silver chloride reference electrode, held at + 0.05 V oxidation potential, and a detector sensitivity of 20 nA full scale.

Injection: 20 μl; inject the test solution and reference solution (b).

System suitability: reference solution (b):
- peak-to-valley ratio: minimum 3, where H_p = height above the baseline of the peak due to cyanide and H_V = height above the baseline of the lowest point of the curve separating this peak from the peak due to ethosuximide.

Limit:
- cyanide: not more than half the height of the corresponding peak in the chromatogram obtained with reference solution (b) (0.5 ppm).

Related substances. Gas chromatography (2.2.28).

Internal standard solution. Dissolve 20 mg of myristyl alcohol R in ethanol R and dilute to 10.0 ml with the same solvent.

Test solution. Dissolve 1.00 g of the substance to be examined in ethanol R, add 1.0 ml of the internal standard solution and dilute to 20.0 ml with ethanol R.

Reference solution (a). Dissolve 20.0 mg of *ethosuximide impurity A CRS* in *ethanol R* and dilute to 10.0 ml with the same solvent. To 0.5 ml of the solution, add 1.0 ml of the internal standard solution and dilute to 20.0 ml with *ethanol R.*

Reference solution (b). Dissolve 0.500 g of the substance to be examined in *ethanol R* and dilute to 10.0 ml with the same solvent. Dilute 1.0 ml to 50.0 ml with *ethanol R.* To 2.0 ml of this solution, add 1.0 ml of the internal standard solution and dilute to 20.0 ml with *ethanol R.*

Column:
— *material*: fused silica,
— *size*: $l = 30$ m, $\varnothing = 0.25$ mm,
— *stationary phase*: *poly(cyanopropyl)(phenylmethyl) siloxane R* (film thickness 0.25 µm).

Carrier gas: *helium for chromatography R.*

Flow rate: 1 ml/min.

Split ratio: 1:67.

Temperature:
— *column*: 175 °C,
— *injection port and detector*: 240 °C.

Detection: flame ionisation.

Injection: 1 µl.

Run time: 1.5 times the retention time of ethosuximide.

Relative retentions with reference to the internal standard (retention time = about 8 min): impurity A = about 0.7; ethosuximide = about 1.1.

System suitability: reference solution (b):
— *resolution*: minimum 5 between the peaks due to the internal standard and to ethosuximide.

Limits:
— *impurity A*: calculate the ratio (*R*) of the area of the peak due to impurity A to the area of the peak due to the internal standard from the chromatogram obtained with reference solution (a); from the chromatogram obtained with the test solution, calculate the ratio of the area of any peak due to impurity A to the area of the peak due to the internal standard: this ratio is not greater than *R* (0.1 per cent),
— *any other impurity*: calculate the ratio (*R*) of half the area of the peak due to ethosuximide to the area of the peak due to the internal standard from the chromatogram obtained with reference solution (b); from the chromatogram obtained with the test solution, calculate the ratio of the area of any peak, apart from the principal peak and the peaks due to impurity A and to the internal standard, to the area of the peak due to the internal standard: this ratio is not greater than *R* (0.1 per cent),
— *total*: calculate the ratio (*R*) of the area of the peak due to ethosuximide to the area of the peak due to the internal standard from the chromatogram obtained with reference solution (b); from the chromatogram obtained with the test solution, calculate the ratio of the sum of the areas of any peaks, apart from the principal peak and the peak due to the internal standard, to the area of the peak due to the internal standard: this ratio is not greater than *R* (0.2 per cent),
— *disregard limit*: calculate the ratio (*R*) of 0.25 times the area of the peak due to impurity A to the area of the peak due to the internal standard from the chromatogram obtained with reference solution (a); from the chromatogram obtained with the test solution, calculate the ratio of the area of any peak, apart from the principal peak and the peak due to the internal

standard, to the area of the peak due to the internal standard: disregard any peak which has a ratio less than *R* (0.025 per cent).

Heavy metals (*2.4.8*): maximum 10 ppm.

12 ml of solution S complies with limit test A. Prepare the standard using *lead standard solution (1 ppm Pb) R.*

Water (*2.5.12*): maximum 0.5 per cent, determined on 1.00 g.

Sulphated ash (*2.4.14*): maximum 0.1 per cent, determined on 1.0 g.

ASSAY

Dissolve 0.120 g in 20 ml of *dimethylformamide R* and carry out a potentiometric titration (*2.2.20*) using *0.1 M tetrabutylammonium hydroxide.* Protect the solution from atmospheric carbon dioxide throughout the titration. Carry out a blank titration.

1 ml of *0.1 M tetrabutylammonium hydroxide* is equivalent to 14.12 mg of $C_7H_{11}NO_2$.

STORAGE

Protected from light.

IMPURITIES

Qualified impurities: A.

A. (2RS)-2-ethyl-2-methylbutanedioic acid.

04/2003:0822

ETHYLCELLULOSE

Ethylcellulosum

DEFINITION

Partly *O*-ethylated cellulose.

Content: 44.0 per cent to 51.0 per cent of ethoxy (-OC$_2$H$_5$) groups (dried substance).

CHARACTERS

Appearance: white or yellowish-white powder or granular powder, odourless or almost odourless.

Solubility: practically insoluble in water, soluble in methylene chloride and in a mixture of 20 g of alcohol and 80 g of toluene, slightly soluble in ethyl acetate and in methanol, practically insoluble in glycerol (85 per cent) and in propylene glycol. The solutions may show a slight opalescence.

IDENTIFICATION

A. Infrared absorption spectrophotometry (*2.2.24*).

Comparison: Ph. Eur. reference spectrum of ethylcellulose.

B. It complies with the limits of the assay.

TESTS

Acidity or alkalinity. To 0.5 g add 25 ml of *carbon dioxide-free water R* and shake for 15 min. Filter through a sintered-glass filter (40). To 10 ml add 0.1 ml of *phenolphthalein solution R* and 0.5 ml of *0.01 M sodium hydroxide*. The solution is pink. To 10 ml add 0.1 ml of *methyl red solution R* and 0.5 ml of *0.01 M hydrochloric acid*. The solution is red.

Viscosity (*2.2.9*). The viscosity, determined at 25 °C and expressed in mPa·s, is not less than 80.0 per cent and not more than 120.0 per cent of that stated on the label for a nominal viscosity greater than 6 mPa·s; and not less than 75.0 per cent and not more than 140.0 per cent of that stated on the label for a nominal viscosity not greater than 6 mPa·s.

Shake a quantity of the substance to be examined equivalent to 5.00 g of the dried substance with 95 g of a mixture of 20 g of *alcohol R* and 80 g of *toluene R* until the substance is dissolved. Determine the viscosity using a capillary viscometer.

Acetaldehyde: maximum 100 ppm.

Introduce 3.0 g into a 250 ml conical flask with a ground-glass stopper, add 10 ml of *water R* and stir mechanically for 1 h. Allow to stand for 24 h, filter and dilute the filtrate to 100.0 ml with *water R*. Transfer 5.0 ml to a 25 ml volumetric flask, add 5 ml of a 0.5 g/l solution of *methylbenzothiazolone hydrazone hydrochloride R* and heat in a water-bath at 60 °C for 5 min. Add 2 ml of *ferric chloride-sulphamic acid reagent R* and heat again at 60 °C for 5 min. Cool and dilute to 25.0 ml with *water R*. The solution is not more intensely coloured than a standard prepared at the same time and in the same manner using instead of the 5.0 ml of filtrate, 5.0 ml of a reference solution prepared by diluting 3.0 ml of *acetaldehyde standard solution (100 ppm C_2H_4O) R1* to 100.0 ml with *water R*.

Chlorides (*2.4.4*): maximum 0.1 per cent.

Disperse 0.250 g in 50 ml of *water R*, heat to boiling and allow to cool, shaking occasionally. Filter and discard the first 10 ml of the filtrate. Dilute 10 ml of the filtrate to 15 ml with *water R*. The solution complies with the limit test for chlorides.

Heavy metals (*2.4.8*): maximum 20 ppm.

1.0 g complies with limit test C. Prepare the standard using 2 ml of *lead standard solution (10 ppm Pb) R*.

Loss on drying (*2.2.32*): maximum 3.0 per cent, determined on 1.000 g by drying in an oven at 100-105 °C for 2 h.

Sulphated ash (*2.4.14*): maximum 0.5 per cent, determined on 1.0 g.

ASSAY

Gas chromatography (*2.2.28*).

CAUTION: hydriodic acid and its reaction by-products are highly toxic. Perform all steps for preparation of the test and reference solutions in a properly functioning hood.

Internal standard solution. Dilute 120 µl of *toluene R* to 10 ml with *o-xylene R*.

Test solution. Transfer 50.0 mg of the substance to be examined, 50.0 mg of *adipic acid R* and 2.0 ml of the internal standard solution into a suitable 5 ml thick-walled reaction vial with a pressure-tight septum-type closure. Cautiously add 2.0 ml of *hydriodic acid R*, immediately close the vial tightly and weigh the contents and the vial accurately. Shake the vial for 30 s, heat to 125 °C for 10 min, allow to cool for 2 min, shake again for 30 s and heat to 125 °C for 10 min. Afterwards allow to cool for 2 min and repeat shaking and

heating for a third time. Allow the vial to cool for 45 min and reweigh. If the loss is greater than 10 mg, discard the mixture and prepare another. Use the upper layer.

Reference solution. Transfer 100.0 mg of *adipic acid R*, 4.0 ml of the internal standard solution and 4.0 ml of *hydriodic acid R* into a suitable 10 ml thick-walled reaction vial with a pressure-tight septum-type closure. Close the vial tightly and weigh the vial and contents accurately. Afterwards inject 50 µl of *iodoethane R* through the septum with a syringe, weigh the vial again and calculate the mass of iodoethane added, by difference. Shake well and allow the layers to separate.

Column:

— *material*: stainless steel,

— *size*: l = 5.0 m, Ø = 2 mm,

— *stationary phase*: *diatomaceous earth for gas chromatography R* (150-180 µm) impregnated with 3 per cent *m/m* of *poly(dimethyl)siloxane R*.

Carrier gas: *nitrogen for chromatography R*.

Flow rate: 15 ml/min.

Temperature:

— *column*: 80 °C,

— *injection port and detector*: 200 °C.

Detection: flame ionisation.

Injection: 1 µl of the upper layer of the test solution and 1 µl of the upper layer of the reference solution.

Relative retention with reference to toluene: iodoethane = about 0.6; *o*-xylene = about 2.3.

System suitability: reference solution:

— *resolution*: minimum 2.0 between the peaks due to iodoethane and toluene.

Calculate the percentage content of ethoxy groups from the following expression:

$$\frac{Q_1 \times m_2 \times 45.1 \times 100 \times 100}{2 \times Q_2 \times m_1 \times 156.0 \times (100 - d)}$$

Q_1 = ratio of iodoethane peak area to toluene peak area in the chromatogram obtained with the test solution,

Q_2 = ratio of iodoethane peak area to toluene peak area in the chromatogram obtained with the reference solution,

m_1 = mass of the substance to be examined used in the test solution, in milligrams,

m_2 = mass of iodoethane used in the reference solution, in milligrams,

d = percentage loss on drying.

LABELLING

The label states the nominal viscosity in millipascal seconds for a 5 per cent *m/m* solution.

F

Monographs
D - K

01/2002:0180
corrected

FRAMYCETIN SULPHATE

Framycetini sulfas

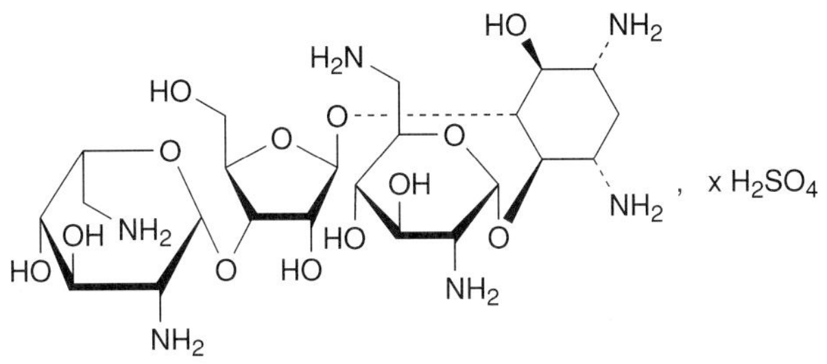

$C_{23}H_{46}N_6O_{13},xH_2SO_4$ M_r 615 (base)

DEFINITION

Sulphate of 2-deoxy-4-O-(2,6-diamino-2,6-dideoxy-α-D-glucopyranosyl)-5-O-[3-O-(2,6-diamino-2,6-dideoxy-β-L-idopyranosyl)-β-D-ribofuranosyl]-D-streptamine (neomycin B), a substance produced by the growth of selected strains of *Streptomyces fradiae* or *Streptomyces decaris* or obtained by any other means.

Content: minimum of 630 IU/mg (dried substance).

CHARACTERS

Appearance: white or yellowish-white powder, hygroscopic.

Solubility: freely soluble in water, very slightly soluble in alcohol, practically insoluble in acetone.

IDENTIFICATION

A. Examine the chromatograms obtained in the test for related substances.

  Results:

    — the retention time of the principal peak in the chromatogram obtained with the test solution is approximately the same as that of the principal peak in the chromatogram obtained with reference solution (a),

    — it complies with the limit given for impurity C.

B. It gives reaction (a) of sulphates (*2.3.1*).

TESTS

pH (*2.2.3*): 6.0 to 7.0.

Dissolve 0.1 g in *carbon dioxide-free water R* and dilute to 10 ml with the same solvent.

Specific optical rotation (*2.2.7*): + 52.5 to + 55.5 (dried substance).

Dissolve 1.00 g in *water R* and dilute to 10.0 ml with the same solvent

Related substances. Liquid chromatography (*2.2.29*).

Test solution. Dissolve 25.0 mg of the substance to be examined in the mobile phase and dilute to 50.0 ml with the mobile phase.

Reference solution (a). Dissolve 25.0 mg of *framycetin sulphate CRS* in the mobile phase and dilute to 50.0 ml with the mobile phase.

Reference solution (b). Dilute 3.0 ml of reference solution (a) to 100.0 ml with the mobile phase.

Reference solution (c). Dilute 1.0 ml of reference solution (a) to 100.0 ml with the mobile phase.

Reference solution (d). Dissolve the contents of a vial of *neamine CRS* (corresponding to 0.5 mg) in the mobile phase and dilute to 100.0 ml with the mobile phase.

Reference solution (e). Dissolve 10 mg of *neomycin sulphate CRS* in the mobile phase and dilute to 100.0 ml with the mobile phase.

Column:

— *size*: l = 0.25 m, Ø = 4.6 mm,

— *stationary phase*: *base-deactivated octadecylsilyl silica gel for chromatography R* (5 μm),

— *temperature*: 25 °C.

Mobile phase: mix 20.0 ml of *trifluoroacetic acid R*, 6.0 ml of *carbonate-free sodium hydroxide solution R* and 500 ml of *water R*, allow to equilibrate, dilute to 1000 ml with *water R* and degas.

Flow rate: 0.7 ml/min.

Post-column solution: *carbonate-free sodium hydroxide solution R* diluted 1 in 25 previously degassed, which is added pulse-less to the column effluent using a 375 μl polymeric mixing coil.

Flow rate: 0.5 ml/min.

Detection: pulsed amperometric detector with a gold working electrode, a silver-silver chloride reference electrode and a stainless steel auxiliary electrode which is the cell body, held at respectively 0.00 V detection, + 0.80 V oxidation and − 0.60 V reduction potentials, with pulse durations according to the instrument used.

Injection: 10 μl.

Run time: 1.5 times the retention time of neomycin B.

Relative retention with reference to neomycin B (retention time = about 10 min): impurity A = about 0.65; impurity C = about 0.9; impurity G = about 1.1.

System suitability:

— *resolution*: minimum 2.0 between the peaks due to impurity C and to neomycin B in the chromatogram obtained with reference solution (e); if necessary, adjust the volume of the carbonate-free sodium hydroxide solution in the mobile phase,

— *signal-to-noise ratio*: minimum 10 for the principal peak in the chromatogram obtained with reference solution (c).

Limits:

— *impurity A*: not more than the area of the principal peak in the chromatogram obtained with reference solution (d) (1.0 per cent),

— *impurity C*: not more than the area of the principal peak in the chromatogram obtained with reference solution (b) (3.0 per cent),

— *total of other impurities*: not more than the area of the principal peak in the chromatogram obtained with reference solution (b) (3.0 per cent),

— *disregard limit*: area of the principal peak in the chromatogram obtained with reference solution (c) (1.0 per cent).

Sulphate: 27.0 per cent to 31.0 per cent (dried substance).

Dissolve 0.250 g in 100 ml of *water R* and adjust the solution to pH 11 using *concentrated ammonia R*. Add 10.0 ml of *0.1 M barium chloride* and about 0.5 mg of *phthalein purple R*. Titrate with *0.1 M sodium edetate* adding 50 ml of *alcohol R* when the colour of the solution begins to change and continuing the titration until the violet-blue colour disappears.

1 ml of *0.1 M barium chloride* is equivalent to 9.606 mg of SO_4.

Loss on drying (2.2.32): maximum 8.0 per cent, determined on 1.000 g by drying at 60 °C over *diphosphorus pentoxide R* at a pressure not exceeding 0.7 kPa for 3 h.

Sulphated ash (2.4.14): maximum 1.0 per cent, determined on 1.0 g.

Sterility (2.6.1). If intended for introduction into body cavities without a further appropriate sterilisation procedure, it complies with the test for sterility.

Bacterial endotoxins (2.6.14, Method D): less than 1.3 IU/mg if intended for introduction into body cavities without a further appropriate procedure for the removal of bacterial endotoxins.

ASSAY

Carry out the microbiological assay of antibiotics (2.7.2). Use *framycetin sulphate CRS* as the reference substance.

STORAGE

In an airtight container, protected from light. If the substance is intended for introduction into body cavities, store in a sterile, tamper-proof container.

LABELLING

The label states:
— where applicable, that the substance is sterile,
— where applicable, that the substance is free from bacterial endotoxins.

IMPURITIES

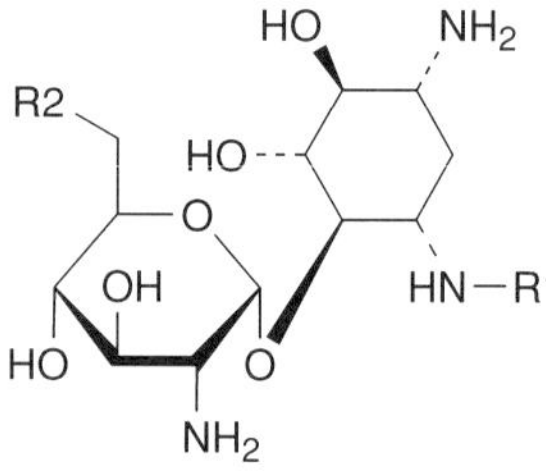

A. R1 = H, R2 = NH$_2$: 2-deoxy-4-O-(2,6-diamino-2,6-dideoxy-α-D-glucopyranosyl)-D-streptamine (neamine or neomycin A-LP),

B. R1 = CO-CH$_3$, R2 = NH$_2$: 3-N-acetyl-2-deoxy-4-O-(2,6-diamino-2,6-dideoxy-α-D-glucopyranosyl)-D-streptamine (3-acetylneamine),

D. R1 = H, R2 = OH: 4-O-(2-amino-2-deoxy-α-D-glucopyranosyl)-2-deoxy-D-streptamine (paromamine or neomycin D),

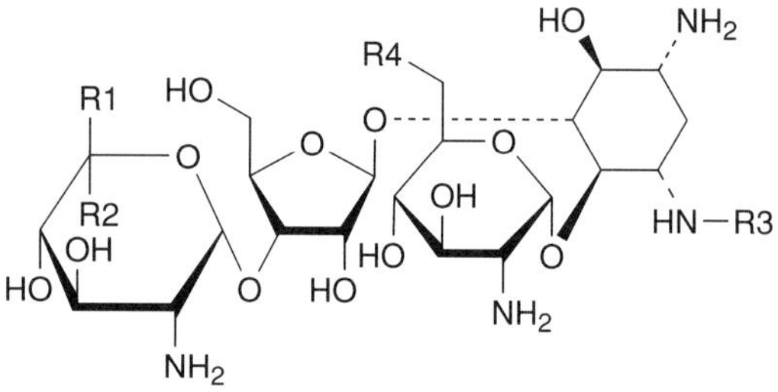

C. R1 = CH$_2$-NH$_2$, R2 = R3 = H, R4 = NH$_2$: 2-deoxy-4-O-(2,6-diamino-2,6-dideoxy-α-D-glucopyranosyl)-5-O-[3-O-(2,6-diamino-2,6-dideoxy-α-D-glucopyranosyl)-β-D-ribofuranosyl]-D-streptamine (neomycin C),

E. R1 = R3 = H, R2 = CH$_2$-NH$_2$, R4 = OH: 4-O-(2-amino-2-deoxy-α-D-glucopyranosyl)-2-deoxy-5-O-[3-O-(2,6-diamino-2,6-dideoxy-β-L-idopyranosyl)-β-D-ribofuranosyl]-D-streptamine (paromomycin I or neomycin E),

F. R1 = CH$_2$-NH$_2$, R2 = R3 = H, R4 = OH: 4-O-(2-amino-2-deoxy-α-D-glucopyranosyl)-2-deoxy-5-O-[3-O-(2,6-diamino-2,6-dideoxy-α-D-glucopyranosyl)-β-D-ribofuranosyl]-D-streptamine (paromomycin II or neomycin F),

G. R1 = H, R2 = CH$_2$-NH$_2$, R3 = CO-CH$_3$, R4 = NH$_2$: 3-N-acetyl-2-deoxy-4-O-(2,6-diamino-2,6-dideoxy-α-D-glucopyranosyl)-5-O-[3-O-(2,6-diamino-2,6-dideoxy-β-L-idopyranosyl)-β-D-ribofuranosyl]-D-streptamine (neomycin B-LP).

G

Monographs
D - K

07/2002:1331
corrected

GLYCERYL TRINITRATE SOLUTION

Glyceroli trinitratis solutio

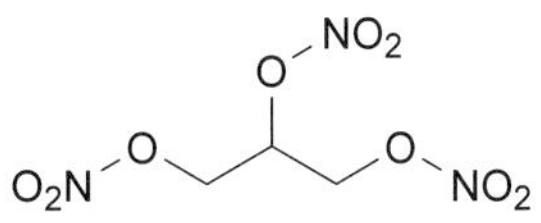

$C_3H_5N_3O_9$ M_r 227.1

DEFINITION

Ethanolic solution of glyceryl trinitrate.

Content: 1 per cent *m/m* to 10 per cent *m/m* of propane-1,2,3-triyl trinitrate and 96.5 per cent to 102.5 per cent of the declared content of glyceryl trinitrate stated on the label.

CHARACTERS

Appearance: clear, colourless or slightly yellow solution.

Solubility: miscible with acetone and with ethanol.

Solubility of pure glyceryl trinitrate: practically insoluble in water, freely soluble in ethanol, miscible with acetone.

IDENTIFICATION

First identification: A, C.

Second identification: B, C.

Upon diluting glyceryl trinitrate solution, care must be taken to always use anhydrous ethanol, otherwise droplets of pure glyceryl trinitrate may precipitate from the solution.

After examination, the residues and the solutions obtained in both the identification and the test sections must be heated on a water-bath for 5 min with dilute sodium hydroxide solution R.

A. Infrared absorption spectrophotometry (*2.2.24*).

   Preparation: place 50 µl of a solution diluted, if necessary, with *ethanol R*, to contain 10 g/l of glyceryl trinitrate, on a disc of *potassium bromide R* and evaporate the solvent *in vacuo*.

   Comparison: *Ph. Eur. reference spectrum of glyceryl trinitrate*.

B. Thin-layer chromatography (*2.2.27*).

   Test solution. Dilute a quantity of the substance to be examined corresponding to 50 mg of glyceryl trinitrate to 100 ml with *acetone R*.

   Reference solution. Dilute 0.05 ml of *glyceryl trinitrate solution CRS* to 1 ml with *acetone R*.

   Plate: *TLC silica gel G plate R*.

   Mobile phase: *ethyl acetate R, toluene R* (20:80 *V/V*).

   Application: 5 µl.

   Development: over 2/3 of the plate.

   Drying: in air.

   Detection: spray with freshly prepared *potassium iodide and starch solution R*. Expose the plate to ultraviolet light at 254 nm for 15 min. Examine in daylight.

   Results: the principal spot in the chromatogram obtained with the test solution is similar in position, colour and size to the principal spot in the chromatogram obtained with the reference solution.

C. It complies with the limits of the assay.

TESTS

Upon diluting glyceryl trinitrate solution, care must be taken always to use anhydrous ethanol, otherwise droplets of pure glyceryl trinitrate may precipitate from the solution.

After examination, the residues and the solutions obtained in both the identification and the test sections must be heated on a water-bath for 5 min with dilute sodium hydroxide solution R.

Appearance of solution. If necessary dilute the solution to be examined to a concentration of 10 g/l with *ethanol R*. The solution is not more intensely coloured than reference solution Y_7 (*2.2.2, Method II*).

Inorganic nitrates. Thin-layer chromatography (*2.2.27*).

Test solution. If necessary dilute the solution to be examined to a concentration of 10 g/l with *ethanol R*.

Reference solution. Dissolve 5 mg of *potassium nitrate R* in 1 ml of *water R* and dilute to 100 ml with *alcohol R*.

Plate: *TLC silica gel plate R*.

Mobile phase: *glacial acetic acid R, acetone R, toluene R* (15:30:60 *V/V/V*).

Application: 10 µl.

Development: over 2/3 of the plate.

Drying: in a current of air until the acetic acid is completely removed.

Detection: spray intensively with freshly prepared *potassium iodide and starch solution R*. Expose the plate to ultraviolet light at 254 nm for 15 min. Examine in daylight.

Limit:

— *nitrate ion*: any spot corresponding to the nitrate ion in the chromatogram obtained with the test solution is not more intense than the spot in the chromatogram obtained with the reference solution (0.5 per cent of the content of glyceryl trinitrate calculated as potassium nitrate).

Related substances. Liquid chromatography (*2.2.29*).

Test solution. Dissolve a quantity of the substance to be examined corresponding to 2 mg of glyceryl trinitrate in the mobile phase and dilute to 20.0 ml with the mobile phase.

Reference solution (a). Dissolve 0.10 g of *glyceryl trinitrate solution CRS* and a quantity of *diluted pentaerythrityl tetranitrate CRS* equivalent to 1.0 mg of pentaerythrityl tetranitrate in the mobile phase and dilute to 100.0 ml with the mobile phase. Sonicate and filter if necessary.

Reference solution (b). Dilute 1.0 ml of the test solution to 100.0 ml with the mobile phase.

Column:

— *size*: l = 0.25 m, Ø = 4.6 mm,

— *stationary phase*: *octadecylsilyl silica gel for chromatography R* (5 µm).

Mobile phase: *acetonitrile R, water R* (50:50 *V/V*).

Flow rate: 1 ml/min.

Detection: spectrophotometer at 210 nm.

Injection: 20 µl.

Run time: 3 times the retention time of the principal peak.

System suitability: reference solution (a):

— *resolution*: minimum 2.0 between the peaks due to glyceryl trinitrate and to pentaerythrityl tetranitrate.

Limits:

— *any impurity*: not more than the area of the principal peak in the chromatogram obtained with reference solution (b) (1 per cent, calculated as glyceryl trinitrate),

— *total*: not more than 3 times the area of the principal peak in the chromatogram obtained with reference solution (b) (3 per cent, calculated as glyceryl trinitrate),

— *disregard limit*: 0.1 times the area of the principal peak in the chromatogram obtained with reference solution (b) (0.1 per cent).

ASSAY

Test solution. Prepare a solution containing 1.0 mg of glyceryl trinitrate in 250.0 ml of *methanol R*.

Reference solution. Dissolve 70.0 mg of *sodium nitrite R* in *methanol R* and dilute to 250.0 ml with the same solvent. Dilute 5.0 ml of the solution to 500.0 ml with *methanol R*.

Into three 50 ml volumetric flasks introduce 10.0 ml of the test solution, 10.0 ml of the reference solution and 10 ml of *methanol R* as a blank. To each flask add 5 ml of *dilute sodium hydroxide solution R*, close the flask, mix and allow to stand at room temperature for 30 min. Add 10 ml of *sulphanilic acid solution R* and 10 ml of *dilute hydrochloric acid R* and mix. After exactly 4 min, add 10 ml of *naphthylethylenediamine dihydrochloride solution R*, dilute to volume with *water R* and mix. After 10 min read the absorbance (*2.2.25*) of the test solution and the reference solution at 540 nm using the blank solution as the compensation liquid.

Calculate the amount of glyceryl trinitrate in milligrams in the test solution from the following expression:

$$\frac{A_T \times m_S \times C}{A_R \times m_T \times 60.8 \times 100}$$

A_T = absorption of the test solution,

m_T = mass of the substance to be examined, in milligrams,

C = percentage content of sodium nitrite used as reference,

A_R = absorption of the reference solution,

m_S = mass of sodium nitrite, in milligrams.

STORAGE

Store diluted solutions (10 g/l) protected from light, at a temperature of 2 °C to 15 °C. Store more concentrated solutions protected from light, at a temperature of 15 °C to 20 °C.

LABELLING

The label states the declared content of glyceryl trinitrate.

IMPURITIES

A. inorganic nitrates,

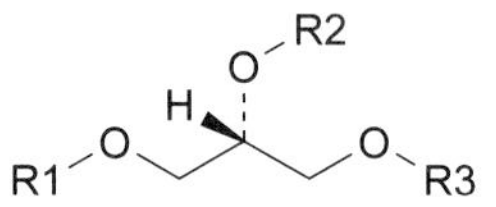

and enantiomer

B. R1 = NO$_2$, R2 = R3 = H: (2*RS*)-2,3-dihydroxypropyl nitrate,

C. R1 = R3 = H, R2 = NO$_2$: 2-hydroxy-1-(hydroxymethyl)ethyl nitrate,

D. R1 = R2 = NO$_2$, R3 = H: (2*RS*)-3-hydroxypropane-1,2-diyl dinitrate,

E. R1 = R3 = NO$_2$, R2 = H: 2-hydroxypropane-1,3-diyl dinitrate.

H

Monographs
D - K

01/2002:0916
corrected

HYDROXYZINE HYDROCHLORIDE

Hydroxyzini hydrochloridum

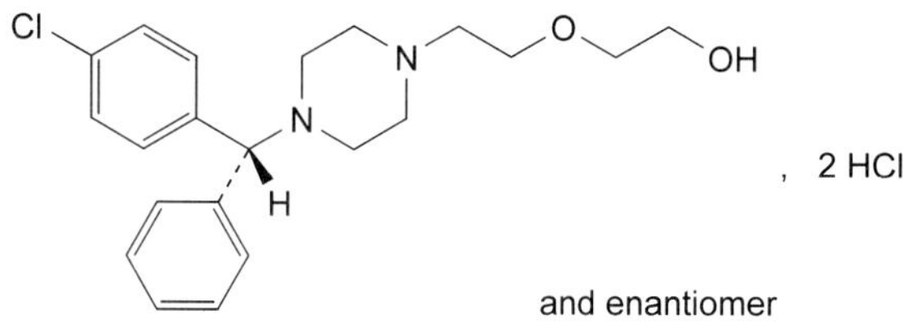

, 2 HCl

and enantiomer

$C_{21}H_{29}Cl_3N_2O_2$ M_r 447.8

DEFINITION

Hydroxyzine hydrochloride contains not less than 99.0 per cent and not more than the equivalent of 101.0 per cent of (RS)-2-[2-[4-[(4-chlorophenyl)phenylmethyl]piperazin-1-yl]ethoxy]ethanol dihydrochloride, calculated with reference to the dried substance.

CHARACTERS

A white or almost white, crystalline powder, hygroscopic, freely soluble in water and in alcohol, very slightly soluble in acetone.

It melts at about 200 °C, with decomposition.

IDENTIFICATION

First identification: A, D.

Second identification: B, C, D.

A. Examine by infrared absorption spectrophotometry (2.2.24), comparing with the spectrum obtained with *hydroxyzine hydrochloride CRS*. Examine the substances prepared as discs.

B. Examine by thin-layer chromatography (2.2.27), using a *TLC silica gel G plate R*.

Test solution. Dissolve 0.50 g of the substance to be examined in a mixture of equal volumes of *methanol R* and *methylene chloride R* and dilute to 10 ml with the same mixture of solvents.

Reference solution (a). Dissolve 0.50 g of *hydroxyzine hydrochloride CRS* in a mixture of equal volumes of *methanol R* and *methylene chloride R* and dilute to 10 ml with the same mixture of solvents.

Reference solution (b). Dissolve 0.50 g of *meclozine hydrochloride R* in a mixture of equal volumes of *methanol R* and *methylene chloride R* and dilute to 10 ml with the same mixture of solvents. Dilute 1 ml to 2 ml with reference solution (a).

Apply to the plate 2 μl of each solution. Develop over a path of 15 cm using a mixture of 1 volume of *concentrated ammonia R*, 24 volumes of *alcohol R* and 75 volumes of *toluene R*. Allow the plate to dry in air. Spray with *potassium iodobismuthate solution R2*. The principal spot in the chromatogram obtained with the test solution is similar in position, colour and size to the principal spot in the chromatogram obtained with reference solution (a). The test is not valid unless the chromatogram obtained with reference solution (b) shows two clearly separated principal spots.

C. Dissolve 0.1 g in *alcohol R* and dilute to 15 ml with the same solvent. Add 15 ml of a saturated solution of *picric acid R* in *alcohol R*. Allow to stand for 15 min. A precipitate is formed. Filter. Recrystallise from *alcohol R*. Initiate crystallisation, if necessary, by scratching the wall of the tube with a glass rod. The crystals melt (2.2.14) at 189 °C to 192 °C.

D. It gives reaction (a) of chlorides (2.3.1).

TESTS

Solution S. Dissolve 2.0 g in *water R* and dilute to 20.0 ml with the same solvent.

Appearance of solution. Solution S is clear (2.2.1) and not more intensely coloured than reference solution Y_7 (2.2.2, *Method II*).

Optical rotation (2.2.7): −0.10° to +0.10°, determined on solution S.

Related substances. Examine by liquid chromatography (2.2.29).

Test solution. Dissolve 10.0 mg of the substance to be examined in the mobile phase and dilute to 10.0 ml with the mobile phase.

Reference solution (a). Dissolve 10.0 mg of *hydroxyzine hydrochloride CRS* in the mobile phase and dilute to 10.0 ml with the mobile phase.

Reference solution (b). Dilute 3.0 ml of the test solution to 200.0 ml with the mobile phase. Dilute 5.0 ml to 25.0 ml with the mobile phase.

The chromatographic procedure may be carried out using:

– a stainless steel column 0.15 m long and 4.6 mm in internal diameter packed with *base-deactivated octadecylsilyl silica gel for chromatography R* (3 μm),

– as mobile phase at a flow rate of 1 ml/min a mixture prepared as follows: dissolve 0.5 g of *sodium methanesulphonate R* in a mixture of 14 volumes of *triethylamine R*, 300 volumes of *acetonitrile R* and 686 volumes of *water R*; adjust to pH 2.7 with *sulphuric acid R*,

– as detector a spectrophotometer set at 230 nm.

Inject 20 μl of reference solution (a) and 20 μl of reference solution (b). Adjust the sensitivity of the system so that the height of the principal peak in the chromatogram obtained with reference solution (b) is at least 50 per cent of the full scale of the recorder.

In the chromatogram obtained with reference solution (a), measure the height (A) above the baseline of the peak immediately before the principal peak and the height (B) above the baseline of the lowest point of the curve (B) separating this peak from the peak due to hydroxyzine. The test is not valid unless A is greater than ten times B.

Inject 20 μl of the test solution and 20 μl of reference solution (b). Continue the chromatography for 2.5 times the retention time of the principal peak. In the chromatogram obtained with the test solution: the area of any peak, apart from the principal peak, is not greater than one third of the area of the principal peak in the chromatogram obtained with reference solution (b) (0.1 per cent); the sum of the areas of all the peaks, apart from the principal peak, is not greater than the area of the principal peak in the chromatogram obtained with reference solution (b) (0.3 per cent). Disregard any peak with an area less than 0.1 times that of the principal peak in the chromatogram obtained with reference solution (b).

Heavy metals (2.4.8). 12 ml of solution S complies with limit test A for heavy metals (10 ppm). Prepare the standard using *lead standard solution (1 ppm Pb) R*.

Loss on drying (2.2.32). Not more than 5.0 per cent, determined on 1.000 g by drying in an oven at 100-105 °C.

Sulphated ash (*2.4.14*). Not more than 0.1 per cent, determined on 1.0 g.

ASSAY

Dissolve 0.200 g in 10 ml of *anhydrous acetic acid R*. Add 40 ml of *acetic anhydride R*. Titrate with *0.1 M perchloric acid*, determining the end-point potentiometrically (*2.2.20*).

1 ml of *0.1 M perchloric acid* is equivalent to 22.39 mg of $C_{21}H_{29}Cl_3N_2O_2$.

STORAGE

Store in an airtight container, protected from light.

IMPURITIES

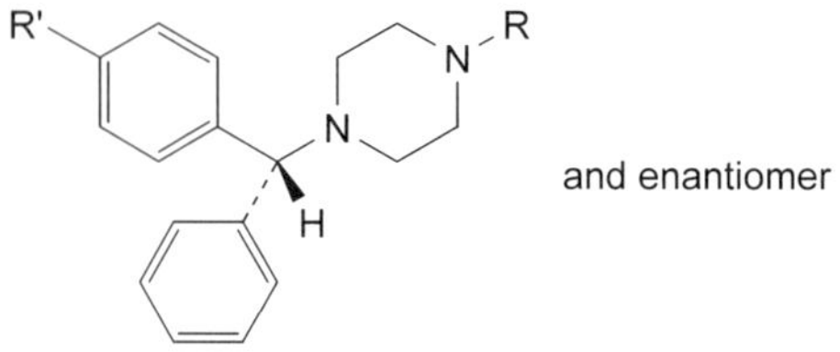

and enantiomer

A. R = H, R′ = Cl: (*RS*)-1-[(4-chlorophenyl)phenylmethyl]piperazine,

B. R = CH_2-CH_2-O-CH_2-CH_2-OH, R′ = H: 2-[2-[4-(diphenylmethyl)piperazin-1-yl]ethoxy]ethanol (decloxizine).

I

04/2003:1018

ISOCONAZOLE

Isoconazolum

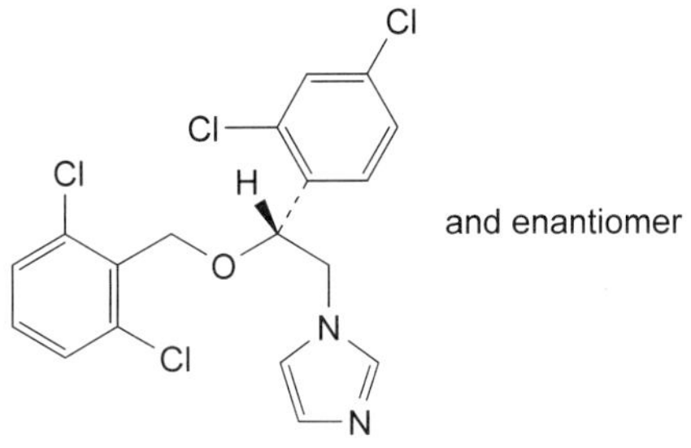

and enantiomer

$C_{18}H_{14}Cl_4N_2O$ M_r 416.1

DEFINITION

Isoconazole contains not less than 99.0 per cent and not more than the equivalent of 101.0 per cent of 1-[(2RS)-2-[(2,6-dichlorobenzyl)oxy]-2-(2,4-dichlorophenyl)ethyl]-1H-imidazole, calculated with reference to the dried substance.

CHARACTERS

A white or almost white powder, practically insoluble in water, very soluble in methanol, freely soluble in alcohol.

IDENTIFICATION

First identification: A, B.

Second identification: A, C, D.

A. Melting point (2.2.14): 111 °C to 115 °C.

B. Examine by infrared absorption spectrophotometry (2.2.24), comparing with the spectrum obtained with isoconazole CRS. Examine the substances prepared as discs.

C. Examine by thin-layer chromatography (2.2.27), using a suitable octadecylsilyl silica gel as the coating substance.

Test solution. Dissolve 30 mg of the substance to be examined in methanol R and dilute to 5 ml with the same solvent.

Reference solution (a). Dissolve 30 mg of isoconazole CRS in methanol R and dilute to 5 ml with the same solvent.

Reference solution (b). Dissolve 30 mg of isoconazole CRS and 30 mg of econazole nitrate CRS in methanol R and dilute to 5 ml with the same solvent.

Apply separately to the plate 5 μl of each solution. Develop over a path of 15 cm using a mixture of 20 volumes of ammonium acetate solution R, 40 volumes of dioxan R and 40 volumes of methanol R. Dry the plate in a current of warm air for 15 min and expose it to iodine vapour until the spots appear. Examine in daylight. The principal spot in the chromatogram obtained with the test solution is similar in position, colour and size to the principal spot in the chromatogram obtained with reference solution (a). The test is not valid unless the chromatogram obtained with reference solution (b) shows 2 clearly separated spots.

D. To about 30 mg in a porcelain crucible add 0.3 g of anhydrous sodium carbonate R. Heat over an open flame for 10 min. Allow to cool. Take up the residue with 5 ml of dilute nitric acid R and filter. To 1 ml of the filtrate add 1 ml of water R. The solution gives reaction (a) of chlorides (2.3.1).

TESTS

Solution S. Dissolve 0.20 g in methanol R and dilute to 20.0 ml with the same solvent.

Appearance of solution. Solution S is clear (2.2.1) and is not more intensely coloured than reference solution Y_6 (2.2.2, Method II).

Optical rotation (2.2.7). The angle of optical rotation, determined on solution S, is −0.10° to + 0.10°.

Related substances. Examine by liquid chromatography (2.2.29).

Test solution. Dissolve 0.100 g of the substance to be examined in 3.2 ml of methanol R. Add 3.0 ml of acetonitrile R and dilute to 10.0 ml with a solution of ammonium acetate R (6.0 g in 380 ml of water R).

Reference solution (a). Dissolve 2.5 mg of isoconazole CRS and 2.5 mg of econazole nitrate CRS in the mobile phase and dilute to 100.0 ml with the mobile phase.

Reference solution (b). Dilute 1.0 ml of the test solution to 100.0 ml with the mobile phase. Dilute 5.0 ml of this solution to 20.0 ml with the mobile phase.

The chromatographic procedure may be carried out using:

− a stainless steel column 0.1 m long and 4.6 mm in internal diameter packed with octadecylsilyl silica gel for chromatography R (3 μm),

− as mobile phase at a flow rate of 2 ml/min a solution of 6.0 g of ammonium acetate R in a mixture of 300 ml of acetonitrile R, 320 ml of methanol R and 380 ml of water R,

− as detector a spectrophotometer set at 235 nm.

Equilibrate the column with the mobile phase at a flow rate of 2 ml/min for about 30 min.

Adjust the sensitivity of the system so that the height of the principal peak in the chromatogram obtained with 10 μl of reference solution (b) is not less than 50 per cent of the full scale of the recorder.

Inject 10 μl of reference solution (a). When the chromatogram is recorded in the prescribed conditions, the retention times are: econazole, about 10 min; isoconazole, about 14 min. The test is not valid unless the resolution between the peaks corresponding to econazole and isoconazole is at least 5.0. If necessary, adjust the composition of the mobile phase.

Inject separately 10 μl of the test solution and 10 μl of reference solution (b). Continue the chromatography for 1.5 times the retention time of the principal peak. In the chromatogram obtained with the test solution: the area of any peak, apart from the principal peak, is not greater than the area of the principal peak in the chromatogram obtained with reference solution (b) (0.25 per cent); the sum of the areas of all the peaks, apart from the principal peak, is not greater than twice the area of the principal peak in the chromatogram obtained with reference solution (b) (0.5 per cent). Disregard any peaks due to the solvent and any peak with an area less than 0.2 times that of the principal peak in the chromatogram obtained with reference solution (b).

Loss on drying (2.2.32). Not more than 0.5 per cent, determined on 1.000 g by drying in an oven at 100 °C to 105 °C for 2 h.

Sulphated ash (2.4.14). Not more than 0.1 per cent, determined on 1.0 g.

ASSAY

Dissolve 0.300 g in 50 ml of a mixture of 1 volume of *anhydrous acetic acid R* and 7 volumes of *methyl ethyl ketone R*. Using 0.2 ml of *naphtholbenzein solution R* as indicator, titrate with *0.1 M perchloric acid* until the colour changes from orange-yellow to green.

1 ml of *0.1 M perchloric acid* is equivalent to 41.61 mg of $C_{18}H_{14}Cl_4N_2O$.

STORAGE

Store protected from light.

IMPURITIES

B. (1RS)-1-(2,4-dichlorophenyl)-2-(1H-imidazol-1-yl)ethanol,

C. (2RS)-2-[(2,6-dichlorobenzyl)oxy]-2-(2,4-dichlorophenyl)ethanamine,

D. 1-[(2RS)-2-[(2,4-dichlorobenzyl)oxy]-2-(2,4-dichlorophenyl)ethyl]-1H-imidazole.

K

04/2003:0921

KETOCONAZOLE

Ketoconazolum

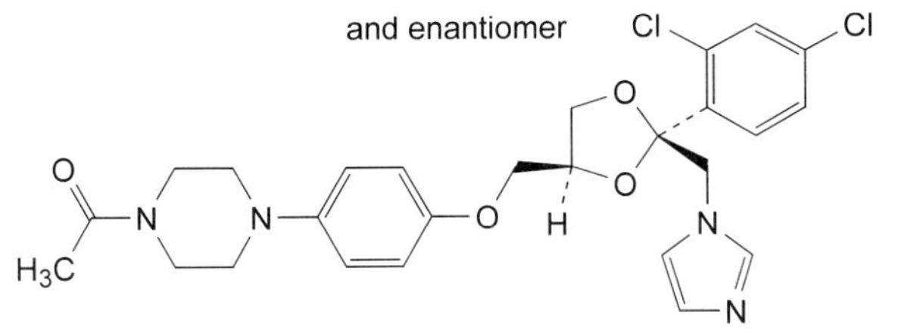

and enantiomer

$C_{26}H_{28}Cl_2N_4O_4$ M_r 531.4

DEFINITION

Ketoconazole contains not less than 99.0 per cent and not more than the equivalent of 101.0 per cent of 1-acetyl-4-[4-[[(2RS,4SR)-2-(2,4-dichlorophenyl)-2-(1H-imidazol-1-ylmethyl)-1,3-dioxolan-4-yl]methoxy]phenyl]piperazine, calculated with reference to the dried substance.

CHARACTERS

A white or almost white powder, practically insoluble in water, freely soluble in methylene chloride, soluble in methanol, sparingly soluble in alcohol.

IDENTIFICATION

First identification: B.

Second identification: A, C, D.

A. Melting point (2.2.14): 148 °C to 152 °C.

B. Examine by infrared absorption spectrophotometry (2.2.24), comparing with the spectrum obtained with *ketoconazole CRS*. Examine the substances prepared as discs.

C. Examine by thin-layer chromatography (2.2.27), using a suitable octadecylsilyl silica gel as the coating substance.

   Test solution. Dissolve 30 mg of the substance to be examined in the mobile phase and dilute to 5 ml with the mobile phase.

   Reference solution (a). Dissolve 30 mg of *ketoconazole CRS* in the mobile phase and dilute to 5 ml with the mobile phase.

   Reference solution (b). Dissolve 30 mg of *ketoconazole CRS* and 30 mg of *econazole nitrate CRS* in the mobile phase and dilute to 5 ml with the mobile phase.

   Apply separately to the plate 5 µl of each solution. Develop over a path of 15 cm using a mixture of 20 volumes of *ammonium acetate solution R*, 40 volumes of *dioxan R* and 40 volumes of *methanol R*. Dry the plate in a current of warm air for 15 min and expose it to iodine vapour until the spots appear. Examine in daylight. The principal spot in the chromatogram obtained with the test solution is similar in position, colour and size to the principal spot in the chromatogram obtained with reference solution (a). The test is not valid unless the chromatogram obtained with reference solution (b) shows two clearly separated spots.

D. To about 30 mg in a porcelain crucible add 0.3 g of *anhydrous sodium carbonate R*. Heat over an open flame for 10 min. Allow to cool. Take up the residue with 5 ml of *dilute nitric acid R* and filter. To 1 ml of the filtrate add 1 ml of *water R*. The solution gives reaction (a) of chlorides (2.3.1).

TESTS

Solution S. Dissolve 1.0 g in *methylene chloride R* and dilute to 10 ml with the same solvent.

Appearance of solution. Solution S is clear (2.2.1) and not more intensely coloured than reference solution BY_4 (2.2.2, *Method II*).

Optical rotation (2.2.7). The angle of optical rotation, determined on solution S, is −0.10° to +0.10°.

Related substances. Examine by liquid chromatography (2.2.29).

Test solution. Dissolve 0.100 g of the substance to be examined in *methanol R* and dilute to 10.0 ml with the same solvent.

Reference solution (a). Dissolve 2.5 mg of *ketoconazole CRS* and 2.5 mg of *loperamide hydrochloride CRS* in *methanol R* and dilute to 50.0 ml with the same solvent.

Reference solution (b). Dilute 5.0 ml of the test solution to 100.0 ml with *methanol R*. Dilute 1.0 ml of this solution to 10.0 ml with *methanol R*.

The chromatographic procedure may be carried out using:

— a stainless steel column 0.10 m long and 4.6 mm in internal diameter packed with *octadecylsilyl silica gel for chromatography R* (3 µm),

— as mobile phase at a flow rate of 2 ml/min a mixture of 0.5 volumes of *acetonitrile R* and 9.5 volumes of a 3.4 g/l solution of *tetrabutylammonium hydrogen sulphate R* changing by linear-gradient elution to a mixture of 5 volumes of *acetonitrile R* and 5 volumes of a 3.4 g/l solution of *tetrabutylammonium hydrogen sulphate R* over 10 min, followed by the final elution mixture for 5 min,

— as detector a spectrophotometer set at 220 nm.

Equilibrate the column for at least 30 min with *acetonitrile R* and then equilibrate at the initial elution composition for at least 5 min.

Adjust the sensitivity of the system so that the height of the principal peak in the chromatogram obtained with 10 µl of reference solution (b) is at least 50 per cent of the full scale of the recorder.

Inject 10 µl of reference solution (a). When the chromatograms are recorded in the prescribed conditions, the retention times are: ketoconazole about 6 min and loperamide hydrochloride about 8 min. The test is not valid unless the resolution between the peaks corresponding to ketoconazole and loperamide hydrochloride is at least 15. If necessary, adjust the final concentration of acetonitrile in the mobile phase or adjust the time programme for the linear-gradient elution.

Inject separately 10 µl of *methanol R* as a blank, 10 µl of the test solution and 10 µl of reference solution (b). In the chromatogram obtained with the test solution, the sum of the areas of all peaks, apart from the principal peak, is not greater than the area of the principal peak in the chromatogram obtained with reference solution (b) (0.5 per cent). Disregard any peak obtained with the blank and any peak with an area less than 0.1 times that of the principal peak in the chromatogram obtained with reference solution (b).

Heavy metals (2.4.8). 1.0 g complies with limit test D for heavy metals (20 ppm). Prepare the standard using 2 ml of *lead standard solution (10 ppm Pb) R*.

Loss on drying (2.2.32). Not more than 0.5 per cent, determined on 1.000 g by drying in an oven at 100 °C to 105 °C.

Sulphated ash (*2.4.14*). Not more than 0.1 per cent, determined on 1.0 g.

ASSAY

Dissolve 0.200 g in 70 ml of a mixture of 1 volume of *anhydrous acetic acid R* and 7 volumes of *methyl ethyl ketone R*. Titrate with *0.1 M perchloric acid*, determining the end-point potentiometrically (*2.2.20*).

1 ml of *0.1 M perchloric acid* is equivalent to 26.57 mg of $C_{26}H_{28}Cl_2N_4O_4$.

STORAGE

Store protected from light.

IMPURITIES

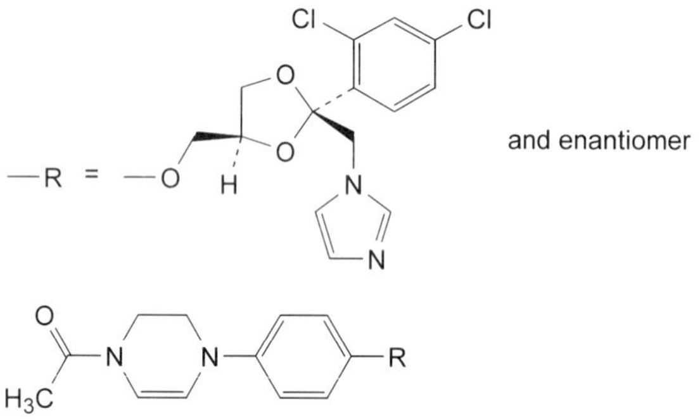

and enantiomer

A. 1-acetyl-4-[4-[[(2*RS*,4*SR*)-2-(2,4-dichlorophenyl)-2-(1*H*-imidazol-1-ylmethyl)-1,3-dioxolan-4-yl]methoxy]phenyl]1,2,3,4-tetrahydropyrazine,

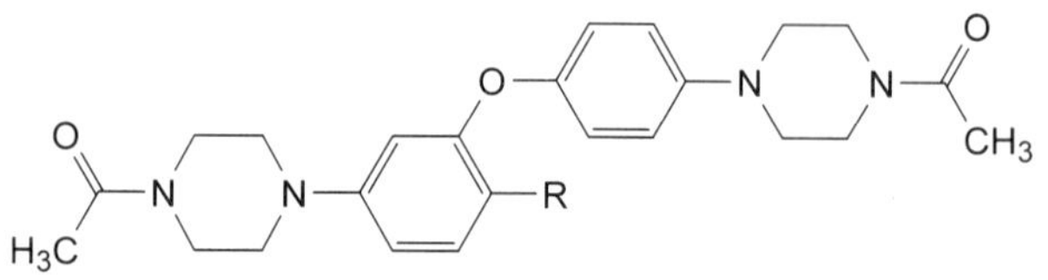

B. 1-acetyl-4-[4-[[(2*RS*,4*SR*)-2-(2,4-dichlorophenyl)-2-(1*H*-imidazol-1-ylmethyl)-1,3-dioxolan-4-yl]methoxy]-3-[4-(4-acetylpiperazin-1-yl)phenoxy]phenyl]piperazine,

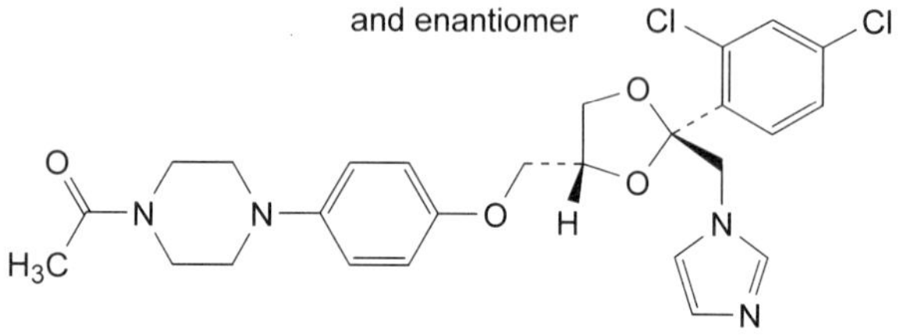

and enantiomer

C. 1-acetyl-4-[4-[[(2*RS*,4*RS*)-2-(2,4-dichlorophenyl)-2-(1*H*-imidazol-1-ylmethyl)-1,3-dioxolan-4-yl]methoxy]phenyl]piperazine,

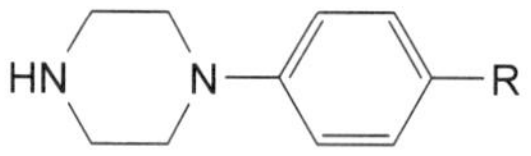

D. 1-[4-[[(2*RS*,4*SR*)-2-(2,4-dichlorophenyl)-2-(1*H*-imidazol-1-ylmethyl)-1,3-dioxolan-4-yl]methoxy]phenyl]piperazine.

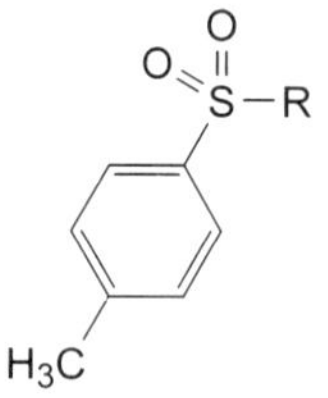

E. [(2*RS*,4*SR*)-2-(2,4-dichlorophenyl)-2-(1*H*-imidazol-1-ylmethyl)-1,3-dioxolan-4-yl]methyl 4-methylbenzenesulphonate.

L

Monographs
L - P

04/2003:1787

LEVOMETHADONE HYDROCHLORIDE

Levomethadoni hydrochloridum

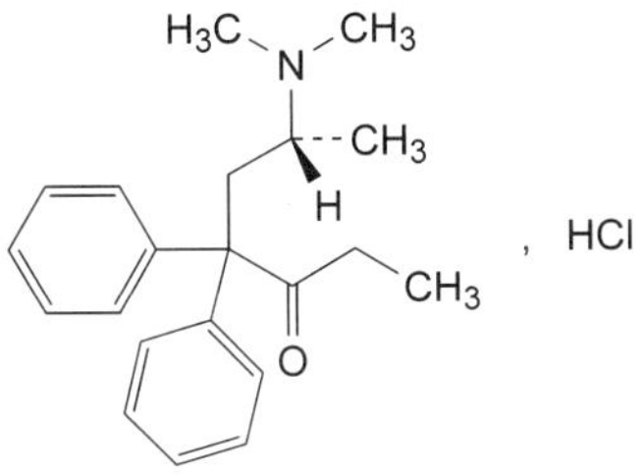

$C_{21}H_{28}ClNO$ M_r 345.9

DEFINITION

(6R)-6-(Dimethylamino)-4,4-diphenylheptan-3-one hydrochloride.

Content: 99.0 per cent to 101.0 per cent (dried substance).

CHARACTERS

Appearance: white, crystalline powder.

Solubility: soluble in water, freely soluble in alcohol.

IDENTIFICATION

First identification: A, C, D.

Second identification: A, B, D.

A. Specific optical rotation (see Tests).

B. Melting point (*2.2.14*): 239 °C to 242 °C.

C. Infrared absorption spectrophotometry (*2.2.24*).

   Comparison: *Ph. Eur. reference spectrum of methadone hydrochloride*.

D. Dilute 1 ml of solution S (see Tests) to 5 ml with *water R* and add 1 ml of *dilute ammonia R1*. Mix, allow to stand for 5 min and filter. The filtrate gives reaction (a) of chlorides (*2.3.1*).

TESTS

Solution S. Dissolve 2.50 g in *carbon dioxide-free water R* and dilute to 50.0 ml with the same solvent.

Appearance of solution. Solution S is clear (*2.2.1*) and colourless (*2.2.2, Method II*).

Acidity or alkalinity. Dilute 10 ml of solution S to 25 ml with *carbon dioxide-free water R*. To 10 ml of the solution add 0.2 ml of *methyl red solution R* and 0.2 ml of *0.01 M sodium hydroxide*. The solution is yellow. Add 0.4 ml of *0.01 M hydrochloric acid*. The solution is red.

Specific optical rotation (*2.2.7*): − 125 to − 135 (dried substance), determined on solution S.

Related substances. Liquid chromatography (*2.2.29*).

Test solution. Dissolve 25.0 mg of the substance to be examined in the mobile phase and dilute to 100.0 ml with the mobile phase.

Reference solution (a). Dilute 1.0 ml of the test solution to 50.0 ml with the mobile phase. Dilute 1.0 ml of the solution to 10.0 ml with the mobile phase.

Reference solution (b). Dissolve 12.0 mg of *imipramine hydrochloride CRS* in the mobile phase and dilute to 10 ml with the mobile phase. To 1 ml of the solution add 5 ml of the test solution and dilute to 10 ml with the mobile phase.

Column:

— *size*: l = 0.125 m, Ø = 4.6 mm,

— *stationary phase*: *octadecylsilyl silica gel for chromatography R* (5 µm),

— *temperature*: 25 °C.

Mobile phase: mix 35 volumes of *acetonitrile R* and 65 volumes of an 11.5 g/l solution of *phosphoric acid R* adjusted to pH 3.6 with *tetraethylammonium hydroxide solution R*.

Flow rate: 1.0 ml/min.

Detection: spectrophotometer at 210 nm.

Equilibration: about 30 min.

Injection: 10 µl.

Run time: 7 times the retention time of levomethadone.

Retention time: levomethadone = about 5 min.

System suitability: reference solution (b):

— *resolution*: minimum 2.5 between the peaks due to imipramine and levomethadone.

Limits:

— *any impurity*: not more than half the area of the principal peak in the chromatogram obtained with reference solution (a) (0.1 per cent),

— *total*: not more than 2.5 times the area of the principal peak in the chromatogram obtained with reference solution (a) (0.5 per cent),

— *disregard limit*: 0.25 times the area of the principal peak in the chromatogram obtained with reference solution (a) (0.05 per cent).

Dextromethadone. Liquid chromatography (*2.2.29*).

Test solution. Dissolve 40.0 mg of the substance to be examined in the mobile phase and dilute to 100.0 ml with the mobile phase.

Reference solution. Dilute 1.0 ml of the test solution to 10.0 ml with the mobile phase. Dilute 1.0 ml of the solution to 20.0 ml with the mobile phase.

Column:

— *size*: l = 0.25 m, Ø = 4.6 mm,

— *stationary phase*: *2-hydroxypropylbetadex for chromatography R* (5 µm),

— *temperature*: 10 °C.

Mobile phase: mix 1 volume of *triethylamine R* adjusted to pH 4.0 with *phosphoric acid R*, 15 volumes of *acetonitrile R* and 85 volumes of a 13.6 g/l solution of *potassium dihydrogen phosphate R*.

Flow rate: 0.7 ml/min.

Detection: spectrophotometer at 210 nm.

Equilibration: about 30 min.

Injection: 10 µl.

Relative retention with reference to levomethadone: dextromethadone = about 1.4.

System suitability: test solution:

— *number of theoretical plates*: minimum 2000, calculated for the peak due to levomethadone,

— *tailing factor*: maximum 3 for the peak due to levomethadone.

Limits:

— *dextromethadone*: not more than the area of the principal peak in the chromatogram obtained with the reference solution (0.5 per cent).

Loss on drying (*2.2.32*): maximum 0.5 per cent, determined on 1.000 g by drying in an oven at 100-105 °C.

Sulphated ash (*2.4.14*): maximum 0.1 per cent, determined on 1.0 g.

ASSAY

Dissolve 0.300 g in a mixture of 40 ml of *water R* and 5 ml of *acetic acid R*. Titrate with *0.1 M silver nitrate*. Determine the end-point potentiometrically (*2.2.20*), using a silver electrode.

1 ml of *0.1 M silver nitrate* is equivalent to 34.59 mg of $C_{21}H_{28}ClNO$.

STORAGE

Protected from light.

IMPURITIES

Qualified impurities: A, B, C, D, E, F.

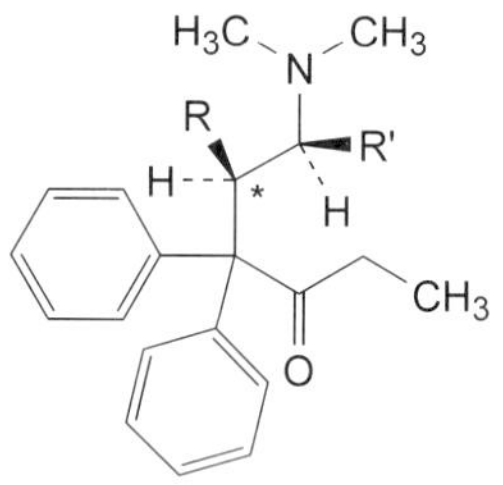

and epimer at C*

A. R = H, R′ = CH₃: (6S)-6-(dimethylamino)-4,4-diphenylheptan-3-one,

D. R = CH₃, R′ = H: (5RS)-6-(dimethylamino)-5-methyl-4,4-diphenylhexan-3-one,

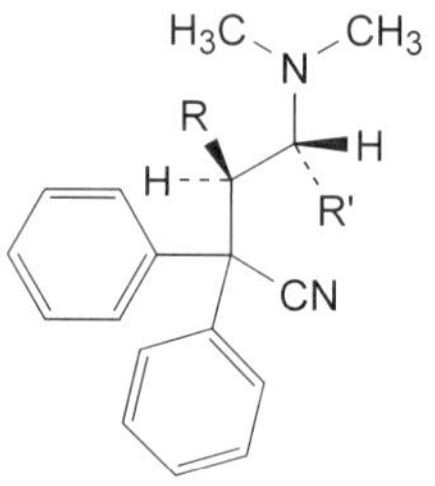

and enantiomer

B. R = H, R′ = CH₃: (4RS)-4-(dimethylamino)-2,2-diphenylpentanenitrile,

C. R = CH₃,R′ = H: (3RS)-4-(dimethylamino)-3-methyl-2,2-diphenylbutanenitrile,

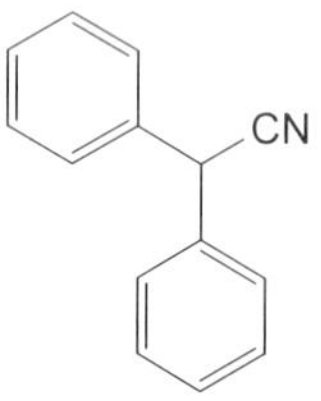

E. diphenylacetonitrile,

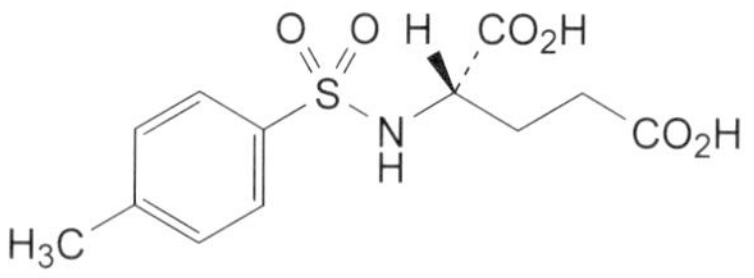

F. (2S)-2-[[(4-methylphenyl)sulphonyl]amino]pentanedioic acid (*N-p*-tosyl-L-glutamic acid).

04/2003:1908

LINSEED OIL, VIRGIN

Lini oleum virginale

DEFINITION

Virgin oil obtained by cold expression from ripe seeds of *Linum usitatissimum* L. A suitable antioxidant may be added.

CHARACTERS

Appearance: clear, yellow or brownish-yellow liquid, on exposure to air turning dark and gradually thickening. When cooled, it becomes a soft mass at about −20 °C.

Solubility: very slightly soluble in alcohol, miscible with light petroleum.

Relative density: about 0.931.

Refractive index: about 1.480.

IDENTIFICATION

First identification: B, C.

Second identification: A, B.

A. Identification of fatty oils by thin-layer chromatography (*2.3.2*). The chromatogram obtained is similar to the type chromatogram for linseed oil.

B. It complies with the test for iodine value (see Tests).

C. It complies with the test for composition of fatty acids (see Tests).

TESTS

Acid value (*2.5.1*): maximum 4.5.

Iodine value (*2.5.4*): 160 to 200.

Peroxide value (*2.5.5*): maximum 15.0.

Saponification value (*2.5.6*): 188 to 195. Carry out the saponification for 1 h.

Unsaponifiable matter (*2.5.7*): maximum 1.5 per cent, determined on 5.0 g.

Composition of fatty acids. Gas chromatography (*2.4.22, Method C*). Use the calibration mixture in Table 2.4.22.-3.

Composition of the fatty-acid fraction of the oil:

— *fatty acids with a chain length less than C_{16}*: maximum 1.0 per cent,

— *palmitic acid*: 3.0 per cent to 8.0 per cent,

— *palmitoleic acid* (equivalent chain length on polyethyleneglycol adipate 16.3): maximum 1.0 per cent,

— *stearic acid*: 2.0 per cent to 8.0 per cent,

— *oleic acid* (equivalent chain length on polyethyleneglycol adipate 18.3): 11.0 per cent to 35.0 per cent,

— *linoleic acid* (equivalent chain length on polyethyleneglycol adipate 18.9): 11.0 per cent to 24.0 per cent,

— *linolenic acid* (equivalent chain length on polyethyleneglycol adipate 19.7): 35.0 per cent to 65.0 per cent,

— *arachidic acid*: maximum 1.0 per cent.

Cadmium (*2.4.27*): maximum 0.5 ppm.

Water (*2.5.32*): maximum 0.1 per cent, determined on 5.00 g.

STORAGE

In an airtight container, protected from light.

LABELLING

The label states the name and concentration of any added antioxidant.

M

Monographs
L - P

04/2003:2035

MAGNESIUM ACETATE TETRAHYDRATE

Magnesii acetas tetrahydricus

$Mg(CH_3COO)_2, 4H_2O$ M_r 214.5

DEFINITION

Content: 98.0 per cent to 101.0 per cent of magnesium acetate (anhydrous substance).

CHARACTERS

Appearance: colourless crystals or white, crystalline powder.

Solubility: freely soluble in water and in alcohol.

IDENTIFICATION

A. Dissolve about 100 mg in 2 ml of *water R*. Add 1 ml of *dilute ammonia R1* and heat. A white precipitate is formed that dissolves slowly on addition of 5 ml of *ammonium chloride solution R*. Add 1 ml of *disodium hydrogen phosphate solution R*. A white crystalline precipitate is formed.

B. It gives reaction (b) of acetates (*2.3.1*).

TESTS

pH (*2.2.3*): 7.5 to 8.5.

Dissolve 2.5 g in *carbon dioxide-free water R* and dilute to 50 ml with the same solvent.

Chlorides (*2.4.4*): maximum 330 ppm.

Dissolve 1.0 g in *water R* and dilute to 100 ml with the same solvent. 15 ml of the solution complies with the limit test for chlorides.

Nitrates: maximum 3 ppm.

Dissolve 1.0 g in *distilled water R* and dilute to 10 ml with the same solvent, add 5 mg of *sodium chloride R*, 0.05 ml of *indigo carmine solution R* and while stirring, 10 ml of *nitrogen-free sulphuric acid R*. A blue colour is produced which persists for at least 10 min.

Sulphates (*2.4.13*): maximum 600 ppm.

Dissolve 0.25 g in *distilled water R* and dilute to 15 ml with the same solvent.

Aluminium (*2.4.17*): maximum 1 ppm.

Prescribed solution. Dissolve 4.0 g in *water R* and dilute to 100 ml with the same solvent. Add 10 ml of *acetate buffer solution pH 6.0 R*.

Reference solution. Mix 2 ml of *aluminium standard solution (2 ppm Al) R*, 10 ml of *acetate buffer solution pH 6.0 R* and 98 ml of *water R*.

Blank solution. Mix 10 ml of *acetate buffer solution pH 6.0 R* and 100 ml of *water R*.

Calcium (*2.4.3*): maximum 100 ppm.

Dissolve 1.0 g in *distilled water R* and dilute to 15 ml with the same solvent.

Potassium: maximum 0.1 per cent.

Atomic emission spectrometry (*2.2.22, Method II*).

Test solution. Dissolve 0.5 g in *water R* and dilute to 100 ml with the same solvent.

Reference solutions. Prepare the reference solutions using *potassium standard solution (600 ppm K) R*, diluted as necessary with *water R*.

Wavelength: 766.5 nm.

Sodium: maximum 0.5 per cent.

Atomic emission spectrometry (*2.2.22, Method II*).

Test solution. Dissolve 1.0 g in *water R* and dilute to 100 ml with the same solvent.

Reference solutions. Prepare the reference solutions using *sodium standard solution (200 ppm Na) R*, diluted as necessary with *water R*.

Wavelength: 589.0 nm.

Heavy metals (*2.4.8*): maximum 40 ppm.

Dissolve 1.0 g in *water R* and dilute to 20 ml with the same solvent. 12 ml of the solution complies with limit test A. Prepare the standard using *lead standard solution (2 ppm Pb) R*.

Readily oxidisable substances. Dissolve 2.0 g in 100 ml of boiling *water R*, add 6 ml of a 150 g/l solution of *sulphuric acid R* and 0.3 ml of *0.02 M potassium permanganate*. Mix and boil gently for 5 min. The pink colour is not completely discharged.

Water (*2.5.12*): 33.0 per cent to 35.0 per cent, determined on 0.100 g.

ASSAY

Dissolve 0.150 g in 300 ml of *water R*. Carry out the complexometric titration of magnesium (*2.5.11*).

1 ml of *0.1 M sodium edetate* is equivalent to 14.24 mg of $C_4H_6MgO_4$.

04/2003:0559

MANNITOL

Mannitolum

$C_6H_{14}O_6$ M_r 182.2

DEFINITION

Mannitol contains not less than 98.0 per cent and not more than the equivalent of 102.0 per cent of D-mannitol, calculated with reference to the anhydrous substance.

CHARACTERS

White or almost white, crystalline powder or free-flowing granules, freely soluble in water, very slightly soluble in alcohol.

It shows polymorphism.

IDENTIFICATION

First identification: A.

Second identification: B, C, D.

A. Examine by infrared absorption spectrophotometry (*2.2.24*), comparing with the spectrum obtained with *mannitol CRS*. Examine the substances prepared as discs. If the spectra obtained show differences, dissolve the substance to be examined and the reference substance separately in *water R*, evaporate to dryness and record new spectra using the residues.

B. Melting point (*2.2.14*): 165 °C to 170 °C.

C. Examine by thin-layer chromatography (*2.2.27*), using a *TLC silica gel G plate R*.

Test solution. Dissolve 25 mg of the substance to be examined in *water R* and dilute to 10 ml with the same solvent.

Reference solution (a). Dissolve 25 mg of *mannitol CRS* in *water R* and dilute to 10 ml with the same solvent.

Reference solution (b). Dissolve 25 mg of *mannitol CRS* and 25 mg of *sorbitol CRS* in *water R* and dilute to 10 ml with the same solvent.

Apply to the plate 2 µl of each solution. Develop over a path of 17 cm using a mixture of 10 volumes of *water R*, 20 volumes of *ethyl acetate R* and 70 volumes of *propanol R*. Allow the plate to dry in air and spray with *4-aminobenzoic acid solution R*. Dry the plate in a current of cold air until the acetone is removed. Heat the plate at 100 °C for 15 min. Allow to cool and spray with a 2 g/l solution of *sodium periodate R*. Dry the plate in a current of cold air. Heat the plate at 100 °C for 15 min. The principal spot in the chromatogram obtained with the test solution is similar in position, colour and size to the principal spot in the chromatogram obtained with reference solution (a). The test is not valid unless the chromatogram obtained with reference solution (b) shows 2 clearly separated spots.

D. Dissolve 2.00 g of the substance to be examined and 2.6 g of *disodium tetraborate R* in about 20 ml of *water R* at a temperature of 30 °C; shake continuously for 15-30 min without further heating. Dilute the resulting clear solution to 25.0 ml with *water R*. The specific optical rotation (*2.2.7*) is + 23 to + 25, calculated with reference to the anhydrous substance.

TESTS

Appearance of solution. Dissolve 5.0 g in *water R* and dilute to 50 ml with the same solvent. The solution is clear (*2.2.1*) and colourless (*2.2.2, Method II*).

Conductivity (*2.2.38*). Not more than 20 µS·cm⁻¹.

Dissolve 20.0 g in *carbon dioxide-free water R* prepared from *distilled water R* and dilute to 100.0 ml with the same solvent. Measure the conductivity of the solution while gently stirring with a magnetic stirrer.

Reducing sugars. Dissolve 5.0 g in 25 ml of *water R* with the aid of gentle heat. Cool and add 20 ml of *cupri-citric solution R* and a few glass beads. Heat so that boiling begins after 4 min and maintain boiling for 3 min. Cool rapidly and add 100 ml of a 2.4 per cent *V/V* solution of *glacial acetic acid R* and 20.0 ml of *0.025 M iodine*. With continuous shaking, add 25 ml of a mixture of 6 volumes of *hydrochloric acid R* and 94 volumes of *water R* and, when the precipitate has dissolved, titrate the excess of iodine with *0.05 M sodium thiosulphate* using 1 ml of *starch solution R*, added towards the end of the titration, as indicator. Not less than 12.8 ml of *0.05 M sodium thiosulphate* is required (0.2 per cent, calculated as glucose equivalent).

Related substances. Examine by liquid chromatography (*2.2.29*) as described under Assay. Inject 20 µl of reference solution (b). Adjust the sensitivity of the system so that the height of the peak due to mannitol is at least 50 per cent of the full scale of the recorder. Inject 20 µl of the test solution and of reference solution (c) and continue the chromatography for twice the retention time of mannitol. In the chromatogram obtained with the test solution: the area of any peak, apart from the principal peak, is not greater than the area of the principal peak in the chromatogram obtained with reference solution (b) (2 per cent); the sum of the areas of all the peaks, apart from the principal peak, is not greater than the area of the principal peak in the chromatogram obtained with reference solution (b) (2 per

cent). Disregard any peak with an area less than the area of the principal peak in the chromatogram obtained with reference solution (c) (0.1 per cent).

Lead (*2.4.10*). It complies with the limit test for lead in sugars (0.5 ppm). Dissolve the substance to be examined in 150.0 ml of the prescribed mixture of solvents.

Nickel (*2.4.15*). It complies with the limit test for nickel in polyols (1 ppm). Dissolve the substance to be examined in 150.0 ml of the prescribed mixture of solvents.

Water (*2.5.12*). Not more than 0.5 per cent, determined on 1.00 g by the semi-micro determination of water.

Microbial contamination. If intended for use in the manufacture of parenteral dosage forms, the total viable aerobic count (*2.6.12*) is not more than 10² bacteria and 10² fungi per gram, determined by plate count. It complies with the tests for *Escherichia coli* and *Salmonella* (*2.6.13*).

Bacterial endotoxins (*2.6.14*): if intended for use in the manufacture of parenteral dosage forms without a further appropriate procedure for the removal of bacterial endotoxins, less than 4 IU/g for parenteral dosage forms having a concentration of 100 g/l or less of mannitol, and less than 2.5 IU/g for parenteral dosage forms having a concentration of more than 100 g/l of mannitol.

ASSAY

Examine by liquid chromatography (*2.2.29*).

Test solution. Dissolve 5.0 g of the substance to be examined in 25 ml of *water R* and dilute to 100.0 ml with the same solvent.

Reference solution (a). Dissolve 0.50 g of *mannitol CRS* in 2.5 ml of *water R* and dilute to 10.0 ml with the same solvent.

Reference solution (b). Dilute 2.0 ml of the test solution to 100.0 ml with *water R*.

Reference solution (c). Dilute 5.0 ml of reference solution (b) to 100.0 ml with *water R*.

Reference solution (d). Dissolve 0.5 g of *mannitol R* and 0.5 g of *sorbitol R* in 5 ml of *water R* and dilute to 10.0 ml with the same solvent.

The chromatography may be carried out using:

– a stainless steel column 0.3 m long and 7.8 mm in internal diameter packed with *strong cation exchange resin (calcium form) R* (9 µm) and maintained at 85 ± 1 °C,

– as mobile phase at a flow rate of 0.5 ml/min, degassed *water R*,

– as detector a refractometer maintained at a constant temperature.

Inject 20 µl of reference solution (d). Continue the chromatography for 3 times the retention time of mannitol. When the chromatograms are recorded in the prescribed conditions, the retention time of mannitol is about 22 min and the relative retention of sorbitol with reference to mannitol is about 1.25. The test is not valid unless the resolution between the peaks due to mannitol and to sorbitol is at least 2 in the chromatogram obtained with reference solution (d).

Inject 20 µl of the test solution and 20 µl of reference solution (a). Continue the chromatography for twice the retention time of mannitol.

Calculate the percentage content of D-mannitol from the areas of the peaks and the declared content of *mannitol CRS*.

LABELLING

The label states:

– where applicable, the maximum concentration of bacterial endotoxins,

— where applicable, that the substance is suitable for use in the manufacture of parenteral dosage forms.

IMPURITIES

A. sorbitol,

B. maltitol,

C. 6-O-α-D-glucopyranosyl-D-glucitol (isomaltitol).

04/2003:1868

MEADOWSWEET

Filipendulae ulmariae herba

DEFINITION

Whole or cut, dried flowering tops of *Filipendula ulmaria* (L.) Maxim. (= *Spiraea ulmaria* L.).

Content: minimum 1 ml/kg of steam-volatile substances (dried drug).

CHARACTERS

Aromatic odour of methyl salicylate, after crushing.

Macroscopic and microscopic characters described under identification tests A and B.

IDENTIFICATION

A. The stem, up to 5 mm in diameter, is greenish-brown, stiff, angular, hollow except at the apex, and has regular, straight, longitudinal furrows. The petiolate leaf, compound imparipinnate, has 2 reddish-brown angular stipules. It consists of 3 to 9 pairs of leaflets, unevenly dentate, some of which are small and fan-shaped. The leaflets are dark green and glabrous on the upper surface, tomentose and lighter, sometimes silvery on the lower surface. The terminal leaflet, the largest, is divided into 3 segments. The veins are prominent and brown on the lower surface. The inflorescence is complex and composed of very numerous flowers arranged in irregular cymose panicles. The flowers are creamish-white and about 3 mm to 6 mm in diameter; the calyx consists of 5 dark green, reflexed and hairy sepals fused at the base to a concave receptacle; the 5 free petals, which are readily detached, are pale yellow, obovate and distinctly narrowed at the base; the stamens are numerous with rounded anthers and they extend beyond the petals; the gynoecium consists of about 4 to 6 carpels, each with a short style and a globular stigma; the carpels become twisted together spirally to form yellowish-brown fruits with a helicoidal twist. Unopened flower buds are frequently present. If the fruit is present, it has a helicoidal twist and contains brownish seeds.

B. Reduce to a powder (355). The powder is yellowish-green. Examine under a microscope using *chloral hydrate solution R*. The powder shows unicellular covering trichomes, some thin-walled, very long and flexuous, with pointed ends, others shorter, thick-walled, conical and thickened at the base; occasional clavate glandular trichomes with a 1- to 3-celled, uniseriate stalk and a multicellular head containing dense brown contents; fragments of the leaves and sepals with sinuous to wavy epidermal cells, anomocytic stomata (*2.8.3*) on the lower surface only and cluster crystals of calcium oxalate in the mesophyll; thin-walled epidermal cells of the petals, some showing rounded papillae; numerous spherical pollen grains with 3 pores and a faintly pitted exine; fragments of the fibrous layer of the anthers with stellate thickenings; groups of small-celled parenchyma from the ovaries containing prism crystals of calcium oxalate; fragments of vascular tissue with spiral and annular vessels from the leaves and stems.

C. Thin-layer chromatography (*2.2.27*).

Test solution. Xylene solution obtained in the assay.

Reference solution. Dissolve 0.1 ml of *methyl salicylate R* and 0.1 ml of *salicylaldehyde R* in *xylene R* and dilute to 5 ml with the same solvent.

Plate: TLC silica gel plate R.

Mobile phase: hexane R, toluene R (50:50 V/V).

Application: 10 µl, as bands.

Development: over a path of 10 cm.

Drying: in air.

Detection: spray the plate with 3 ml of *ferric chloride solution R3* and examine in daylight.

Results: see below the sequence of the zones present in the chromatograms obtained with the reference solution and the test solution. Furthermore, other zones are present in the chromatogram obtained with the test solution.

Top of the plate	
————	————
Methyl salicylate: a violet-brown zone	A violet-brown zone (methyl salicylate)
Salicylaldehyde: a violet-brown zone	A violet-brown zone (salicylaldehyde)
————	————
Reference solution	**Test solution**

TESTS

Foreign matter (*2.8.2*): maximum 5.0 per cent of stems with a diameter greater than 5 mm and maximum 2.0 per cent of foreign matter.

Loss on drying (*2.2.32*): maximum 12.0 per cent, determined on 1.000 g of the powdered drug (355) by drying in an oven at 100-105 °C for 2 h.

Total ash (*2.4.16*): maximum 7.0 per cent.

ASSAY

Examine according to the method described for the determination of essential oils in vegetable drugs (*2.8.12*). Use 50.0 g, a 1000 ml flask and 300 ml of *dilute hydrochloric acid R* as distillation liquid and 0.5 ml of *xylene R* in the graduated tube. Distil at a rate of 2-3 ml/min for 2 h.

04/2003:0931

METFORMIN HYDROCHLORIDE

Metformini hydrochloridum

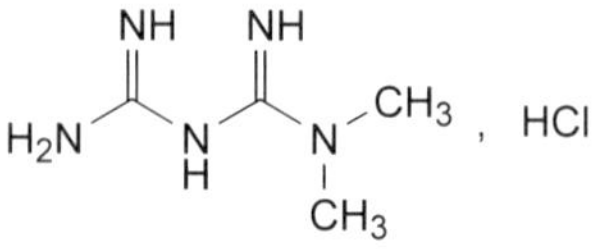

$$H_2N \overset{NH}{\underset{N}{\mid}} \overset{NH}{\underset{\mid}{N}} \overset{CH_3}{\underset{CH_3}{N}} , \; HCl$$

$C_4H_{12}ClN_5$ M_r 165.6

DEFINITION

1,1-Dimethylbiguanide hydrochloride.

Content: 98.5 per cent to 101.0 per cent (dried substance).

CHARACTERS

Appearance: white crystals.

Solubility: freely soluble in water, slightly soluble in alcohol, practically insoluble in acetone and in methylene chloride.

IDENTIFICATION

First identification: B, E.

Second identification: A, C, D, E.

A. Melting point (*2.2.14*): 222 °C to 226 °C.

B. Infrared absorption spectrophotometry (*2.2.24*).

   Preparation: discs of *potassium chloride R*.

   Comparison: *metformin hydrochloride CRS*.

C. Thin-layer chromatography (*2.2.27*).

   Test solution. Dissolve 20 mg of the substance to be examined in *water R* and dilute to 5 ml with the same solvent.

   Reference solution. Dissolve 20 mg of *metformin hydrochloride CRS* in *water R* and dilute to 5 ml with the same solvent.

   Plate: *TLC silica gel G plate R*.

   Mobile phase: upper layer of a mixture of 10 volumes of *glacial acetic acid R*, 40 volumes of *butanol R* and 50 volumes of *water R*.

   Application: 5 μl.

   Development: over a path of 15 cm.

   Drying: at 100-105 °C for 15 min.

   Detection: spray with a mixture of equal volumes of a 100 g/l solution of *sodium nitroprusside R*, a 100 g/l solution of *potassium ferricyanide R* and a 100 g/l solution of *sodium hydroxide R*, prepared 20 min before use.

   Results: the principal spot in the chromatogram obtained with the test solution is similar in position, colour and size to the principal spot in the chromatogram obtained with the reference solution.

D. Dissolve about 5 mg in *water R* and dilute to 100 ml with the same solvent. To 2 ml of the solution add 0.25 ml of *strong sodium hydroxide solution R* and 0.10 ml of *α-naphthol solution R*. Mix and allow to stand in iced water for 15 min. Add 0.5 ml of *sodium hypobromite solution R* and mix. A pink colour develops.

E. It gives reaction (a) of chlorides (*2.3.1*).

TESTS

Solution S. Dissolve 2.0 g in *water R* and dilute to 20 ml with the same solvent.

Appearance of solution. Solution S is clear (*2.2.1*) and colourless (*2.2.2, Method II*).

Related substances. Liquid chromatography (*2.2.29*).

Test solution. Dissolve 0.50 g of the substance to be examined in the mobile phase and dilute to 100.0 ml with the mobile phase.

Reference solution (a). Dissolve 20.0 mg of *cyanoguanidine R* in *water R* and dilute to 100.0 ml with the same solvent. Dilute 1.0 ml to 200.0 ml with the mobile phase.

Reference solution (b). Dilute 1.0 ml of the test solution to 50.0 ml with the mobile phase. Dilute 1.0 ml of this solution to 20.0 ml with the mobile phase.

Reference solution (c). Dissolve 10.0 mg of *melamine R* in about 90 ml of *water R*. Add 5.0 ml of the test solution and dilute to 100.0 ml with *water R*. Dilute 1.0 ml of this solution to 50.0 ml with the mobile phase.

Column:

— *size*: $l = 0.25$ m, Ø = 4.6 mm,

— *stationary phase*: irregular, porous silica gel to which benzenesulphonic acid groups have been chemically bonded (10 μm),

or

— *size*: $l = 0.11$ m, Ø = 4.7 mm,

— *stationary phase*: regular, porous silica gel to which benzenesulphonic acid groups have been chemically bonded (5 μm).

Mobile phase: 17 g/l solution of *ammonium dihydrogen phosphate R* adjusted to pH 3.0 with *phosphoric acid R*.

Flow rate: 1 ml/min.

Detection: spectrophotometer at 218 nm.

Injection: 20 μl.

Run time: twice the retention time of metformin hydrochloride.

System suitability: reference solution (c):

— *resolution*: minimum of 10 between the peaks due to melamine and to metformin hydrochloride.

Limits:

— *impurity A*: not more than the area of the corresponding peak in the chromatogram obtained with reference solution (a) (0.02 per cent),

— *any other impurity*: not more than the area of the principal peak in the chromatogram obtained with reference solution (b) (0.1 per cent).

Heavy metals (*2.4.8*): maximum 10 ppm.

12 ml of solution S complies with limit test A. Prepare the standard using *lead standard solution (1 ppm Pb) R*.

Loss on drying (*2.2.32*): maximum 0.5 per cent, determined on 1.000 g by drying in an oven at 100-105 °C for 5 h.

Sulphated ash (*2.4.14*): maximum 0.1 per cent, determined on 1.0 g.

ASSAY

Dissolve 0.100 g in 4 ml of *anhydrous formic acid R*. Add 80 ml of *acetonitrile R*. Carry out the titration immediately. Titrate with *0.1 M perchloric acid*, determining the end-point potentiometrically (*2.2.20*).

1 ml of *0.1 M perchloric acid* is equivalent to 16.56 mg of $C_4H_{12}ClN_5$.

IMPURITIES

Qualified impurities: A.

Other detectable impurities: B, C, D, E, F.

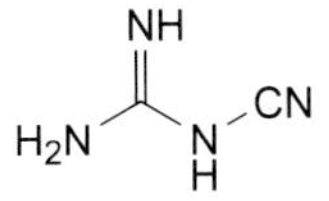

A. cyanoguanidine,

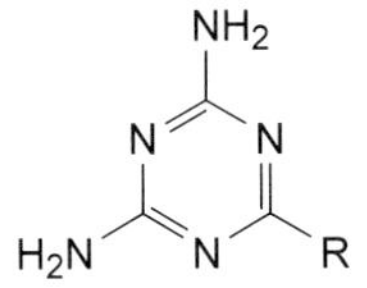

B. R = NH-C(=NH)-NH$_2$: (4,6-diamino-1,3,5-triazin-2-yl)guanidine,

C. R = N(CH$_3$)$_2$: N,N-dimethyl-1,3,5-triazine-2,4,6-triamine,

D. R = NH$_2$: 1,3,5-triazine-2,4,6-triamine (melamine),

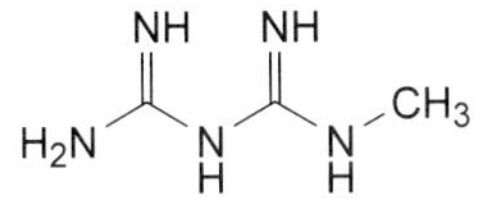

E. 1-methylbiguanide,

F. CH$_3$-NH-CH$_3$: N-methylmethanamine.

01/2002:1128
corrected

METHACRYLIC ACID - ETHYL ACRYLATE COPOLYMER (1:1)

Acidum methacrylicum et ethylis acrylas polymerisatum 1:1

DEFINITION

Methacrylic acid - ethyl acrylate copolymer (1:1) is a copolymer of methacrylic acid and ethyl acrylate having a mean relative molecular mass of about 250 000. The ratio of carboxylic groups to ester groups is about 1:1. It may contain suitable surface-active agents such as sodium dodecyl sulphate and polysorbate 80. It contains not less than 46.0 per cent m/m and not more than 50.6 per cent m/m of methacrylic acid units, calculated with reference to the dried substance.

CHARACTERS

A white, free-flowing powder, practically insoluble in water, freely soluble in ethanol and in 2-propanol, practically insoluble in ethyl acetate. It is freely soluble in a 40 g/l solution of sodium hydroxide.

IDENTIFICATION

A. Examine by infrared absorption spectrophotometry (2.2.24), comparing with the *Ph. Eur. reference spectrum of methacrylic acid - ethyl acrylate copolymer (1:1)*.

B. It complies with the limits of the assay.

TESTS

Apparent viscosity. Dissolve a quantity of substance to be examined corresponding to 37.5 g of the dried substance in a mixture of 7.9 g of *water R* and 254.6 g of *2-propanol R*. Determine the viscosity (2.2.10) using a rotating viscometer at 20 °C. At a shear rate of 10 s^{-1}, the apparent viscosity is not less than 100 mPa·s and not more than 200 mPa·s.

Appearance of a film. Place 1 ml of the solution prepared for the apparent viscosity test on a glass plate and allow to dry. A clear brittle film is formed.

Ethyl acrylate and methacrylic acid. Total content: not more than 0.1 per cent, determined by liquid chromatography (2.2.29).

Blank solution. To 50.0 ml of *methanol R* add 25.0 ml of mobile phase.

Test solution. Dissolve 40 mg of the substance to be examined in 50.0 ml of *methanol R* and add 25.0 ml of mobile phase.

Reference solution. Dissolve 10 mg each of *ethyl acrylate R* and *methacrylic acid R* in *methanol R* and dilute to 50.0 ml with the same solvent. Dilute 0.1 ml of this solution to 50.0 ml with *methanol R* and add 25.0 ml of mobile phase.

The chromatographic procedure may be carried out using:

— a stainless steel column 0.10 m long and 4 mm in internal diameter packed with *octadecylsilyl silica gel for chromatography R* (5 µm),

— as mobile phase at a flow rate of 2.5 ml/min a mixture of 30 volumes of *methanol R* and 70 volumes of *phosphate buffer solution pH 2.0 R*,

— as detector a spectrophotometer set at 202 nm.

Inject 50 µl of each solution. The test is not valid unless the resolution between the peaks corresponding to ethyl acrylate and methacrylic acid in the chromatogram obtained with the reference solution is at least 2.0. The test is not valid if the chromatogram obtained with the blank solution shows peaks with the same retention times as ethyl acrylate or methacrylic acid.

Calculate the percentage content of monomers from the area of the peaks in the chromatograms obtained with the test solution and the reference solution and from the content of monomers in the reference solution.

Loss on drying (2.2.32). Not more than 5.0 per cent, determined on 1.000 g by drying at 100 °C to 105 °C for 6 h.

Sulphated ash (2.4.14). Not more than 0.4 per cent, determined on 1.0 g.

ASSAY

Dissolve 1.000 g in a mixture of 40 ml of *water R* and 60 ml of *2-propanol R*. Titrate slowly while stirring with *0.5 M sodium hydroxide*, using *phenolphthalein solution R* as indicator.

1 ml of *0.5 M sodium hydroxide* is equivalent to 43.05 mg of C$_4$H$_6$O$_2$ (methacrylic acid units).

LABELLING

The label states, where applicable, the name and concentration of any surface-active agents.

01/2002:1129
corrected

METHACRYLIC ACID - ETHYL ACRYLATE COPOLYMER (1:1) DISPERSION 30 PER CENT

Acidum methacrylicum et ethylis acrylas polymerisatum 1:1 dispersio 30 per centum

DEFINITION

Methacrylic acid - ethyl acrylate copolymer (1:1) dispersion 30 per cent is a dispersion in water of a copolymer of methacrylic acid and ethyl acrylate having a mean relative molecular mass of about 250 000. The ratio of carboxylic groups to ester groups is about 1:1. It may contain suitable surface-active agents such as sodium dodecyl sulphate and

Monographs
L - P

polysorbate 80. It contains not less than 46.0 per cent m/m and not more than 50.6 per cent m/m of methacrylic acid units, calculated with reference to the residue on evaporation.

CHARACTERS

An opaque, white, slightly viscous liquid, miscible with water. On addition of solvents such as acetone, ethanol or 2-propanol, a precipitate is formed which dissolves on addition of excess solvent. It is miscible with a 40 g/l solution of sodium hydroxide.

It is sensitive to spoilage by microbial contaminants.

IDENTIFICATION

A. Examine by infrared absorption spectrophotometry (*2.2.24*), comparing with the *Ph. Eur. reference spectrum of methacrylic acid - ethyl acrylate copolymer (1:1) dispersion 30 per cent.*

B. It complies with the limits of the assay.

TESTS

Apparent viscosity. Determine the viscosity (*2.2.10*) using a rotating viscometer at 20 °C. At a shear rate of 50 s⁻¹, the apparent viscosity is not more than 15 mPa·s.

Appearance of a film. Place 1 ml on a glass plate and allow to dry. A clear, brittle film is formed.

Particulate matter. Filter 100.0 g through a tared stainless steel sieve (90). Rinse with *water R* until a clear filtrate is obtained and dry at 100 °C to 105 °C. The mass of the residue is not more than 1.00 g.

Ethyl acrylate and methacrylic acid. Total content not more than 0.1 per cent, determined by liquid chromatography (*2.2.29*) and calculated with reference to the dried substance.

Blank solution. To 50.0 ml of *methanol R* add 25.0 ml of mobile phase.

Test solution. Dissolve 40 mg of the substance to be examined in 50.0 ml of *methanol R* and add 25.0 ml of mobile phase.

Reference solution. Dissolve 10 mg each of *ethyl acrylate R* and *methacrylic acid R* in *methanol R* and dilute to 50.0 ml with the same solvent. Dilute 0.1 ml of this solution to 50.0 ml with *methanol R* and add 25.0 ml of mobile phase.

The chromatographic procedure may be carried out using:

— a stainless steel column 0.10 m long and 4 mm in internal diameter packed with *octadecylsilyl silica gel for chromatography R* (5 µm),

— as mobile phase at a flow rate of 2.5 ml/min a mixture of 30 volumes of *methanol R* and 70 volumes of *phosphate buffer solution pH 2.0 R*,

as detector a spectrophotometer set at 202 nm.

Inject 50 µl of each solution. The test is not valid unless the resolution between the peaks corresponding to ethyl acrylate and methacrylic acid in the chromatogram obtained with the reference solution is at least 2.0. The test is not valid if the chromatogram obtained with the blank solution shows peaks with the same retention times as ethyl acrylate or methacrylic acid.

Calculate the percentage content of monomers from the area of the peaks in the chromatograms obtained with the test solution and the reference solution and from the content of monomers in the reference solution.

Residue on evaporation. Dry 1.000 g at 110 °C for 5 h. The residue weighs not less than 0.285 g and not more than 0.315 g.

Sulphated ash (*2.4.14*). Not more than 0.2 per cent, determined on 1.0 g.

Microbial contamination. Total viable aerobic count (*2.6.12*) not more than 10³ micro-organisms per gram, determined by plate count.

ASSAY

Dissolve 1.500 g in a mixture of 40 ml of *water R* and 60 ml of *2-propanol R*. Titrate slowly while stirring with *0.5 M sodium hydroxide*, using *phenolphthalein solution R* as indicator.

1 ml of *0.5 M sodium hydroxide* is equivalent to 43.05 mg of $C_4H_6O_2$ (methacrylic acid units).

STORAGE

Store protected from freezing. Handle the substance so as to minimise microbial contamination.

LABELLING

The label states, where applicable, the name and concentration of any surface-active agents.

01/2002:1127
corrected

METHACRYLIC ACID - METHYL METHACRYLATE COPOLYMER (1:1)

Acidum methacrylicum et methylis methacrylas polymerisatum 1:1

DEFINITION

Methacrylic acid - methyl methacrylate copolymer (1:1) is a copolymer of methacrylic acid and methyl methacrylate having a mean relative molecular mass of about 135 000. The ratio of carboxylic groups to ester groups is about 1:1. It contains not less than 46.0 per cent m/m and not more than 50.6 per cent of methacrylic acid units, calculated with reference to the dried substance.

CHARACTERS

A white, free-flowing powder, practically insoluble in water, freely soluble in ethanol and in 2-propanol, practically insoluble in ethyl acetate. It is freely soluble in a 40 g/l solution of sodium hydroxide.

IDENTIFICATION

A. Examine by infrared absorption spectrophotometry (*2.2.24*), comparing with the *Ph. Eur. reference spectrum of methacrylic acid - methyl methacrylate copolymer (1:1)*.

B. It complies with the limits of the assay.

TESTS

Apparent viscosity. Dissolve a quantity of substance to be examined corresponding to 37.5 g of the dried substance in a mixture of 7.9 g of *water R* and 254.6 g of *2-propanol R*. Determine the viscosity (*2.2.10*) using a rotating viscometer at 20 °C. At a shear rate of 10 s⁻¹, the apparent viscosity is not less than 50 mPa·s and not more than 200 mPa·s.

Appearance of a film. Place 1 ml of the solution prepared for the viscosity test on a glass plate and allow to dry. A clear brittle film is formed.

Methyl methacrylate and methacrylic acid. Total content: not more than 0.1 per cent, determined by liquid chromatography (*2.2.29*).

Blank solution. To 50.0 ml of *methanol R* add 25.0 ml of mobile phase.

Test solution. Dissolve 40 mg of the substance to be examined in 50.0 ml of *methanol R* and add 25.0 ml of mobile phase.

Reference solution. Dissolve 10 mg each of *methyl methacrylate R* and *methacrylic acid R* in *methanol R* and dilute to 50.0 ml with the same solvent. Dilute 0.1 ml of this solution to 50.0 ml with *methanol R* and add 25.0 ml of mobile phase.

The chromatographic procedure may be carried out using:

— a stainless steel column 0.10 m long and 4 mm in internal diameter packed with *octadecylsilyl silica gel for chromatography R* (5 μm),

— as mobile phase at a flow rate of 2.5 ml/min a mixture of 30 volumes of *methanol R* and 70 volumes of *phosphate buffer solution pH 2.0 R*,

— as detector a spectrophotometer set at 202 nm.

Inject 50 μl of each solution. The test is not valid unless the resolution between the peaks corresponding to methyl methacrylate and methacrylic acid in the chromatogram obtained with the reference solution is at least 2.0. The test is not valid if the chromatogram obtained with the blank solution shows peaks with the same retention times as methyl methacrylate or methacrylic acid.

Calculate the percentage content of monomers from the area of the peaks in the chromatograms obtained with the test solution and the reference solution and from the content of monomers in the reference solution.

Loss on drying (*2.2.32*). Not more than 5.0 per cent, determined on 1.000 g by drying at 100 °C to 105 °C for 6 h.

Sulphated ash (*2.4.14*). Not more than 0.1 per cent, determined on 1.0 g.

ASSAY

Dissolve 1.000 g in a mixture of 40 ml of *water R* and 60 ml of *2-propanol R*. Titrate slowly while stirring with *0.5 M sodium hydroxide*, using *phenolphthalein solution R* as indicator.

1 ml of *0.5 M sodium hydroxide* is equivalent to 43.05 mg of $C_4H_6O_2$ (methacrylic acid units).

01/2002:1130
corrected

METHACRYLIC ACID - METHYL METHACRYLATE COPOLYMER (1:2)

Acidum methacrylicum et methylis methacrylas polymerisatum 1:2

DEFINITION

Methacrylic acid - methyl methacrylate copolymer (1:2) is a copolymer of methacrylic acid and methyl methacrylate having a mean relative molecular mass of about 135 000. The ratio of carboxylic groups to ester groups is about 1:2. It contains not less than 27.6 per cent *m/m* and not more than 30.7 per cent *m/m* of methacrylic acid units, calculated with reference to the dried substance.

CHARACTERS

A white, free-flowing powder, practically insoluble in water, freely soluble in ethanol and in 2-propanol, practically insoluble in ethyl acetate. It is freely soluble in a 40 g/l solution of sodium hydroxide.

IDENTIFICATION

A. Examine by infrared absorption spectrophotometry (*2.2.24*), comparing with the *Ph. Eur. reference spectrum of methacrylic acid - methyl methacrylate copolymer (1:2)*.

B. It complies with the limits of the assay.

TESTS

Apparent viscosity. Dissolve a quantity of substance to be examined corresponding to 37.5 g of the dried substance in a mixture of 7.9 g of *water R* and 254.6 g of *2-propanol R*. Determine the viscosity (*2.2.10*) using a rotating viscometer at 20 °C. At a shear rate of 10 s^{-1}, the apparent viscosity is not less than 50 mPa·s and not more than 200 mPa·s.

Appearance of a film. Place 1 ml of the solution prepared for the viscosity test on a glass plate and allow to dry. A clear brittle film is formed.

Methyl methacrylate and methacrylic acid. Total content: not more than 0.1 per cent, determined by liquid chromatography (*2.2.29*).

Blank solution. To 50.0 ml of *methanol R* add 25.0 ml of mobile phase.

Test solution. Dissolve 40 mg of the substance to be examined in 50.0 ml of *methanol R* and add 25.0 ml of mobile phase.

Reference solution. Dissolve 10 mg each of *methyl methacrylate R* and *methacrylic acid R* in *methanol R* and dilute to 50.0 ml with the same solvent. Dilute 0.1 ml of this solution to 50.0 ml with *methanol R* and add 25.0 ml of mobile phase.

The chromatographic procedure may be carried out using:

— a stainless steel column 0.10 m long and 4 mm in internal diameter packed with *octadecylsilyl silica gel for chromatography R* (5 μm),

— as mobile phase at a flow rate of 2.5 ml/min a mixture of 30 volumes of *methanol R* and 70 volumes of *phosphate buffer solution pH 2.0 R*,

— as detector a spectrophotometer set at 202 nm.

Inject 50 μl of each solution. The test is not valid unless the resolution between the peaks corresponding to methyl methacrylate and methacrylic acid in the chromatogram obtained with the reference solution is at least 2.0. The test is not valid if the chromatogram obtained with the blank solution shows peaks with the same retention times as methyl methacrylate or methacrylic acid.

Calculate the percentage content of monomers from the area of the peaks in the chromatograms obtained with the test solution and the reference solution and from the content of monomers in the reference solution.

Loss on drying (*2.2.32*). Not more than 5.0 per cent, determined on 1.000 g by drying in an oven at 100 °C to 105 °C for 6 h.

Sulphated ash (*2.4.14*). Not more than 0.1 per cent, determined on 1.0 g.

ASSAY

Dissolve 1.000 g in a mixture of 40 ml of *water R* and 60 ml of *2-propanol R*. Titrate slowly while stirring with *0.5 M sodium hydroxide*, using *phenolphthalein solution R* as indicator.

1 ml of *0.5 M sodium hydroxide* is equivalent to 43.05 mg of $C_4H_6O_2$ (methacrylic acid units).

N

**Monographs
L - P**

01/2002:1594
corrected

NAFTIDROFURYL HYDROGEN OXALATE

Naftidrofuryli hydrogenooxalas

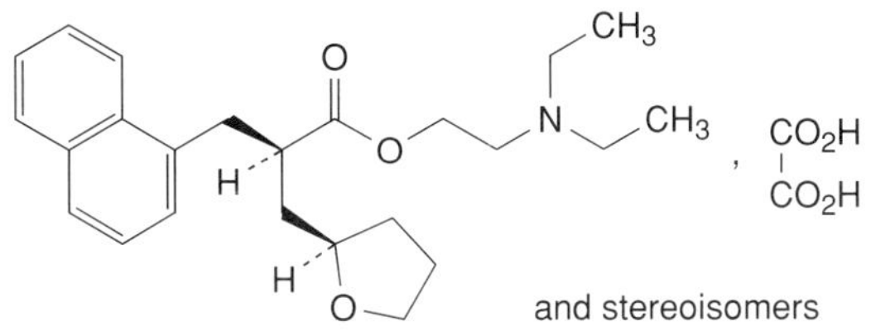

and stereoisomers

$C_{26}H_{35}NO_7$ M_r 473.6

DEFINITION

Mixture of 4 stereoisomers of 2-(diethylaminoethyl)ethyl-2-[(naphthalen-1-yl)methyl]-3-(tetrahydrofuran-2-yl)propanoate hydrogen oxalate.

Content: 99.0 per cent to 101.0 per cent (dried substance).

CHARACTERS

Appearance: white or almost white powder.

Solubility: freely soluble in water and in alcohol, slightly or sparingly soluble in acetone.

IDENTIFICATION

First identification: C.

Second identification: A, B, D.

A. Melting point (*2.2.14*): 109 °C to 113 °C.

B. Dissolve 0.100 g in *water R* and dilute to 100.0 ml with the same solvent. Dilute 5.0 ml of the solution to 100.0 ml with *water R* (solution A). Dilute 8.0 ml of solution A to 100.0 ml with *water R* (solution B). Examined between 220 nm and 350 nm (*2.2.25*), solution A shows an absorption maximum at 283 nm, an absorption maximum at 272 nm and an absorption minimum at 241 nm. The specific absorbance at the maximum at 283 nm is 133 to 147. Examined between 210 nm and 350 nm (*2.2.25*), solution B shows 2 absorption maxima, at 223 nm and 283 nm.

C. Infrared absorption spectrophotometry (*2.2.24*).

Comparison: Ph. Eur. reference spectrum of naftidrofuryl hydrogen oxalate.

D. Dissolve 0.5 g in *water R* and dilute to 10 ml with the same solvent. Add 2.0 ml of *calcium chloride solution R*. A white precipitate is formed. The precipitate dissolves after the addition of 3.0 ml of *hydrochloric acid R*.

TESTS

Optical rotation (*2.2.7*): −0.10° to + 0.10°.

Dissolve 2.50 g in *water R* and dilute to 25.0 ml with the same solvent.

Absorbance (*2.2.25*): maximum 0.1 at 430 nm.

Dissolve 1.5 g in *water R* and dilute to 10 ml with the same solvent. If necessary use an ultrasonic bath.

Related substances. Liquid chromatography (*2.2.29*).

Test solution. Dissolve 80.0 mg of the substance to be examined in the mobile phase and dilute to 20.0 ml with the mobile phase. Treat in an ultrasonic bath for 10 s. A precipitate is formed. Filter through a 0.45 μm membrane filter, discarding the first 5 ml. *Use this solution within 5 min of preparation.*

Reference solution. Dissolve 10.0 mg of *naftidrofuryl impurity A CRS*, 5.0 mg of *naftidrofuryl impurity B CRS* and 20.0 mg of *naftidrofuryl impurity C CRS* in *acetonitrile R* and dilute to 25.0 ml with the same solvent. Dilute 1.0 ml of the solution to 100.0 ml with the mobile phase.

Column:

– *size*: l = 0.25 m, Ø = 4.6 mm,

– *stationary phase*: spherical *octadecylsilyl silica gel for chromatography R* (5 μm) with a carbon loading of 16 per cent, a specific surface of 330 m²/g and a pore size of 7.5 nm.

Mobile phase: mix 150 ml of *tetrabutylammonium buffer solution pH 7.0 R* with 60 ml of *methanol R* and dilute to 1000 ml with *acetonitrile R*.

Flow rate: 1 ml/min.

Detection: spectrophotometer at 283 nm.

Injection: 20 μl.

Relative retention with reference to naftidrofuryl (retention time = about 17 min); impurity A = about 0.2; impurity B = about 0.3; impurity C = about 1.6.

System suitability: reference solution:

– *resolution*: minimum 1.5 between the peaks due to impurity A and impurity B.

Limits:

– *impurity A*: not more than the area of the corresponding peak in the chromatogram obtained with the reference solution (0.1 per cent),

– *impurity B*: not more than the area of the corresponding peak in the chromatogram obtained with the reference solution (0.05 per cent),

– *impurity C*: not more than the area of the corresponding peak in the chromatogram obtained with the reference solution (0.2 per cent),

– *any other impurity*: not more than 0.25 times the area of the peak due to impurity A in the chromatogram obtained with the reference solution (0.025 per cent),

– *total of all other impurities*: not more than the area of the peak due to impurity A in the chromatogram obtained with the reference solution (0.1 per cent),

– *disregard limit*: 0.1 times the area of the peak due to impurity A in the chromatogram obtained with the reference solution (0.01 per cent).

Heavy metals (*2.4.8*): maximum 10 ppm.

In a silica crucible, mix thoroughly 1.0 g of the substance to be examined with 0.5 g of *magnesium oxide R1*. Ignite to dull redness until a homogeneous white or greyish-white mass is obtained. If after 30 min of ignition the mixture remains coloured, allow to cool, mix using a fine glass rod and repeat the ignition. If necessary repeat the operation. Heat at 800 °C for about 1 h. Take up the residue in 2 quantities, each of 5 ml, of a mixture of equal volumes of *hydrochloric acid R1* and *water R*. Add 0.1 ml of *phenolphthalein solution R* and then *concentrated ammonia R* until a pink colour is obtained. Cool, add *glacial acetic acid R* until the solution is decolorised and add 0.5 ml in excess. Filter if necessary and wash the filter. Dilute to 20 ml with *water R*. The solution complies with limit test E. Prepare the standard using 1 ml of *lead standard solution (1 ppm Pb) R*.

Loss on drying (*2.2.32*): maximum 0.5 per cent, determined on 1.000 g by drying in an oven at 100-105 °C.

Sulphated ash (*2.4.14*): maximum 0.1 per cent, determined on 1.0 g.

ASSAY

Dissolve 0.350 g in 50 ml of *anhydrous acetic acid R*. Titrate with *0.1 M perchloric acid*, determining the end-point potentiometrically (*2.2.20*).

1 ml of *0.1 M perchloric acid* is equivalent to 47.36 mg of $C_{26}H_{35}NO_7$.

IMPURITIES

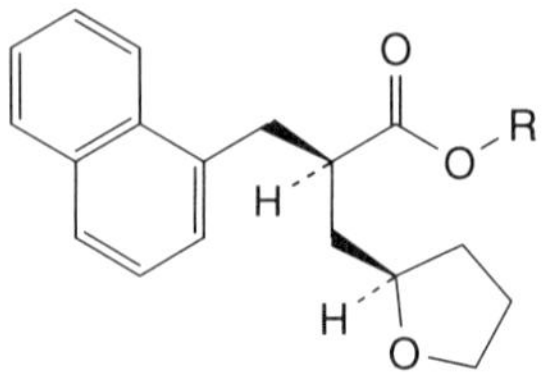

A. R = H: 2-[(naphthalen-1-yl)methyl]-3-(tetrahydrofuran-2-yl)propanoic acid,

B. R = CH$_2$-CH$_3$: ethyl 2-[(naphthalen-1-yl)methyl]-3-(tetrahydrofuran-2-yl)propanoate,

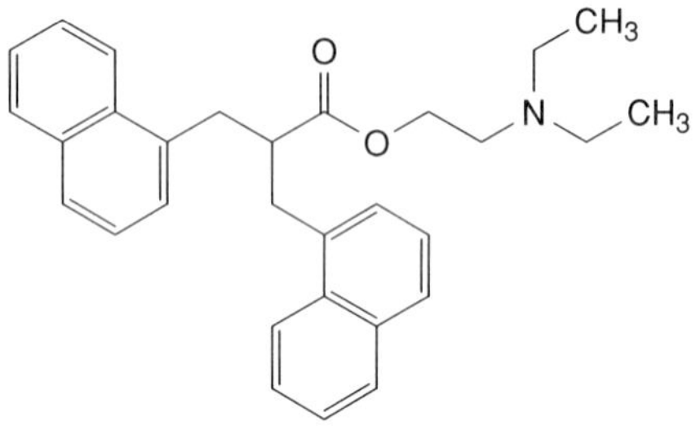

C. 2-(diethylamino)ethyl 3-(naphthalen-1-yl)-2-[(naphthalen-1-yl)methyl]propanoate,

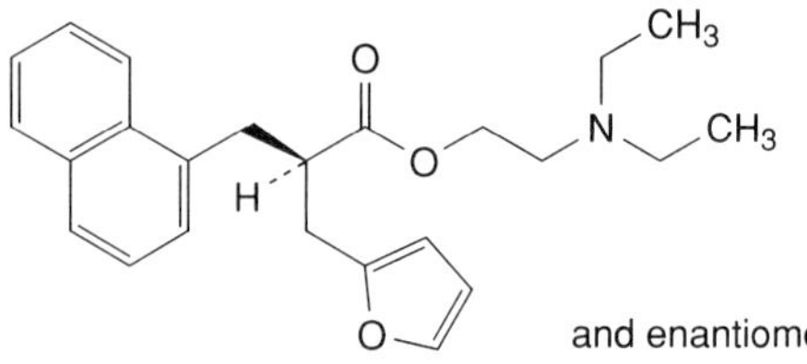

D. 2-(diethylamino)ethyl (2RS)-2-[(furan-2-yl)methyl]-3-(naphthalen-1-yl)propanoate.

01/2002:0197
corrected

NEOMYCIN SULPHATE

Neomycini sulfas

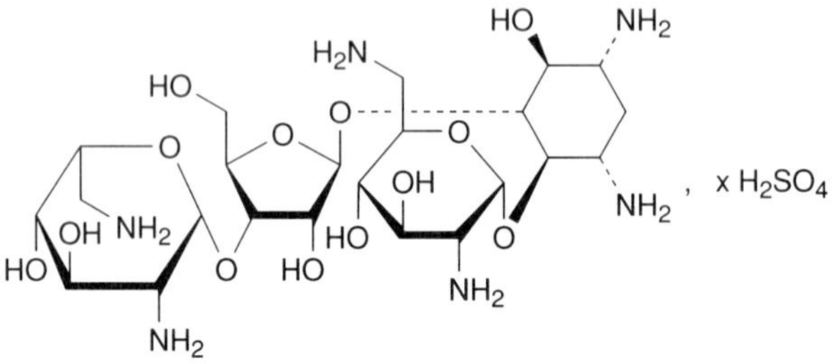

$C_{23}H_{46}N_6O_{13}, xH_2SO_4$ M_r 615 (base)

DEFINITION

Mixture of sulphates of substances produced by the growth of certain selected strains of *Streptomyces fradiae*, the main component being the sulphate of 2-deoxy-4-O-(2,6-diamino-2,6-dideoxy-α-D-glucopyranosyl)-5-O-[3-O-(2,6-diamino-2,6-dideoxy-β-L-idopyranosyl)-β-D-ribofuranosyl]-D-streptamine (neomycin B).

Content: minimum of 680 IU/mg (dried substance).

CHARACTERS

Appearance: white or yellowish-white powder, hygroscopic.

Solubility: very soluble in water, very slightly soluble in alcohol, practically insoluble in acetone.

IDENTIFICATION

A. Examine the chromatograms obtained in the test for related substances.

   Results:

   – the retention time of the principal peak in the chromatogram obtained with the test solution is approximately the same as that of the principal peak in the chromatogram obtained with reference solution (e),

   – it complies with the limits given for impurity C.

B. It gives reaction (a) of sulphates (*2.3.1*).

TESTS

pH (*2.2.3*): 5.0 to 7.5.

Dissolve 0.1 g in *carbon dioxide-free water R* and dilute to 10 ml with the same solvent.

Specific optical rotation (*2.2.7*): + 53.5 to + 59.0 (dried substance).

Dissolve 1.00 g in *water R* and dilute to 10.0 ml with the same solvent.

Related substances. Liquid chromatography (*2.2.29*).

Test solution. Dissolve 25.0 mg of the substance to be examined in the mobile phase and dilute to 50.0 ml with the mobile phase.

Reference solution (a). Dissolve 25.0 mg of *framycetin sulphate CRS* in the mobile phase and dilute to 50.0 ml with the mobile phase.

Reference solution (b). Dilute 5.0 ml of reference solution (a) to 100.0 ml with the mobile phase.

Reference solution (c). Dilute 1.0 ml of reference solution (a) to 100.0 ml with the mobile phase.

Reference solution (d). Dissolve the contents of a vial of *neamine CRS* (corresponding to 0.5 mg) in the mobile phase and dilute to 50.0 ml with the mobile phase.

Reference solution (e). Dissolve 10 mg of *neomycin sulphate CRS* in the mobile phase and dilute to 100.0 ml with the mobile phase.

Column:

– *size*: l = 0.25 m, Ø = 4.6 mm,

– *stationary phase*: base-deactivated octadecylsilyl silica gel for chromatography R (5 μm),

– *temperature*: 25 °C.

Mobile phase: mix 20.0 ml of *trifluoroacetic acid R*, 6.0 ml of *carbonate-free sodium hydroxide solution R* and 500 ml of *water R*, allow to equilibrate, dilute to 1000 ml with *water R* and degas.

Flow rate: 0.7 ml/min.

Post-column solution: carbonate-free sodium hydroxide solution R diluted 1 in 25 previously degassed, which is added pulse-less to the column effluent using a 375 μl polymeric mixing coil.

Flow rate: 0.5 ml/min.

Detection: pulsed amperometric detector with a gold indicator electrode, a silver-silver chloride reference electrode and a stainless steel auxiliary electrode which is the cell body, held at respectively 0.00 V detection, + 0.80 V oxidation and − 0.60 V reduction potentials, with pulse durations according to the instrument used.

Injection: 10 µl; inject the test solution and the reference solutions (b), (c), (d) and (e).

Run time: 1.5 times the retention time of neomycin B.

Relative retention with reference to neomycin B (retention time = about 10 min): impurity A = about 0.65; impurity C = about 0.9; impurity G = about 1.1.

System suitability:

— *resolution*: minimum of 2.0 between the peaks due to impurity C and to neomycin B in the chromatogram obtained with reference solution (e); if necessary, adjust the volume of the carbonate-free sodium hydroxide solution in the mobile phase,

— *signal-to-noise ratio*: minimum 10 for the principal peak in the chromatogram obtained with reference solution (c).

Limits:

— *impurity A*: not more than the area of the principal peak in the chromatogram obtained with reference solution (d) (2.0 per cent),

— *impurity C*: not more than 3 times the area of the principal peak in the chromatogram obtained with reference solution (b) (15.0 per cent) and not less than 0.6 times the area of the principal peak in the chromatogram obtained with reference solution (b) (3.0 per cent),

— *any other impurity*: not more than the area of the principal peak in the chromatogram obtained with reference solution (b) (5.0 per cent),

— *total of other impurities*: not more than 3 times the area of the principal peak in the chromatogram obtained with reference solution (b) (15.0 per cent),

— *disregard limit*: area of the principal peak in the chromatogram obtained with reference solution (c) (1.0 per cent).

Sulphate: 27.0 per cent to 31.0 per cent (dried substance).

Dissolve 0.250 g in 100 ml of *water R* and adjust the solution to pH 11 using *concentrated ammonia R*. Add 10.0 ml of *0.1 M barium chloride* and about 0.5 mg of *phthalein purple R*. Titrate with *0.1 M sodium edetate* adding 50 ml of *alcohol R* when the colour of the solution begins to change, continuing the titration until the violet-blue colour disappears.

1 ml of *0.1 M barium chloride* is equivalent to 9.606 mg of SO_4.

Loss on drying (*2.2.32*): maximum 8.0 per cent, determined on 1.000 g by drying at 60 °C over *diphosphorus pentoxide R* at a pressure not exceeding 0.7 kPa for 3 h.

Sulphated ash (*2.4.14*): maximum 1.0 per cent, determined on 1.0 g.

ASSAY

Carry out the microbiological assay of antibiotics (*2.7.2*). Use *neomycin sulphate for microbiological assay CRS* as the reference substance.

STORAGE

In an airtight container, protected from light.

IMPURITIES

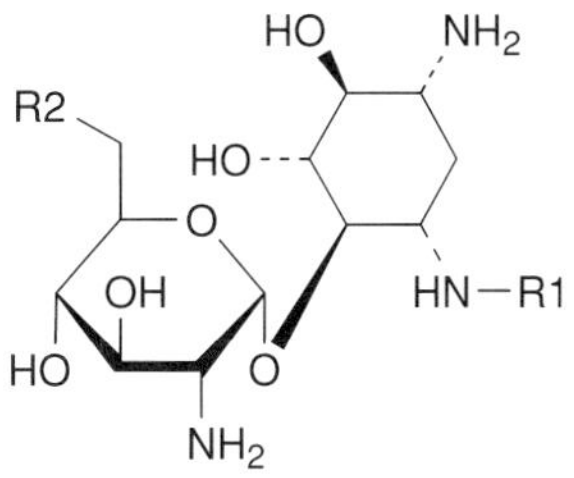

A. R1 = H, R2 = NH$_2$: 2-deoxy-4-*O*-(2,6-diamino-2,6-dideoxy-α-D-glucopyranosyl)-D-streptamine (neamine or neomycin A-LP),

B. R1 = CO-CH$_3$, R2 = NH$_2$: 3-*N*-acetyl-2-deoxy-4-*O*-(2,6-diamino-2,6-dideoxy-α-D-glucopyranosyl)-D-streptamine (3-acetylneamine),

D. R1 = H, R2 = OH: 4-*O*-(2-amino-2-deoxy-α-D-glucopyranosyl)-2-deoxy-D-streptamine (paromamine or neomycin D),

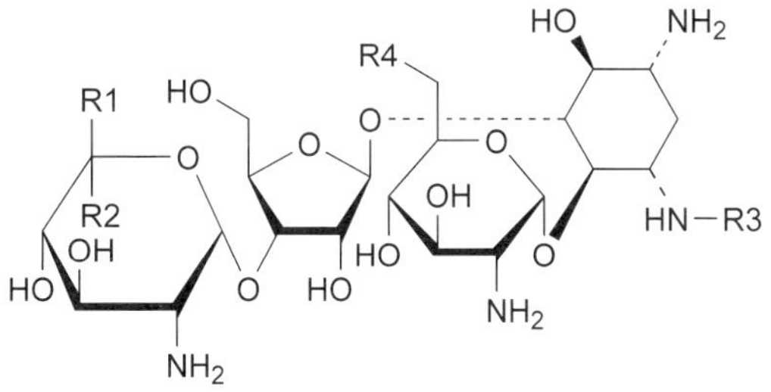

C. R1 = CH$_2$-NH$_2$, R2 = R3 = H, R4 = NH$_2$: 2-deoxy-4-*O*-(2,6-diamino-2,6-dideoxy-α-D-glucopyranosyl)-5-*O*-[3-*O*-(2,6-diamino-2,6-dideoxy-α-D-glucopyranosyl]-β-D-ribofuranosyl]-D-streptamine (neomycin C),

E. R1 = R3 = H, R2 = CH$_2$-NH$_2$, R4 = OH: 4-*O*-(2-amino-2-deoxy-α-D-glucopyranosyl)-2-deoxy-5-*O*-[3-*O*-(2,6-diamino-2,6-dideoxy-β-L-idopyranosyl)-β-D-ribofuranosyl]-D-streptamine (paromomycin I or neomycin E),

F. R1 = CH$_2$-NH$_2$, R2 = R3 = H, R4 = OH: 4-*O*-(2-amino-2-deoxy-α-D-glucopyranosyl)-2-deoxy-5-*O*-[3-*O*-(2,6-diamino-2,6-dideoxy-α-D-glucopyranosyl)-β-D-ribofuranosyl]-D-streptamine (paromomycin II or neomycin F),

G. R1 = H, R2 = CH$_2$-NH$_2$, R3 = CO-CH$_3$, R4 = NH$_2$: 3-*N*-acetyl-2-deoxy-4-*O*-(2,6-diamino-2,6-dideoxy-α-D-glucopyranosyl)-5-*O*-[3-*O*-(2,6-diamino-2,6-dideoxy-β-L-idopyranosyl)-β-D-ribofuranosyl]-D-streptamine (neomycin B-LP).

04/2003:1792

NICOTINE RESINATE

Nicotini resinas

DEFINITION

Complex of nicotine (3-[(2*S*)-1-methylpyrrolidin-2-yl]pyridine) with a weak cationic exchange resin.

Content: 95.0 per cent to 115.0 per cent of the declared content of nicotine stated on the label (anhydrous susbtance). It may contain glycerol.

CHARACTERS

Appearance: white or slightly yellowish powder.

Solubility: practically insoluble in water.

IDENTIFICATION

A. Infrared absorption spectrophotometry (*2.2.24*).

Preparation: shake a quantity of the substance to be examined equivalent to 100 mg of nicotine with a mixture of 10 ml of *dilute ammonia R2*, 10 ml of *water R*, 5 ml of *strong sodium hydroxide solution R* and 20 ml of *hexane R* for 5 min. Transfer the upper layer to a beaker and evaporate to produce an oily residue. Record the spectrum of the oily residue as a thin film between *sodium chloride R* plates.

Comparison: *Ph. Eur. reference spectrum of nicotine.*

B. It complies with the test for nicotine release (see Tests).

TESTS

Nicotine release: minimum 70 per cent of the content determined under Assay in 10 min.

Transfer an accurately weighed quantity of the substance to be examined equivalent to about 4 mg of nicotine, to a glass-stoppered test-tube, add 10.0 ml of a 9 g/l solution of *sodium chloride R* previously heated to 37 °C and shake vigorously for 10 min. Immediately filter the liquid through a dry filter paper discarding the first millilitre of filtrate. Transfer 1.0 ml of the filtrate to a 20 ml volumetric flask, dilute to volume with *0.1 M hydrochloric acid* and mix. Determine the absorbance (*2.2.25*) at the minima at about 236 nm and 282 nm and at the maximum at 259 nm using 1.0 ml of a 9 g/l solution of *sodium chloride R* diluted to 20 ml with *0.1 M hydrochloric acid* as compensation liquid.

Calculate the percentage of nicotine release from the expression:

$$\frac{20 \cdot 10^6 \times \left(A_{259} - 0.5 A_{236} - 0.5 A_{282}\right)}{323\, C\, m}$$

323	=	specific absorbance of nicotine at 259 nm,
C	=	percentage of nicotine in the substance to be examined on the basis of the amount determined in the assay,
m	=	mass of the substance to be examined, in milligrams,
$A_{259}, A_{236}, A_{282}$	=	absorbances of the solution at the wavelength indicated by the subscript.

Related substances. Liquid chromatography (*2.2.29*).

Test solution. Accurately weigh a quantity of the substance to be examined equivalent to 20 mg of nicotine into a glass-stoppered test-tube, add 5.0 ml of *dilute ammonia R2*, 5.0 ml of *water R* and shake vigorously for 10 min. Centrifuge at about 2000 r/min for 10 min and dilute 3.0 ml of the clear solution to 10.0 ml with a 39.5 g/l solution of *phosphoric acid R*.

Reference solution (a). Weigh 60.0 mg of *nicotine ditartrate CRS* into a glass-stoppered test-tube, add 5.0 ml of *dilute ammonia R2*, 5.0 ml of *water R* and shake until dissolution is complete. Dilute 3.0 ml of the clear solution to 10.0 ml with a 39.5 g/l solution of *phosphoric acid R*.

The following chromatogram is published for information.

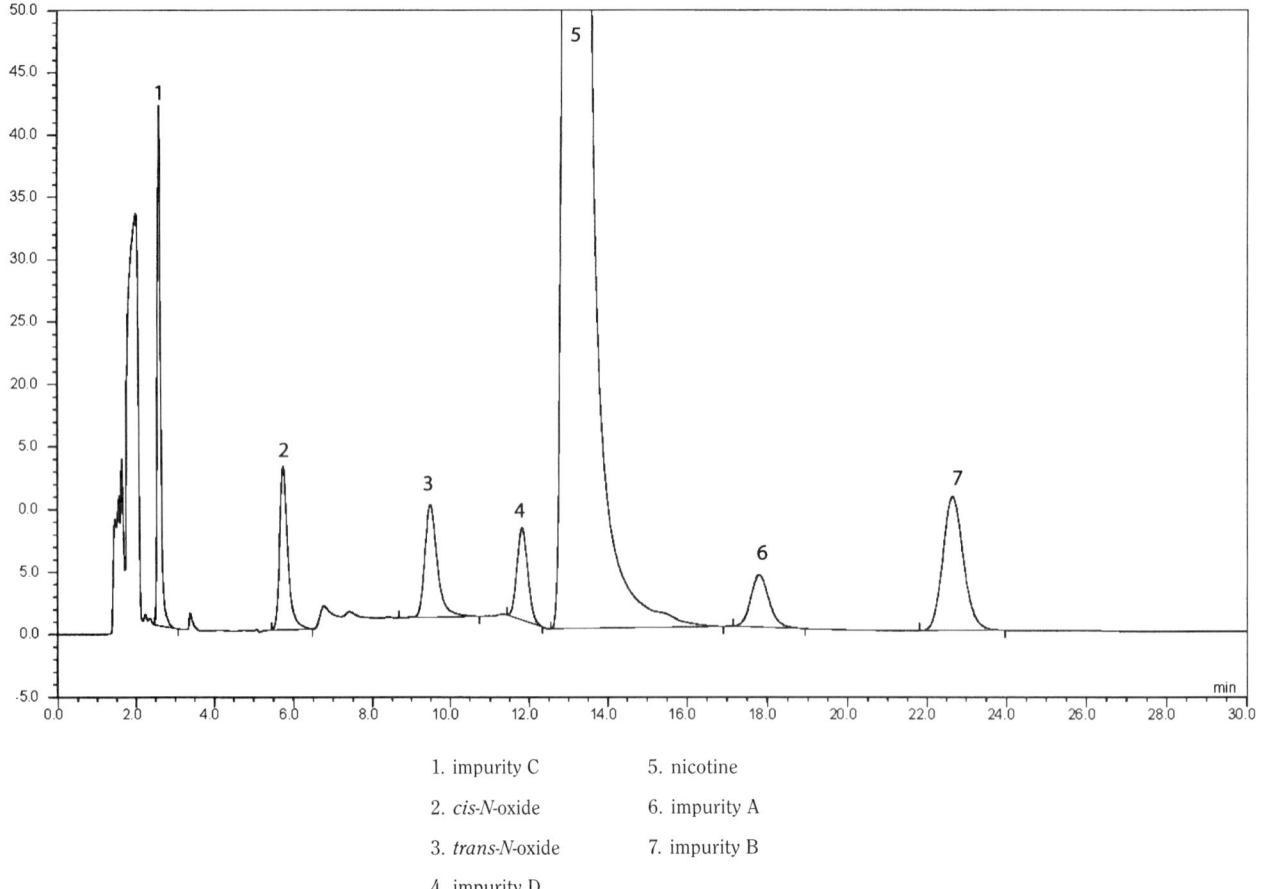

1. impurity C

2. *cis-N*-oxide

3. *trans-N*-oxide

4. impurity D

5. nicotine

6. impurity A

7. impurity B

Figure 1792.-1. – *Chromatogram for the test for related substances of nicotine resinate*

Reference solution (b). Dissolve 5 mg of *myosmine R* in *acetonitrile R* and dilute to 5.0 ml with the same solvent. To 2.0 ml add 1.0 ml of the clear solution obtained during preparation of reference solution (a) and dilute to 10.0 ml with a 39.5 g/l solution of *phosphoric acid R*.

Reference solution (c). Dilute 1.0 ml of the test solution to 10.0 ml with a 39.5 g/l solution of *phosphoric acid R*. Dilute 1.0 ml to 20.0 ml with the mobile phase.

Column:

– *size*: *l* = 0.10 m, Ø = 8 mm,

– *stationary phase*: *octadecylsilyl silica gel for chromatography R* (4 μm).

Mobile phase: dissolve 2.31 g of *sodium dodecyl sulphate R* in a mixture of 250 ml of *acetonitrile R* and 750 ml of a 13.6 g/l solution of *potassium dihydrogen phosphate R* adjusted to pH 4.5 with *dilute sodium hydroxide R* or *dilute phosphoric acid R*.

Flow rate: 1.5 ml/min.

Detection: spectrophotometer at 254 nm.

Injection: 50 μl.

Run time: twice the retention time of nicotine.

System suitability: reference solution (b):

– *resolution*: minimum 1.5 between the peaks due to impurity D and nicotine.

Limits:

– *any impurity*: not more than the area of the principal peak in the chromatogram obtained with reference solution (c) (0.5 per cent),

– *total*: not more than twice the area of the principal peak in the chromatogram obtained with reference solution (c) (1.0 per cent),

– *disregard limit*: 0.1 times the area of the principal peak in the chromatogram obtained with reference solution (c) (0.05 per cent).

Water (*2.5.12*): maximum 5.0 per cent.

Suspend 1.0 g in 20.0 ml of *methanol R*, shake for 30 min and allow to stand for 30 min. Use 10 ml of the methanol layer for the titration. Carry out a blank titration.

ASSAY

Liquid chromatography (*2.2.29*) as described in the test for related substances.

Calculate the percentage content of nicotine using the chromatograms obtained with the test solution and reference solution (a) taking into account the declared content of *nicotine ditartrate CRS*.

STORAGE

In an airtight container, protected from light.

LABELLING

The label states the content of nicotine.

IMPURITIES

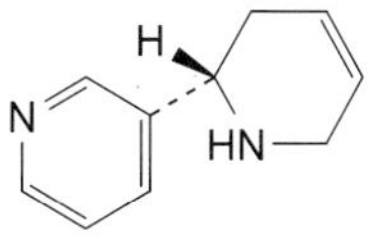

A. (2S)-1,2,3,6-tetrahydro-2,3′-bipyridyl (anatabine),

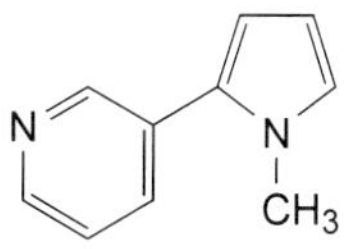

B. 3-(1-methyl-1*H*-pyrrol-2-yl)pyridine (β-nicotyrine),

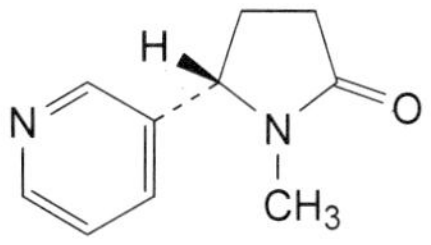

C. (5S)-1-methyl-5-(pyridin-3-yl)pyrrolidin-2-one (cotinine),

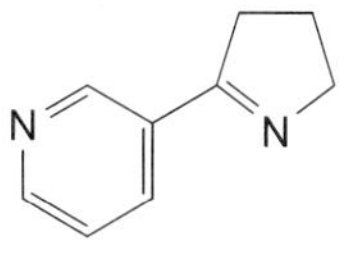

D. 3-(4,5-dihydro-3*H*-pyrrol-2-yl)pyridine (myosmine),

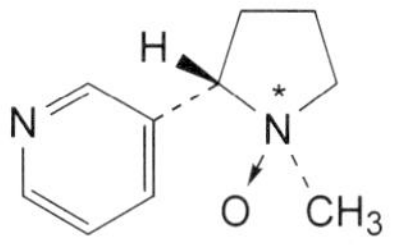

E. (1*RS*,2*S*)-1-methyl-2-(pyridin-3-yl)pyrrolidine 1-oxide (nicotine *N*-oxide).

04/2003:1999

NIFUROXAZIDE

Nifuroxazidum

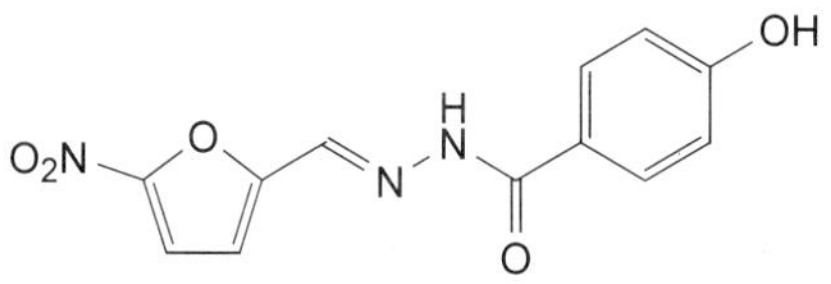

$C_{12}H_9N_3O_5$ M_r 275.2

DEFINITION

1-(4-Hydroxybenzoyl)-2-[(5-nitrofuran-2-yl)methylene]diazane.

Content: 98.5 per cent to 101.5 per cent (dried substance).

CHARACTERS

Appearance: bright yellow, crystalline powder.

Solubility: practically insoluble in water, slightly soluble in alcohol and in methylene chloride.

IDENTIFICATION

Infrared absorption spectrophotometry (*2.2.24*).

Comparison: *Ph. Eur. reference spectrum of nifuroxazide*.

TESTS

Specific absorbance (*2.2.25*): 940 to 1000 at the absorbance maximum at 367 nm.

Protected from light, dissolve 10.0 mg in 10 ml of *ethylene glycol monomethyl ether R* and dilute to 100.0 ml with *methanol R*. Dilute 5.0 ml of this solution to 100.0 ml with *methanol R*.

Impurity A: maximum 0.05 per cent.

Test solution (a). Dissolve 1.0 g of the substance to be examined in *dimethyl sulphoxide R* and dilute to 10.0 ml with the same solvent.

Test solution (b). To 5.5 ml of test solution (a) add 50.0 ml of *water R* while stirring. Allow to stand for 15 min and filter.

Reference solution. To 0.5 ml of test solution (a), add 5.0 ml of a 50 mg/l solution of *4-hydroxybenzohydrazide R* in *dimethyl sulphoxide R*. Add 50.0 ml of *water R* while stirring. Allow to stand for 15 min and filter.

Add 0.5 ml of *phosphomolybdotungstic reagent R* and 10.0 ml of *sodium carbonate solution R* to 10.0 ml of test solution (b) and to 10.0 ml of the reference solution. Allow to stand for 1 h. Examine the 2 solutions at 750 nm. The absorbance (*2.2.25*) of the solution obtained with test solution (b) is not greater than that obtained with reference solution.

Related substances. Liquid chromatography (*2.2.29*). *Use freshly prepared solutions, protected from light.*

Test solution. Dissolve 0.100 g of the substance to be examined in 5.0 ml of *dimethylformamide R* and dilute to 100.0 ml with the mobile phase.

Reference solution (a). Dissolve 10.0 mg of *methyl parahydroxybenzoate R* (impurity B) in 2.0 ml of *dimethylformamide R* and dilute to 20.0 ml with the mobile phase. Dilute 1.0 ml of this solution to 100.0 ml with the mobile phase.

Reference solution (b). Dissolve 5 mg of the substance to be examined and 10 mg of *methyl parahydroxybenzoate R* in 2 ml of *dimethylformamide R* and dilute to 20 ml with the mobile phase. Dilute 1 ml to 100 ml with the mobile phase.

Column:
- *size*: $l = 0.25$ m, $\varnothing = 4.6$ mm,
- *stationary phase*: spherical *octadecylsilyl silica gel for chromatography R* (5 μm) with a specific surface of 340 m^2/g, a pore size of 10 nm and a carbon loading of 19 per cent.

Mobile phase: acetonitrile R, water R (35:65 *V/V*).

Flow rate: 1 ml/min.

Detection: spectrophotometer at 280 nm.

Injection: 20 μl.

Run time: 6 times the retention time of the principal peak.

Relative retention with reference to nifuroxazide (retention time = about 6.5 min): impurity A = about 0.4; impurity B = about 1.2; impurity C = about 2.8; impurity D = about 5.2.

System suitability: reference solution (b):
- *resolution*: minimum 4 between the peaks due to nifuroxazide and impurity B.

Limits:
- *any impurity*: not more than 0.6 times the area of the principal peak in the chromatogram obtained with reference solution (a) (0.3 per cent) not more than 1, and such peak has an area greater than 0.2 times the area of the principal peak in the chromatogram obtained with reference solution (a) (0.1 per cent),
- *total*: not more than the area of the principal peak in the chromatogram obtained with reference solution (a) (0.5 per cent),
- *disregard limit*: 0.1 times the area of the principal peak in the chromatogram obtained with reference solution (a) (0.05 per cent).

Heavy metals (*2.4.8*): maximum 20 ppm.

1.0 g complies with limit test D. Prepare the standard using 2 ml of *lead standard solution (10 ppm Pb) R*.

Loss on drying (*2.2.32*): maximum 0.5 per cent, determined on 1.000 g by drying in an oven at 100-105 °C for 3 h.

Sulphated ash (*2.4.14*): maximum 0.1 per cent, determined on 1.0 g.

ASSAY

Dissolve 0.200 g, if necessary, with heating in 30 ml of *dimethylformamide R* and add 20 ml of *water R*. Titrate with *0.1 M sodium hydroxide* determining the end-point potentiometrically (*2.2.20*).

1 ml of *0.1 M sodium hydroxide* is equivalent to 27.52 mg of $C_{12}H_9N_3O_5$.

STORAGE

Protected from light.

IMPURITIES

Qualified impurities: A, B, C, D.

A. R = NH-NH$_2$: (4-hydroxybenzoyl)diazane (*p*-hydroxybenzohydrazide),

B. R = OCH$_3$: methyl 4-hydroxybenzoate,

C. (5-nitrofuran-2-yl)methylene diacetate,

D. 1,2-bis[(5-nitrofuran-2-yl)methylene]diazane (5-nitrofurfural azine).

04/2003:1454

NONOXINOL 9

Nonoxinolum 9

DEFINITION

α-(4-Nonylphenyl)-ω-hydroxynona(oxyethylene).

Mixture consisting mainly of mononnonylphenyl ethers of macrogols corresponding to the formula: $C_9H_{19}C_6H_4$-[OCH$_2$-CH$_2$]$_n$-OH where the average value of *n* is 9. It may contain free macrogols.

CHARACTERS

Appearance: clear, colourless or light yellow, viscous liquid.

Solubility: miscible with water, with alcohol and with vegetable oils.

IDENTIFICATION

A. Infrared absorption spectrophotometry (*2.2.24*).

   Comparison: Ph. Eur. reference spectrum of nonoxinol 9.

   Preparation: film between *sodium chloride R* plates.

B. It complies with the test for cloud point (see Tests).

TESTS

Acidity or alkalinity. Boil 1.0 g with 20 ml of *carbon dioxide-free water R* for 1 min, with constant stirring. Cool and filter. To 10 ml of the filtrate, add 0.05 ml of *bromothymol blue solution R1*. Not more than 0.5 ml of *0.01 M hydrochloric acid* or *0.01 M sodium hydroxide* is required to change the colour of the indicator.

Hydroxyl value (*2.5.3, Method A*): 84 to 94.

Cloud point: 52 °C to 58 °C.

Dissolve 1.0 g in 99 g of *water R*. Transfer about 30 ml of this solution into a test-tube, heat on a water-bath and stir continuously until the solution becomes cloudy. Remove the test-tube from the water-bath (ensuring that the temperature does not increase more than 2 °C) and continue to stir. The cloud point is the temperature at which the solution becomes sufficiently clear that the entire thermometer bulb is plainly seen.

Ethylene oxide and dioxan (*2.4.25*): maximum 1 ppm of ethylene oxide and maximum 10 ppm of dioxan.

Heavy metals (*2.4.8*): maximum 10 ppm.

Dissolve 2.0 g in *distilled water R* and dilute to 20.0 ml with the same solvent. 12 ml of this solution complies with limit test A. Prepare the standard using *lead standard solution (1 ppm Pb) R*.

Water (*2.5.12*): maximum 0.5 per cent, determined on 2.00 g.

Total ash (*2.4.16*): maximum 0.4 per cent, determined on 1.0 g.

STORAGE

In an airtight container.

04/2003:0516

NOSCAPINE

Noscapinum

$C_{22}H_{23}NO_7$ M_r 413.4

DEFINITION

(3S)-6,7-Dimethoxy-3-[(5R)-4-methoxy-6-methyl-5,6,7,8-tetrahydro-1,3-dioxolo[4,5-g]isoquinolin-5-yl]isobenzofuran-1(3H)-one.

Content: 99.0 per cent to 101.0 per cent (dried substance).

CHARACTERS

Appearance: white, crystalline powder or colourless crystals.

Solubility: practically insoluble in water, soluble in acetone, slightly soluble in alcohol. It dissolves in strong acids; on dilution of the solution with water, the base may be precipitated.

IDENTIFICATION

First identification: *C, E*.

Second identification: *A, B, D, E*.

A. It complies with the test for specific optical rotation (see Tests).

B. Melting point (*2.2.14*): 174 °C to 177 °C.

C. Infrared absorption spectrophotometry (*2.2.24*).
   Comparison: noscapine CRS.

D. Thin-layer chromatography (*2.2.27*).
   Test solution. Dissolve 25 mg of the substance to be examined in *acetone R* and dilute to 100 ml with the same solvent.
   Reference solution. Dissolve 25 mg of *noscapine CRS* in *acetone R* and dilute to 100 ml with the same solvent.
   Plate: TLC silica gel plate R.
   Mobile phase: concentrated ammonia R, alcohol R, acetone R, toluene R (1:3:20:20 V/V/V/V).
   Application: 10 µl.
   Development: over 2/3 of the plate.
   Drying: in air.
   Detection: spray with *dilute potassium iodobismuthate solution R*.
   Results: the principal spot in the chromatogram obtained with the test solution is similar in position, colour and size to the principal spot in the chromatogram obtained with the reference solution.

E. To 20 mg add 10 ml of *water R* and shake. It does not dissolve.

TESTS

Appearance of solution. The solution is clear (*2.2.1*) and not more intensely coloured than reference solution Y_6 (*2.2.2, Method II*).

Dissolve 0.2 g in *acetone R* and dilute to 10 ml with the same solvent. Examine immediately after preparation.

Specific optical rotation (*2.2.7*): + 42 to + 48 (dried substance).

Dissolve 0.500 g in *0.1 M hydrochloric acid* and dilute to 25.0 ml with the same acid.

Related substances. Liquid chromatography (*2.2.29*).

Test solution. Dissolve 20.0 mg of the substance to be examined with gentle heating in 14 ml of *methanol R*, cool the solution and dilute to 20.0 ml with *phosphate buffer solution pH 6.0 R1*.

Reference solution (a). Dilute 1.0 ml of the test solution to 20.0 ml with the mobile phase. Dilute 1.0 ml of the solution to 10.0 ml with the mobile phase.

Reference solution (b). Dissolve 5 mg of *papaverine hydrochloride R* in the mobile phase and dilute to 50.0 ml with the mobile phase. Dilute 1.0 ml of the solution to 20.0 ml with the mobile phase.

Reference solution (c). Dissolve 1.5 mg of *papaverine hydrochloride R* in 10 ml of the test solution and dilute to 50 ml with the mobile phase.

Column:
- *size*: $l = 0.125$ m, Ø = 4.6 mm,
- *stationary phase*: nitrile silica gel for chromatography R (5 µm).

Mobile phase: methanol R, phosphate buffer solution pH 6.0 R1 (350:650 V/V).

Flow rate: 1 ml/min.

Detection: spectrophotometer at 240 nm.

Injection: 20 µl.

Run time: 2.5 times the retention time of noscapine.

Relative retention with reference to noscapine (retention time = about 10 min): impurity A = about 1.3.

System suitability: reference solution (c):

— *resolution*: minimum 2 between the peaks due to noscapine and to impurity A.

Limits:

— *impurity A*: not more than the area of the principal peak in the chromatogram obtained with reference solution (b) (0.5 per cent),

— *any other impurity*: not more than 0.4 times the area of the principal peak in the chromatogram obtained with reference solution (a) (0.2 per cent),

— *total of other impurities*: not more than the area of the principal peak in the chromatogram obtained with reference solution (a) (0.5 per cent),

— *disregard limit*: 0.1 times the area of the principal peak in the chromatogram obtained with reference solution (a) (0.05 per cent).

Loss on drying (*2.2.32*): maximum 1.0 per cent, determined on 0.500 g by drying in an oven at 100-105 °C.

Sulphated ash (*2.4.14*): maximum 0.1 per cent, determined on 1.0 g.

ASSAY

Dissolve 0.350 g in 40 ml of *anhydrous acetic acid R*, warming gently. Titrate with *0.1 M perchloric acid*, determining the end-point potentiometrically (*2.2.20*).

1 ml of *0.1 M perchloric acid* is equivalent to 41.34 mg of $C_{22}H_{23}NO_7$.

STORAGE

Protected from light.

IMPURITIES

A. papaverine.

04/2003:0515

NOSCAPINE HYDROCHLORIDE

Noscapini hydrochloridum

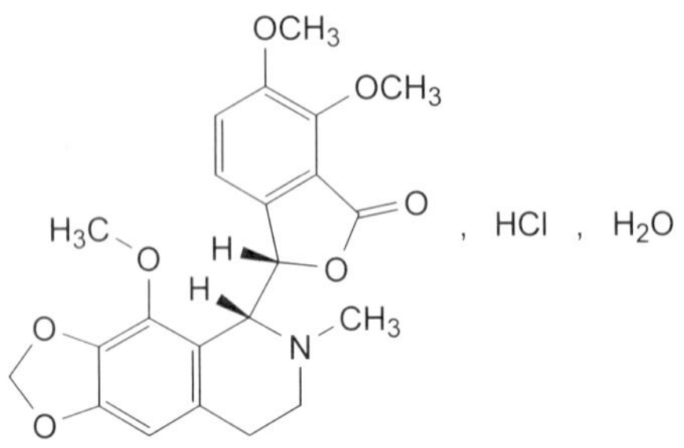

$C_{22}H_{24}ClNO_7,H_2O$ M_r 467.9

DEFINITION

(3*S*)-6,7-Dimethoxy-3-[(5*R*)-4-methoxy-6-methyl-5,6,7,8-tetrahydro-1,3-dioxolo[4,5-*g*]isoquinolin-5-yl]isobenzofuran-1(3*H*)-one hydrochloride monohydrate.

Content: 99.0 per cent to 101.0 per cent (dried substance).

CHARACTERS

Appearance: white, crystalline powder or colourless crystals, hygroscopic.

Solubility: freely soluble in water and in alcohol. Aqueous solutions are faintly acid; the base may be precipitated when the solutions are allowed to stand.

mp: about 200 °C, with decomposition.

IDENTIFICATION

First identification: C, E.

Second identification: A, B, D, E.

A. It complies with the test for specific optical rotation (see Tests).

B. Melting point (*2.2.14*) of the precipitate obtained in identification test E: 174 °C to 177 °C.

C. Infrared absorption spectrophotometry (*2.2.24*).

Preparation: examine the precipitate obtained in identification test E.

Comparison: noscapine CRS.

D. Thin-layer chromatography (*2.2.27*).

Test solution. Dissolve 25 mg of the substance to be examined in *alcohol R* and dilute to 100 ml with the same solvent.

Reference solution. Dissolve 22 mg of *noscapine CRS* in *acetone R* and dilute to 100 ml with the same solvent.

Plate: *TLC silica gel plate R*.

Mobile phase: *concentrated ammonia R, alcohol R, acetone R, toluene R* (1:3:20:20 *V/V/V/V*).

Application: 10 µl.

Development: over 2/3 of the plate.

Drying: in air.

Detection: spray with *dilute potassium iodobismuthate solution R*.

Results: the principal spot in the chromatogram obtained with the test solution is similar in position, colour and size to the principal spot in the chromatogram obtained with the reference solution.

E. Dissolve about 40 mg in a mixture of 2 ml of *water R* and 3 ml of *alcohol R* and add 1 ml of *dilute ammonia R2*. Heat until dissolution is complete. Allow to cool, scratching the wall of the tube with a glass rod. Filter. The filtrate gives reaction (a) of chlorides (*2.3.1*). Wash the precipitate with *water R*, dry at 100-105 °C and reserve for identification tests B and C.

TESTS

Appearance of solution. The solution is clear (*2.2.1*) and not more intensely coloured than reference solution Y_6 or BY_6 (*2.2.2, Method II*).

Dissolve 0.5 g in *water R*, add 0.3 ml of *0.1 M hydrochloric acid* and dilute to 25 ml with *water R*.

pH (*2.2.3*): minimum 3.0.

Dissolve 0.2 g in 10 ml of *carbon dioxide-free water R*.

Specific optical rotation (*2.2.7*): + 38.5 to + 44.0 (dried substance).

Dissolve 0.500 g in *0.01 M hydrochloric acid* and dilute to 25.0 ml with the same acid.

Related substances. Liquid chromatography (*2.2.29*).

Test solution. Dissolve 20.0 mg of the substance to be examined with gentle heating in 14 ml of *methanol R*, cool the solution and dilute to 20.0 ml with *phosphate buffer solution pH 6.0 R1*.

Reference solution (a). Dilute 1.0 ml of the test solution to 20.0 ml with the mobile phase. Dilute 1.0 ml of the solution to 10.0 ml with the mobile phase.

Reference solution (b). Dissolve 5 mg of *papaverine hydrochloride R* in the mobile phase and dilute to 50.0 ml with the mobile phase. Dilute 1.0 ml of the solution to 20.0 ml with the mobile phase.

Reference solution (c). Dissolve 1.5 mg of *papaverine hydrochloride R* in 10 ml of the test solution and dilute to 50 ml with the mobile phase.

Column:
- *size*: l = 0.125 m, Ø = 4.6 mm,
- *stationary phase*: *nitrile silica gel for chromatography R* (5 µm).

Mobile phase: *methanol R, phosphate buffer solution pH 6.0 R1* (350:650 *V/V*).

Flow rate: 1 ml/min.

Detection: spectrophotometer at 240 nm.

Injection: 20 µl.

Run time: 2.5 times the retention time of noscapine.

Relative retention with reference to noscapine (retention time = about 10 min): impurity A = about 1.3.

System suitability: reference solution (c):
- *resolution*: minimum 2 between the peaks due to noscapine and to impurity A.

Limits:
- *impurity A*: not more than the area of the principal peak in the chromatogram obtained with reference solution (b) (0.5 per cent),

- *any other impurity*: not more than 0.4 times the area of the principal peak in the chromatogram obtained with reference solution (a) (0.2 per cent),
- *total of other impurities*: not more than the area of the principal peak in the chromatogram obtained with reference solution (a) (0.5 per cent),
- *disregard limit*: 0.1 times the area of the principal peak in the chromatogram obtained with reference solution (a) (0.05 per cent).

Loss on drying (*2.2.32*): 2.5 per cent to 6.5 per cent, determined on 0.200 g by drying in an oven at 100-105 °C.

Sulphated ash (*2.4.14*): maximum 0.1 per cent, determined on 1.0 g.

ASSAY

Dissolve 0.400 g in a mixture of 5.0 ml of *0.01 M hydrochloric acid* and 50 ml of *alcohol R*. Carry out a potentiometric titration (*2.2.20*), using *0.1 M sodium hydroxide*. Read the volume added between the 2 points of inflexion.

1 ml of *0.1 M sodium hydroxide* is equivalent to 44.99 mg of $C_{22}H_{24}ClNO_7$.

STORAGE

In an airtight container, protected from light.

IMPURITIES

A. papaverine.

O

04/2003:1553

OCTOXINOL 10

Octoxinolum 10

DEFINITION

α-[4-(1,1,3,3-Tetramethylbutyl)phenyl]-ω-hydroxydeca(oxy-ethylene).

Mixture consisting mainly of mono-octylphenyl ethers of macrogols corresponding to the formula $C_8H_{17}C_6H_4$-[OCH_2-CH_2]$_n$-OH where the average value of n is 10. It may contain free macrogols.

CHARACTERS

Appearance: clear, colourless or light yellow, viscous liquid.

Solubility: miscible with water, with ethanol and with vegetable oils.

IDENTIFICATION

A. Infrared absorption spectrophotometry (*2.2.24*).

    Comparison: *Ph. Eur. reference spectrum of octoxinol 10.*

    Preparation: film between *sodium chloride R* plates.

B. It complies with the test for cloud point (see Tests).

TESTS

Acidity or alkalinity. Boil 1.0 g with 20 ml of *carbon dioxide-free water R* for 1 min, with constant stirring. Cool and filter. To 10 ml of the filtrate, add 0.05 ml of *bromothymol blue solution R1*. Not more than 0.5 ml of *0.01 M hydrochloric acid* or *0.01 M sodium hydroxide* is required to change the colour of the indicator.

Hydroxyl value (*2.5.3, Method A*): 85 to 101.

Cloud point: 63 °C to 70 °C.

Dissolve 1.0 g in 99 g of *water R*. Transfer about 30 ml of this solution to a test-tube, heat on a water-bath and stir continuously until the solution becomes cloudy. Remove the test-tube from the water-bath (ensuring that the temperature does not increase more than 2 °C), and continue to stir. The cloud point is the temperature at which the solution becomes sufficiently clear that the entire thermometer bulb is plainly seen.

Ethylene oxide and dioxan (*2.4.25*): maximum 1 ppm of ethylene oxide and maximum 10 ppm of dioxan.

Heavy metals (*2.4.8*): maximum 10 ppm.

Dissolve 2.0 g in *distilled water R* and dilute to 20.0 ml with the same solvent. 12 ml of this solution complies with limit test A. Prepare the standard using *lead standard solution (1 ppm Pb) R*.

Water (*2.5.12*): maximum 0.5 per cent, determined on 2.00 g.

Total ash (*2.4.16*): maximum 0.4 per cent, determined on 1.0 g.

STORAGE

In an airtight container.

01/2003:2016
corrected

ONDANSETRON HYDROCHLORIDE DIHYDRATE

Ondansetroni hydrochloridum dihydricum

and enantiomer

$C_{18}H_{20}ClN_3O,2H_2O$ M_r 365.9

DEFINITION

(3*RS*)-9-Methyl-3-[(2-methyl-1*H*-imidazol-1-yl)methyl]-1,2,3,9-tetrahydro-4*H*-carbazol-4-one hydrochloride dihydrate.

Content: 97.5 per cent to 102.0 per cent (anhydrous substance).

CHARACTERS

Appearance: white or almost white powder.

Solubility: sparingly soluble in water and in alcohol, soluble in methanol, slightly soluble in methylene chloride.

IDENTIFICATION

A. Infrared absorption spectrophotometry (*2.2.24*).
    Comparison: *ondansetron hydrochloride dihydrate CRS*.

B. It gives reaction (a) of chlorides (*2.3.1*).

TESTS

Impurity B. Thin-layer chromatography (*2.2.27*).

Test solution. Dissolve 0.125 g of the substance to be examined in a mixture of 0.5 volumes of *concentrated ammonia R*, 100 volumes of *alcohol R* and 100 volumes of *methanol R*, and dilute to 10.0 ml with the same mixture of solvents.

Reference solution (a). Dissolve 12.5 mg of *ondansetron for TLC system suitability CRS* in a mixture of 0.5 volumes of *concentrated ammonia R*, 100 volumes of *alcohol R* and 100 volumes of *methanol R*, and dilute to 1.0 ml with the same mixture of solvents.

Reference solution (b). Dilute 1 ml of the test solution to 100 ml with a mixture of 0.5 volumes of *concentrated ammonia R*, 100 volumes of *alcohol R* and 100 volumes of *methanol R*. Dilute 4.0 ml to 10.0 ml with a mixture of 0.5 volumes of *concentrated ammonia R*, 100 volumes of *alcohol R* and 100 volumes of *methanol R*.

Plate: *TLC silica gel F$_{254}$ plate R*.

Mobile phase: concentrated ammonia R, methanol R, ethyl acetate R, methylene chloride R (2:40:50:90 *V/V/V/V*).

Application: 20 μl.

Development: over 3/4 of the plate.

Drying: in air.

Detection: examine in ultraviolet light at 254 nm.

Order of elution: ondansetron, impurity B, impurity A.

System suitability: the chromatogram obtained with reference solution (a) shows 3 clearly separated spots.

Limits:

— *impurity B*: any spot corresponding to impurity B in the chromatogram obtained with the test solution is not more intense than the principal spot in the chromatogram obtained with reference solution (b) (0.4 per cent).

Related substances. Liquid chromatography (*2.2.29*).

Test solution (a). Dissolve 50.0 mg of the substance to be examined in the mobile phase and dilute to 100.0 ml with the mobile phase.

Test solution (b). Dissolve 90.0 mg of the substance to be examined in the mobile phase and dilute to 100.0 ml with the mobile phase. Dilute 10.0 ml to 100.0 ml with the mobile phase.

Reference solution (a). Dilute 2.0 ml of test solution (a) to 100.0 ml with the mobile phase. Dilute 10.0 ml to 100.0 ml with the mobile phase.

Reference solution (b). Dissolve 10.0 mg of *imidazole R* and 10.0 mg of *2-methylimidazole R* in the mobile phase and dilute to 100.0 ml with the mobile phase. Dilute 1.0 ml to 100.0 ml with the mobile phase.

Reference solution (c). Dissolve 5.0 mg of *ondansetron for LC system suitability CRS* in the mobile phase and dilute to 10.0 ml with the mobile phase.

Reference solution (d). Dissolve 5.0 mg of *ondansetron impurity D CRS* in the mobile phase and dilute to 100.0 ml with the mobile phase. Dilute 1.0 ml to 100.0 ml with the mobile phase.

Reference solution (e). Dissolve 90.0 mg of *ondansetron hydrochloride dihydrate CRS* in the mobile phase and dilute to 100.0 ml with the mobile phase. Dilute 10.0 ml to 100.0 ml with the mobile phase.

Column:
— *size*: $l = 0.25$ m, $\varnothing = 4.6$ mm,
— *stationary phase*: spherical *nitrile silica gel for chromatography R* (5 µm) with a specific surface area of 220 m^2/g and a pore size of 8 nm.

Mobile phase: mix 20 volumes of *acetonitrile R* and 80 volumes of a 2.8 g/l solution of *sodium dihydrogen phosphate monohydrate R* previously adjusted to pH 5.4 with a 40 g/l solution of *sodium hydroxide R*.

Flow rate: 1.5 ml/min.

Detection: spectrophotometer at 216 nm.

Injection: 20 µl; inject test solution (a) and reference solutions (a), (b), (c) and (d).

Run time: 1.5 times the retention time of ondansetron.

Relative retentions with reference to ondansetron (retention time = about 18 min): impurity E = about 0.1; impurity F = about 0.2; impurity C = about 0.4; impurity D = about 0.5; impurity H = about 0.7; impurity A = about 0.8; impurity G = about 0.9.

System suitability:
— *resolution*: minimum of 1.3 between the peak due to impurity E (first peak) and the peak due to impurity F (second peak) in the chromatogram obtained with reference solution (b) and minimum of 2.5 between the peak due to impurity C (first peak) and the peak due to impurity D (second peak) in the chromatogram obtained with reference solution (c).

Limits:
— *correction factor*: for the calculation of contents, multiply the peak area of impurity C by 0.6,
— *impurity C*: not more than the area of the principal peak in the chromatogram obtained with reference solution (a) (0.2 per cent),

— *impurity D*: not more than the area of the principal peak in the chromatogram obtained with reference solution (d) (0.1 per cent),
— *impurity E*: not more than the area of the corresponding peak in the chromatogram obtained with reference solution (b) (0.2 per cent),
— *impurity F*: not more than the area of the corresponding peak in the chromatogram obtained with reference solution (b) (0.2 per cent),
— *any other impurity*: not more than the area of the principal peak in the chromatogram obtained with reference solution (a) (0.2 per cent),
— *total*: not more than twice the area of the principal peak in the chromatogram obtained with reference solution (a) (0.4 per cent),
— *disregard limit*: 0.2 times the area of the principal peak in the chromatogram obtained with reference solution (a) (0.04 per cent).

Water (*2.5.12*): 9.0 per cent to 10.5 per cent, determined on 0.200 g.

Sulphated ash (*2.4.14*): maximum 0.1 per cent, determined on 1.0 g.

ASSAY

Liquid chromatography (*2.2.29*) as described in the test for related substances with the following modification.

Injection: test solution (b) and reference solution (e).

Calculate the percentage content of $C_{18}H_{20}ClN_3O$.

STORAGE

Protected from light.

IMPURITIES

A. (3*RS*)-3-[(dimethylamino)methyl]-9-methyl-1,2,3,9-tetrahydro-4*H*-carbazol-4-one,

B. 6,6′-methylenebis[(3*RS*)-9-methyl-3-[(2-methyl-1*H*-imidazol-1-yl)methyl]-1,2,3,9-tetrahydro-4*H*-carbazol-4-one],

C. R1 = R2 = H: 9-methyl-1,2,3,9-tetrahydro-4*H*-carbazol-4-one,

D. R1 + R2 = CH$_2$: 9-methyl-3-methylene-1,2,3,9-tetrahydro-4*H*-carbazol-4-one,

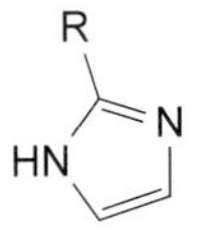

E. R = H: 1*H*-imidazole,

F. R = CH$_3$: 2-methyl-1*H*-imidazole,

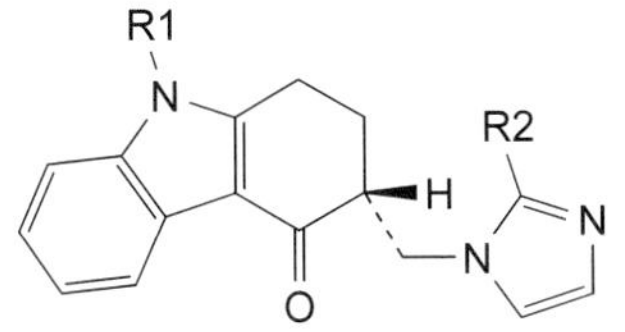

and enantiomer

G. R1 = CH$_3$, R2 = H: (3*RS*)-3-[(1*H*-imidazol-1-yl)methyl(-9-methyl-1,2,3,9-tetrahydro-4*H*-carbazol-4-one (*C*-demethylondansetron),

H. R1 = H, R2 = CH$_3$: (3*RS*)-3-[(2-methyl-1*H*-imidazol-1-yl)methyl]-1,2,3,9-tetrahydro-4*H*-carbazol-4-one (*N*-demethylondansetron).

04/2003:2017

OXALIPLATIN

Oxaliplatinum

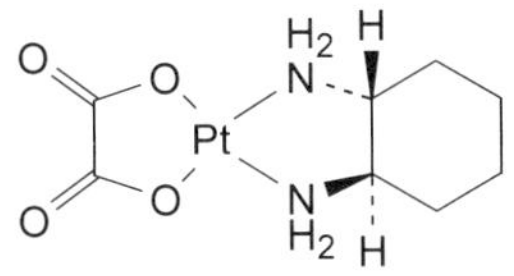

C$_8$H$_{14}$N$_2$O$_4$Pt   *M*$_r$ 397.3

DEFINITION

(*SP*-4-2)-[(1*R*,2*R*)-Cyclohexane-1,2-diamine-κ*N*,κ*N'*] [ethanedioato(2-)-κ*O¹*,κ*O²*]platinum.

Content: 98.0 per cent to 102.0 per cent (dried substance).

CHARACTERS

Appearance: white or almost white, crystalline powder.

Solubility: slightly soluble in water, very slightly soluble in methanol, practically insoluble in ethanol.

IDENTIFICATION

A. Infrared absorption spectrophotometry (*2.2.24*).

   Comparison: oxaliplatin CRS.

B. It complies with the test for specific optical rotation (see Tests).

TESTS

Appearance of solution. The solution is clear (*2.2.1*) and colourless (*2.2.2, Method II*).

Dissolve 0.10 g in *water R* and dilute to 50 ml with the same solvent.

Acidity. Dissolve 0.10 g in *carbon dioxide-free water R*, dilute to 50 ml with the same solvent and add 0.5 ml of *phenolphthalein solution R1*. The solution is colourless. Not more than 0.60 ml of *0.01 M sodium hydroxide* is required to change the colour of the indicator to pink.

Specific optical rotation (*2.2.7*): + 74.5 to + 78.0 (dried substance).

Dissolve 0.250 g in *water R* and dilute to 50.0 ml with the same solvent.

Related substances

A. Impurity A. Liquid chromatography (*2.2.29*). *Use vigorous shaking and very brief sonication to dissolve the substance to be examined. Inject the test solution within 20 min of preparation.*

Test solution. Dissolve 0.100 g of the substance to be examined in *water R* and dilute to 50.0 ml with the same solvent.

Reference solution (a). Dissolve 14.0 mg of *oxalic acid R* (impurity A) in *water R* and dilute to 250.0 ml with the same solvent.

Reference solution (b). Dilute 5.0 ml of reference solution (a) to 200.0 ml with *water R*.

Reference solution (c). Dissolve 12.5 mg of *sodium nitrate R* in *water R* and dilute to 250.0 ml with the same solvent. Dilute a mixture of 2.0 ml of this solution and 25.0 ml of reference solution (a) to 100.0 ml with *water R*.

Column:

– *size*: *l* = 25 cm, Ø = 4.6 mm,

– *stationary phase*: *base-deactivated octadecylsilyl silica gel for chromatography R* (5 µm).

Temperature: 40 °C.

Mobile phase: mix 20 volumes of *acetonitrile R* with 80 volumes of a solution prepared as follows: to 10 ml of a 320 g/l solution of *tetrabutylammonium hydroxide R* add 1.36 g of *potassium dihydrogen phosphate R* and dilute to 1000 ml with *water R*; adjust this solution to pH 6.0 with *phosphoric acid R*.

Flow rate: 2 ml/min.

Detection: spectrophotometer at 205 nm.

Injection: 20 µl; inject the test solution and reference solutions (b) and (c).

Run time: twice the retention time of impurity A.

Retention times: nitrate = about 2.7 min; impurity A = about 4.7 min.

System suitability:

– *resolution*: minimum 9 between the peaks due to nitrate and impurity A in the chromatogram obtained with reference solution (c),

– *signal-to-noise ratio*: minimum of 10 for the peak due to impurity A in the chromatogram obtained with reference solution (b).

Limits:

– *impurity A*: not more than twice the area of the principal peak in the chromatogram obtained with reference solution (b) (0.1 per cent).

B. Impurity B. Liquid chromatography (*2.2.29*). *Use vigorous shaking and very brief sonication to dissolve the substance to be examined. Inject the test solution within 20 min of preparation. Use suitable polypropylene containers for the preparation and injection of all solutions. Glass pipettes may be used for diluting solutions.*

Test solution. Dissolve 0.100 g of the substance to be examined in *water R* and dilute to 50.0 ml with the same solvent.

Reference solution (a). Dissolve 12.5 mg of *oxaliplatin impurity B CRS* in 63 ml of *methanol R* and dilute to 250.0 ml with *water R*. Dilute 3.0 ml to 200.0 ml with *water R*.

Reference solution (b). In order to prepare *in situ* the degradation compound (impurity E) dissolve 12.5 mg of *oxaliplatin impurity B CRS* in 63 ml of *methanol R* and dilute to 250 ml with *water R*. Adjust to pH 6.0 with a 0.2 g/l solution of *sodium hydroxide R*. Heat for 4 h at 70 °C and allow to cool.

Monographs
L - P

Column:
- *size*: l = 25 cm, Ø = 4.6 mm,
- *stationary phase*: *base-deactivated octadecylsilyl silica gel for chromatography R* (5 µm).

Temperature: 40 °C.

Mobile phase: mix 20 volumes of *acetonitrile R* with 80 volumes of a solution prepared as follows: dissolve 1.36 g of *potassium dihydrogen phosphate R* and 1 g of *sodium heptanesulphonate R* in 1000 ml of *water R*; adjust this solution to pH 3.0 ± 0.05 with *phosphoric acid R*.

Flow rate: 2.0 ml/min.

Detection: spectrophotometer at 215 nm.

Injection: 20 µl.

Run time: 2.5 times the retention time of impurity B.

Retention times: impurity B = about 4.3 min; impurity E = about 6.4 min.

System suitability:
- *resolution*: minimum 7 between the peaks due to impurity B and impurity E in the chromatogram obtained with reference solution (b),
- *signal-to-noise ratio*: minimum of 10 for the peak due to impurity B in the chromatogram obtained with reference solution (a).

Limits:
- *impurity B*: not more than 3.3 times the area of the principal peak in the chromatogram obtained with reference solution (a) (0.1 per cent).

C. Impurity C and other related substances. Liquid chromatography (*2.2.29*). *Use vigorous shaking and very brief sonication to dissolve the substance to be examined. Inject the test solution within 20 min of preparation.*

Test solution (a). Dissolve 0.100 g of the substance to be examined in *water R* and dilute to 50.0 ml with the same solvent.

Test solution (b). Dissolve 50.0 mg of the substance to be examined in *water R* and dilute to 500.0 ml with the same solvent.

Reference solution (a). Dissolve 10 mg of *oxaliplatin impurity C CRS* and 10 mg of *oxaliplatin CRS* in *water R* and dilute to 100.0 ml with the same solvent.

Reference solution (b). Dilute 1.0 ml of reference solution (a) to 100.0 ml with *water R*.

Reference solution (c). Dissolve 5 mg of *dichlorodiaminocyclohexaneplatinum CRS* in *methanol R* and dilute to 50.0 ml with the same solvent. To 10.0 ml of this solution add 10.0 ml of reference solution (a) and dilute to 100.0 ml with *water R*.

Reference solution (d). Dissolve 50.0 mg of *oxaliplatin CRS* in *water R* and dilute to 500.0 ml with the same solvent.

Reference solution (e). Dissolve 5.0 mg of *dichlorodiaminocyclohexaneplatinum CRS* in reference solution (d) and dilute to 50.0 ml with the same solvent.

Reference solution (f). To 0.100 g of the substance to be examined add 1.0 ml of reference solution (a) and dilute to 50.0 ml with *water R*.

Column:
- *size*: l = 25 cm, Ø = 4.6 mm,
- *stationary phase*: *octadecylsilyl silica gel for chromatography R* (5 µm).

Temperature: 40 °C.

Mobile phase: mixture of solutions A and B (99:1 *V/V*).

- *solution A*: dilute 0.6 ml of *dilute phosphoric acid R* in 1000 ml of *water R* and adjust to pH 3.0 with either *sodium hydroxide solution R* or *phosphoric acid R*,
- *solution B*: *acetonitrile R*.

Flow rate: 1.2 ml/min.

Detection: spectrophotometer at 210 nm.

Injection: 10 µl; inject test solution (a) and reference solutions (b), (c) and (f).

Run time: 3 times the retention time of oxaliplatin.

Retention times: impurity C = about 4.4 min; dichlorodiaminocyclohexaneplatinum = about 6.9 min; oxaliplatin = about 8.0 min.

System suitability:
- *resolution*: minimum 2.0 between the peaks due to dichlorodiaminocyclohexaneplatinum and oxaliplatin in the chromatogram obtained with reference solution (c),
- *signal-to-noise ratio*: minimum 50 for the peak due to impurity C and minimum 10 for the peak due to oxaliplatin in the chromatogram obtained with reference solution (b).

Limits:
- *impurity C*: not more than half the area of the peak due to impurity C in the chromatogram obtained with reference solution (f) (0.1 per cent),
- *any other impurity*: not more than twice the area of the peak due to oxaliplatin in the chromatogram obtained with reference solution (b) (0.1 per cent),
- *total of other impurities*: not more than twice the area of the peak due to oxaliplatin in the chromatogram obtained with reference solution (b) (0.1 per cent),
- *disregard limit*: the area of the peak due to oxaliplatin in the chromatogram obtained with reference solution (b) (0.05 per cent); disregard any peak with a retention time less than 2 min.

D. *Total of impurities*: the sum of impurities A, B, C and other related impurities is not greater than 0.30 per cent.

Impurity D. Liquid chromatography (*2.2.29*).

Test solution. Dissolve 30 mg of the substance to be examined in *methanol R* and dilute to 50.0 ml with the same solvent.

Reference solution (a). Dissolve 5 mg of *oxaliplatin impurity D CRS* in *methanol R* and dilute to 100.0 ml with the same solvent.

Reference solution (b). Dilute 15.0 ml of reference solution (a) to 50.0 ml with *methanol R*.

Reference solution (c). Dissolve 150.0 mg of *oxaliplatin CRS* in *methanol R* and dilute to 200.0 ml with the same solvent.

Reference solution (d). Dilute 5.0 ml of reference solution (c) to 100.0 ml with *methanol R*.

Reference solution (e). To 40 ml of reference solution (c) add 1.0 ml of reference solution (b) and dilute to 50.0 ml with *methanol R*.

Reference solution (f). Mix 4.0 ml of reference solution (a) and 5.0 ml of reference solution (d) and dilute to 50.0 ml with *methanol R*.

Column:
- *size*: l = 25 cm, Ø = 4.6 mm,
- *stationary phase*: *silica gel OC for chiral separations R*.

Temperature: 40 °C.

Mobile phase: ethanol R, methanol R (3:7 *V/V*).

Flow rate: 0.3 ml/min.

Detection: spectrophotometer at 254 nm.

Injection: 20 μl; inject the test solution and reference solutions (e) and (f).

Run time: twice the retention time of oxaliplatin.

Retention times: oxaliplatin = about 14 min; impurity D = about 16 min.

System suitability:

— *resolution*: minimum 1.5 between the peaks due to oxaliplatin and impurity D in the chromatogram obtained with reference solution (f),

— *signal-to-noise ratio*: minimum 10 for the peak due to impurity D in the chromatogram obtained with reference solution (e).

Limits:

— *impurity D*: not more than twice the peak height of the corresponding peak in the chromatogram obtained with reference solution (e) (0.1 per cent).

Silver: maximum 5 ppm.

Atomic absorption spectrometry (*2.2.23, Method II*).

Test solution. Dissolve 0.1000 g of the substance to be examined in *water R* and dilute to 50.0 ml with the same solvent. Dilute 20 μl of this solution to 40 μl with *0.5 M nitric acid*.

Reference solution (a). Dilute a solution of *silver nitrate R* containing 1000 ppm of silver in *0.5 M nitric acid* with *0.5 M nitric acid* to obtain a solution which contains 10 ppb of silver.

Reference solution (b). Mix 20 μl of the test solution and 8 μl of reference solution (a) and dilute to 40 μl with *0.5 M nitric acid*.

Reference solution (c). Mix 20 μl of the test solution and 16 μl of reference solution (a) and dilute to 40 μl with *0.5 M nitric acid*.

Source: silver hollow-cathode lamp.

Wavelength: 328.1 nm.

Atomisation device: furnace.

Measure the absorbance of the test solution and reference solutions (b) and (c).

Loss on drying (*2.2.32*): maximum 0.5 per cent, determined on 1.000 g by drying in an oven at 100-105 °C for 2 h.

Bacterial endotoxins (*2.6.14*): less than 1.0 IU/mg, if intended for use in the manufacture of parenteral dosage forms without a further appropriate procedure for the removal of bacterial endotoxins.

ASSAY

Liquid chromatography (*2.2.29*) as described in the test for impurity C and other related substances with the following modifications.

Injection: 20 μl; inject test solution (b) and reference solutions (d) and (e).

System suitability:

— *resolution*: minimum 2.0 between the peaks due to dichlorodiaminocyclohexaneplatinum and oxaliplatin in the chromatogram obtained with reference solution (e),

— *repeatability*: reference solution (d).

Calculate the percentage content of oxaliplatin using the chromatogram obtained with reference solution (d).

LABELLING

The label states where applicable, that the substance is free from bacterial endotoxins.

IMPURITIES

Qualified impurities: A, B, C, D.

Other detectable impurities: E.

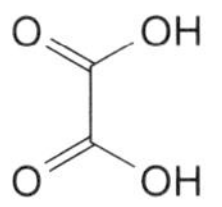

A. ethanedioic acid (oxalic acid),

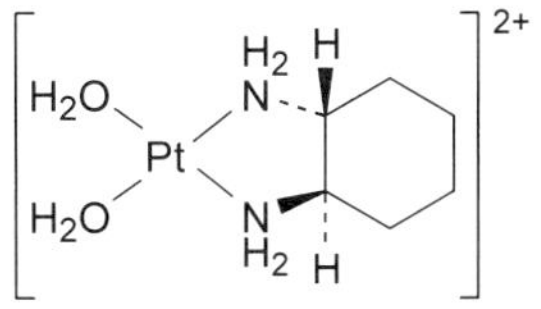

B. (*SP*-4-2)-diaqua[(1*R*,2*R*)-cyclohexane-1,2-diamine-κ*N*,κ*N'*]platinum (diaquodiaminocyclohexaneplatinum),

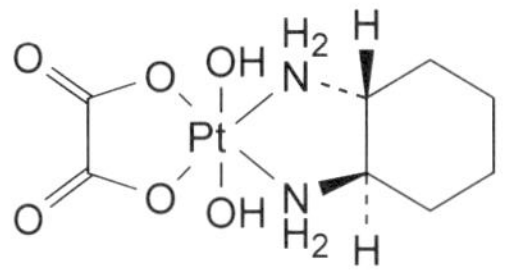

C. (*OC*-6-33)-[(1*R*,2*R*)-cyclohexane-1,2-diamine-κ*N*,κ*N'*][ethanedioato(2-)-κ*O¹*,κ*O²*]dihydroxyplatinum,

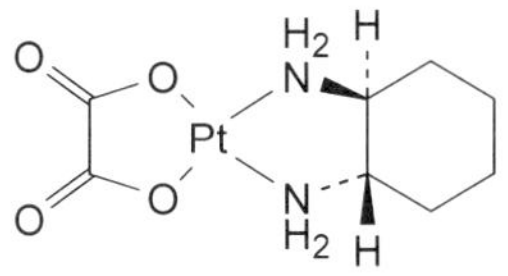

D. (*SP*-4-2)-[(1*S*,2*S*)-cyclohexane-1,2-diamine-κ*N*,κ*N'*][ethanedioato(2-)-κ*O¹*,κ*O²*]platinum (*S*,*S*-enantiomer of oxaliplatin),

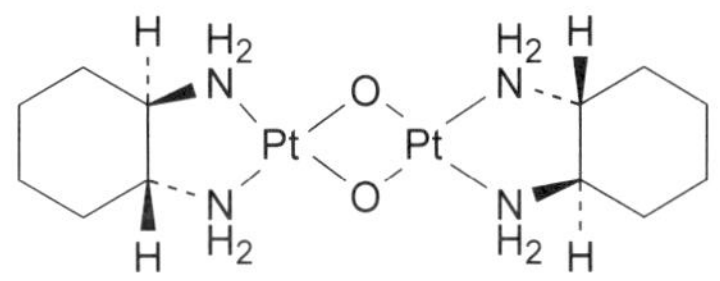

E. (*SP*-4-2)-di-μ-oxobis[(1*R*,2*R*)-cyclohexane-1,2-diamine-κ*N*,κ*N'*]diplatinum (diaquodiaminocyclohexaneplatinum dimer).

04/2003:1458

OXFENDAZOLE FOR VETERINARY USE

Oxfendazolum ad usum veterinarium

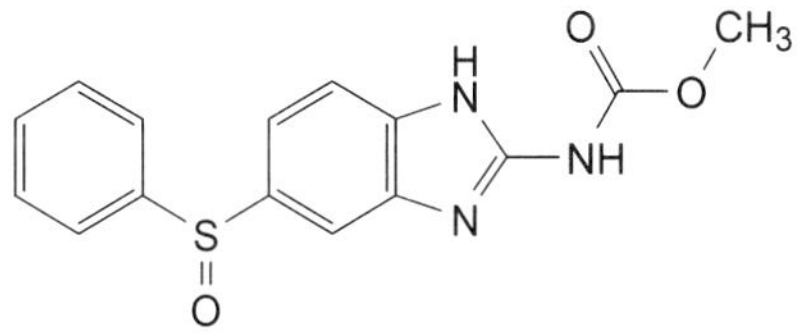

$C_{15}H_{13}N_3O_3S$ M_r 315.4

DEFINITION

Methyl [5-(phenylsulphinyl)-1*H*-benzimidazol-2-yl]carbamate.

Content: 97.5 per cent to 100.5 per cent (dried substance).

CHARACTERS

Appearance: white or almost white powder.

Solubility: practically insoluble in water, slightly soluble in alcohol and in methylene chloride.

It shows polymorphism.

IDENTIFICATION

Infrared absorption spectrophotometry (2.2.24).

Comparison: oxfendazole CRS.

If the spectra obtained in the solid state show differences, dissolve the substance to be examined and the reference substance separately in *alcohol R*, evaporate to dryness and record new spectra using the residues.

TESTS

Related substances. Liquid chromatography (2.2.29).

Test solution. Dissolve 25.0 mg of the substance to be examined in the mobile phase and dilute to 100.0 ml with the mobile phase.

Reference solution (a). Dilute 1.0 ml of the test solution to 100.0 ml with the mobile phase.

Reference solution (b). To 10 ml of the test solution, add 0.25 ml of *strong hydrogen peroxide solution R* and dilute to 25 ml with the mobile phase.

Reference solution (c). Dissolve 5.0 mg of *fenbendazole CRS* and 10.0 mg of *oxfendazole impurity B CRS* in the mobile phase and dilute to 100.0 ml with the mobile phase. Dilute 1.0 ml to 20.0 ml with the mobile phase.

Reference solution (d). Dissolve 5 mg of *oxfendazole with impurity D CRS* in the mobile phase and dilute to 20 ml with the mobile phase (solution used for identification of impurity D).

Column:

— *size*: l = 0.25 m, Ø = 4.6 mm,

— *stationary phase*: spherical *end-capped octadecylsilyl silica gel for chromatography R* (5 μm) with a specific surface area of 350 m^2/g, a pore size of 10 nm and a carbon loading of 14 per cent.

Mobile phase: mix 36 volumes of *acetonitrile R* and 64 volumes of a 2 g/l solution of *sodium pentanesulphonate R* adjusted to pH 2.7 with a 2.8 per cent V/V solution of *sulphuric acid R*.

Flow rate: 1 ml/min.

Detection: spectrophotometer at 254 nm.

Injection: 20 μl.

Run time: 4 times the retention time of oxfendazole.

Retention time: oxfendazole = about 6.5 min.

System suitability: reference solution (b):

— *resolution*: minimum 4.0 between the 2 principal peaks corresponding to impurity C (1st peak) and oxfendazole (2nd peak).

Limits:

— *impurity A*: not more than the area of the corresponding peak in the chromatogram obtained with reference solution (c) (1.0 per cent),

— *impurity B*: not more than the area of the corresponding peak in the chromatogram obtained with reference solution (c) (2.0 per cent),

— *impurity C or D*: for each impurity, not more than the area of the principal peak in the chromatogram obtained with reference solution (a) (1.0 per cent),

— *any other impurity*: not more than 0.1 times the area of the principal peak in the chromatogram obtained with reference solution (a) (0.1 per cent),

— *total*: not more than 3 times the area of the principal peak in the chromatogram obtained with reference solution (a) (3.0 per cent),

— *disregard limit*: 0.05 times the area of the principal peak in the chromatogram obtained with reference solution (a) (0.05 per cent).

Loss on drying (2.2.32): maximum 0.5 per cent, determined on 1.000 g by drying in an oven at 100-105 °C at a pressure not exceeding 0.7 kPa for 2 h.

Sulphated ash (2.4.14): maximum 0.2 per cent, determined on 1.0 g.

ASSAY

Dissolve 0.250 g in 3 ml of *anhydrous formic acid R*. Add 40 ml of *anhydrous acetic acid R*. Titrate with *0.1 M perchloric acid*, determining the end-point potentiometrically (2.2.20).

1 ml of *0.1 M perchloric acid* is equivalent to 31.54 mg of $C_{15}H_{13}N_3O_3S$.

STORAGE

Protected from light.

IMPURITIES

A. fenbendazole,

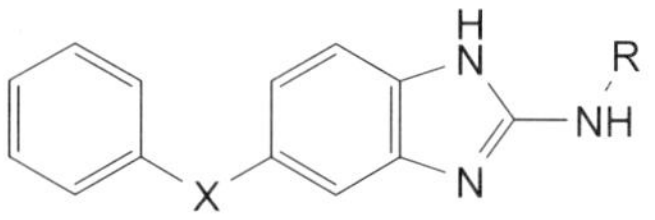

B. X = SO_2, R = CO_2-CH_3: methyl [5-(phenylsulphonyl)-1*H*-benzimidazol-2-yl]carbamate,

C. X = SO, R = H: 5-(phenylsulphinyl)-1*H*-benzimidazol-2-amine,

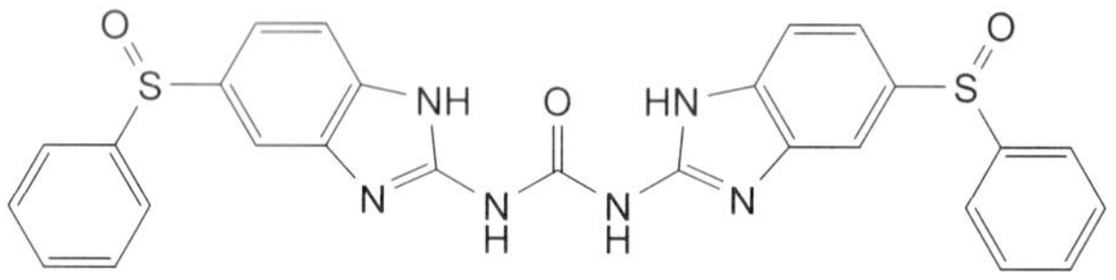

D. *N,N'*-bis[5-(phenylsulphinyl)-1*H*-benzimidazol-2-yl]urea.

04/2003:0199

OXYTETRACYCLINE DIHYDRATE

Oxytetraclinum dihydricum

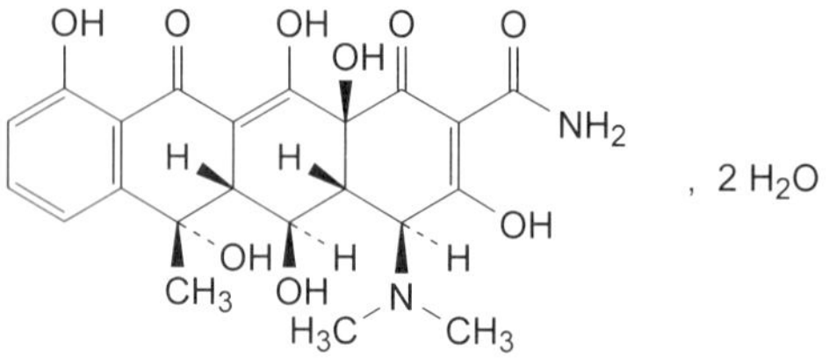

$C_{22}H_{24}N_2O_9$,2 H_2O M_r 496.4

DEFINITION

(4S,4aR,5S,5aR,6S,12aS)-4-(Dimethylamino)-3,5,6,10,12,12a-hexahydroxy-6-methyl-1,11-dioxo-1,4,4a,5,5a,6,11,12a-octahydrotetracene-2-carboxamide dihydrate.

Substance produced by the growth of certain strains of *Streptomyces rimosus* or obtained by any other means.

Content: 95.0 per cent to 102.0 per cent (anhydrous substance).

CHARACTERS

Appearance: yellow, crystalline powder.

Solubility: very slightly soluble in water. It dissolves in dilute acid and alkaline solutions.

IDENTIFICATION

A. Thin-layer chromatography (*2.2.27*).

Test solution. Dissolve 5 mg of the substance to be examined in *methanol R* and dilute to 10 ml with the same solvent.

Reference solution (a). Dissolve 5 mg of oxytetracycline CRS in *methanol R* and dilute to 10 ml with the same solvent.

Reference solution (b). Dissolve 5 mg of oxytetracycline CRS, 5 mg of *tetracycline hydrochloride R* and 5 mg of *minocycline hydrochloride R* in *methanol R* and dilute to 10 ml with the same solvent.

Plate: TLC octadecylsilyl silica gel F_{254} plate R.

Mobile phase: mix 20 volumes of *acetonitrile R*, 20 volumes of *methanol R* and 60 volumes of a 63 g/l solution of *oxalic acid R* previously adjusted to pH 2 with *concentrated ammonia R*.

Application: 1 µl.

Development: over 3/4 of the plate.

Drying: in air.

Detection: examine in ultraviolet light at 254 nm.

System suitability: the chromatogram obtained with reference solution (b) shows 3 clearly separated spots.

Results: the principal spot in the chromatogram obtained with the test solution is similar in position and size to the principal spot in the chromatogram obtained with reference solution (a).

B. To about 2 mg add 5 ml of *sulphuric acid R*. A deep red colour develops. Add the solution to 2.5 ml of *water R*. The colour becomes yellow.

C. Dissolve about 10 mg in a mixture of 1 ml of *dilute nitric acid R* and 5 ml of *water R*. Shake and add 1 ml of *silver nitrate solution R2*. Any opalescence in the solution is not more intense than that in a mixture of 1 ml of *dilute nitric acid R*, 5 ml of a 0.021 g/l solution of *potassium chloride R* and 1 ml of *silver nitrate solution R2*.

TESTS

pH (*2.2.3*): 4.5 to 7.5.

Suspend 0.1 g in 10 ml of *carbon dioxide-free water R*.

Specific optical rotation (*2.2.7*): -203 to -216 (anhydrous substance).

Dissolve 0.250 g in *0.1 M hydrochloric acid* and dilute to 25.0 ml with the same acid.

Specific absorbance (*2.2.25*): 290 to 310 determined at 353 nm (anhydrous substance).

Dissolve 20.0 mg in *buffer solution pH 2.0 R* and dilute to 100.0 ml with the same buffer solution. Dilute 10.0 ml of the solution to 100.0 ml with *buffer solution pH 2.0 R*.

Light-absorbing impurities. *Carry out the measurements within 1 h of preparing the solutions.*

Dissolve 20.0 mg in a mixture of 1 volume of *1 M hydrochloric acid* and 99 volumes of *methanol R* and dilute to 10.0 ml with the same mixture of solvents. The absorbance (*2.2.25*), determined at 430 nm has a maximum of 0.25 (anhydrous substance).

Dissolve 0.100 g in a mixture of 1 volume of *1 M hydrochloric acid* and 99 volumes of *methanol R* and dilute to 10.0 ml with the same mixture of solvents. The absorbance (*2.2.25*) determined at 490 nm has a maximum of 0.20 (anhydrous substance).

Related substances. Liquid chromatography (*2.2.29*).

Test solution. Dissolve 20.0 mg of the substance to be examined in *0.01 M hydrochloric acid* and dilute to 25.0 ml with the same acid.

Reference solution (a). Dissolve 20.0 mg of oxytetracycline CRS in *0.01 M hydrochloric acid* and dilute to 25.0 ml with the same acid.

Reference solution (b). Dissolve 20.0 mg of 4-epioxytetracycline CRS in *0.01 M hydrochloric acid* and dilute to 25.0 ml with the same acid.

Reference solution (c). Dissolve 20.0 mg of *tetracycline hydrochloride CRS* in *0.01 M hydrochloric acid* and dilute to 25.0 ml with the same acid.

Reference solution (d). Mix 1.5 ml of reference solution (a), 1.0 ml of reference solution (b) and 3.0 ml of reference solution (c) and dilute to 25.0 ml with *0.01 M hydrochloric acid*.

Reference solution (e). Mix 1.0 ml of reference solution (b) and 4.0 ml of reference solution (c) and dilute to 200.0 ml with *0.01 M hydrochloric acid*.

Column:
- *size*: l = 0.25 m, Ø = 4.6 mm,
- *stationary phase*: *styrene-divinylbenzene copolymer R* (8 µm),
- *temperature*: 60 °C.

Mobile phase: weigh 60.0 g of *2-methyl-2-propanol R* and transfer to a 1000 ml volumetric flask with the aid of 200 ml of *water R*; add 60 ml of *0.33 M phosphate buffer solution pH 7.5 R*, 50 ml of a 10 g/l solution of *tetrabutylammonium hydrogen sulphate R* adjusted to pH 7.5 with *dilute sodium hydroxide solution R* and 10 ml of a 0.4 g/l solution of *sodium edetate R* adjusted to pH 7.5 with *dilute sodium hydroxide solution R*; dilute to 1000 ml with *water R*.

Flow rate: 1.0 ml/min.

Detection: spectrophotometer at 254 nm.

Injection: 20 µl; inject the test solution and reference solutions (d) and (e).

System suitability: reference solution (d):
- *resolution*: minimum 4.0 between the peaks due to impurity A (1st peak) and oxytetracycline (2nd peak) and minimum 5.0 between the peaks and due to oxytetracycline and impurity B (3rd peak); adjust the 2-methyl-2-propanol content in the mobile phase if necessary,
- *symmetry factor*: maximum 1.25 for the peak due to oxytetracycline.

Limits:
- *impurity A*: not more than the area of the corresponding peak in the chromatogram obtained with reference solution (e) (0.5 per cent),
- *impurity B*: not more than the area of the corresponding peak in the chromatogram obtained with reference solution (e) (2.0 per cent),
- *impurity C (eluting on the tail of the principal peak)*: not more than 4 times the area of the peak due to impurity A in the chromatogram obtained with reference solution (e) (2.0 per cent),
- *disregard limit*: 0.02 times the area of the peak due to oxytetracycline in the chromatogram obtained with reference solution (d) (0.1 per cent).

Heavy metals (*2.4.8*): maximum 50 ppm.

0.5 g complies with limit test F. Prepare the standard using 2.5 ml of *lead standard solution (10 ppm Pb) R*.

Water (*2.5.12*): 6.0 per cent to 9.0 per cent, determined on 0.250 g.

Sulphated ash (*2.4.14*): maximum 0.5 per cent, determined on 1.0 g.

ASSAY

Liquid chromatography (*2.2.29*) as described in the test for related substances with the following modification.

Injection: test solution and reference solution (a).

Calculate the percentage content of $C_{22}H_{24}N_2O_9$.

STORAGE

In an airtight container, protected from light.

IMPURITIES

A. R1 = NH$_2$, R2 = N(CH$_3$)$_2$, R3 = R4 = H, R5 = OH: (4*R*,4a*R*,5*S*,5a*R*,6*S*,12a*S*)-4-(dimethylamino)-3,5,6,10,12,12a-hexahydroxy-6-methyl-1,11-dioxo-1,4,4a,5,5a,6,11,12a-octahydrotetracene-2-carboxamide (4-epioxytetracycline),

B. R1 = NH$_2$, R2 = R4 = R5 = H, R3 = N(CH$_3$)$_2$: tetracycline,

C. R1 = CH$_3$, R2 = R4 = H, R3 = N(CH$_3$)$_2$, R5 = OH: (4*S*,4a*R*,5*S*,5a*R*,6*S*,12a*S*)-2-acetyl-4-(dimethylamino)-3,5,6,10,12,12a-hexahydroxy-6-methyl-4a,5a,6,12a-tetrahydrotetracene-1,11(4*H*,5*H*)-dione (2-acetyl-2-decarbamoyloxytetracycline).

04/2003:0198

OXYTETRACYCLINE HYDROCHLORIDE

Oxytetracyclini hydrochloridum

$C_{22}H_{25}ClN_2O_9$ M_r 496.9

DEFINITION

(4*S*,4a*R*,5*S*,5a*R*,6*S*,12a*S*)-4-(Dimethylamino)-3,5,6,10,12,12a-hexahydroxy-6-methyl-1,11-dioxo-1,4,4a,5,5a,6,11,12a-octahydrotetracene-2-carboxamide hydrochloride.

Substance produced by the growth of certain strains of *Streptomyces rimosus* or obtained by any other means.

Content: 95.0 per cent to 102.0 per cent (anhydrous substance).

CHARACTERS

Appearance: yellow, crystalline powder, hygroscopic.

Solubility: freely soluble in water, sparingly soluble in alcohol. Solutions in water become turbid on standing, owing to the precipitation of oxytetracycline.

IDENTIFICATION

A. Thin-layer chromatography (*2.2.27*).

Test solution. Dissolve 5 mg of the substance to be examined in *methanol R* and dilute to 10 ml with the same solvent.

Reference solution (a). Dissolve 5 mg of *oxytetracycline hydrochloride CRS* in *methanol R* and dilute to 10 ml with the same solvent.

Reference solution (b). Dissolve 5 mg of *oxytetracycline hydrochloride CRS*, 5 mg of *tetracycline hydrochloride R* and 5 mg of *minocycline hydrochloride R* in *methanol R* and dilute to 10 ml with the same solvent.

Plate: TLC octadecylsilyl silica gel F$_{254}$ plate R.

Mobile phase: mix 20 volumes of *acetonitrile R*, 20 volumes of *methanol R* and 60 volumes of a 63 g/l solution of *oxalic acid R* previously adjusted to pH 2 with *concentrated ammonia R*.

Application: 1 µl.

Development: over 3/4 of the plate.

Drying: in air.

Detection: examine in ultraviolet light at 254 nm.

System suitability: the chromatogram obtained with reference solution (b) shows 3 clearly separated spots.

Results: the principal spot in the chromatogram obtained with the test solution is similar in position and size to the principal spot in the chromatogram obtained with reference solution (a).

B. To about 2 mg add 5 ml of *sulphuric acid R*. A deep red colour develops. Add the solution to 2.5 ml of *water R*. The colour becomes yellow.

C. It gives reaction (a) of chlorides (*2.3.1*).

TESTS

pH (*2.2.3*): 2.3 to 2.9.

Dissolve 0.1 g in 10 ml of *carbon dioxide-free water R*.

Specific optical rotation (*2.2.7*): − 188 to − 200 (anhydrous substance).

Dissolve 0.250 g in *0.1 M hydrochloric acid* and dilute to 25.0 ml with the same acid.

Specific absorbance (*2.2.25*): 270 to 290 determined at 353 nm (anhydrous substance).

Dissolve 20.0 mg in *buffer solution pH 2.0 R* and dilute to 100.0 ml with the same buffer solution. Dilute 10.0 ml of the solution to 100.0 ml with *buffer solution pH 2.0 R*.

Light-absorbing impurities. *Carry out the measurements within 1 h of preparing the solutions.*

Dissolve 20.0 mg in a mixture of 1 volume of *1 M hydrochloric acid* and 99 volumes of *methanol R* and dilute to 10.0 ml with the same mixture of solvents. The absorbance (*2.2.25*) determined at 430 nm has a maximum of 0.50 (anhydrous substance).

Dissolve 0.100 g in a mixture of 1 volume of *1 M hydrochloric acid* and 99 volumes of *methanol R* and dilute to 10.0 ml with the same mixture of solvents. The absorbance (*2.2.25*) determined at 490 nm has a maximum of 0.20 (anhydrous substance).

Related substances. Liquid chromatography (*2.2.29*).

Test solution. Dissolve 20.0 mg of the substance to be examined in *0.01 M hydrochloric acid* and dilute to 25.0 ml with the same acid.

Reference solution (a). Dissolve 20.0 mg of *oxytetracycline CRS* in *0.01 M hydrochloric acid* and dilute to 25.0 ml with the same acid.

Reference solution (b). Dissolve 20.0 mg of *4-epioxytetracycline CRS* in *0.01 M hydrochloric acid* and dilute to 25.0 ml with the same acid.

Reference solution (c). Dissolve 20.0 mg of *tetracycline hydrochloride CRS* in *0.01 M hydrochloric acid* and dilute to 25.0 ml with the same acid.

Reference solution (d). Dissolve 8.0 mg of *α-apo-oxytetracycline CRS* in 5 ml of *0.01 M sodium hydroxide* and dilute to 100.0 ml with *0.01 M hydrochloric acid.*

Reference solution (e). Dissolve 8.0 mg of *β-apo-oxytetracycline CRS* in 5 ml of *0.01 M sodium hydroxide* and dilute to 100.0 ml with *0.01 M hydrochloric acid.*

Reference solution (f). Mix 1.5 ml of reference solution (a), 1.0 ml of reference solution (b), 3.0 ml of reference solution (c), 3.0 ml of reference solution (d) and 3.0 ml of reference solution (e) and dilute to 25.0 ml with *0.01 M hydrochloric acid.*

Reference solution (g). Mix 1.0 ml of reference solution (b), 4.0 ml of reference solution (c) and 40.0 ml of reference solution (e) and dilute to 200.0 ml with *0.01 M hydrochloric acid.*

Column:

— *size*: l = 0.25 m, Ø = 4.6 mm,

— *stationary phase*: *styrene-divinylbenzene copolymer R* (8 μm),

— *temperature*: 60 °C.

Mobile phase: weigh 30.0 g (for mobile phase A) and 100.0 g (for mobile phase B) of *2-methyl-2-propanol R* and transfer separately to 1000 ml volumetric flasks with the aid of 200 ml of *water R*; to each flask add 60 ml of *0.33 M phosphate buffer solution pH 7.5 R*, 50 ml of a 10 g/l solution of *tetrabutylammonium hydrogen sulphate R* adjusted to pH 7.5 with *dilute sodium hydroxide solution R* and 10 ml of a 0.4 g/l solution of *sodium edetate R* adjusted to pH 7.5 with *dilute sodium hydroxide solution R*; dilute each solution to 1000 ml with *water R,*

Time (min)	Mobile phase A (per cent *V/V*)	Mobile phase B (per cent *V/V*)
0 - 15	70	30
15 - 30	30	70
30 - 45	70	30

Flow rate: 1 ml/min.

Detection: spectrophotometer at 254 nm.

Injection: 20 μl; inject the test solution and reference solutions (f) and (g).

System suitability: reference solution (f):

— *resolution*: minimum 4.0 between the peaks due to impurity A (1st peak) and oxytetracycline (2nd peak), minimum 5.0 between the peaks due to oxytetracycline and impurity B (3rd peak) and minimum 3.5 between the peaks due to impurity D (4th peak) and impurity E (5th peak); if necessary, adapt the ratio mobile phase A: mobile phase B and/or adjust the time programme used to produce the one-step gradient elution,

— *symmetry factor*: maximum 1.25 for the peak due to oxytetracycline.

Limits:

— *impurity A*: not more than the area of the corresponding peak in the chromatogram obtained with reference solution (g) (0.5 per cent),

— *impurity B*: not more than the area of the corresponding peak in the chromatogram obtained with reference solution (g) (2.0 per cent),

— *impurity C (eluting on the tail of the main peak)*: not more than 4 times the area of the peak due to impurity A in the chromatogram obtained with reference solution (g) (2.0 per cent),

— *total of impurities D, E and F (eluting between the latter two)*: not more than the area of the peak due to impurity E in the chromatogram obtained with reference solution (g) (2.0 per cent),

— *disregard limit*: 0.02 times the area of the peak due to oxytetracycline in the chromatogram obtained with reference solution (f) (0.1 per cent).

Heavy metals (*2.4.8*): maximum 50 ppm.

0.5 g complies with limit test F. Prepare the standard using 2.5 ml of *lead standard solution (10 ppm Pb) R*.

Water (*2.5.12*): maximum 2.0 per cent, determined on 0.500 g.

Sulphated ash (*2.4.14*): maximum 0.5 per cent, determined on 1.0 g.

Sterility (*2.6.1*). If intended for use in the manufacture of parenteral dosage forms without a further appropriate sterilisation procedure, it complies with the test for sterility.

Bacterial endotoxins (*2.6.14*): less than 0.4 IU/mg, if intended for use in the manufacture of parenteral dosage forms without a further appropriate procedure for the removal of bacterial endotoxins.

ASSAY

Liquid chromatography (*2.2.29*) as described in the test for related substances with the following modification.

Injection: test solution and reference solution (a).

Calculate the percentage content of $C_{22}H_{25}ClN_2O_9$ taking 1 mg of oxytetracycline as equivalent to 1.079 mg of oxytetracycline hydrochloride.

STORAGE

In an airtight container, protected from light. If the substance is sterile, store in a sterile, airtight, tamper-proof container.

LABELLING

The label states:

— where applicable, that the substance is sterile,

— where applicable, that the substance is free from bacterial endotoxins.

IMPURITIES

A. R1 = NH$_2$, R2 = N(CH$_3$)$_2$, R3 = R4 = H, R5 = OH:
(4R,4aR,5S,5aR,6S,12aS)-4-(dimethylamino)-
3,5,6,10,12,12a-hexahydroxy-6-methyl-1,11-dioxo-
1,4,4a,5,5a,6,11,12a-octahydrotetracene-2-carboxamide
(4-epioxytetracycline),

B. R1 = NH$_2$, R2 = R4 = R5 = H, R3 = N(CH$_3$)$_2$: tetracycline,

C. R1 = CH$_3$, R2 = R4 = H, R3 = N(CH$_3$)$_2$, R5 = OH:
(4S,4aR,5S,5aR,6S,12aS)-2-acetyl-4-(dimethylamino)-
3,5,6,10,12,12a-hexahydroxy-6-methyl-4a,5a,6,12a-
tetrahydrotetracene-1,11(4H,5H)-dione (2-acetyl-2-
decarbamoyloxytetracycline),

D. R = OH, R′ = H: (3S,4S,5S)-4-[(1R)-4,5-dihydroxy-9-
methyl-3-oxo-1,3-dihydronaphtho[2,3-c]furan-1-yl]-
3-(dimethylamino)-2,5-dihydroxy-6-oxocyclohex-1-
enecarboxamide (α-apo-oxytetracycline),

E. R = H, R′ = OH: (3S,4S,5R)-4-[(1R)-4,5-dihydroxy-
9-methyl-3-oxo-1,3-dihydronaphtho[2,3-c]furan-1-yl]-
3-(dimethylamino)-2,5-dihydroxy-6-oxocyclohex-1-
enecarboxamide (β-apo-oxytetracycline),

F. (4S,4aR,5R,12aS)-4-(dimethylamino)-3,5,10,11,12a-
pentahydroxy-6-methyl-1,12-dioxo-1,4,4a,5,12,12a-
hexahydrotetracene-2-carboxamide (anhydro-
oxytetracycline).

01/2002:0780
corrected

OXYTOCIN

Oxytocinum

H-Cys—Tyr—Ile—Gln—Asn—Cys—Pro—Leu—Gly-NH$_2$

$C_{43}H_{66}N_{12}O_{12}S_2$ M_r 1007

DEFINITION

Oxytocin is a cyclic nonapeptide having the structure of the hormone produced by the posterior lobe of the pituitary gland that stimulates contraction of the uterus and milk ejection in receptive mammals. It is obtained by chemical synthesis and is available in the freeze-dried form as an acetate. It contains not less than 93.0 per cent and not more than the equivalent of 102.0 per cent of the peptide $C_{43}H_{66}N_{12}O_{12}S_2$, calculated with reference to the anhydrous, acetic acid-free substance.

By convention, for the purpose of labelling oxytocin preparations, 1 mg of oxytocin peptide ($C_{43}H_{66}N_{12}O_{12}S_2$) is equivalent to 600 IU of biological activity.

CHARACTERS

A white or almost white powder, hygroscopic, very soluble in water and in dilute solutions of acetic acid and of ethanol.

IDENTIFICATION

Examine the chromatograms obtained in the assay. The retention time of the principal peak in the chromatogram obtained with the test solution is approximately the same as that of the principal peak in the chromatogram obtained with the reference solution.

TESTS

pH (*2.2.3*). Dissolve 0.200 g in *carbon dioxide-free water R* and dilute to 10.0 ml with the same solvent. The pH of the solution is 3.0 to 6.0.

Amino acids. Examine by means of an amino-acid analyser. Standardise the apparatus with a mixture containing equimolar amounts of ammonia, glycine and the L-form of the following amino acids:

lysine	threonine	alanine	leucine
histidine	serine	valine	tyrosine
arginine	glutamic acid	methionine	phenylalanine
aspartic acid	proline	isoleucine	

together with half the equimolar amount of L-cystine. For the validation of the method, an appropriate internal standard, such as DL-*norleucine R*, is used.

Test solution. Place 1.0 mg of the substance to be examined in a rigorously cleaned hard-glass tube 100 mm long and 6 mm in internal diameter. Add a suitable amount of a 50 per cent *V/V* solution of *hydrochloric acid R*. Immerse the tube in a freezing mixture at −5 °C, reduce the pressure to below 133 Pa and seal. Heat at 110 °C to 115 °C for 16 h. Cool, open the tube, transfer the contents to a 10 ml flask with the aid of five quantities, each of 0.2 ml, of *water R* and evaporate to dryness over *potassium hydroxide R* under reduced pressure. Take up the residue in *water R* and evaporate to dryness over *potassium hydroxide R* under reduced pressure; repeat these operations once. Take up the residue in a buffer solution suitable for the amino-acid analyser used and dilute to a suitable volume with the same buffer solution. Apply a suitable volume to the amino-acid analyser.

Express the content of each amino acid in moles. Calculate the relative proportions of the amino acids, taking one-sixth of the sum of the number of moles of aspartic acid, glutamic acid, proline, glycine, isoleucine and leucine as equal to one. The values fall within the following limits: aspartic acid 0.95 to 1.05; glutamic acid 0.95 to 1.05; proline 0.95 to 1.05; glycine 0.95 to 1.05; leucine 0.90 to 1.10; isoleucine 0.90 to 1.10; tyrosine 0.7 to 1.05; half-cystine 1.4 to 2.1; not more than traces of other amino acids are present.

Related peptides. Examine by liquid chromatography (*2.2.29*) as described under Assay.

Inject 50 µl of the test solution. In the chromatogram obtained the area of any peak, apart from the principal peak, is not greater than 1.5 per cent of the total area of the peaks; the sum of the areas of all the peaks, apart from the principal peak, is not greater than 5 per cent of the total area of the peaks. Disregard any peak due to the solvent and any peak with an area less than 0.1 per cent of that of the principal peak.

Acetic acid (2.5.34): 6.0 per cent to 10.0 per cent.

Test solution. Dissolve 15.0 mg of the substance to be examined in a mixture of 5 volumes of mobile phase B and 95 volumes of mobile phase A and dilute to 10.0 ml with the same mixture of solvents.

Water (2.5.12). Not more than 5.0 per cent, determined on at least 50 mg by the semi-micro determination of water.

Sterility (2.6.1). If intended for use in the manufacture of parenteral dosage forms without a further appropriate sterilisation procedure, it complies with the test for sterility.

Bacterial endotoxins (2.6.14): less than 300 IU/mg, if intended for use in the manufacture of parenteral dosage forms without a further appropriate procedure for removal of bacterial endotoxins.

ASSAY

Examine by liquid chromatography (2.2.29).

Test solution. Prepare a 0.25 mg/ml solution of the substance to be examined in a 15.6 g/l solution of *sodium dihydrogen phosphate R*.

Reference solution. Dissolve the contents of a vial of *oxytocin CRS* in a 15.6 g/l solution of *sodium dihydrogen phosphate R* to obtain a concentration of 0.25 mg/ml.

Resolution solution. Dissolve the contents of a vial of *oxytocin/desmopressin validation mixture CRS* in 500 µl of a 15.6 g/l solution of *sodium dihydrogen phosphate R*.

The chromatographic procedure may be carried out using:

- a stainless steel column 0.125 m long and 4.6 mm in internal diameter packed with *octadecylsilyl silica gel for chromatography R* (5 µm),

- as mobile phase at a flow rate of 1 ml/min:

  Mobile phase A. A 15.6 g/l solution of *sodium dihydrogen phosphate R*,

  Mobile phase B. Mix 1 volume of *acetonitrile for chromatography R* with 1 volume of *water R*,

Time (min)	Mobile phase A (per cent *V/V*)	Mobile phase B (per cent *V/V*)	Comment
0 - 30	70 → 40	30 → 60	linear gradient
30 - 30.1	40 → 70	60 → 30	switch to initial eluent composition
30.1 - 45	70	30	re-equilibration

- as detector a spectrophotometer set at 220 nm.

Equilibrate the column with a mixture of 30 volumes of mobile phase B and 70 volumes of mobile phase A.

Inject 25 µl of the resolution solution. When the chromatograms are recorded in the prescribed conditions, the retention times are: oxytocin about 7.5 min and desmopressin about 10 min. The test is not valid unless the resolution between the peaks corresponding to desmopressin and oxytocin is at least 5.0.

Inject 25 µl of the test solution and 25 µl of the reference solution.

Calculate the content of oxytocin ($C_{43}H_{66}N_{12}O_{12}S_2$) from the peak areas in the chromatograms obtained with the test solution and the reference solution and the declared content of $C_{43}H_{66}N_{12}O_{12}S_2$ in *oxytocin CRS*.

STORAGE

Store in an airtight container, protected from light, at a temperature of 2 °C to 8 °C. If the substance is sterile, store in a sterile, airtight, tamper-proof container.

LABELLING

The label states:

- the oxytocin peptide content ($C_{43}H_{66}N_{12}O_{12}S_2$),

- where applicable, that the substance is sterile,

- where applicable, that the substance is free from bacterial endotoxins.

01/2002:0779
corrected

OXYTOCIN BULK SOLUTION

Oxytocini solutio

DEFINITION

Oxytocin bulk solution is a solution of oxytocin, a cyclic nonapeptide having the structure of the hormone produced by the posterior lobe of the pituitary gland that stimulates contraction of the uterus and milk ejection in receptive mammals. It is obtained by chemical synthesis. It is available as a bulk solution with a stated concentration of not less than 0.25 mg of oxytocin per millilitre, in a solvent that may contain an appropriate antimicrobial preservative. It contains not less than 95.0 per cent and not more than 105.0 per cent of the amount of the peptide $C_{43}H_{66}N_{12}O_{12}S_2$ stated per millilitre.

By convention, for the purpose of labelling oxytocin preparations, 1 mg of oxytocin peptide ($C_{43}H_{66}N_{12}O_{12}S_2$) is equivalent to 600 IU of biological activity.

CHARACTERS

A clear, colourless liquid.

IDENTIFICATION

Examine the chromatograms obtained under Assay. The retention time of the principal peak in the chromatogram obtained with the test solution is similar to that of the principal peak in the chromatogram obtained with the reference solution.

TESTS

pH (2.2.3). The pH of the preparation to be examined is 3.0 to 5.0.

Amino acids. Examine by means of an amino-acid analyser. Standardise the apparatus with a mixture containing equimolar amounts of ammonia, glycine and the L-form of the following amino acids:

lysine	threonine	alanine	leucine
histidine	serine	valine	tyrosine
arginine	glutamic acid	methionine	phenylalanine
aspartic acid	proline	isoleucine	

together with half the equimolar amount of L-cystine. For the validation of the method, an appropriate internal standard, such as DL-*norleucine R*, is used.

Test solution. Place a volume of the preparation to be examined containing 0.25 mg of peptide in a rigorously cleaned hard-glass tube 100 mm long and 6 mm in internal diameter. Evaporate to dryness. Add a suitable amount of a 50 per cent *V/V* solution of *hydrochloric acid R*. Immerse the tube in a freezing mixture at −5 °C, reduce the pressure to below 133 Pa and seal. Heat at 110 °C to 115 °C for 16 h. Cool, open the tube, transfer the contents to a 10 ml flask with the aid of five quantities, each of 0.2 ml, of *water R* and evaporate to dryness over *potassium hydroxide R* under reduced pressure. Take up the residue in *water R* and evaporate to dryness over *potassium hydroxide R* under reduced pressure; repeat these operations once. Take up the residue in a buffer solution suitable for the amino-acid analyser used and dilute to a suitable volume with the same buffer solution.

Apply to the amino-acid analyser a suitable, accurately measured volume of the test solution such that the peak given by the amino acid present in the largest amount occupies most of the available chart height of the recorder.

Express the content of each amino acid in moles. Calculate the relative proportions of the amino acids taking one sixth of the sum of the number of moles of aspartic acid, glutamic acid, proline, glycine, isoleucine and leucine as equal to 1. The values fall within the following limits: aspartic acid 0.95 to 1.05; glutamic acid 0.95 to 1.05; proline 0.95 to 1.05; glycine 0.95 to 1.05; leucine 0.90 to 1.10; isoleucine 0.90 to 1.10; tyrosine 0.7 to 1.05; half cystine 1.4 to 2.1; not more than traces of other amino acids are present.

Related peptides. Examine by liquid chromatography (*2.2.29*) as described under Assay.

Inject 50 µl of the test solution. In the chromatogram obtained, the area of any peak apart from the principal peak is not greater than 1.5 per cent of the total area of the peaks; the sum of the areas of all peaks, apart from the principal peak, is not greater than 5 per cent of the total area of the peaks. Disregard any peak due to the solvent or to the antimicrobial preservative and any peak with an area less than 0.1 per cent of that of the principal peak.

Sterility (*2.6.1*). If intended for use in the manufacture of parenteral dosage forms without a further appropriate sterilisation procedure, it complies with the test for sterility.

Bacterial endotoxins (*2.6.14*): less than 300 IU in the volume that contains 1 mg of oxytocin, if intended for use in the manufacture of parenteral dosage forms without a further appropriate procedure for the removal of bacterial endotoxins.

ASSAY

Examine by liquid chromatography (*2.2.29*).

Test solution. Use the preparation to be examined.

Reference solution. Dissolve the contents of a vial of *oxytocin CRS* in a 15.6 g/l solution of *sodium dihydrogen phosphate R* to obtain a concentration of 0.25 mg/ml.

Resolution solution. Dissolve the contents of a vial of *oxytocin/desmopressin validation mixture CRS* with 500 µl of a 15.6 g/l solution of *sodium dihydrogen phosphate R*.

The chromatographic procedure may be carried out using:

— a stainless steel column 0.125 m long and 4.6 mm in internal diameter packed with *octadecylsilyl silica gel for chromatography R* (5 µm),

— as mobile phases at a flow rate of 1 ml/min:

   Mobile phase A. A 15.6 g/l solution of *sodium dihydrogen phosphate R*,

   Mobile phase B. Mix 1 volume of *acetonitrile for chromatography R* with 1 volume of *water R*,

Time (min)	Mobile phase A (per cent *V/V*)	Mobile phase B (per cent *V/V*)	Comment
0 - 30	70 → 40	30 → 60	linear gradient
30 - 30.1	40 → 70	60 → 30	return to initial conditions
30.1 - 45	70	30	re-equilibration

— as detector a spectrophotometer set at 220 nm.

Equilibrate the column with a mixture of 30 volumes of mobile phase B and 70 volumes of mobile phase A.

Inject 25 µl of the resolution solution. When the chromatograms are recorded in the prescribed conditions, the retention times are: oxytocin about 7.5 min and desmopressin about 10 min. The test is not valid unless the resolution between the desmopressin peak and the oxytocin peak is at least 5.0.

Inject 25 µl of the reference solution and 25 µl of the test solution. Calculate the content of oxytocin ($C_{43}H_{66}N_{12}O_{12}S_2$) from the peak areas in the chromatograms obtained with the test solution and the reference solution and the declared content of $C_{43}H_{66}N_{12}O_{12}S_2$ in *oxytocin CRS*.

STORAGE

Store at a temperature between 2 °C and 8 °C, protected from light. If the substance is sterile, store in a sterile, airtight, tamper-proof container.

LABELLING

The label states:

— the oxytocin peptide content in milligrams of $C_{43}H_{66}N_{12}O_{12}S_2$ per millilitre,

— where applicable, that the preparation is sterile,

— where applicable, that the preparation is free from bacterial endotoxins,

— the name of any added antimicrobial preservative.

P

04/2003:0049

PARACETAMOL

Paracetamolum

$C_8H_9NO_2$ M_r 151.2

DEFINITION

N-(4-Hydroxyphenyl)acetamide.

Content: 99.0 per cent to 101.0 per cent (dried substance).

CHARACTERS

Appearance: white, crystalline powder.

Solubility: sparingly soluble in water, freely soluble in alcohol, very slightly soluble in methylene chloride.

IDENTIFICATION

First identification: A, C.

Second identification: A, B, D, E.

A. Melting point (*2.2.14*): 168 °C to 172 °C.

B. Dissolve 0.1 g in *methanol R* and dilute to 100.0 ml with the same solvent. To 1.0 ml of the solution add 0.5 ml of a 10.3 g/l solution of *hydrochloric acid R* and dilute to 100.0 ml with *methanol R*. Protect the solution from bright light and immediately measure the absorbance (*2.2.25*) at the absorption maximum at 249 nm. The specific absorbance at the maximum is 860 to 980.

C. Infrared absorption spectrophotometry (*2.2.24*).

Preparation: discs.

Comparison: paracetamol CRS.

D. To 0.1 g add 1 ml of *hydrochloric acid R*, heat to boiling for 3 min, add 1 ml of *water R* and cool in an ice bath. No precipitate is formed. Add 0.05 ml of a 4.9 g/l solution of *potassium dichromate R*. A violet colour develops which does not change to red.

E. It gives the reaction of acetyl (*2.3.1*). Heat over a naked flame.

TESTS

Related substances. Liquid chromatography (*2.2.29*).

Prepare the solutions immediately before use.

Test solution. Dissolve 0.200 g of the substance to be examined in 2.5 ml of *methanol R* containing 4.6 g/l of a 400 g/l solution of *tetrabutylammonium hydroxide R* and dilute to 10.0 ml with a mixture of equal volumes of a 17.9 g/l solution of *disodium hydrogen phosphate R* and of a 7.8 g/l solution of *sodium dihydrogen phosphate R*.

Reference solution (a). Dilute 1.0 ml of the test solution to 50.0 ml with the mobile phase. Dilute 5.0 ml of this solution to 100.0 ml with the mobile phase.

Reference solution (b). Dilute 1.0 ml of reference solution (a) to 10.0 ml with the mobile phase.

The following chromatogram is published for information.

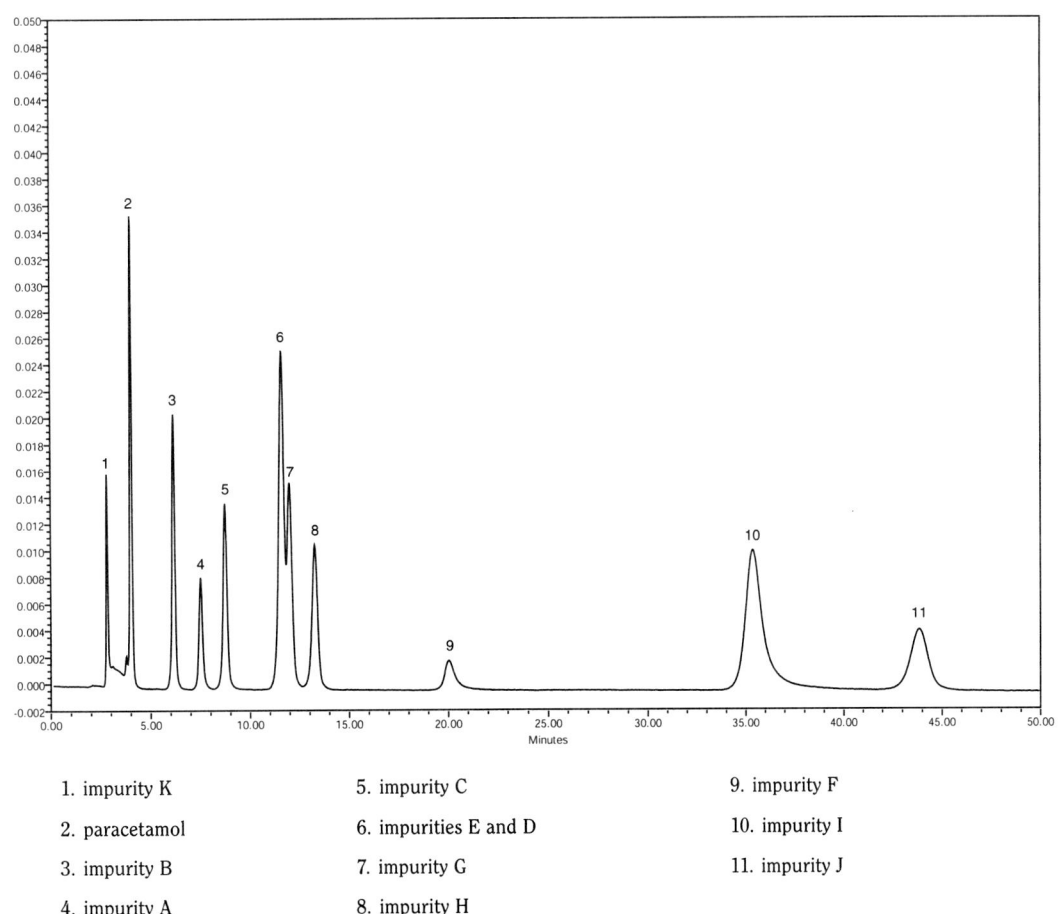

1. impurity K
2. paracetamol
3. impurity B
4. impurity A
5. impurity C
6. impurities E and D
7. impurity G
8. impurity H
9. impurity F
10. impurity I
11. impurity J

Figure 0049.-1. – *Chromatogram for the test for related substances: paracetamol solution spiked with the impurities*

Reference solution (c). Dissolve 5.0 mg of *4-aminophenol R*, 5 mg of *paracetamol CRS* and 5.0 mg of *chloroacetanilide R* in *methanol R* and dilute to 20.0 ml with the same solvent. Dilute 1.0 ml to 250.0 ml with the mobile phase.

Reference solution (d). Dissolve 20.0 mg of *4-nitrophenol R* in *methanol R* and dilute to 50.0 ml with the same solvent. Dilute 1.0 ml to 20.0 ml with the mobile phase.

Column:

– *size*: l = 0.25 m, $\varnothing$ = 4.6 mm,

– *stationary phase*: *octylsilyl silica gel for chromatography R* (5 μm),

– *temperature*: 35 °C.

Mobile phase: mix 375 volumes of a 17.9 g/l solution of *disodium hydrogen phosphate R*, 375 volumes of a 7.8 g/l solution of *sodium dihydrogen phosphate R* and 250 volumes of *methanol R* containing 4.6 g/l of a 400 g/l solution of *tetrabutylammonium hydroxide R*.

Flow rate: 1.5 ml/min.

Detection: spectrophotometer at 245 nm.

Injection: 20 μl.

Run time: 12 times the retention time of paracetamol.

Relative retentions with reference to paracetamol (retention time = about 4 min): impurity K = about 0.8; impurity F = about 3; impurity J = about 7.

System suitability: reference solution (c):

– *resolution*: minimum 4.0 between the peaks due to impurity K and to paracetamol,

– *signal-to-noise ratio*: minimum 50 for the peak due to impurity J.

Limits:

– *impurity J*: not more than 0.2 times the area of the corresponding peak in the chromatogram obtained with reference solution (c) (10 ppm),

– *impurity K*: not more than the area of the corresponding peak in the chromatogram obtained with reference solution (c) (50 ppm),

– *impurity F*: not more than half the area of the corresponding peak in the chromatogram obtained with reference solution (d) (0.05 per cent),

– *any other impurity*: not more than half the area of the principal peak in the chromatogram obtained with reference solution (a) (0.05 per cent),

– *total of other impurities*: not more than the area of the principal peak in the chromatogram obtained with reference solution (a) (0.1 per cent),

– *disregard limit* for the calculation of the total of other impurities: the area of the principal peak in the chromatogram obtained with reference solution (b) (0.01 per cent).

Heavy metals (*2.4.8*): maximum 20 ppm.

Dissolve 1.0 g in a mixture of 15 volumes of *water R* and 85 volumes of *acetone R* and dilute to 20 ml with the same mixture of solvents. 12 ml of the solution complies with limit test B. Prepare the standard using lead standard solution (1 ppm Pb) obtained by diluting *lead standard solution (100 ppm Pb) R* with a mixture of 15 volumes of *water R* and 85 volumes of *acetone R*.

Loss on drying (*2.2.32*): maximum 0.5 per cent, determined on 1.000 g by drying in an oven at 100-105 °C.

Sulphated ash (*2.4.14*): maximum 0.1 per cent, determined on 1.0 g.

ASSAY

Dissolve 0.300 g in a mixture of 10 ml of *water R* and 30 ml of *dilute sulphuric acid R*. Boil under a reflux condenser for 1 h, cool and dilute to 100.0 ml with *water R*. To 20.0 ml of the solution add 40 ml of *water R*, 40 g of ice, 15 ml of *dilute hydrochloric acid R* and 0.1 ml of *ferroin R*. Titrate with *0.1 M cerium sulphate* until a greenish-yellow colour is obtained. Carry out a blank titration.

1 ml of *0.1 M cerium sulphate* is equivalent to 7.56 mg of $C_8H_9NO_2$.

STORAGE

Protected from light.

IMPURITIES

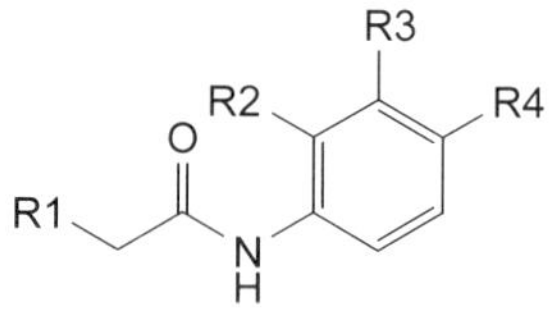

A. R1 = R3 = R4 = H, R2 = OH: *N*-(2-hydroxyphenyl)acetamide,

B. R1 = CH$_3$, R2 = R3 = H, R4 = OH: *N*-(4-hydroxyphenyl)propanamide,

C. R1 = R2 = H, R3 = Cl, R4 = OH: *N*-(3-chloro-4-hydroxyphenyl)acetamide,

D. R1 = R2 = R3 = R4 = H: *N*-phenylacetamide,

H. R1 = R2 = R3 = H, R4 = O-CO-CH$_3$: 4-(acetylamino)phenyl acetate,

J. R1 = R2 = R3 = H, R4 = Cl: *N*-(4-chlorophenyl)acetamide (chloroacetanilide),

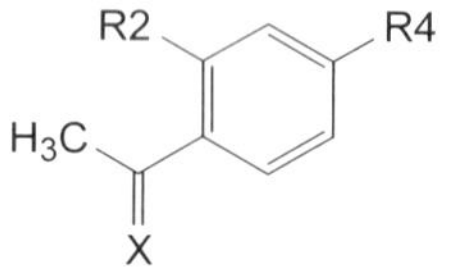

E. X = O, R2 = H, R4 = OH: 1-(4-hydroxyphenyl)ethanone,

G. X = N-OH, R2 = H, R4 = OH: 1-(4-hydroxyphenyl)ethanone oxime,

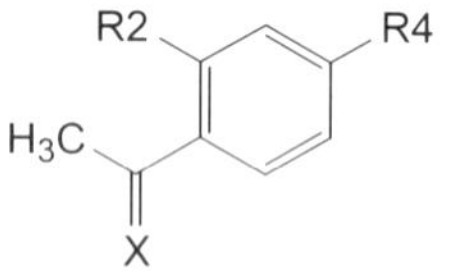

I. X = O, R2 = OH, R4 = H: 1-(2-hydroxyphenyl)ethanone,

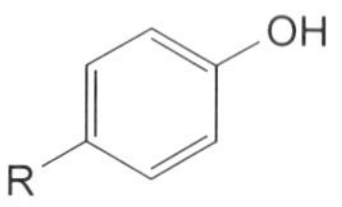

F. R = NO$_2$: 4-nitrophenol,

K. R = NH$_2$: 4-aminophenol.

04/2003:1621

PENTOXYVERINE HYDROGEN CITRATE

Pentoxyverini hydrogenocitras

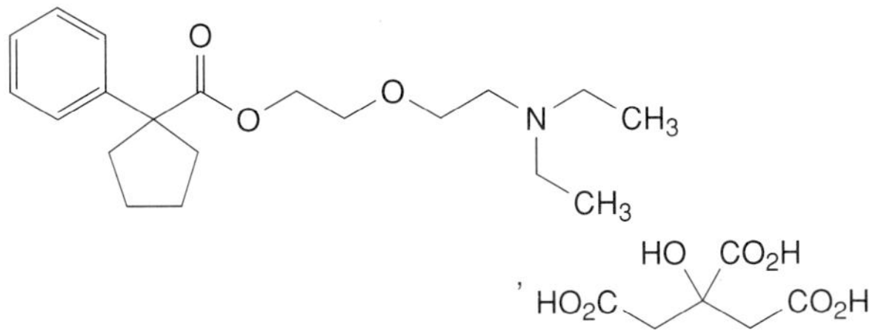

$C_{26}H_{39}NO_{10}$ M_r 525.6

DEFINITION

2-[2-(Diethylamino)ethoxy]ethyl 1-phenylcyclopentanecarboxylate dihydrogen 2-hydroxypropane-1,2,3-tricarboxylate.

Content: 98.5 per cent to 101.0 per cent (dried substance).

CHARACTERS

Appearance: white or almost white, crystalline powder.

Solubility: freely soluble in water, very soluble in glacial acetic acid, freely soluble in methanol, soluble in alcohol and in methylene chloride.

mp: about 93 °C.

IDENTIFICATION

A. Infrared absorption spectrophotometry (2.2.24).

Comparison: Ph. Eur. reference spectrum of pentoxyverine hydrogen citrate.

B. Dissolve 0.25 g in 5 ml of water R. The solution gives the reaction of citrates (2.3.1).

TESTS

Solution S. Dissolve 5.0 g in carbon dioxide-free water R and dilute to 50 ml with the same solvent.

Appearance of solution. Solution S is clear (2.2.1) and not more intensely coloured than reference solution Y_6 (2.2.2, Method II).

pH (2.2.3): 3.3 to 3.7 for solution S.

Related substances. Liquid chromatography (2.2.29).

Test solution. Dissolve 25.0 mg of the substance to be examined in the mobile phase and dilute to 25.0 ml with the mobile phase.

Reference solution. Introduce 5.0 mg of pentoxyverine impurity A CRS and 5.0 mg of pentoxyverine impurity B CRS in a conical flask, add 5.0 ml of the test solution and dilute to 100.0 ml with the mobile phase. Dilute 3.0 ml of the solution to 50.0 ml with the mobile phase.

Column:

— size: l = 0.15 m, Ø = 3.9 mm,

— stationary phase: end-capped octylsilyl silica gel for chromatography R (5 µm) with a pore size of 10 nm and a carbon loading of 12 per cent,

— temperature: 50 °C.

Mobile phase: mix 35 volumes of acetonitrile R and 65 volumes of a 0.15 per cent (m/V) solution of sodium heptanesulphonate R adjusted to pH 3.0 with dilute sulphuric acid R.

Flow rate: 1.0 ml/min.

Detection: spectrophotometer at 205 nm.

Injection: 20 µl.

Run time: 3 times the retention time of pentoxyverine.

Relative retention with reference to pentoxyverine (retention time = about 6 min): impurity B = about 0.8; impurity A = about 1.5.

System suitability: reference solution:

— resolution: minimum of 5.0 between the peaks due to pentoxyverine and to impurity A,

— signal-to-noise ratio: minimum of 100 for the peak due to pentoxyverine,

— symmetry factor: maximum of 2.0 for the peak due to pentoxyverine.

Limits:

— impurity A: not more than the area of the corresponding peak in the chromatogram obtained with the reference solution (0.3 per cent),

— impurity B: not more than the area of the corresponding peak in the chromatogram obtained with the reference solution (0.3 per cent),

— any other impurity: not more than one-third of the area of the peak due to pentoxyverine in the chromatogram obtained with the reference solution (0.1 per cent),

— total of any other impurity: not more than the area of the peak due to pentoxyverine in the chromatogram obtained with the reference solution (0.3 per cent),

— disregard limit: 0.1 times the area of the peak due to pentoxyverine in the chromatogram obtained with the reference solution (0.03 per cent); disregard any peak with a retention time less than or equal to 2.5 min.

Loss on drying (2.2.32): maximum 0.5 per cent, determined on 1.000 g by drying in vacuo at 60 °C for 4 h.

Sulphated ash (2.4.14): maximum 0.1 per cent, determined on 1.0 g.

ASSAY

Dissolve 0.400 g in 70 ml of anhydrous acetic acid R. Titrate with 0.1 M perchloric acid, determining the end-point potentiometrically (2.2.20).

1 ml of 0.1 M perchloric acid is equivalent to 52.56 mg of $C_{26}H_{39}NO_{10}$.

STORAGE

Protected from light.

IMPURITIES

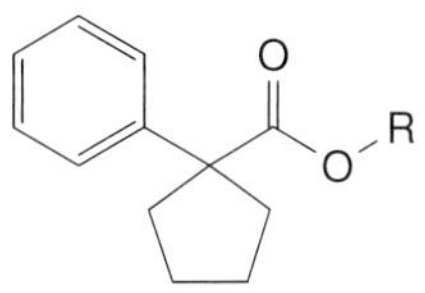

A. R = H: 1-phenylcyclopentanecarboxylic acid,

B. R = CH_2-CH_2-N(CH_2-CH_3)$_2$: 2-(diethylamino)ethyl 1-phenylcyclopentanecarboxylate (caramiphen).

04/2003:0422

PHENYLBUTAZONE

Phenylbutazonum

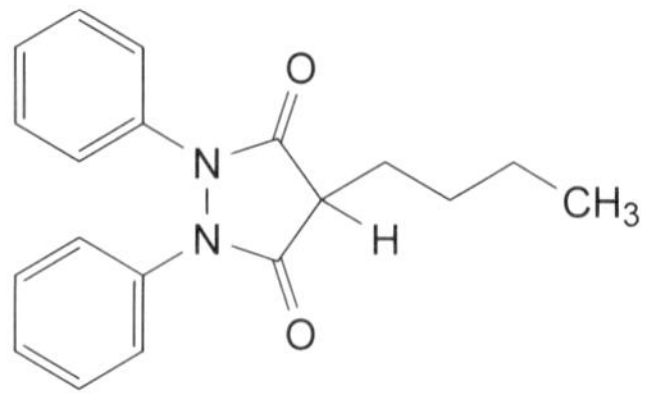

$C_{19}H_{20}N_2O_2$ M_r 308.4

DEFINITION

4-Butyl-1,2-diphenylpyrazolidine-3,5-dione.

Content: 99.0 per cent to 101.0 per cent (dried substance).

CHARACTERS

Appearance: white or almost white, crystalline powder.

Solubility: practically insoluble in water, sparingly soluble in alcohol. It dissolves in alkaline solutions.

IDENTIFICATION

First identification: A, C.

Second identification: A, B, D.

A. Melting point (*2.2.14*): 104 °C to 107 °C.

B. Thin-layer chromatography (*2.2.27*).

Test solution. Dissolve 25 mg of the substance to be examined in a mixture of equal volumes of *ethanol R* and *methylene chloride R* and dilute to 25 ml with the same mixture of solvents.

Reference solution. Dissolve 25 mg of *phenylbutazone CRS* in a mixture of equal volumes of *ethanol R* and *methylene chloride R* and dilute to 25 ml with the same mixture of solvents.

Plate: TLC silica gel GF$_{254}$ plate R.

Mobile phase: acetone R, methylene chloride R (20:80 V/V).

Application: 5 µl.

Development: over a path of 10 cm.

Drying: in air.

Detection: examine in ultraviolet light at 254 nm.

Results: the principal spot in the chromatogram obtained with the test solution is similar in position and size to the principal spot in the chromatogram obtained with the reference solution.

C. Infrared absorption spectrophotometry (*2.2.24*).

Comparison: phenylbutazone CRS.

D. To 0.1 g add 1 ml of *glacial acetic acid R* and 2 ml of *hydrochloric acid R* and heat the mixture under a reflux condenser for 30 min. Cool, add 10 ml of *water R* and filter. To the filtrate add 3 ml of a 7 g/l solution of *sodium nitrite R*. A yellow colour is produced. To 1 ml of the solution add a solution of 10 mg of *β-naphthol R* in 5 ml of *sodium carbonate solution R*. A brownish-red to violet-red precipitate is formed.

TESTS

Solution S. Dissolve 1.0 g with shaking in 20 ml of *dilute sodium hydroxide solution R* and maintain the solution at 25 °C for 3 h.

Appearance of solution. Solution S is clear (*2.2.1*).

Acidity or alkalinity. Heat to boiling 1.0 g in 50 ml of *water R*, cool with shaking in a closed flask and filter. To 25 ml of the filtrate add 0.5 ml of *phenolphthalein solution R*. The solution is colourless. Not more than 0.5 ml of *0.01 M sodium hydroxide* is required to change the colour of the indicator. Add 0.6 ml of *0.01 M hydrochloric acid* and 0.1 ml of *methyl red solution R*; the solution is red or orange.

Absorbance (*2.2.25*): maximum 0.20 for solution S at 420 nm in a 4 cm cell.

Related substances. Liquid chromatography (*2.2.29*). *Prepare the solutions immediately before use.*

Test solution. Dissolve 100.0 mg of the substance to be examined in *acetonitrile R* and dilute to 10.0 ml with the same solvent.

Reference solution (a). Dilute 1.0 ml of the test solution to 100.0 ml with *acetonitrile R*. Dilute 1.0 ml to 10.0 ml with *acetonitrile R*.

Reference solution (b). Dissolve 5 mg of *phenylbutazone impurity B CRS* and 5 mg of *1,2-diphenylhydrazine R* in *acetonitrile R*, add 0.5 ml of the test solution and dilute to 50 ml with *acetonitrile R*. Dilute 2.5 ml to 10 ml with *acetonitrile R*.

Reference solution (c). Dissolve 1.0 mg of *benzidine R* in *acetonitrile R* and dilute to 100.0 ml with the same solvent. Dilute 1.0 ml to 100.0 ml with *acetonitrile R*. Dilute 5.0 ml to 10.0 ml with *acetonitrile R*.

Column:

— *size*: l = 0.125 m, Ø = 4.0 mm,

— *stationary phase*: octadecylsilyl silica gel for chromatography R (5 µm),

— *temperature*: 30 °C.

Mobile phase:

— *mobile phase A*: dissolve 1.36 g of *sodium acetate R* in *water R*, adjust to pH 5.2 with a 52.5 g/l solution of *citric acid R* and dilute to 1000 ml with *water R*,

— *mobile phase B*: acetonitrile R,

Time (min)	Mobile phase A (per cent *V/V*)	Mobile phase B (per cent *V/V*)
0 - 10	70	30
10 - 20	70 → 40	30 → 60
20 - 35	40	60
35 - 40	40 → 70	60 → 30

Flow rate: 1.5 ml/min.

Detection: spectrophotometer at 240 nm.

Injection: 20 µl; inject the test solution and reference solutions (a) and (b).

Relative retentions with reference to phenylbutazone (retention time = about 13 min): impurity E = about 0.2; impurity A = about 0.5; impurity B = about 1.2; impurity C = about 1.3; impurity D = about 1.7.

System suitability: reference solution (b):

— *resolution*: minimum 2.0 between the peaks due to phenylbutazone and to impurity B.

Limits:

— *correction factor*: for the calculation of content, multiply the peak area of impurity C by 0.55,

— *impurity A or B*: for each impurity, not more than 2.5 times the area of the principal peak in the chromatogram obtained with reference solution (a) (0.25 per cent),

The following chromatogram is published for information.

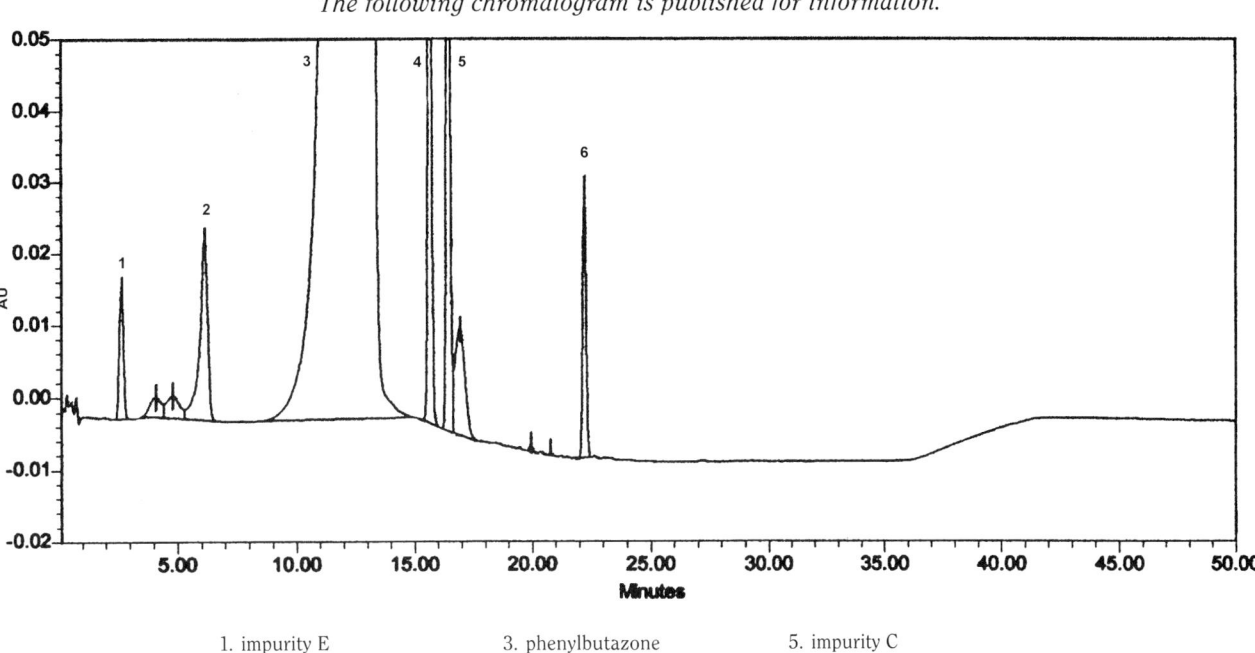

Figure 0422.-1. – *Chromatogram for the test for related substances of phenylbutazone: test solution spiked with the impurities*

1. impurity E   3. phenylbutazone   5. impurity C

2. impurity A   4. impurity B   6. impurity D

— *impurity C*: not more than twice the area of the principal peak in the chromatogram obtained with reference solution (a) (0.20 per cent),

— *any other impurity*: not more than the area of the principal peak in the chromatogram obtained with reference solution (a) (0.1 per cent),

— *total*: not more than 5 times the area of the principal peak in the chromatogram obtained with reference solution (a) (0.5 per cent),

— *disregard limit*: 0.25 times the area of the principal peak in the chromatogram obtained with reference solution (a) (0.025 per cent); disregard any peak due to impurity E.

Impurity E. Liquid chromatography (*2.2.29*) as described in the test for related substances with the following modifications.

Detection: spectrophotometer at 280 nm.

Injection: test solution and reference solution (c).

System suitability: reference solution (c):

— *signal-to-noise ratio*: minimum 10 for the principal peak.

Limit:

— *impurity E*: not more than the area of the principal peak in the chromatogram obtained with reference solution (c) (5 ppm).

Heavy metals (*2.4.8*): maximum 20 ppm.

1.0 g complies with limit test C. Prepare the standard using 2 ml of *lead standard solution (10 ppm Pb) R*.

Loss on drying (*2.2.32*): maximum 0.2 per cent, determined on 1.000 g by drying *in vacuo* at 80 °C for 4 h.

Sulphated ash (*2.4.14*): maximum 0.1 per cent, determined on 1.0 g.

ASSAY

Dissolve 0.250 g in 25 ml of *acetone R* and add 0.5 ml of *bromothymol blue solution R1*. Titrate with *0.1 M sodium hydroxide* until a blue colour is obtained which persists for 15 s. Carry out a blank titration.

1 ml of *0.1 M sodium hydroxide* is equivalent to 30.84 mg of $C_{19}H_{20}N_2O_2$.

STORAGE

Protected from light.

IMPURITIES

A. (2RS)-2-[(1,2-diphenyldiazanyl)carbonyl]hexanoic acid,

B. 4-butyl-4-hydroxy-1,2-diphenylpyrazolidine-3,5-dione,

C. C_6H_5-NH-NH-C_6H_5: 1,2-diphenyldiazane, (1,2-diphenylhydrazine),

D. C_6H_5-N=N-C_6H_5: 1,2-diphenyldiazene,

E. biphenyl-4,4′-diamine (benzidine).

04/2003:2042

PHENYLMERCURIC ACETATE

Phenylhydrargyri acetas

$C_8H_8HgO_2$ M_r 336.7

DEFINITION

Content: 98.0 per cent to 100.5 per cent (dried substance).

CHARACTERS

Appearance: white or yellowish, crystalline powder or small, colourless crystals.

Solubility: slightly soluble in water, soluble in acetone and in alcohol.

IDENTIFICATION

First identification: A.

Second identification: B, C.

A. Infrared absorption spectrophotometry (*2.2.24*).

   Comparison: Ph. Eur. reference spectrum of phenylmercuric acetate.

B. To 5 ml of solution S (see Tests) add 5 ml of *water R* and 0.1 ml of *sodium sulphide solution R*. A white precipitate is formed that darkens slowly on heating.

C. To 10 ml of solution S add 2 ml of *potassium iodide solution R* and shake vigorously. Filter. The filtrate gives reaction (b) of acetates (*2.3.1*).

TESTS

Solution S. Dissolve 0.250 g in 40 ml of *water R* by heating to boiling. Allow to cool and dilute to 50 ml with *water R*. Prepare the solution immediately before use.

Appearance of solution. Solution S is not more opalescent than reference suspension II (*2.2.1*) and is colourless (*2.2.2, Method II*).

Ionised mercury: maximum 0.2 per cent.

To 2 ml of solution S add 8 ml of *water R*, 2 ml of *potassium iodide solution R* and 3 ml of *dilute hydrochloric acid R*. Filter. The filtrate is not more coloured than the potassium iodide solution used. Wash the precipitate with 3 ml of *water R*. Combine the filtrate and the washings, add 2 ml of *dilute sodium hydroxide solution R* and dilute to 20 ml with *water R*. 12 ml of this solution complies with limit test A for heavy metals (*2.4.8*). Prepare the standard using *lead standard solution (1 ppm Pb) R*.

Polymercuric benzene compounds: maximum 1.5 per cent.

Shake 0.2 g with 10 ml of *acetone R*. Filter. Wash the residue twice with 5 ml of *acetone R*. Dry the residue at 105 °C for 1 h. The residue weighs a maximum of 3 mg.

Loss on drying (*2.2.32*): maximum 0.5 per cent, determined on 0.500 g by drying in an oven at 45 °C for 15 h.

ASSAY

Dissolve with heating 0.300 g in 100 ml of *water R*. Cool and add 3 ml of *nitric acid R*. Titrate with *0.1 M ammonium thiocyanate* using 2 ml of *ferric ammonium sulphate solution R2* as indicator, until a persistent reddish-yellow colour is obtained.

1 ml of *0.1 M ammonium thiocyanate* is equivalent to 33.67 mg of phenylmercuric acetate.

STORAGE

Protected from light.

07/2002:1140
corrected

POTASSIUM CLAVULANATE

Kalii clavulanas

$C_8H_8KNO_5$ M_r 237.3

DEFINITION

Potassium (2R,3Z,5R)-3-(2-hydroxyethylidene)-7-oxo-4-oxa-1-azabicyclo[3.2.0]heptane-2-carboxylate, the potassium salt of a substance produced by the growth of certain strains of *Streptomyces clavuligerus* or obtained by any other means.

Content: 96.5 per cent to 102.0 per cent (anhydrous substance).

CHARACTERS

Appearance: white or almost white, crystalline powder, hygroscopic.

Solubility: freely soluble in water, slightly soluble in alcohol, very slightly soluble in acetone.

PRODUCTION

The method of production, extraction and purification are such that clavam-2-carboxylate is eliminated or present at a level not exceeding 0.01 per cent.

IDENTIFICATION

A. Infrared absorption spectrophotometry (*2.2.24*).

   Comparison: Ph. Eur. reference spectrum of potassium clavulanate.

B. It gives reaction (b) of potassium (*2.3.1*).

TESTS

Solution S. Dissolve 0.400 g in *carbon dioxide-free water R* and dilute to 20.0 ml with the same solvent.

pH (*2.2.3*): 5.5 to 8.0.

Dilute 5 ml of solution S in *carbon dioxide-free water R* and dilute to 10 ml with the same solvent.

Specific optical rotation (*2.2.7*): + 53 to + 63 (anhydrous substance), determined on solution S.

Absorbance (*2.2.25*): maximum 0.40 at 278 nm.

Dissolve 50.0 mg in *0.1 M phosphate buffer solution pH 7.0 R* and dilute to 50.0 ml with the same solution. Measure immediately the absorbance of this solution.

Related substances. Liquid chromatography (*2.2.29*). *Prepare the solutions immediately before use.*

Test solution. Dissolve 0.250 g of the substance to be examined in mobile phase A and dilute to 25.0 ml with mobile phase A.

Reference solution (a). Dilute 1.0 ml of the test solution to 100.0 ml with mobile phase A.

Reference solution (b). Dissolve 10 mg of *lithium clavulanate CRS* and 10 mg of *amoxicillin trihydrate CRS* in mobile phase A and dilute to 100 ml with mobile phase A.

Column:

- *size: l* = 0.10 m, Ø = 4.6 mm,
- *stationary phase: octadecylsilyl silica gel for chromatography R* (5 µm),
- *temperature:* 40 °C.

Mobile phase:

- *mobile phase A*: a 7.8 g/l solution of *sodium dihydrogen phosphate R* adjusted to pH 4.0 with *phosphoric acid R* and filtered through a 0.5 µm filter,
- *mobile phase B*: a mixture of equal volumes of mobile phase A and *methanol R*,

Time (min)	Mobile phase A (per cent *V/V*)	Mobile phase B (per cent *V/V*)
0 - 4	100	0
4 - 15	100 → 50	0 → 50
15 - 18	50	50
18 - 24	50 → 100	50 → 0
24 - 39	100	0

Flow rate: 1 ml/min.

Detection: spectrophotometer at 230 nm.

Injection: 20 µl.

System suitability: reference solution (b):

- *resolution:* minimum 13 between the first peak (clavulanate) and the second peak (amoxicillin).

Limits:

- *any impurity:* not more than the area of the principal peak in the chromatogram obtained with reference solution (a) (1.0 per cent),
- *total:* not more than twice the area of the principal peak in the chromatogram obtained with reference solution (a) (2.0 per cent),
- *disregard limit:* 0.05 times the area of the principal peak in the chromatogram obtained with reference solution (a) (0.05 per cent).

Aliphatic amines. Gas chromatography (*2.2.28*).

The method shown below can be used to determine the following aliphatic amines: 1,1-dimethylethylamine; diethylamine; *N,N,N´,N´*-tetramethylethylenediamine; 1,1,3,3-tetramethylbutylamine; *N,N´*-diisopropylethylenediamine; 2,2´-oxydi(*N,N*)dimethylethylamine.

Internal standard solution: dissolve 50 µl of *3-methylpentan-2-one R* in *water R* and dilute to 100.0 ml with the same solvent.

Test solution. Weigh 1.00 g of the substance to be examined into a centrifuge tube. Add 5.0 ml of the internal standard solution, 5.0 ml of *dilute sodium hydroxide solution R*, 10.0 ml of *water R*, 5.0 ml of *2-methylpropanol R* and 5 g of *sodium chloride R*. Shake vigorously for 1 min. Centrifuge to separate the layers.

Reference solution. Dissolve 80.0 mg of each of the following amines *1,1-dimethylethylamine R*; *diethylamine R*; *tetramethylethylenediamine R*; *1,1,3,3-tetramethylbutylamine R*; *N,N´-diisopropylethylenediamine R* and *2,2´-oxybis(N,N-dimethylethylamine) R* in *dilute hydrochloric acid R* and dilute to 200.0 ml with the same acid. Introduce 5.0 ml of this solution into a centrifuge tube. Add 5.0 ml of the internal standard solution, 10.0 ml of *dilute

sodium hydroxide solution R*, 5.0 ml of *2-methylpropanol R* and 5 g of *sodium chloride R*. Shake vigorously for 1 min. Centrifuge to separate the layers.

Column:

- *material:* fused silica,
- *size: l* = 50 m, Ø = 0.53 mm,
- *stationary phase: poly(dimethyl)(diphenyl)siloxane R* (film thickness 5 µm).

Carrier gas: helium for chromatography R.

Flow rate: 8 ml/min.

Split ratio: 1:10.

Temperature:

	Time (min)	Temperature (°C)
Column	0 - 7	35
	7 - 10.8	35 → 150
	10.8 - 25.8	150
Injection port		200
Detector		250

Detection: flame ionisation.

Injection: 1 µl of the upper layers obtained from test solution and reference solution.

Relative retention with reference to 3-methylpentan-2-one (retention time = about 11.4 min): impurity H = about 0.55; impurity I = about 0.76; impurity J = about 1.07; impurity K = about 1.13; impurity L = about 1.33; impurity M = about 1.57.

Limit:

- *aliphatic amines:* maximum 0.2 per cent.

2-Ethylhexanoic acid (*2.4.28*): maximum 0.8 per cent.

Water (*2.5.12*): maximum 0.5 per cent, determined on 1.00 g.

Sterility (*2.6.1*). If intended for use in the manufacture of parenteral dosage forms without a further appropriate sterilisation procedure, it complies with the test for sterility.

Bacterial endotoxins (*2.6.14*): less than 0.03 IU/mg if intended for use in the manufacture of parenteral dosage forms without a further appropriate procedure for the removal of bacterial endotoxins.

ASSAY

Liquid chromatography (*2.2.29*). *Prepare the solutions immediately before use.*

Test solution. Dissolve 50.0 mg of the substance to be examined in a 4.1 g/l solution of *sodium acetate R* previously adjusted to pH 6.0 with *glacial acetic acid R*, and dilute to 50.0 ml with the same solution.

Reference solution (a). Dissolve 50.0 mg of *lithium clavulanate CRS* in a 4.1 g/l solution of *sodium acetate R* previously adjusted to pH 6.0 with *glacial acetic acid R* and dilute to 50.0 ml with the same solution.

Reference solution (b). Dissolve 50.0 mg of *lithium clavulanate CRS* and 50.0 mg of *amoxicillin trihydrate CRS* in a 4.1 g/l solution of *sodium acetate R* previously adjusted to pH 6.0 with *glacial acetic acid R* and dilute to 50.0 ml with the same solution.

Column:

- *size: l* = 0.3 m, Ø = 4.6 mm,
- *stationary phase: octadecylsilyl silica gel for chromatography R* (5 µm).

Mobile phase: mix 5 volumes of *methanol R1* and 95 volumes of a 15 g/l solution of *sodium dihydrogen phosphate R* previously adjusted to pH 4.0 with *dilute phosphoric acid R*,

Flow rate: 1 ml/min.

Detection: spectrophotometer at 230 nm.

Injection: 20 µl.

System suitability: reference solution (b):

— *resolution*: minimum 3.5 between the first peak (clavulanate) and the second peak (amoxicillin).

1 mg of clavulanate ($C_8H_9NO_5$) is equivalent to 1.191 mg of $C_8H_8KNO_5$.

STORAGE

In an airtight container, at a temperature of 2 °C to 8 °C. If the substance is sterile, store in a sterile, airtight, tamper-proof container.

LABELLING

The label states:

— where applicable, that the substance is sterile,

— where applicable, that the substance is free from bacterial endotoxins.

IMPURITIES

Qualified impurities: A, B, C, D, G, H, I, J, K, L, M.

Other detectable impurities: E, F.

By liquid chromatography: A, B, C, D, E, F, G.

By gas chromatography: H, I, J, K, L, M.

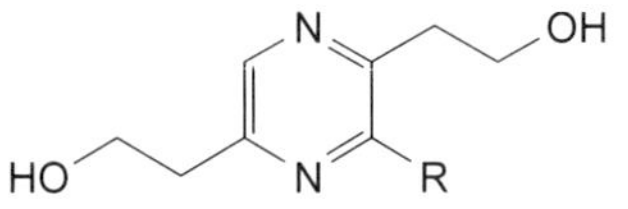

A. R = H: 2,2'-(pyrazine-2,5-diyl)diethanol,

B. R = CH_2-CH_2-CO_2H: 3-[3,6-bis(2-hydroxyethyl)pyrazin-2-yl]propanoic acid,

C. R = CH_2-CH_3: 2,2'-(3-ethylpyrazine-2,5-diyl)diethanol,

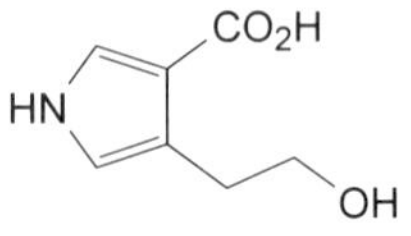

D. 4-(2-hydroxyethyl)pyrrole-3-carboxylic acid,

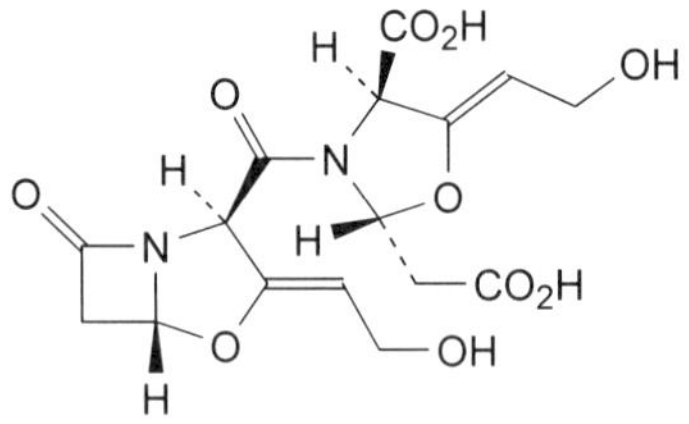

E. (2R,4R,5Z)-2-(carboxymethyl)-5-(2-hydroxyethylidene)-3-[[(2R,3Z,5R)-3-(2-hydroxyethylidene)-7-oxo-4-oxa-1-azabicyclo[3.2.0]hept-2-yl]carbonyl]oxazolidine-4-carboxylic acid,

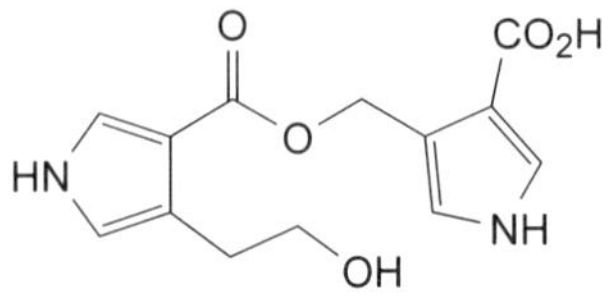

F. 4-[[[[4-(2-hydroxyethyl)-1H-pyrrol-3-yl]carbonyl]oxy]methyl]-1H-pyrrole-3-carboxylic acid,

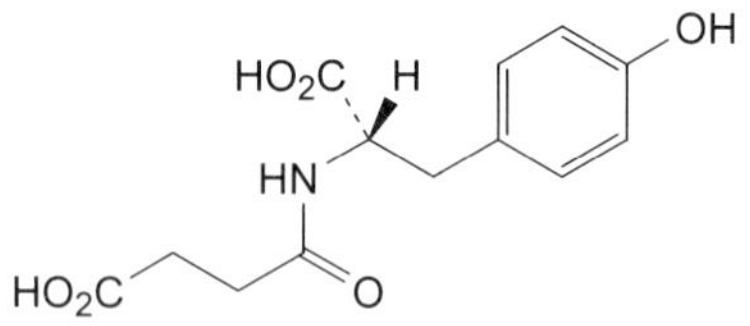

G. 4-[[(1S)-1-carboxy-2-(4-hydroxyphenyl)ethyl]amino]-4-oxobutanoic acid (N-succinyltyrosine),

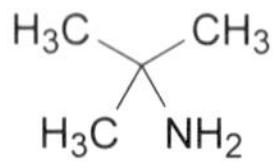

H. 2-amino-2-methylpropane (1,1-dimethylethylamine),

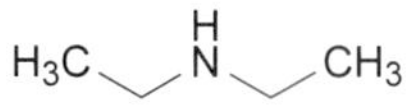

I. diethylamine,

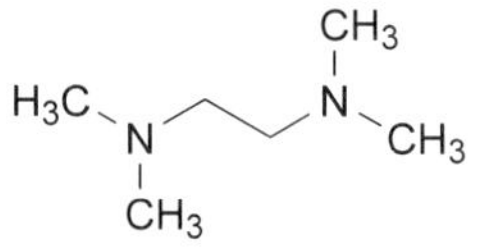

J. 1,2-bis(dimethylamino)ethane (N,N,N',N'-tetramethylethylenediamine),

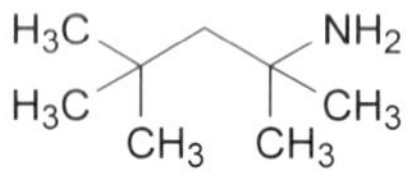

K. 2-amino-2,4,4-trimethylpentane (1,1,3,3-tetramethylbutylamine),

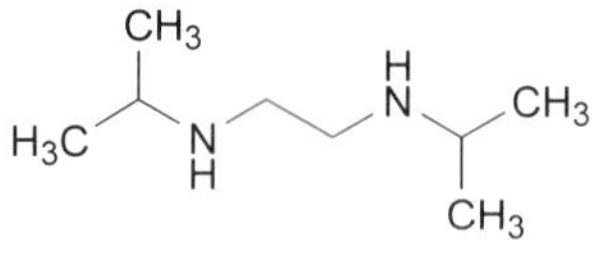

L. N,N'-bis(1-methylethyl)-1,2-ethanediamine (N,N'-diisopropylethylenediamine),

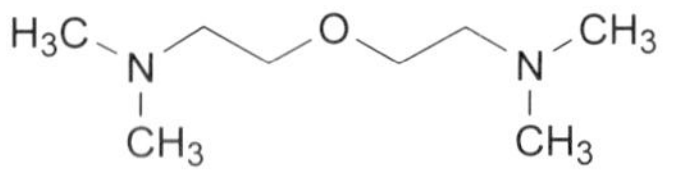

M. bis(2-dimethylamino)ethyl ether [2,2'-oxybis(N,N-dimethylethylamine)].

04/2003:1653

POTASSIUM CLAVULANATE, DILUTED

Kalii clavulanas dilutus

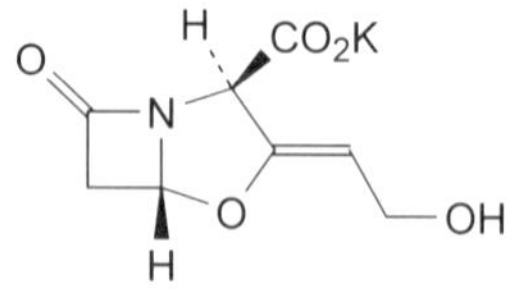

$C_8H_8KNO_5$ M_r 237.3

DEFINITION

Dry mixture of *Potassium clavulanate (1140)* and *Cellulose, microcrystalline (0316)* or *Silica, colloidal anhydrous (0434)* or *Silica, colloidal hydrated (0738)*.

Content: 91.2 per cent to 107.1 per cent of the content of potassium clavulanate stated on the label.

CHARACTERS

Appearance of diluted potassium clavulanate: white or almost white powder, hygroscopic.

Solubility of potassium clavulanate: freely soluble in water, slightly soluble in alcohol, very slightly soluble in acetone.

The solubility of the diluted product depends on the diluent and its concentration.

IDENTIFICATION

A. Examine the chromatograms obtained in the assay.

    Results: the principal peak in the chromatogram obtained with the test solution is similar in retention time to the principal peak in the chromatogram obtained with reference solution (a).

B. It gives reaction (b) of potassium (*2.3.1*).

C. Depending on the diluent used, carry out the corresponding identification test (a) or (b).

    (a) A quantity of the substance to be examined, corresponding to 20 mg of cellulose, when placed on a watch-glass and dispersed in 4 ml of *iodinated zinc chloride solution R*, becomes violet-blue.

    (b) It gives the reaction of silicates (*2.3.1*).

TESTS

pH (*2.2.3*): 4.8 to 8.0.

Suspend a quantity of the substance to be examined corresponding to 0.200 g of potassium clavulanate in 20 ml of *carbon dioxide-free water R*.

Absorbance (*2.2.25*): maximum 0.40 measured immediately at 278 nm.

Disperse a quantity of the substance to be examined corresponding to 50.0 mg of potassium clavulanate in 10 ml of *0.1 M phosphate buffer solution pH 7.0 R*, dilute to 50.0 ml with the same buffer solution and filter.

Related substances. Liquid chromatography (*2.2.29*). *Prepare the solutions immediately before use.*

Test solution. Disperse a quantity of the substance to be examined corresponding to 0.250 g of potassium clavulanate in 5 ml of mobile phase A, dilute to 25.0 ml with mobile phase A and filter.

Reference solution (a). Dilute 1.0 ml of the test solution to 100.0 ml with mobile phase A.

Reference solution (b). Dissolve 10 mg of *amoxicillin trihydrate CRS* in 1 ml of the test solution and dilute to 100 ml with mobile phase A.

Column:

— *size*: l = 0.10 m, $\emptyset$ = 4.6 mm,

— *stationary phase*: *octadecylsilyl silica gel for chromatography R* (5 µm),

— *temperature*: 40 °C.

Mobile phase:

— *mobile phase A*: 7.8 g/l solution of *sodium dihydrogen phosphate R* adjusted to pH 4.0 with *dilute phosphoric acid R*,

— *mobile phase B*: mixture of equal volumes of mobile phase A and *methanol R*,

Time (min)	Mobile phase A (per cent *V/V*)	Mobile phase B (per cent *V/V*)
0 - 4	100	0
4 - 15	100 → 50	0 → 50
15 - 18	50	50
18 - 24	50 → 100	50 → 0
24 - 39	100	0

Flow rate: 1 ml/min.

Detection: spectrophotometer at 230 nm.

Injection: 20 µl.

System suitability: reference solution (b):

— *resolution*: minimum of 13 between the peak due to clavulanate (1st peak) and the peak due to amoxicillin (2nd peak).

Limits:

— *any impurity*: not more than the area of the principal peak in the chromatogram obtained with reference solution (a) (1.0 per cent),

— *total*: not more than twice the area of the principal peak in the chromatogram obtained with reference solution (a) (2.0 per cent),

— *disregard limit*: 0.05 times the area of the principal peak in the chromatogram obtained with reference solution (a) (0.05 per cent).

Water (*2.5.12*): maximum 2.5 per cent, determined on 1.000 g.

ASSAY

Liquid chromatography (*2.2.29*). *Prepare the solutions immediately before use.*

Test solution. Disperse a quantity of the substance to be examined corresponding to 50.0 mg of potassium clavulanate in a 4.1 g/l solution of *sodium acetate R* previously adjusted to pH 6.0 with *glacial acetic acid R*, dilute to 50.0 ml with the same solution and filter.

Reference solution (a). Dissolve 50.0 mg of *lithium clavulanate CRS* in a 4.1 g/l solution of *sodium acetate R* previously adjusted to pH 6.0 with *glacial acetic acid R* and dilute to 50.0 ml with the same solution.

Reference solution (b). Dissolve 10 mg of *amoxicillin trihydrate CRS* in 10 ml of reference solution (a).

Column:

— *size*: l = 0.3 m, $\emptyset$ = 4.6 mm,

— *stationary phase*: *octadecylsilyl silica gel for chromatography R* (10 µm).

Mobile phase: mix 5 volumes of *methanol R1* and 95 volumes of a 15 g/l solution of *sodium dihydrogen phosphate R* previously adjusted to pH 4.0 with *dilute phosphoric acid R*.

Flow rate: 1 ml/min.

Detection: spectrophotometer at 230 nm.

Injection: 20 µl.

System suitability: reference solution (b):

— *resolution*: minimum 3.5 between the peak due to clavulanate (1st peak) and the peak due to amoxicillin (2nd peak).

1 mg of $C_8H_9NO_5$ is equivalent to 1.191 mg of $C_8H_8KNO_5$.

STORAGE

In an airtight container.

LABELLING

The label states the *m/m* percentage content of potassium clavulanate and the diluent used to prepare the mixture.

IMPURITIES

Qualified impurities: A, B, C, D, G.

Other detectable impurities: E, F.

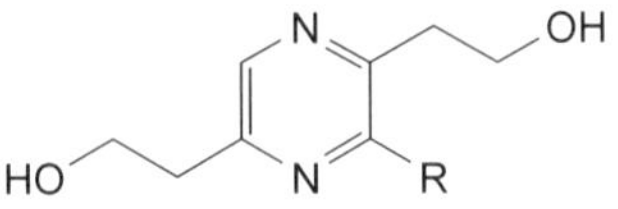

A. R = H: 2,2′-(pyrazine-2,5-diyl)diethanol,

B. R = CH$_2$-CH$_2$-CO$_2$H: 3-[3,6-bis(2-hydroxyethyl)pyrazin-2-yl]propanoic acid,

C. R = CH$_2$-CH$_3$: 2,2′-(3-ethylpyrazine-2,5-diyl)diethanol,

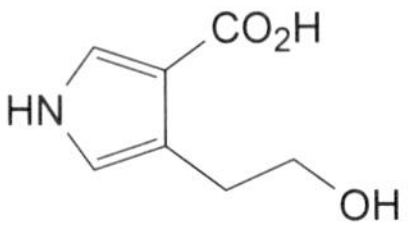

D. 4-(2-hydroxyethyl)-1*H*-pyrrole-3-carboxylic acid,

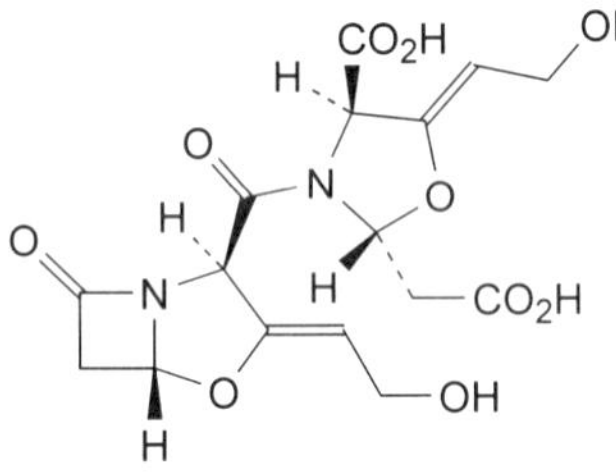

E. (2*R*,4*R*,5*Z*)-2-(carboxymethyl)-5-(2-hydroxyethylidene)-3-[[(2*R*,3*Z*,5*R*)-3-(2-hydroxyethylidene)-7-oxo-4-oxa-1-azabicyclo[3.2.0]hept-2-yl]carbonyl]oxazolidine-4-carboxylic acid,

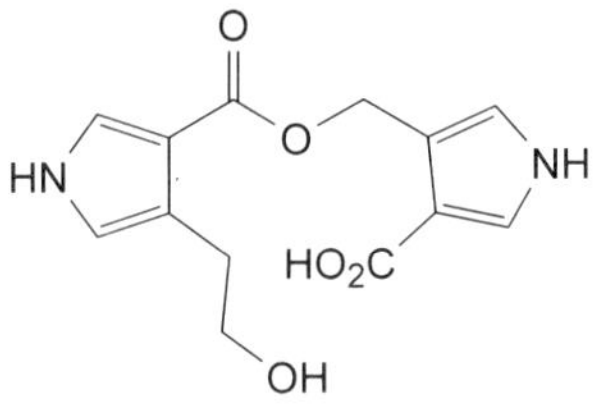

F. 4-[[[[4-(2-hydroxyethyl)-1*H*-pyrrol-3-yl]carbonyl]oxy]methyl]-1*H*-pyrrole-3-carboxylic acid,

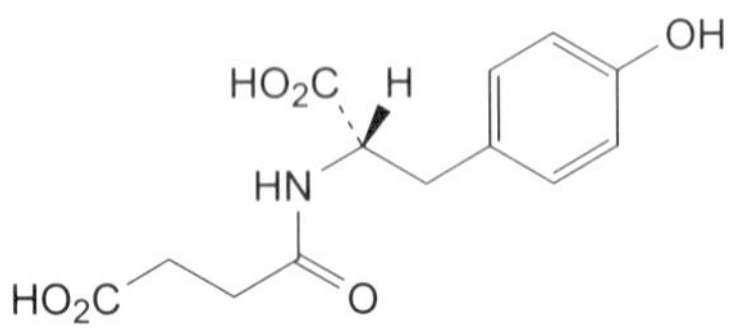

G. 4-[[(1*S*)-1-carboxy-2-(4-hydroxyphenyl)ethyl]amino]-4-oxobutanoic acid (*N*-succinyltyrosine).

04/2003:2002

PROGUANIL HYDROCHLORIDE

Proguanili hydrochloridum

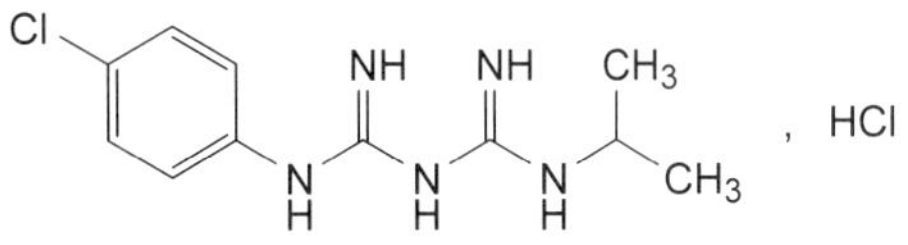

C$_{11}$H$_{17}$Cl$_2$N$_5$ M_r 290.2

DEFINITION

1-(4-Chlorophenyl)-5-(1-methylethyl)biguanide hydrochloride.

Content: 98.5 per cent to 101.0 per cent (dried substance).

CHARACTERS

Appearance: white, crystalline powder.

Solubility: slightly soluble in water, sparingly soluble in ethanol, practically insoluble in methylene chloride.

IDENTIFICATION

First identification: A, D.

Second identification: B, C, D.

A. Infrared absorption spectrophotometry (*2.2.24*).

   Comparison: Ph. Eur. reference spectrum of proguanil hydrochloride.

B. Dissolve 0.4 g in 50 ml of *water R* (solution A). To 15 ml of solution A add 2 ml of *dilute sodium hydroxide solution R*. Extract with 20 ml of *ethyl acetate R*. Wash the organic layer with *water R*, evaporate to dryness and dry at 105 °C. The melting point (*2.2.14*) of the residue is 130 °C to 133 °C.

C. To 10 ml of solution A, add 1 drop of *copper sulphate solution R* and 2 ml of *dilute ammonia R1*. Add 5 ml of *toluene R* and stir. Allow to stand until separation of the layers is obtained. The upper layer is violet-red.

D. It gives reaction (a) of chlorides (*2.3.1*).

TESTS

Acidity or alkalinity. To 35 ml of *water R* maintained at 60-65 °C, add 0.2 ml of *methyl red mixed solution R*. Neutralise to a grey colour with either *0.01 M sodium hydroxide* or *0.01 M hydrochloric acid*. Add 0.4 g of the substance to be examined and stir until completely dissolved. The solution is grey or green. Not more than 0.2 ml of *0.01 M hydrochloric acid* is required to change the colour of the solution to reddish-violet.

Chloroaniline: maximum 250 ppm.

Dissolve 0.10 g in 1 ml of *2 M hydrochloric acid* and dilute to 20 ml with *water R*. Cool to 5 °C. Add 1 ml of a 3.45 g/l solution of *sodium nitrite R* and allow to stand at 5 °C for 5 min. Add 2 ml of a 50 g/l solution of *ammonium sulphamate R* and allow to stand for 10 min. Add 2 ml of *naphthylethylenediamine dihydrochloride solution R*, dilute to 50 ml with *water R* and allow to stand for 30 min. Any red colour produced is not more intense than that of a standard prepared at the same time and in the same manner, using 20 ml of a 1.25 mg/l solution of *chloroaniline R*.

Related substances. Liquid chromatography (*2.2.29*).

Test solution. Dissolve 10.0 mg of the substance to be examined in the mobile phase and dilute to 100.0 ml with the mobile phase.

Reference solution (a). Dilute 1.0 ml of the test solution to 50.0 ml with the mobile phase. Dilute 1.0 ml of this solution to 10.0 ml with the mobile phase.

Reference solution (b). Dissolve 5 mg of *proguanil impurity C CRS* in the mobile phase and dilute to 100 ml with the mobile phase. Dilute 0.1 ml to 10 ml with the mobile phase.

Reference solution (c). Dissolve 5 mg of *proguanil impurity D CRS* in the mobile phase and dilute to 100 ml with the mobile phase. Dilute 0.1 ml to 10 ml with the mobile phase.

Reference solution (d). Dilute 1 ml of the test solution to 200 ml with the mobile phase. To 1 ml add 1 ml of reference solution (c) and mix.

Column:

— *size*: l = 0.125 m, Ø = 4.6 mm,
— *stationary phase*: octadecylsilyl silica gel for chromatography R (5 µm).

Mobile phase: dissolve 3.78 g of *sodium hexanesulphonate R* in a mixture of 10 volumes of *glacial acetic acid R*, 800 volumes of *water R* and 1200 volumes of *methanol R*.

Flow rate: 1 ml/min.

Detection: spectrophotometer at 230 nm and 254 nm.

Injection: 20 µl.

Run time: 5 times the retention time of proguanil.

Retention time: proguanil = about 6 min.

System suitability: reference solution (d) at 230 nm:

— *resolution*: minimum 5 between the peaks due to impurity D and proguanil.

Limits:

— *impurity C*: not more than 3.5 times the area of the principal peak in the chromatogram obtained with reference solution (a) at 230 nm (0.7 per cent),

— *impurity D*: not more than the area of the principal peak in the chromatogram obtained with reference solution (a) at 230 nm (0.2 per cent),

— *any other impurity*: not more than 0.5 times the area of the principal peak in the chromatogram obtained with reference solution (a) at 230 nm and at 254 nm (0.1 per cent),

— *total*: the sum of the calculated percentage contents of known and unknown impurities is not greater than 1 per cent, considering each peak at the wavelength at which the peak shows the higher value,

— *disregard limit*: 0.25 times the area of the principal peak in the chromatogram obtained with reference solution (a) (0.05 per cent).

Loss on drying (*2.2.32*): maximum 0.5 per cent, determined on 1.000 g by drying in an oven at 100-105 °C.

Sulphated ash (*2.4.14*): maximum 0.1 per cent, determined on 1.0 g.

ASSAY

Suspend 0.100 g in 20 ml of *anhydrous acetic acid R*, shake and heat at 50 °C for 5 min. Cool to room temperature and add 40 ml of *acetic anhydride R*. Titrate with *0.1 M perchloric acid*, determining the end-point potentiometrically (*2.2.20*).

1 ml of *0.1 M perchloric acid* is equivalent to 14.51 mg of $C_{11}H_{17}Cl_2N_5$.

STORAGE

Protected from light.

IMPURITIES

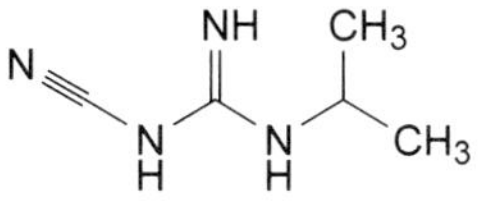

A. 1-cyano-3-(1-methylethyl)guanidine,

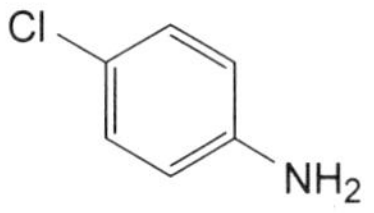

B. 4-chloroaniline,

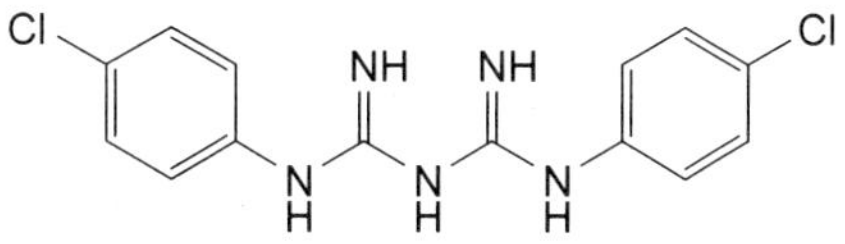

C. 1,5-bis(4-chlorophenyl)biguanide,

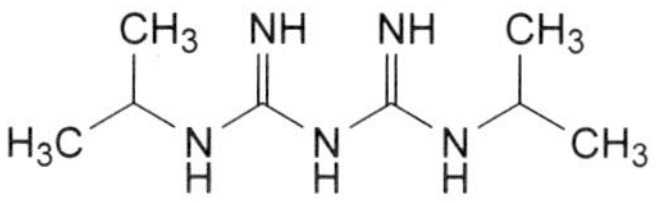

D. 1,5-bis(1-methylethyl)biguanide.

R

Monographs
Q - Z

04/2003:1884

RIBWORT PLANTAIN

Plantaginis lanceolatae folium

DEFINITION

Whole or fragmented, dried leaf of *Plantago lanceolata* L. s. l.

Content: minimum 1.5 per cent of total *ortho*-dihydroxycinnamic acid derivatives expressed as acteoside ($C_{29}H_{36}O_{15}$; M_r 624.6) (dried drug).

CHARACTERS

Macroscopic and microscopic characters described under identification tests A and B.

IDENTIFICATION

A. The leaf is up to 30 cm long and 4 cm wide, yellowish-green to brownish-green, with a prominent, whitish-green, almost parallel venation on the abaxial surface. It consists of a lanceolate lamina narrowing at the base into a channelled petiole. The margin is indistinctly dentate and often undulate. It has 3, 5 or 7 primary veins, nearly equal in length and running almost parallel. Hairs may be almost absent, sparsely scattered or sometimes abundant, especially on the lower surface and over the veins.

B. Reduce to a powder (355). The powder is yellowish-green. Examine under a microscope using *chloral hydrate solution R*. The powder shows fragments of epidermis, composed of cells with irregular sinuous anticlinal walls with stomata mostly of the diacytic type (*2.8.3*) and sometimes anomocytic. The multicellular, uniseriate, conical covering trichomes are highly characteristic, with a basal cell larger than the other epidermal cells followed by a short cell supporting 2 or more elongated thick-walled cells; the terminal cell has an acute apex and a filiform lumen. The glandular trichomes have a unicellular cylindrical stalk and a multicellular, elongated, conical head consisting of several rows of small cells and a single terminal cell.

C. Examine the chromatograms obtained for *Digitalis lanata* leaves.

Results A: see below the sequence of the zones present in the chromatograms obtained with the reference solution and the test solution. Furthermore, other zones may be present in the chromatograms obtained with the test solution.

Top of the plate	
Acteoside: a yellow zone	A yellow zone (acteoside)
Aucubin: a blue zone	A blue zone (aucubin)
Reference solution	**Test solution**

TESTS

Digitalis lanata leaves. Thin layer chromatography (*2.2.27*).

Test solution. Use a freshly prepared solution. To 1 g of the powdered drug (355) in a 25 ml flask, add 10 ml of a mixture of 30 volumes of *water R* and 70 volumes of *methanol R*

and shake for 30 min. Filter, rinse the flask and filter with 2 quantities, each of 5 ml, with the mixture of 30 volumes of *water R* and 70 volumes of *methanol R*. Dilute to 25 ml with a mixture of 30 volumes of *water R* and 70 volumes of *methanol R*.

Reference solution. Dissolve 1 mg of *acteoside R* and 1 mg of *aucubin R* in 1 ml of a mixture of 30 volumes of *water R* and 70 volumes of *methanol R*.

Plate: TLC silica gel F_{254} *plate R*.

Mobile phase: acetic acid R, anhydrous formic acid R, water R, ethyl acetate R (11:11:27:100 V/V/V/V).

Application: 10 µl, as bands.

Developement: over a path of 8 cm.

Detection A: examine in daylight.

Detection B: heat immediately after development at about 120 °C for 5-10 min. Examine in ultraviolet light at 365 nm.

Results B: the chromatogram obtained with the test solution shows no bright blue fluorescent zone just below the reddish-brown fluorescent zone corresponding to aucubin in the chromatogram obtained with the reference solution.

Foreign matter (*2.8.2*): maximum 5 per cent of leaves of different colour and maximum 2 per cent of other foreign matter.

Loss on drying (*2.2.32*): maximum 10.0 per cent, determined on 1.000 g of the powdered drug (355) by drying in an oven at 100-105 °C for 2 h.

Total ash (*2.4.16*): maximum 14.0 per cent.

ASSAY

Stock solution. In a flask, place 1.000 g of the powdered drug (355) and add 90 ml of *alcohol (50 per cent V/V) R*. Boil in a water-bath under a reflux condenser for 30 min. Allow to cool and filter into a 100 ml volumetric flask. Rinse the flask and the filter with 10 ml of *alcohol (50 per cent V/V) R*. Combine the filtrate and the rinsings and dilute to 100.0 ml with *alcohol (50 per cent V/V) R*.

Test solution. To a 10 ml volumetric flask add, mixing after each addition, 1.0 ml of stock solution, 2 ml of *0.5 M hydrochloric acid*, 2 ml of a solution prepared by dissolving 10 g of *sodium nitrite R* and 10 g of *sodium molybdate R* in 100 ml of *water R* and then add 2 ml of *dilute sodium hydroxide solution R*. Dilute to 10.0 ml with *water R*.

Immediately measure the absorbance (*2.2.25*) of test solution at 525 nm using as compensation liquid a solution prepared as follows: to a 10 ml volumetric flask, add 1.0 ml of stock solution, 2 ml of *0.5 M hydrochloric acid*, 2 ml of *dilute sodium hydroxide solution R* and dilute to 10.0 ml with *water R*.

Calculate the percentage content of total *ortho*-dihydroxycinnamic acid derivatives, expressed as acteoside, from the expression:

$$\frac{A \times 1000}{185 \times m}$$

i.e. taking the specific absorbance to be 185 for acteoside at 525 nm.

A = absorbance of the test solution at 525 nm,

m = mass of the substance to be examined, in grams.

07/2002:1657
corrected

RIFABUTIN

Rifabutinum

$C_{46}H_{62}N_4O_{11}$ M_r 847

DEFINITION

(9S,12E,14S,15R,16S,17R,18R,19R,20S,21S,22E,24Z)-6,18,20-trihydroxy-14-methoxy-7,9,15,17,19,21,25-heptamethyl-1′-(2-methylpropyl)-5,10,26-trioxo-3,5,9,10-tetrahydrospiro[9,4-(epoxypentadecal[1,11,13]trienimino)-2H-furo[2′,3′:7,8]naphtho[1,2-d]imidazole-2,4′-piperidine]-16-yl acetate.

Content: 96.0 per cent to 102.0 per cent (anhydrous substance).

CHARACTERS

Appearance: reddish-violet amorphous powder.

Solubility: slightly soluble in water, soluble in methanol, slightly soluble in alcohol.

IDENTIFICATION

A. Infrared absorption spectrophotometry (2.2.24).
   Preparation: discs.
   Comparison: rifabutin CRS.

B. Examine the chromatograms obtained in the test for related substances.
   Results: the principal peak in the chromatogram obtained with the test solution is similar in retention time and size to the principal peak in the chromatogram obtained with reference solution (a).

TESTS

Impurity A. Thin-layer chromatography (2.2.27).

Test solution. Dissolve 0.100 g of the substance to be examined in a mixture of equal volumes of methanol R and methylene chloride R and dilute to 10 ml with the same mixture of solvents.

Reference solution. Dissolve 10 mg of rifabutin impurity A CRS in a mixture of equal volumes of methanol R and methylene chloride R and dilute to 10 ml with the same mixture of solvents. Dilute 3 ml of the solution to 100 ml with a mixture of equal volumes of methanol R and methylene chloride R.

Plate: TLC silica gel F_{254} plate R.

Mobile phase: acetone R, light petroleum R (23:77 V/V).

Application: 10 µl.

Development: over 2/3 of the plate.

Drying: in air.

Detection: expose the plate to iodine vapour for about 5 min, then spray with potassium iodide and starch solution R and allow to stand for 5 min.

Limits:
— impurity A: any spot corresponding to impurity A is not more intense than the spot in the chromatogram obtained with the reference solution (0.3 per cent).

Related substances. Liquid chromatography (2.2.29).

Test solution. Dissolve 50.0 mg of the substance to be examined in the mobile phase and dilute to 50.0 ml with the mobile phase.

Reference solution (a). Dissolve 50.0 mg of rifabutin CRS in the mobile phase and dilute to 50.0 ml with the mobile phase.

Reference solution (b). Dilute 1.0 ml of reference solution (a) to 100.0 ml with the mobile phase.

Reference solution (c). Dissolve about 10 mg of rifabutin CRS in 2 ml of methanol R, add 1 ml of dilute sodium hydroxide solution R and allow to stand for about 4 min. Add 1 ml of dilute hydrochloric acid R and dilute to 50 ml with the mobile phase.

Column:
— size: l = 0.110 m, Ø = 4.6 mm,
— stationary phase: octylsilyl silica gel for chromatography R (5 µm).

Mobile phase: mix equal volumes of acetonitrile R and a 13.6 g/l solution of potassium dihydrogen phosphate R adjusted to pH 6.5 with dilute sodium hydroxide solution R.

Flow rate: 1 ml/min.

Detection: spectrophotometer at 254 nm.

Injection: 20 µl.

Run time: 2.5 times the retention time of rifabutin.

Relative retention with reference to rifabutin (retention time = about 9 min): impurity E = about 0.5; impurity B = about 0.6; impurity D = about 0.9; impurity C = about 1.3.

System suitability: reference solution (c):
— resolution: minimum 2.0 between the second peak of the 3 peaks due to degradation products and the peak due to rifabutin.

Limits:
— any impurity: not more than the area of the principal peak in the chromatogram obtained with reference solution (b) (1.0 per cent); not more than 1 such peak has an area greater than half the area of the principal peak in the chromatogram obtained with reference solution (b) (0.5 per cent),
— total: not more than 3 times the area of the principal peak in the chromatogram obtained with reference solution (b) (3.0 per cent),
— disregard limit: 0.05 times the area of the principal peak in the chromatogram obtained with reference solution (b) (0.05 per cent).

Water (2.5.12): maximum 2.5 per cent, determined on 0.200 g.

Sulphated ash (2.4.14): maximum 0.3 per cent, determined on 1.0 g.

ASSAY

Liquid chromatography (2.2.29) as described in the test for related substances with the following modification.

Injection: test solution and reference solution (a).

Calculate the percentage content of ribabutin.

IMPURITIES

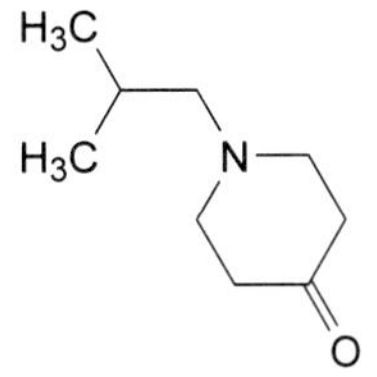

A. 1-(2-methylpropyl)piperidin-4-one,

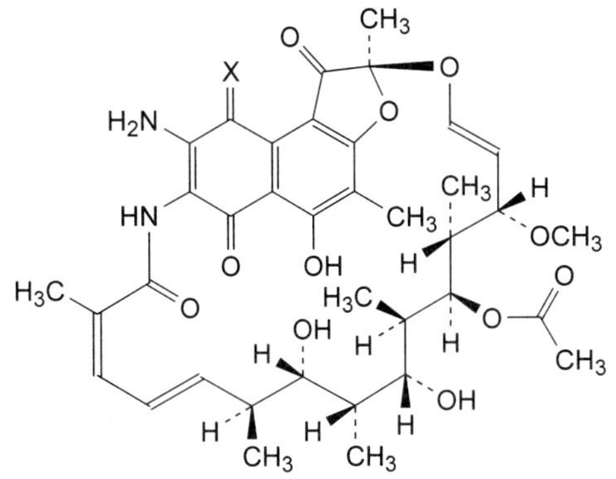

B. X = O: 3-aminorifamycin S,

D. X = NH: 3-amino-4-imidorifamycin S,

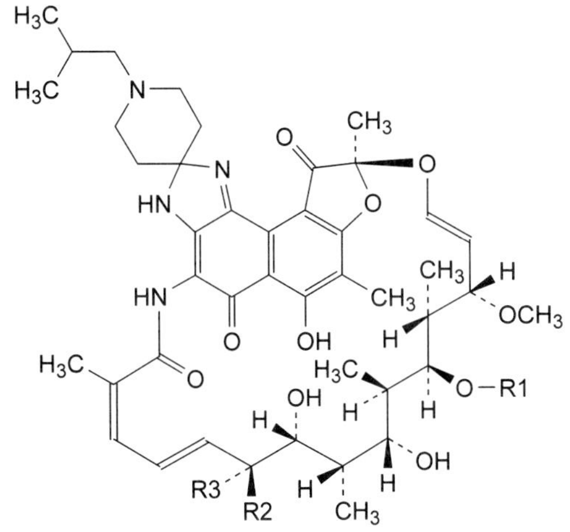

C. R1 = CO-CH₃, R2 + R3 = CH₂: 20,31-didehydrorifabutin,

E. R1 = R3 = H, R2 = CH₃: 25-deacetylrifabutin.

04/2003:2020

RILMENIDINE DIHYDROGEN PHOSPHATE

Rilmenidini dihydrogenophosphas

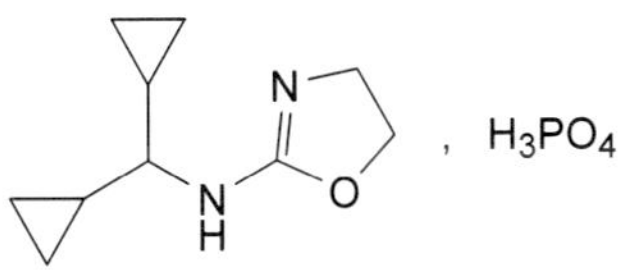

, H_3PO_4

$C_{10}H_{19}N_2O_5P$ M_r 278.2

DEFINITION

N-(Dicyclopropylmethyl)-4,5-dihydro-oxazol-2-amine dihydrogen phosphate.

Content: 99.0 per cent to 101.0 per cent (dried substance).

CHARACTERS

Appearance: white or almost white powder.

Solubility: freely soluble in water, slightly soluble in alcohol, practically insoluble in methylene chloride.

IDENTIFICATION

A. Infrared absorption spectrophotometry (*2.2.24*).

Preparation: mulls in *liquid paraffin R*.

Comparison: *Ph. Eur. reference spectrum of rilmenidine dihydrogen phosphate*.

B. Dissolve 10 mg in *water R* and dilute to 1 ml with the same solvent. The solution gives reaction (b) of phosphates (*2.3.1*).

TESTS

Related substances. Liquid chromatography (*2.2.29*).

Test solution. Dissolve 60.0 mg of the substance to be examined in *water R* and dilute to 20.0 ml with the same solvent.

Reference solution (a). Dilute 1.0 ml of the test solution to 100.0 ml with *water R* and dilute 10.0 ml of this solution to 50.0 ml with the same solvent.

Reference solution (b). Dilute 5.0 ml of reference solution (a) to 20.0 ml with *water R*.

Reference solution (c). Dissolve 15.0 mg of *rilmenidine for system suitability CRS* in *water R* and dilute to 5.0 ml with the same solvent.

Column:

– *size*: l = 0.15 m, Ø = 3 mm,

– *stationary phase*: *base-deactivated octadecylsilyl silica gel for chromatography R* (5 µm) with a pore size of 10 nm and a carbon loading of 25 per cent,

– *temperature*: 40 °C.

Mobile phase:

– *mobile phase A*: dissolve 3 g of *sodium heptanesulphonate R* in *water R* and dilute to 860 ml with the same solvent; add 130 ml of *methanol R2*, 10 ml of *tetrahydrofuran for chromatography R* and 1.0 ml of *phosphoric acid R*,

– *mobile phase B*: dissolve 3 g of *sodium heptanesulphonate R* in *water R* and dilute to 600 ml with the same solvent; add 350 ml of *acetonitrile for chromatography R*, 50 ml of *tetrahydrofuran for chromatography R* and 1.0 ml of *phosphoric acid R*,

Time (min)	Mobile phase A (per cent *V/V*)	Mobile phase B (per cent *V/V*)
0 - 14	100 → 0	0 → 100
14 - 15	0 → 100	100 → 0
15 - 30	100	0

Flow rate: 1 ml/min.

Detection: spectrophotometer at 205 nm.

Injection: 20 µl.

Relative retention with reference to rilmenidine (retention time = about 13 min): impurity A = about 0.6; impurity B = about 0.9; impurity C = about 1.4.

With these conditions the inflexion of the baseline, corresponding to the beginning of the gradient, appears on the recorder after a minimum time t of 5 min. If this is not the case (t < 5 min) modify the chromatographic sequence by adding an isocratic elution with 100 per cent of mobile phase A for a time corresponding to (5-t) min before the linear gradient.

System suitability: reference solution (c):

– *peak-to-valley ratio*: minimum 3, where H_p = height above the baseline of the peak due to impurity B and H_v = height above the baseline of the lowest point of the curve separating this peak from the peak due to rilmenidine.

Limits:

– *any impurity*: not more than 0.5 times the area of the principal peak in the chromatogram obtained with reference solution (a) (0.1 per cent),

– *total*: not more than the area of the principal peak in the chromatogram obtained with reference solution (a) (0.2 per cent),

– *disregard limit*: the area of the principal peak in the chromatogram obtained with reference solution (b) (0.05 per cent).

Loss on drying (*2.2.32*): maximum 0.5 per cent, determined on 1.000 g by drying in an oven *in vacuo* at 50 °C over *diphosphorus pentoxide R* for 2 h.

ASSAY

Dissolve 0.200 g in 50 ml of *anhydrous acetic acid R*. Titrate with *0.1 M perchloric acid*, determining the end-point potentiometrically (*2.2.20*).

1 ml of *0.1 M perchloric acid* is equivalent to 27.82 mg of $C_{10}H_{19}N_2O_5P$.

IMPURITIES

Qualified impurities: A, B, C.

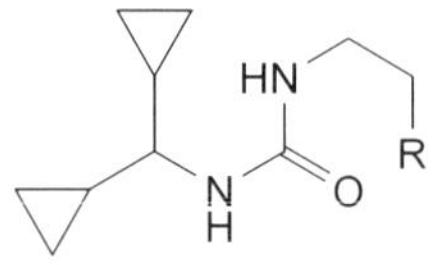

A. R = OH: 1-(dicyclopropylmethyl)-3-(2-hydroxyethyl)urea,

B. R = Cl: 1-(2-chloroethyl)-3-(dicyclopropylmethyl)urea,

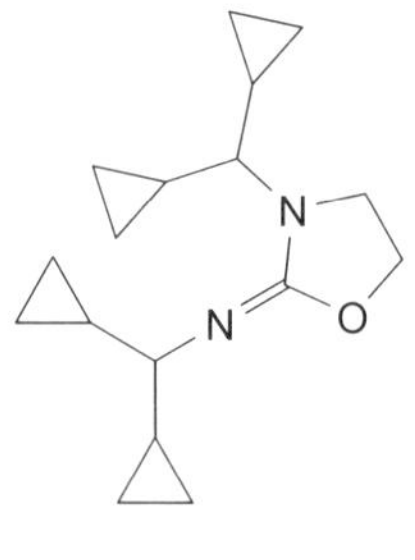

C. *N*,3-bis(dicyclopropylmethyl)oxazolidin-2-imine.

01/2002:1623
corrected

ROSELLE

Hibisci sabdariffae flos

DEFINITION

Whole or cut dried calyces and epicalyces of *Hibiscus sabdariffa* L. collected during fruiting.

Content: minimum 13.5 per cent of acids, expressed as citric acid ($C_6H_8O_7$; M_r 192.1) (dried drug).

CHARACTERS

Acidic taste.

Macroscopic and microscopic characters described under identification tests A and B.

IDENTIFICATION

A. The calyx is joined in the lower half to form an urceolate structure, the upper half dividing to form 5 long acuminate recurved tips. The tips have a prominent, slightly protruding midrib and a large, thick nectary gland about 1 mm in diameter. The epicalyx consist of 8 to 12 small, obovate leaflets which are adnate to the base of the calyx. The calyx and epicalyx are fleshy, dry, easily fragmented and coloured bright-red to deep-purple, somewhat lighter at the base of the inner side.

B. Reduce to a powder (355). The powder is red to purplish-red. Examine under a microscope using *chloral hydrate solution R*. The powder shows predominantly red coloured fragments of the parenchyme containing numerous crystal clusters of calcium oxalate and, sporadically, mucilage filled cavities, sometimes associated with polygonal epidermal cells and anisocytic stomata (*2.8.3*); numerous fragments of vascular bundles with spiral and reticulate vessels; sclerenchymatous fibres with a wide lumen; rarely, rectangular, pitted parenchymatous cells; fragments of unicellular, smooth, bent covering trichomes and occasional glandular trichomes; rounded pollen grains with spiny exine.

C. Thin-layer chromatography (*2.2.27*).

Test solution. To 1.0 g of the powdered drug (355) add 10 ml of *alcohol (60 per cent) V/V R*. Shake for 15 min and filter.

Reference solution. Dissolve 2.5 mg of *quinaldine red R* in 10 ml of *alcohol R*.

Plate: *TLC silica gel plate R*.

Mobile phase: *acetic acid R*, *water R*, *butanol R* (15:30:60 *V/V/V*).

Application: 20 µl, as bands.

Development: over a path of 10 cm.

Drying: in air.

Detection: examine in daylight.

Results: see below the sequence of the zones present in the chromatograms obtained with the reference and test solutions.

Top of the plate	
Quinaldine red: an orange red zone	
	A pale violet zone
	A violet-blue zone
	A violet-blue zone
	A violet-blue zone
Reference solution	**Test solution**

TESTS

Foreign matter (*2.8.2*): maximum 2 per cent of fragments of fruits: red funicles and parts of the 5 caverned capsule with yellowish-grey pericarp, whose thin walls consist of several layers of differently directed fibres; flattened, reniform seeds with a dotted surface.

Loss on drying (*2.2.32*): maximum 11.0 per cent, determined on 1.000 g of the powdered drug (355) by drying in an oven at 100-105 °C for 2 h.

Total ash (*2.4.16*): maximum 10.0 per cent.

Colouring power: reduce the drug to a coarse powder (1400) and mix 100 g of drug. Reduce about 10 g of this mixture to a powder (355). To 1.0 g of the powdered drug (355) add 25 ml of boiling *water R* in a 100 ml flask and heat for 15 min on a water-bath with frequent shaking. Filter the hot mixture into a 50 ml graduated flask; rinse successively the 100 ml flask and the filter 3 times with 5 ml of warm *water R*. After cooling dilute to 50 ml with *water R*.

Dilute 5 ml of this solution to 50 ml with *water R*. Measure the absorbance (*2.2.25*) at 520 nm using *water R* as the compensation liquid. The absorbance is not less than 0.350 for the whole drug and not less than 0.250 for the cut drug.

ASSAY

Shake 1.000 g of the powdered drug (355) with 100 ml of *carbon dioxide free water R* for 15 min. Filter. To 50.0 ml of the filtrate add 100 ml of *carbon dioxide free water R*. Titrate with *0.1 M sodium hydroxide* until pH 7.0, determining the end-point potentiometrically (*2.2.20*).

1 ml of *0.1 M sodium hydroxide* is equivalent to 6.4 mg of citric acid.

S

Monographs Q - Z

01/2002:1563
corrected

SIMVASTATIN

Simvastatinum

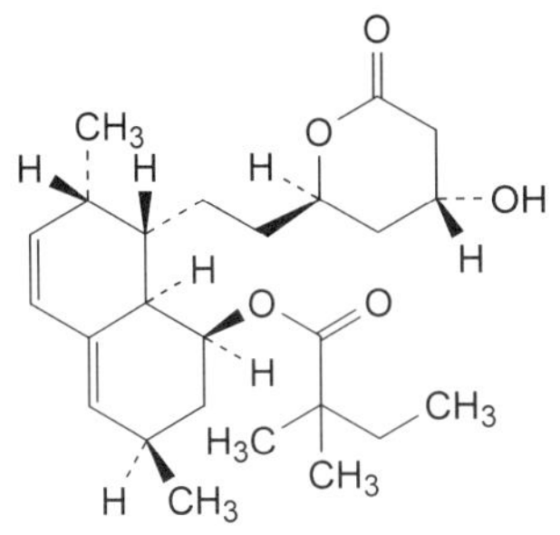

C₂₅H₃₈O₅ M_r 418.6

$C_{25}H_{38}O_5$ M_r 418.6

DEFINITION

Simvastatin contains not less than 97.0 per cent and not more than the equivalent of 102.0 per cent of (1S,3R,7S,8S,8aR)-8-[2-[(2R,4R)-4-hydroxy-6-oxotetrahydro-2H-pyran-2-yl]ethyl]-3,7-dimethyl-1,2,3,7,8,8a-hexahydronaphthalen-1-yl 2,2-dimethylbutanoate, calculated with reference to the dried substance. A suitable antioxidant may be added.

CHARACTERS

A white or almost white, crystalline powder, practically insoluble in water, very soluble in methylene chloride, freely soluble in alcohol.

IDENTIFICATION

A. It complies with the test for specific optical rotation (see Tests).

B. Examine by infrared absorption spectrophotometry (2.2.24), comparing with the spectrum obtained with simvastatin CRS. Examine the substances prepared as discs.

TESTS

Appearance of solution. Dissolve 0.200 g in methanol R and dilute to 20 ml with the same solvent. The solution is clear (2.2.1) and not more intensely coloured than reference solution BY₇ (2.2.2, Method II).

Specific optical rotation (2.2.7). Dissolve 0.125 g in acetonitrile R and dilute to 25.0 ml with the same solvent. The specific optical rotation is + 285 to + 300, calculated with reference to the dried substance.

Related substances. Examine by liquid chromatography (2.2.29) as prescribed under Assay.

Inject 5 µl of reference solution (b). Adjust the sensitivity of the system so that the height of the principal peak in the chromatogram obtained is at least 20 per cent of the full scale of the recorder. Inject 5 µl of test solution (a) and continue the chromatography for five times the retention time of simvastatin. When the chromatograms are recorded under the prescribed conditions the relative retentions are: impurity A about 0.45, lovastatin (impurity E) and epilovastatin (impurity F) about 0.60, impurity G about 0.80, impurity B about 2.38, impurity C about 2.42 and impurity D about 3.80 (retention time of simvastatin: about 2.6 min). In the chromatogram obtained with test solution (a): the area of the peak due to lovastatin and epilovastatin is not greater than twice the area of the principal peak in the chromatogram obtained with reference solution (b) (1.0 per

cent); the area of any peak apart from the principal peak and the peak due to lovastatin and epilovastatin is not greater than 0.8 times the area of the principal peak in the chromatogram obtained with reference solution (b) (0.4 per cent); the sum of the areas of all peaks, apart from the principal peak and the peak due to lovastatin and epilovastatin, is not greater than twice the area of the principal peak in the chromatogram obtained with reference solution (b) (1.0 per cent). Disregard any peak with an area less than 0.1 times the area of the principal peak in the chromatogram obtained with reference solution (b) (0.05 per cent).

Heavy metals (2.4.8). 1.0 g complies with limit test C for heavy metals (20 ppm). Prepare the standard using 2 ml of lead standard solution (10 ppm Pb) R.

Loss on drying (2.2.32). Not more than 0.5 per cent, determined on 1.000 g by drying in a desiccator under high vacuum at 60 °C for 3 h.

Sulphated ash (2.4.14). Not more than 0.1 per cent, determined on 1.0 g.

ASSAY

Examine by liquid chromatography (2.2.29). *Prepare the solutions immediately before use.*

Solvent mixture. Prepare a mixture of 40 volumes of a solution of a 1.4 g/l solution of *potassium dihydrogen phosphate R*, adjusted to pH 4.0 with *phosphoric acid R*, and 60 volumes of *acetonitrile R*. Filter.

Test solution (a). Dissolve 75.0 mg of the substance to be examined in the solvent mixture and dilute to 50.0 ml with the solvent mixture.

Test solution (b). Dissolve 40.0 mg of the substance to be examined in the solvent mixture and dilute to 50.0 ml with the solvent mixture.

Reference solution (a). Dissolve 1.0 mg of *simvastatin CRS* and 1.0 mg of *lovastatin CRS* in the solvent mixture and dilute to 50.0 ml with the solvent mixture.

Reference solution (b). Dilute 0.5 ml of test solution (a) to 100.0 ml with the solvent mixture.

Reference solution (c). Dissolve 40.0 mg of *simvastatin CRS* in the solvent mixture and dilute to 50.0 ml with the solvent mixture.

The chromatographic procedure may be carried out using:

— a stainless steel column 0.033 m long and 4.6 mm in internal diameter packed with *end-capped octadecylsilyl silica gel for chromatography R* (3 µm),

— as mobile phase at a flow rate of 3.0 ml/min:

Mobile phase A. Mix 50 volumes of *acetonitrile R* and 50 volumes of a 0.1 per cent V/V solution of *phosphoric acid R*,

Mobile phase B. A 0.1 per cent V/V solution of *phosphoric acid R* in *acetonitrile R*,

Time (min)	Mobile phase A (per cent V/V)	Mobile phase B (per cent V/V)	Comment
0 - 4.5	100	0	isocratic
4.5 - 4.6	100 → 95	0 → 5	linear gradient
4.6 - 8.0	95 → 25	5 → 75	linear gradient
8.0 - 11.5	25	75	isocratic
11.5 - 11.6	25 → 100	75 → 0	linear gradient
11.6 - 13	100	0	re-equilibration

— as detector a spectrophotometer set at 238 nm.

Inject 5 µl of reference solution (a). The test and the assay are not valid unless, in the chromatogram obtained, the resolution between the peak corresponding to lovastatin and epilovastatin and the peak corresponding to simvastatin is at least 5.0. When the chromatograms are recorded under the prescribed conditions the retention times are: lovastatin and epilovastatin about 1.6 min and simvastatin about 2.6 min. Inject 5 µl of reference solution (c). Adjust the sensitivity of the system so that the height of the principal peak is at least 50 per cent of the full scale of the recorder. Inject 5 µl of test solution (b).

Calculate the content of simvastatin from the peak areas in the chromatograms obtained with test solution (b) and reference solution (c) and the declared content of *simvastatin CRS*.

STORAGE

Store under nitrogen, in an airtight container, protected from light.

LABELLING

The label states the name and concentration of any added antioxidant.

IMPURITIES

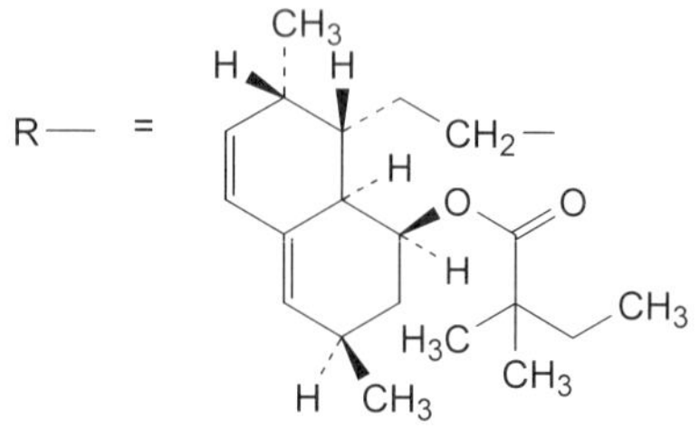

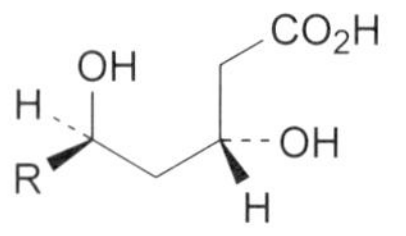

A. (3R,5R)-7-[(1S,2S,6R,8S,8aR)-8-[(2,2-dimethylbutanoyl)oxy]-2,6-dimethyl-1,2,6,7,8,8a-hexahydronaphthalen-1-yl]-3,5-dihydroxyheptanoic acid (hydroxy acid),

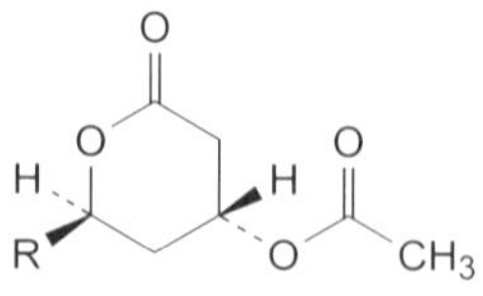

B. (1S,3R,7S,8S,8aR)-8-[2-[(2R,4R)-4-(acetyloxy)-6-oxotetrahydro-2H-pyran-2-yl]ethyl]-3,7-dimethyl-1,2,3,7,8,8a-hexahydronaphthalen-1-yl 2,2-dimethylbutanoate (acetate ester),

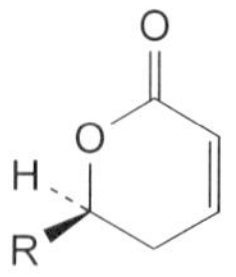

C. (1S,3R,7S,8S,8aR)-3,7-dimethyl-8-[2-[(2R)-6-oxo-3,6-dihydro-2H-pyran-2-yl]ethyl]-1,2,3,7,8,8a-hexahydronaphthalen-1-yl 2,2-dimethylbutanoate (anhydrosimvastatin),

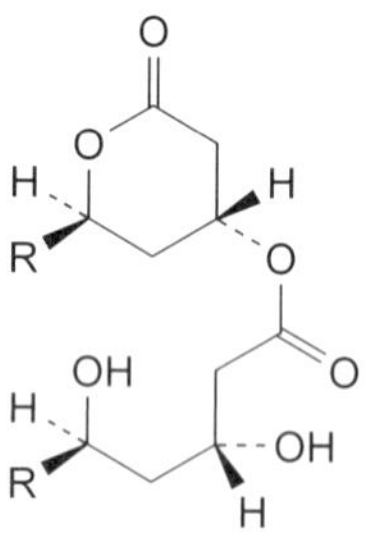

D. (2R,4R)-2-[[(1S,2S,6R,8S,8aR)-8-[(2,2-dimethylbutanoyl)oxy]-2,6-dimethyl-1,2,6,7,8,8a-hexahydronaphthalen-1-yl]ethyl]-6-oxotetrahydro-2H-pyran-4-yl (3R,5R)-7-[(1S,2S,6R,8S,8aR)-8-[(2,2-dimethylbutanoyl)oxy]-2,6-dimethyl-1,2,6,7,8,8a-hexahydronaphthalen-1-yl]-3,5-dihydroxyheptanoate (dimer),

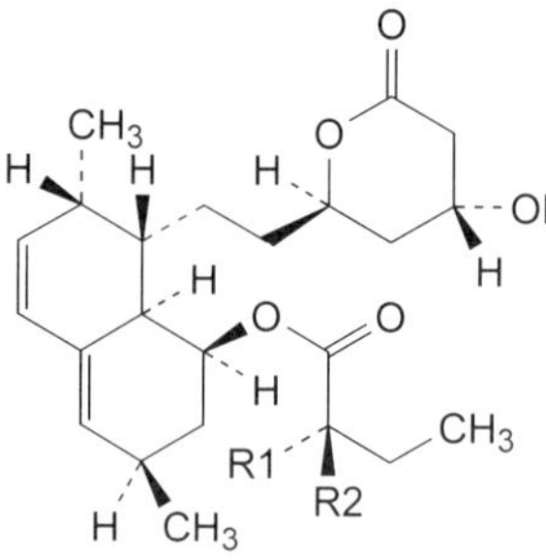

E. R1 = CH₃, R2 = H: (1S,3R,7S,8S,8aR)-8-[2-[(2R,4R)-4-hydroxy-6-oxotetrahydro-2H-pyran-2-yl]ethyl]-3,7-dimethyl-1,2,3,7,8,8a-hexahydronaphthalen-1-yl (2S)-2-methylbutanoate (lovastatin),

F. R1 = H, R2 = CH₃: (1S,3R,7S,8S,8aR)-8-[2-[(2R,4R)-4-hydroxy-6-oxotetrahydro-2H-pyran-2-yl]ethyl]-3,7-dimethyl-1,2,3,7,8,8a-hexahydronaphthalen-1-yl (2R)-2-methylbutanoate (epilovastatin),

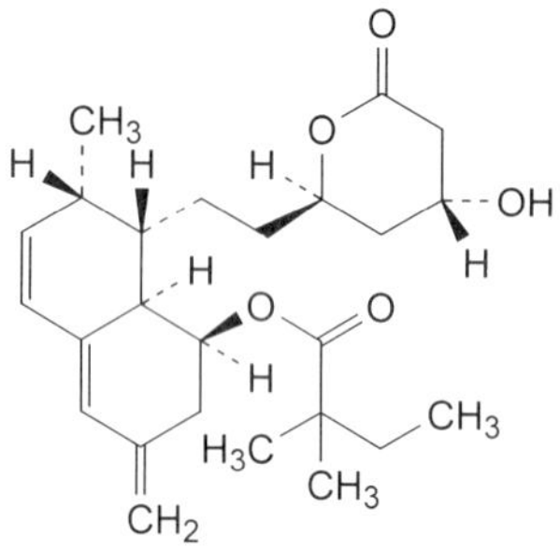

G. (1S,7S,8S,8aR)-8-[2-[(2R,4R)-4-hydroxy-6-oxotetrahydro-2H-pyran-2-yl]ethyl]-7-methyl-3-methylene-1,2,3,7,8,8a-hexahydronaphthalen-1-yl 2,2-dimethylbutanoate.

01/2002:1564
corrected

SODIUM ALENDRONATE

Natrii alendronas

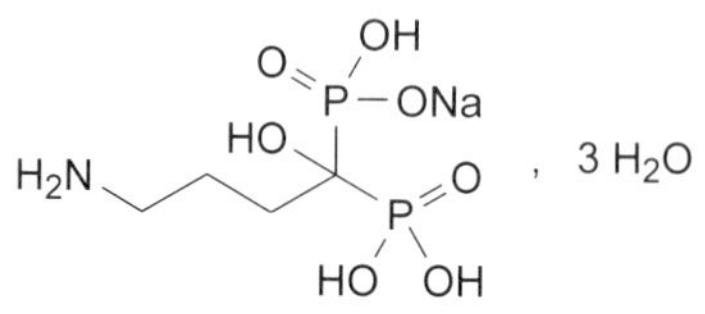

$C_4H_{12}NNaO_7P_2,3H_2O$

M_r 325.1

DEFINITION

Sodium alendronate contains not less than 98.0 per cent and not more than the equivalent of 102.0 per cent of (4-amino-1-hydroxybutylidene)bisphosphonic acid monosodium salt trihydrate, calculated with reference to the dried substance.

CHARACTERS

A white or almost white, crystalline powder, soluble in water, very slightly soluble in methanol, practically insoluble in methylene chloride.

IDENTIFICATION

A. Examine by infrared absorption spectrophotometry (*2.2.24*), comparing with the spectrum obtained with *sodium alendronate CRS*. Examine the substances prepared as discs.

B. It gives reaction (a) of sodium (*2.3.1*).

TESTS

Solution S. Dissolve 0.5 g in *carbon dioxide-free water R* prepared from *distilled water R* and dilute to 50 ml with the same solvent.

Appearance of solution. Solution S is clear (*2.2.1*) and not more intensely coloured than reference solution B_7 or BY_7 (*2.2.2, Method II*).

pH (*2.2.3*). The pH of solution S is 4.0 to 5.0.

4-aminobutanoic acid. Examine by thin-layer chromatography (*2.2.27*), using a *TLC silica gel plate R*.

Test solution. Dissolve 0.10 g of the substance to be examined in *water R* and dilute to 10 ml with the same solvent.

Reference solution (a). Dissolve 0.10 g of *4-aminobutanoic acid R* in *water R* and dilute to 200 ml with the same solvent.

Reference solution (b). Dilute 1 ml of reference solution (a) to 10 ml with *water R*.

Apply to the plate 5 µl of the test solution and 5 µl of reference solution (b). Allow the plate to dry in air. Develop over a path of 15 cm using a mixture of 20 volumes of *water R*, 20 volumes of *glacial acetic acid R* and 60 volumes of *butanol R*. Dry the plate in a current of warm air. Spray with *ninhydrin solution R* and heat at 100 °C to 105 °C for 15 min. Any spots corresponding to 4-aminobutanoic acid in the chromatogram obtained with the test solution are not more intense than the spot in the chromatogram obtained with reference solution (b) (0.5 per cent).

Phosphate and phosphite. Examine the chromatograms obtained in the assay. In the chromatogram obtained with the test solution: the area of any peak corresponding to phosphate is not greater than that of the peak due to phosphate in the chromatogram obtained with reference solution (d) (0.5 per cent); the area of any peak corresponding to phosphite is not greater than that of the peak due to phosphite in the chromatogram obtained with reference solution (d) (0.5 per cent).

Heavy metals (*2.4.8*). 1.0 g complies with limit test F for heavy metals (20 ppm). Prepare the standard using 2 ml of *lead standard solution (10 ppm Pb) R*.

Loss on drying (*2.2.32*): 16.1 per cent to 17.1 per cent, determined on 1.000 g by drying in an oven at 140 °C to 145 °C.

ASSAY

Examine by liquid chromatography (*2.2.29*).

Test solution. Dissolve 50.0 mg of the substance to be examined in *water R* and dilute to 25.0 ml with the same solvent.

Reference solution (a). Dissolve 50.0 mg of *sodium alendronate CRS* in *water R* and dilute to 25.0 ml with the same solvent.

Reference solution (b). Dissolve 3.0 g of *phosphoric acid R* in *water R* and dilute to 100.0 ml with the same solvent. Dilute 1.0 ml of the solution to 100.0 ml with *water R*.

Reference solution (c). Dissolve 2.5 g of *phosphorous acid R* in *water R* and dilute to 100.0 ml with the same solvent. Dilute 1.0 ml of the solution to 100.0 ml with *water R*.

Reference solution (d). Mix 2.0 ml of reference solution (b) and 2.0 ml of reference solution (c) and dilute to 50.0 ml with *water R*.

The chromatographic procedure may be carried out using:

– a column 0.15 m long and 4.6 mm in internal diameter packed with *anion exchange resin R1* (7 µm),

– as mobile phase at a flow rate of 1.2 ml/min a solution of 0.2 ml of *anhydrous formic acid R* in 1000 ml of *water R*, adjusted to pH 3.5 with *2 M sodium hydroxide solution*,

– as detector a refractometer,

– a 100 µl loop injector,

maintaining the temperature of the column at 35 °C.

Inject reference solution (a) six times. The assay is not valid unless the relative standard deviation of the peak area of sodium alendronate is at most 1.0 per cent. Inject the test solution, reference solution (a) and reference solution (d). The retention time of sodium alendronate is about 16 min and the relative retention times are: phosphate about 1.3 and phosphite about 1.6. Record the chromatograms for twice the retention time of the principal peak in the chromatogram obtained with the test solution.

Calculate the percentage content of $C_4H_{12}NNaO_7P_2$ from the peak areas and the declared content of *sodium alendronate CRS*.

IMPURITIES

$H_2N\diagup\diagdown\diagup CO_2H$

A. 4-aminobutanoic acid,

B. phosphate,

C. phosphite.

04/2003:2041

SODIUM PROPIONATE

Natrii propionas

$H_3C\diagup\diagdown\diagup ONa$ (with =O)

$C_3H_5NaO_2$ $\qquad$ M_r 96.1

DEFINITION

Sodium propanoate.

Content: 99.0 per cent to 101.0 per cent (dried substance).

CHARACTERS

Appearance: colourless crystals or white powder, slightly hygroscopic.

Solubility: freely soluble in water, sparingly soluble in alcohol, practically insoluble in methylene chloride.

IDENTIFICATION

First identification: A, D.

Second identification: B, C, D.

A. Infrared absorption spectrophotometry (*2.2.24*).

Comparison: Ph. Eur. reference spectrum of sodium propionate.

B. Dissolve 0.1 g in a mixture of 2 ml of *copper sulphate solution R* and 2 ml of *methylene chloride R*. Shake vigorously and allow to stand. Both the upper and the lower layer show a blue colour.

C. To 5 ml of solution S (see Tests) add 2 ml of *0.1 M silver nitrate*. A white precipitate is formed.

D. Solution S gives reaction (a) of sodium (*2.3.1*).

TESTS

Solution S. Dissolve 10 g in *carbon dioxide-free water R* prepared from *distilled water R* and dilute to 100 ml with the same solvent.

Appearance of solution. Solution S is clear (*2.2.1*) and colourless (*2.2.2, Method II*).

pH (*2.2.3*): 7.8 to 9.2.

Dilute 1 ml of solution S to 5 ml with *water R*.

Related substances. Liquid chromatography (*2.2.29*).

Test solution. Dissolve 0.250 g of the substance to be examined in *water R* and dilute to 100 ml with the same solvent.

Reference solution (a). Dissolve 10 mg of the substance to be examined and 10 mg of *sodium acetate R* in *water R* and dilute to 100 ml with the same solvent.

Reference solution (b). Dilute 1.0 ml of the test solution to 100 ml with *water R*.

Column:

− *size*: $l = 0.25$ m, $\emptyset = 4.6$ mm,

− *stationary phase*: *octadecylsilyl silica gel for chromatography R* (5 μm).

Mobile phase: dilute 1 ml of *phosphoric acid R* to 1000 ml with *water R*.

Flow rate: 1 ml/min.

Detection: spectrophotometer at 210 nm.

Injection: 20 μl.

System suitability: reference solution (a):

− *resolution*: minimum 5 between the peaks due to sodium acetate and sodium propionate.

Limits:

− *any impurity*: not more than 0.1 times the area of the principal peak in the chromatogram obtained with reference solution (b) (0.1 per cent),

− *total*: not more than half the area of the principal peak in the chromatrogram obtained with reference solution (b) (0.5 per cent),

− *disregard limit*: 0.05 times the area of the principal peak in the chromatogram obtained with reference solution (b) (0.05 per cent).

Readily oxidisable substances. In a ground-glass-stoppered conical flask introduce 10 g of the substance to be examined. Add 100 ml of *water R* and stir to dissolve. Add 25 ml of *sodium hypobromite solution R* and 10 ml of a 200 g/l solution of *sodium acetate R*, stopper the flask and allow to stand for 15 min. Add 10 ml of *potassium iodide solution R* and 20 ml of *hydrochloric acid R* while cooling. Titrate with *0.2 M sodium thiosulphate*, adding 2 ml of *starch solution R*

towards the end of the titration. Carry out a blank titration. The difference between the volumes used in the 2 titrations is not greater than 2.2 ml.

Iron (*2.4.9*): maximum 10 ppm.

10 ml of solution S complies with the limit test for iron.

Heavy metals (*2.4.8*): maximum 10 ppm.

12 ml of solution S complies with limit test A. Prepare the standard using *lead standard solution (1 ppm Pb) R*.

Loss on drying (*2.2.32*): maximum 0.5 per cent, determined on 1.000 g by heating in an oven at 100-105 °C for 3 h.

ASSAY

Dissolve 80.0 mg in 30 ml of *anhydrous acetic acid R*. Titrate with *0.1 M perchloric acid*, determining the end-point potentiometrically (*2.2.20*).

1 ml of *0.1 M perchloric acid* is equivalent to 9.61 mg of $C_3H_5NaO_2$.

STORAGE

In an airtight container.

04/2003:0436

SORBITOL, LIQUID (CRYSTALLISING)

Sorbitolum liquidum cristallisabile

DEFINITION

Aqueous solution of a hydrogenated, partly hydrolysed starch.

Content:

− anhydrous substance: 68.0 per cent *m/m* to 72.0 per cent *m/m*,

− D-glucitol (D-sorbitol, $C_6H_{14}O_6$): 92.0 per cent to 101.0 per cent (anhydrous substance).

CHARACTERS

Appearance: clear, colourless, syrupy liquid, miscible with water.

IDENTIFICATION

A. Examine the chromatograms obtained in the assay.

Results: the principal peak in the chromatogram obtained with the test solution is similar in retention time to the principal peak in the chromatogram obtained with reference solution (a).

B. To 7.0 g add 40 ml of *water R* and 6.4 g of *disodium tetraborate R*, allow to stand for 1 h, shaking occasionally, and dilute to 50.0 ml with *water R*. Filter if necessary. The angle of rotation (*2.2.7*) is 0° to + 1.5°.

C. It is a clear, syrupy liquid at a temperature of 25 °C.

TESTS

Appearance of solution. The solution is clear (*2.2.1*) and colourless (*2.2.2, Method II*).

Dilute 7.0 g to 50 ml with *water R*.

Conductivity (*2.2.38*): maximum 10 μS·cm⁻¹ measured on the undiluted liquid sorbitol (crystallising) while gently stirring with a magnetic stirrer.

Reducing sugars: maximum 0.2 per cent calculated as glucose equivalent.

To 5.0 g add 6 ml of *water R*, 20 ml of *cupri-citric solution R* and a few glass beads. Heat so that boiling begins after 4 min and maintain boiling for 3 min. Cool rapidly and add 100 ml of a 2.4 per cent *V/V* solution of *glacial acetic acid R* and 20.0 ml of *0.025 M iodine*. With continuous shaking, add 25 ml of a mixture of 6 volumes of *hydrochloric acid R* and 94 volumes of *water R* and, when the precipitate has dissolved, titrate the excess of iodine with *0.05 M sodium thiosulphate* using 1 ml of *starch solution R*, added towards the end of the titration, as indicator. Not less than 12.8 ml of *0.05 M sodium thiosulphate* is required.

Lead (*2.4.10*): maximum 0.5 ppm.

Nickel (*2.4.15*): maximum 1 ppm.

Water (*2.5.12*): 28.0 per cent to 32.0 per cent *m/m*, determined on 0.1 g.

ASSAY

Liquid chromatography (*2.2.29*).

Test solution. Mix 1.00 g of the substance to be examined with 20 ml of *water R* and dilute to 50.0 ml with the same solvent.

Reference solution (a). Dissolve 65.0 mg of *sorbitol CRS* in 2 ml of *water R* and dilute to 5.0 ml with the same solvent.

Reference solution (b). Dissolve 65 mg of *mannitol CRS* and 65 mg of *sorbitol CRS* in 2 ml of *water R* and dilute to 5.0 ml with the same solvent.

Column:
– *size*: l = 0.3 m, Ø = 7.8 mm,
– *stationary phase*: *strong cation exchange resin (calcium form) R* (9 µm),
– *temperature*: 85 ± 1 °C.

Mobile phase: degassed *water R*.

Flow rate: 0.5 ml/min.

Detection: refractometer maintained at a constant temperature.

Injection: 20 µl.

Run time: 3 times the retention time of sorbitol.

Relative retention with reference to sorbitol (retention time = about 27 min): mannitol = about 0.8.

System suitability: reference solution (b):
– *resolution*: minimum 2 between the peaks due to mannitol and to sorbitol.

Calculate the percentage content of D-sorbitol from the areas of the peaks and the declared content of *sorbitol CRS*.

04/2003:0437

SORBITOL, LIQUID (NON-CRYSTALLISING)

Sorbitolum liquidum non cristallisabile

DEFINITION

Aqueous solution of a hydrogenated, partly hydrolysed starch.

Content:
– anhydrous substance: 68.0 per cent *m/m* to 72.0 per cent *m/m*,

– D-glucitol (D-sorbitol, $C_6H_{14}O_6$): 72.0 per cent to 92.0 per cent (anhydrous substance).

CHARACTERS

Appearance: clear, colourless, syrupy liquid, miscible with water.

IDENTIFICATION

A. Examine the chromatograms obtained in the assay.
   Results: the principal peak in the chromatogram obtained with the test solution is similar in retention time to the principal peak in the chromatogram obtained with reference solution (a).

B. To 7.0 g add 40 ml of *water R* and 6.4 g of *disodium tetraborate R*. Allow to stand for 1 h, shaking occasionally, and dilute to 50.0 ml with *water R*. Filter if necessary. The angle of rotation (*2.2.7*) is + 1.5° to + 3.5°.

C. It is a clear, syrupy liquid at 25 °C.

TESTS

Appearance of solution. The solution is clear (*2.2.1*) and colourless (*2.2.2, Method II*).

Dilute 7.0 g to 50 ml with *water R*.

Conductivity (*2.2.38*): maximum 10 µS·cm⁻¹ measured on the undiluted liquid sorbitol (non crystallising) while gently stirring with a magnetic stirrer.

Reducing sugars: maximum 0.2 per cent calculated as glucose equivalent.

To 5.0 g add 6 ml of *water R*, 20 ml of *cupri-citric solution R* and a few glass beads. Heat so that boiling begins after 4 min and maintain boiling for 3 min. Cool rapidly and add 100 ml of a 2.4 per cent *V/V* solution of *glacial acetic acid R* and 20.0 ml of *0.025 M iodine*. With continuous shaking, add 25 ml of a mixture of 6 volumes of *hydrochloric acid R* and 94 volumes of *water R* and, when the precipitate has dissolved, titrate the excess of iodine with *0.05 M sodium thiosulphate* using 1 ml of *starch solution R*, added towards the end of the titration, as indicator. Not less than 12.8 ml of *0.05 M sodium thiosulphate* is required.

Reducing sugars after hydrolysis: maximum 9.3 per cent calculated as glucose equivalent.

To 6.0 g add 35 ml of *water R*, 40 ml of *1 M hydrochloric acid* and a few glass beads. Boil under a reflux condenser for 4 h. Cool and neutralise with *dilute sodium hydroxide solution R* using 0.2 ml of *bromothymol blue solution R1* as indicator. Cool and dilute to 100.0 ml with *water R*. To 3.0 ml of the solution add 5 ml of *water R*, 20 ml of *cupri-citric solution R* and a few glass beads. Heat so that boiling begins after 4 min and maintain boiling for 3 min. Cool rapidly and add 100 ml of a 2.4 per cent *V/V* solution of *glacial acetic acid R* and 20.0 ml of *0.025 M iodine*. With continuous shaking, add 25 ml of a mixture of 6 volumes of *hydrochloric acid R* and 94 volumes of *water R*. When the precipitate has dissolved, titrate the excess of iodine with *0.05 M sodium thiosulphate* using 1 ml of *starch solution R*, added towards the end of the titration, as indicator. Not less than 8.0 ml of *0.05 M sodium thiosulphate* is required.

Lead (*2.4.10*): maximum 0.5 ppm.

Nickel (*2.4.15*): maximum 1 ppm.

Water (*2.5.12*): 28.0 per cent to 32.0 per cent *m/m*, determined on 0.1 g.

ASSAY

Liquid chromatography (*2.2.29*).

Test solution. Mix 1.00 g of the substance to be examined with 20 ml of *water R* and dilute to 50.0 ml with the same solvent.

Reference solution (a). Dissolve 55.0 mg of *sorbitol CRS* in 2 ml of *water R* and dilute to 5.0 ml with the same solvent.

Reference solution (b). Dissolve 55 mg of *mannitol CRS* and 55 mg of *sorbitol CRS* in 2 ml of *water R* and dilute to 5.0 ml with the same solvent.

Column:

− *size*: l = 0.3 m, Ø = 7.8 mm,

− *stationary phase*: *strong cation exchange resin (calcium form) R* (9 µm),

− *temperature*: 85 ± 1 °C.

Mobile phase: degassed *water R*.

Flow rate: 0.5 ml/min.

Detection: refractometer maintained at a constant temperature.

Injection: 20 µl.

Run time: 3 times the retention time of sorbitol.

Relative retention with reference to sorbitol (retention time = about 27 min): mannitol = about 0.8.

System suitability: reference solution (b):

− *resolution*: minimum 2 between the peaks due to mannitol and to sorbitol.

Calculate the percentage content of D-sorbitol from the areas of the peaks and the declared content of *sorbitol CRS*.

04/2003:1630

SQUALANE

Squalanum

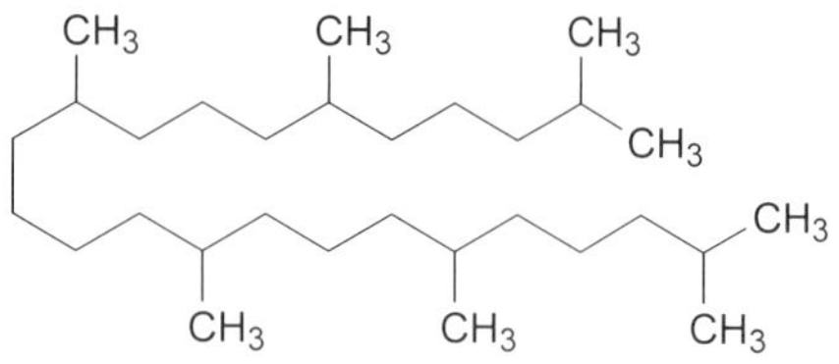

$C_{30}H_{62}$

M_r 422.8

DEFINITION

2,6,10,15,19,23-Hexamethyltetracosane (perhydrosqualene). It may be of vegetable (unsaponifiable matter of olive oil) or animal (shark liver oil) origin.

Content: 96.0 per cent to 103.0 per cent.

CHARACTERS

Appearance: clear, colourless, oily liquid.

Solubility: practically insoluble in water, miscible with most fats and oils, freely soluble in acetone and in cyclohexane, practically insoluble in alcohol.

Relative density: about 0.815.

IDENTIFICATION

A. Infrared absorption spectrophotometry (*2.2.24*).

 Comparison: *squalane CRS*.

B. It complies with the test for refractive index (see Tests).

C. Examine the chromatograms obtained in the assay.

Results: the principal peak in the chromatogram obtained with the test solution is similar in retention time and size to the principal peak in the chromatogram obtained with reference solution (a).

The chromatogram obtained with squalane of vegetable origin shows a peak corresponding to cyclosqualane (Figure 1630.-1 and Figure 1630.-2).

TESTS

Appearance. The substance to be examined is clear (*2.2.1*) and colourless (*2.2.2, Method II*).

Refractive index (*2.2.6*): 1.450 to 1.454.

Acid value (*2.5.1*): maximum 0.2.

Iodine value (*2.5.4*): maximum 4.0.

Saponification value (*2.5.6*): maximum 3.0.

Nickel (*2.4.27*): maximum 1 ppm.

Total ash (*2.4.16*): maximum 0.5 per cent, determined on 1.000 g.

ASSAY

Gas chromatography (*2.2.28*).

Internal standard solution. To 1.0 ml of *dimethylacetamide R*, add 100.0 ml of *heptane R*.

Test solution. Dissolve 0.100 g in the internal standard solution and dilute to 25.0 ml with the same solution.

Reference solution (a). Dissolve 0.100 g of *squalane CRS* in the internal standard solution and dilute to 25.0 ml with the same solution.

Reference solution (b). To 0.1 ml of *methyl erucate R* add 0.100 g of the substance to be examined, dissolve in the internal standard solution and dilute to 25.0 ml with the same solution.

Column:

− *material*: fused silica,

− *size*: l = 30 m, Ø = 0.32 mm,

− *stationary phase*: *poly(dimethyl)siloxane R* (film thickness 1 µm).

Carrier gas: *helium for chromatography R*.

Flow rate: 1.7 ml/min.

Split ratio: 1:12.

Temperature:

	Time (min)	Temperature (°C)
Column	0 - 39	60 - 290
	39 - 50	290
Injection port		275
Detector		300

Detection: flame ionisation.

Injection: 1 µl.

Relative retentions with reference to squalane (retention time = about 41 min): internal standard = about 0.2; methyl erucate = about 0.9; cyclosqualane = 1.05.

System suitability: reference solution (b):

− *resolution*: minimum 5 between the peaks due to methyl erucate and squalane.

Calculate the percentage content of squalane from the areas of the peaks and the declared content of *squalane CRS*.

LABELLING

The label states the origin of squalane (vegetable or animal).

The following chromatogram is published for information.

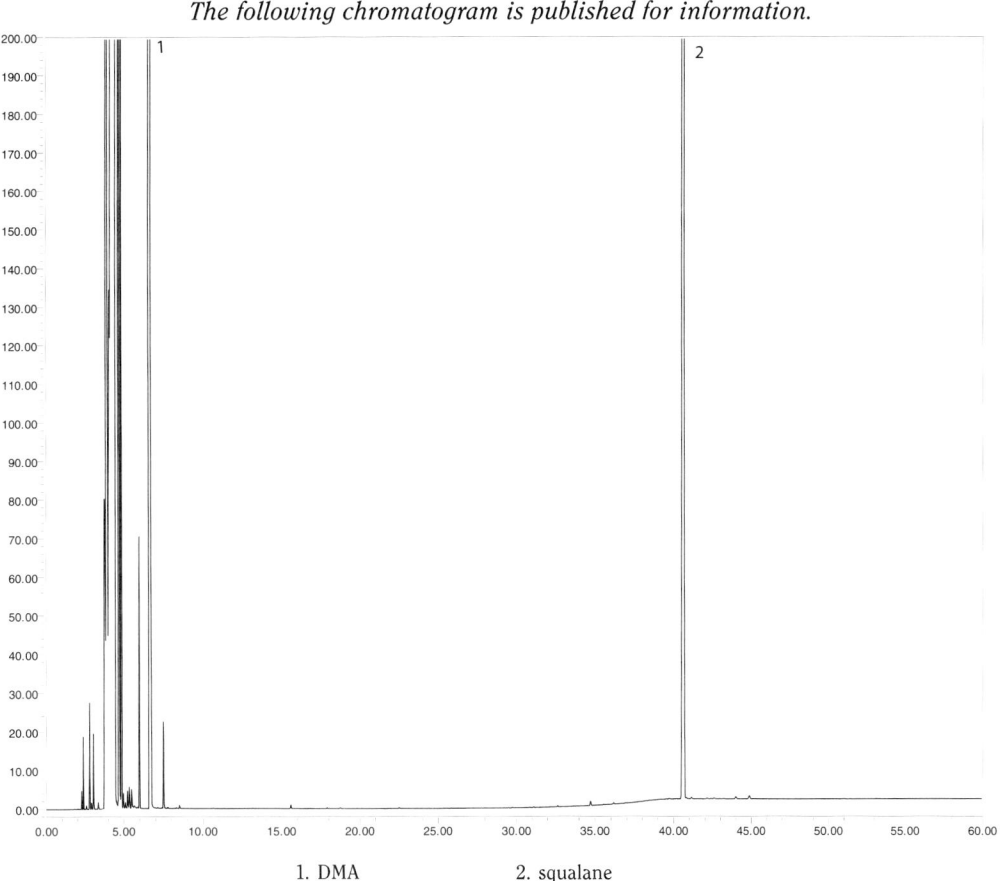

1. DMA   2. squalane

Figure 1630.-1. – *Chromatogram of squalane of animal origin*

The following chromatogram is published for information.

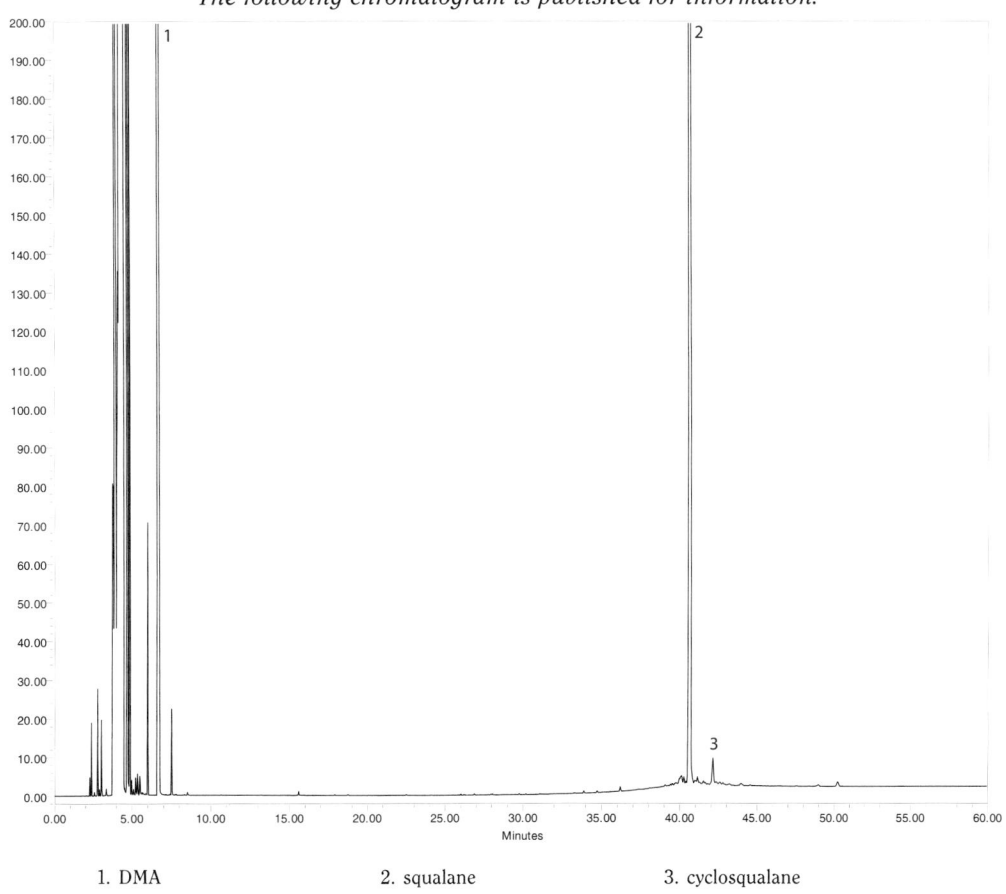

1. DMA   2. squalane   3. cyclosqualane

Figure 1630.-2. – *Chromatogram of squalane of vegetable origin*

T

Monographs
Q - Z

04/2003:0211

TETRACYCLINE

Tetracyclinum

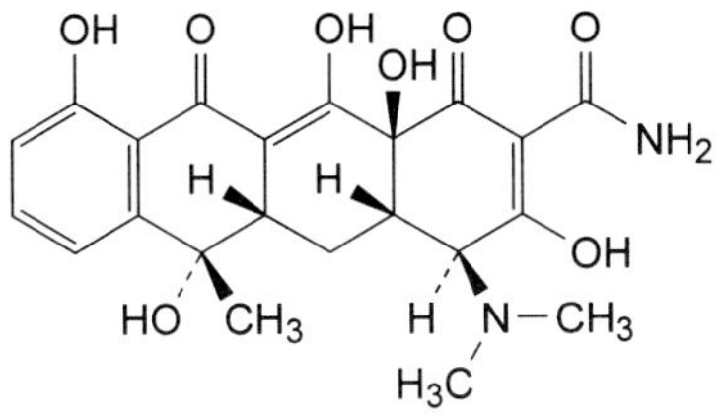

$C_{22}H_{24}N_2O_8$ M_r 444.4

DEFINITION

(4S,4aS,5aS,6S,12aS)-4-(Dimethylamino)-3,6,10,12,12a-pentahydroxy-6-methyl-1,11-dioxo-1,4,4a,5,5a,6,11,12a-octahydrotetracene-2-carboxamide.

Content: 88.0 per cent to 102.0 per cent (dried substance).

CHARACTERS

Appearance: yellow, crystalline powder.

Solubility: very slightly soluble in water, soluble in alcohol and in methanol, sparingly soluble in acetone. It dissolves in dilute acid and alkaline solutions.

IDENTIFICATION

A. Thin-layer chromatography (*2.2.27*).

Test solution. Dissolve 5 mg of the substance to be examined in *methanol R* and dilute to 10 ml with the same solvent.

Reference solution (a). Dissolve 5 mg of *tetracycline hydrochloride CRS* in *methanol R* and dilute to 10 ml with the same solvent.

Reference solution (b). Dissolve 5 mg of *tetracycline hydrochloride CRS*, 5 mg of *demeclocycline hydrochloride R* and 5 mg of *oxytetracycline hydrochloride R* in *methanol R* and dilute to 10 ml with the same solvent.

Plate: TLC octadecylsilyl silica gel F_{254} plate R.

Mobile phase: mix 20 volumes of *acetonitrile R*, 20 volumes of *methanol R* and 60 volumes of a 63 g/l solution of *oxalic acid R* previously adjusted to pH 2 with *concentrated ammonia R*.

Application: 1 µl.

Development: over 3/4 of the plate.

Drying: in air.

Detection: examine in ultraviolet light at 254 nm.

System suitability: the chromatogram obtained with reference solution (b) shows 3 clearly separated spots.

Results: the principal spot in the chromatogram obtained with the test solution is similar in position and size to the principal spot in the chromatogram obtained with reference solution (a).

B. To about 2 mg add 5 ml of *sulphuric acid R*. A violet-red colour develops. Add the solution to 2.5 ml of *water R*. The colour becomes yellow.

C. Dissolve about 10 mg in a mixture of 1 ml of *dilute nitric acid R* and 5 ml of *water R*. Shake and add 1 ml of *silver nitrate solution R2*. Any opalescence in the solution is not more intense than that in a mixture of 1 ml of *dilute nitric acid R*, 5 ml of *water R* and 1 ml of *silver nitrate solution R2*.

TESTS

pH (*2.2.3*): 3.5 to 6.0.

Suspend 0.1 g in 10 ml of *carbon dioxide-free water R*.

Specific optical rotation (*2.2.7*): −260 to −280 (dried substance).

Dissolve 0.250 g in *0.1 M hydrochloric acid* and dilute to 50.0 ml with the same acid.

Related substances. Liquid chromatography (*2.2.29*).

Test solution. Dissolve 25.0 mg of the substance to be examined in *0.01 M hydrochloric acid* and dilute to 25.0 ml with the same acid.

Reference solution (a). Dissolve 25.0 mg of *tetracycline hydrochloride CRS* in *0.01 M hydrochloric acid* and dilute to 25.0 ml with the same acid.

Reference solution (b). Dissolve 12.5 mg of *4-epitetracycline hydrochloride CRS* in *0.01 M hydrochloric acid* and dilute to 50.0 ml with the same acid.

Reference solution (c). Dissolve 10.0 mg of *anhydrotetracycline hydrochloride CRS* in *0.01 M hydrochloric acid* and dilute to 100.0 ml with the same acid.

Reference solution (d). Dissolve 10.0 mg of *4-epianhydrotetracycline hydrochloride CRS* in *0.01 M hydrochloric acid* and dilute to 50.0 ml with the same acid.

Reference solution (e). Mix 1.0 ml of reference solution (a), 2.0 ml of reference solution (b) and 5.0 ml of reference solution (d) and dilute to 25.0 ml with *0.01 M hydrochloric acid*.

Reference solution (f). Mix 40.0 ml of reference solution (b), 20.0 ml of reference solution (c) and 5.0 ml of reference solution (d) and dilute to 200.0 ml with *0.01 M hydrochloric acid*.

Reference solution (g). Dilute 1.0 ml of reference solution (c) to 50.0 ml with *0.01 M hydrochloric acid*.

Column:

− *size*: l = 0.25 m, Ø = 4.6 mm,

− *stationary phase*: *styrene-divinylbenzene copolymer R* (8 µm),

− *temperature*: 60 °C.

Mobile phase: weigh 80.0 g of *2-methyl-2-propanol R* and transfer to a 1000 ml volumetric flask with the aid of 200 ml of *water R*; add 100 ml of a 35 g/l solution of *dipotassium hydrogen phosphate R* adjusted to pH 9.0 with *dilute phosphoric acid R*, 200 ml of a 10 g/l solution of *tetrabutylammonium hydrogen sulphate R* adjusted to pH 9.0 with *dilute sodium hydroxide solution R* and 10 ml of a 40 g/l solution of *sodium edetate R* adjusted to pH 9.0 with *dilute sodium hydroxide solution R*; dilute to 1000.0 ml with *water R*.

Flow rate: 1.0 ml/min.

Detection: spectrophotometer at 254 nm.

Injection: 20 µl; inject the test solution and reference solutions (e), (f) and (g).

System suitability:

− *resolution*: minimum 2.5 between the peaks due to impurity A (1st peak) and tetracycline (2nd peak) and minimum 8.0 between the peaks due to tetracycline and impurity D (3rd peak) in the chromatogram obtained with reference solution (e); if necessary, adjust the concentration of 2-methyl-2-propanol in the mobile phase,

− *signal-to-noise ratio*: minimum 3 for the principal peak in the chromatogram obtained with reference solution (g),

— *symmetry factor*: maximum 1.25 for the peak due to tetracycline in the chromatogram obtained with reference solution (e).

Limits:

— *impurity A*: not more than the area of the corresponding peak in the chromatogram obtained with reference solution (f) (5.0 per cent),

— *impurity B* (eluting on the tail of the principal peak): not more than 0.4 times the area of the peak due to impurity A in the chromatogram obtained with reference solution (f) (2.0 per cent),

— *impurity C*: not more than the area of the corresponding peak in the chromatogram obtained with reference solution (f) (1.0 per cent),

— *impurity D*: not more than the area of the corresponding peak in the chromatogram obtained with reference solution (f) (0.5 per cent).

Heavy metals (*2.4.8*): maximum 50 ppm.

0.5 g complies with limit test C. Prepare the standard using 2.5 ml of *lead standard solution (10 ppm Pb) R*.

Loss on drying (*2.2.32*): maximum 13.0 per cent, determined on 1.000 g by drying in an oven at 100-105 °C.

Sulphated ash (*2.4.14*): maximum 0.5 per cent, determined on 1.0 g.

ASSAY

Liquid chromatography (*2.2.29*) as described in the test for related substances with the following modification.

Injection: test solution and reference solution (a).

Calculate the percentage content of $C_{22}H_{24}N_2O_8$.

STORAGE

Protected from light.

IMPURITIES

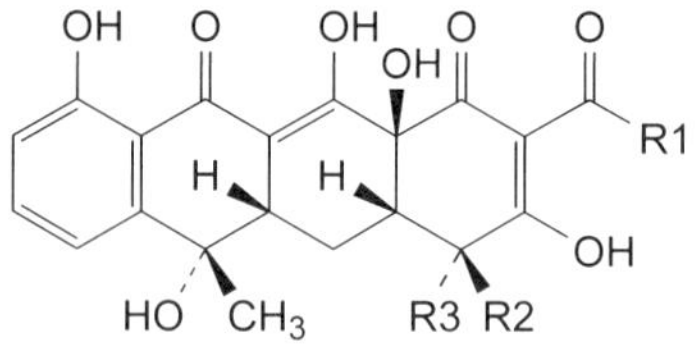

A. R1 = NH$_2$, R2 = H, R3 = N(CH$_3$)$_2$: (4*R*,4a*S*,5a*S*,6*S*,12a*S*)-4-(dimethylamino)-3,6,10,12,12a-pentahydroxy-6-methyl-1,11-dioxo-1,4,4a,5,5a,6,11,12a-octahydrotetracene-2-carboxamide (4-epitetracycline),

B. R1 = CH$_3$, R2 = N(CH$_3$)$_2$, R3 = H: (4*S*,4a*S*,5a*S*,6*S*,12a*S*)-2-acetyl-4-(dimethylamino)-3,6,10,12,12a-pentahydroxy-6-methyl-4a,5,5a,6,12a-tetrahydrotetracene-1,11(4*H*,5*H*)-dione (2-acetyl-2-decarbamoyltetracycline),

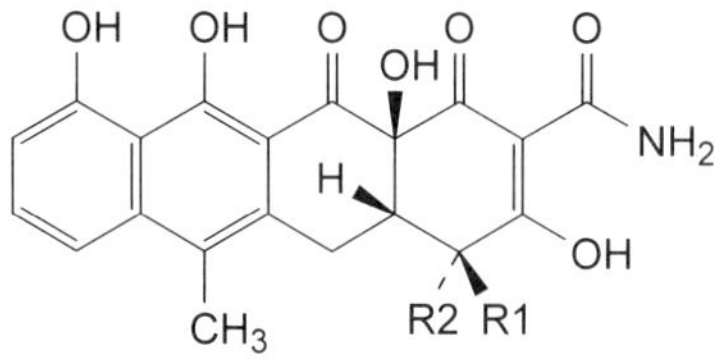

C. R1 = N(CH$_3$)$_2$, R2 = H: (4*S*,4a*S*,12a*S*)-4-(dimethylamino)-3,10,11,12a-tetrahydroxy-6-methyl-1,12-dioxo-1,4,4a,5,12,12a-hexahydrotetracene-2-carboxamide (anhydrotetracycline),

D. R1 = H, R2 = N(CH$_3$)$_2$: (4*R*,4a*S*,12a*S*)-4-(dimethylamino)-3,10,11,12a-tetrahydroxy-6-methyl-1,12-dioxo-1,4,4a,5,12,12a-hexahydrotetracene-2-carboxamide (4-epianhydrotetracycline).

04/2003:0210

TETRACYCLINE HYDROCHLORIDE

Tetracyclini hydrochloridum

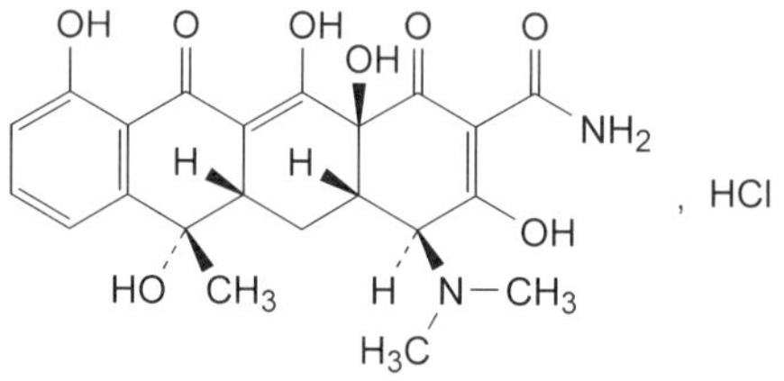

$C_{22}H_{25}ClN_2O_8$ M_r 480.9

DEFINITION

(4*S*,4a*S*,5a*S*,6*S*,12a*S*)-4-(Dimethylamino)-3,6,10,12,12a-pentahydroxy-6-methyl-1,11-dioxo-1,4,4a,5,5a,6,11,12a-octahydrotetracene-2-carboxamide hydrochloride.

Content: 95.0 per cent to 102.0 per cent (dried substance).

CHARACTERS

Appearance: yellow, crystalline powder.

Solubility: soluble in water, slightly soluble in alcohol, practically insoluble in acetone. It dissolves in solutions of alkali hydroxides and carbonates. Solutions in water become turbid on standing, owing to the precipitation of tetracycline.

IDENTIFICATION

A. Thin-layer chromatography (*2.2.27*).

Test solution. Dissolve 5 mg of the substance to be examined in *methanol R* and dilute to 10 ml with the same solvent.

Reference solution (a). Dissolve 5 mg of *tetracycline hydrochloride CRS* in *methanol R* and dilute to 10 ml with the same solvent.

Reference solution (b). Dissolve 5 mg of *tetracycline hydrochloride CRS*, 5 mg of *demeclocycline hydrochloride R* and 5 mg of *oxytetracycline hydrochloride R* in *methanol R* and dilute to 10 ml with the same solvent.

Plate: TLC octadecylsilyl silica gel F$_{254}$ plate R.

Mobile phase: mix 20 volumes of *acetonitrile R*, 20 volumes of *methanol R* and 60 volumes of a 63 g/l solution of *oxalic acid R* previously adjusted to pH 2 with *concentrated ammonia R*.

Application: 1 µl.

Development: over 3/4 of the plate.

Drying: in air.

Detection: examine in ultraviolet light at 254 nm.

System suitability: the chromatogram obtained with reference solution (b) shows 3 clearly separated spots.

Results: the principal spot in the chromatogram obtained with the test solution is similar in position and size to the principal spot in the chromatogram obtained with reference solution (a).

B. To about 2 mg add 5 ml of *sulphuric acid R*. A violet-red colour develops. Add the solution to 2.5 ml of *water R*. The colour becomes yellow.

C. It gives reaction (a) of chlorides (*2.3.1*).

TESTS

pH (*2.2.3*): 1.8 to 2.8.

Dissolve 0.1 g in 10 ml of *carbon dioxide-free water R*.

Specific optical rotation (*2.2.7*): −240 to −255 (dried substance).

Dissolve 0.250 g in *0.1 M hydrochloric acid* and dilute to 25.0 ml with the same acid.

Related substances. Liquid chromatography (*2.2.29*).

Test solution. Dissolve 25.0 mg of the substance to be examined in *0.01 M hydrochloric acid* and dilute to 25.0 ml with the same acid.

Reference solution (a). Dissolve 25.0 mg of *tetracycline hydrochloride CRS* in *0.01 M hydrochloric acid* and dilute to 25.0 ml with the same acid.

Reference solution (b). Dissolve 15.0 mg of *4-epitetracycline hydrochloride CRS* in *0.01 M hydrochloric acid* and dilute to 50.0 ml with the same acid.

Reference solution (c). Dissolve 10.0 mg of *anhydrotetracycline hydrochloride CRS* in *0.01 M hydrochloric acid* and dilute to 100.0 ml with the same acid.

Reference solution (d). Dissolve 10.0 mg of *4-epianhydrotetracycline hydrochloride CRS* in *0.01 M hydrochloric acid* and dilute to 50.0 ml with the same acid.

Reference solution (e). Mix 1.0 ml of reference solution (a), 2.0 ml of reference solution (b) and 5.0 ml of reference solution (d) and dilute to 25.0 ml with *0.01 M hydrochloric acid*.

Reference solution (f). Mix 20.0 ml of reference solution (b), 10.0 ml of reference solution (c) and 5.0 ml of reference solution (d) and dilute to 200.0 ml using *0.01 M hydrochloric acid*.

Reference solution (g). Dilute 1.0 ml of reference solution (c) to 50.0 ml with *0.01 M hydrochloric acid*.

Column:

— *size*: l = 0.25 m, Ø = 4.6 mm,

— *stationary phase*: *styrene-divinylbenzene copolymer R* (8 µm),

— *temperature*: 60 °C.

Mobile phase: weigh 80.0 g of *2-methyl-2-propanol R* and transfer to a 1000 ml volumetric flask with the aid of 200 ml of *water R*; add 100 ml of a 35 g/l solution of *dipotassium hydrogen phosphate R* adjusted to pH 9.0 with *dilute phosphoric acid R*, 200 ml of a 10 g/l solution of *tetrabutylammonium hydrogen sulphate R* adjusted to pH 9.0 with *dilute sodium hydroxide solution R* and 10 ml of a 40 g/l solution of *sodium edetate R* adjusted to pH 9.0 with *dilute sodium hydroxide solution R*; dilute to 1000.0 ml with *water R*.

Flow rate: 1.0 ml/min.

Detection: spectrophotometer at 254 nm.

Injection: 20 µl; inject the test solution and reference solutions (e), (f) and (g).

System suitability:

— *resolution*: minimum 2.5 between the peaks due to impurity A (1st peak) and tetracycline (2nd peak) and minimum 8.0 between the peaks due to tetracycline and impurity D (3rd peak) in the chromatogram obtained with reference solution (e); if necessary, adjust the concentration of 2-methyl-2-propanol in the mobile phase,

— *signal-to-noise ratio*: minimum 3 for the principal peak in the chromatogram obtained with reference solution (g),

— *symmetry factor*: maximum 1.25 for the peak due to tetracycline in the chromatogram obtained with reference solution (e).

Limits:

— *impurity A*: not more than the area of the corresponding peak in the chromatogram obtained with reference solution (f) (3.0 per cent),

— *impurity B* (eluting on the tail of the principal peak): not more than half the area of the peak due to impurity A in the chromatogram obtained with reference solution (f) (1.5 per cent),

— *impurity C*: not more than the area of the corresponding peak in the chromatogram obtained with reference solution (f) (0.5 per cent),

— *impurity D*: not more than the area of the corresponding peak in the chromatogram obtained with reference solution (f) (0.5 per cent).

Heavy metals (*2.4.8*): maximum 50 ppm.

0.5 g complies with limit test C. Prepare the standard using 2.5 ml of *lead standard solution (10 ppm Pb) R*.

Loss on drying (*2.2.32*): maximum 2.0 per cent, determined on 1.000 g by drying at 60 °C over *diphosphorus pentoxide R* at a pressure not exceeding 670 Pa for 3 h.

Sulphated ash (*2.4.14*): maximum 0.5 per cent, determined on 1.0 g.

Sterility (*2.6.1*). If intended for use in the manufacture of parenteral dosage forms without a further appropriate sterilisation procedure, it complies with the test for sterility.

Bacterial endotoxins (*2.6.14*): less than 0.5 IU/mg, if intended for use in the manufacture of parenteral dosage forms without a further appropriate procedure for the removal of bacterial endotoxins.

ASSAY

Liquid chromatography (*2.2.29*) as described in the test for related substances with the following modification.

Injection: test solution and reference solution (a).

Calculate the percentage content of $C_{22}H_{25}ClN_2O_8$.

STORAGE

Protected from light. If the substance is sterile, store in a sterile, tamper-proof container.

LABELLING

The label states:

— where applicable, that the substance is sterile,

— where applicable, that the substance is free from bacterial endotoxins.

IMPURITIES

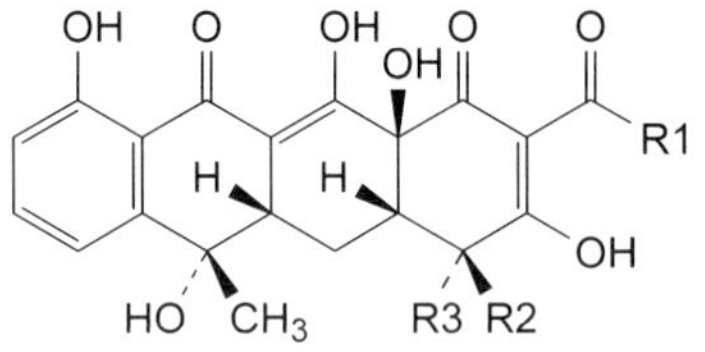

A. R1 = NH$_2$, R2 = H, R3 = N(CH$_3$)$_2$: (4R,4aS,5aS,6S,12aS)-
4-(dimethylamino)-3,6,10,12,12a-pentahydroxy-6-methyl-
1,11-dioxo-1,4,4a,5,5a,6,11,12a-octahydrotetracene-2-
carboxamide (4-epitetracycline),

B. R1 = CH$_3$, R2 = N(CH$_3$)$_2$, R3 = H: (4S,4aS,5aS,6S,12aS)-
2-acetyl-4-(dimethylamino)-3,6,10,12,12a-pentahydroxy-6-
methyl-4a,5a,6,12a-tetrahydrotetracene-1,11(4H,5H)-dione
(2-acetyl-2-decarbamoyltetracycline),

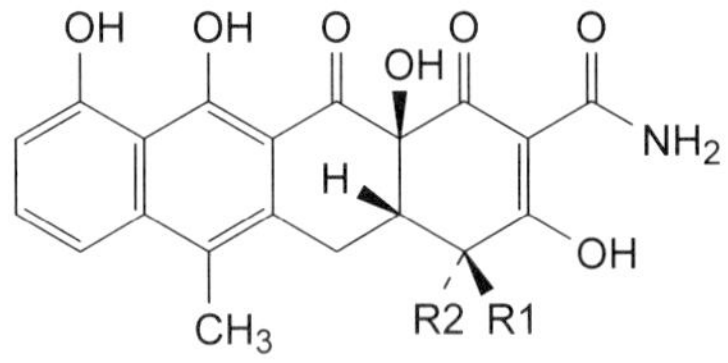

C. R1 = N(CH$_3$)$_2$, R2 = H: (4S,4aS,12aS)-4-(dimethylamino)-
3,10,11,12a-tetrahydroxy-6-methyl-1,12-dioxo-
1,4,4a,5,12,12a-hexahydrotetracene-2-carboxamide
(anhydrotetracycline),

D. R1 = H, R2 = N(CH$_3$)$_2$: (4R,4aS,12aS)-4-(dimethylamino)-
3,10,11,12a-tetrahydroxy-6-methyl-1,12-dioxo-
1,4,4a,5,12,12a-hexahydrotetracene-2-carboxamide
(4-epianhydrotetracycline).

07/2002:1740
corrected

TRIBENOSIDE

Tribenosidum

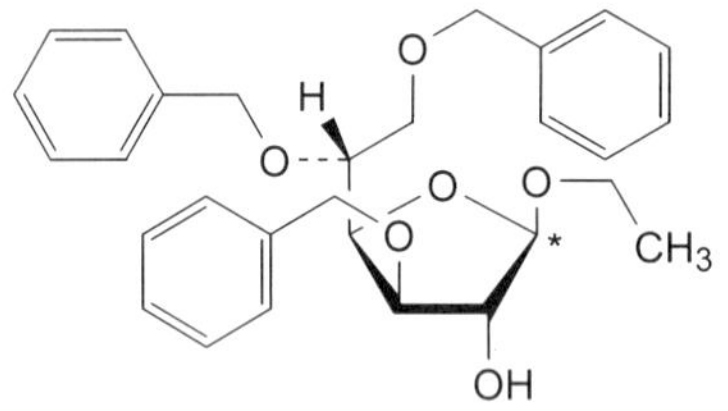

and anomer at C*

C$_{29}$H$_{34}$O$_6$ M_r 478.6

DEFINITION

Mixture of α- and β-anomers of ethyl 3,5,6-tri-O-benzyl-D-
glucofuranoside.

Content: 96.0 per cent to 102.0 per cent.

CHARACTERS

Appearance: yellowish to pale yellow, clear, viscous liquid.

Solubility: practically insoluble in water, very soluble in
acetone, in methanol and in methylene chloride.

IDENTIFICATION

Infrared absorption spectrophotometry (*2.2.24*).

Preparation: discs.

Comparison: tribenoside CRS.

TESTS

Solution S. Dissolve 4.00 g in *methanol R* and dilute to
20 ml with the same solvent.

Appearance of solution. Solution S is clear (*2.2.1*) and its
absorbance (*2.2.25*) at 420 nm has a maximum of 0.10.

Specific optical rotation (*2.2.7*): −31.0 to −40.0.

Dilute 2.0 ml of solution S to 20.0 ml with *methanol R*.

Related substances. Liquid chromatography (*2.2.29*).

Test solution (a). Dissolve 1.000 g of the substance to
be examined in a mixture of 5 volumes of *water R* and
95 volumes of *acetonitrile R* and dilute to 25.0 ml with the
same mixture of solvents.

Test solution (b). Dissolve 50.0 mg of the substance to
be examined in a mixture of 5 volumes of *water R* and
95 volumes of *acetonitrile R* and dilute to 50.0 ml with the
same mixture of solvents.

Reference solution (a). Dilute 25.0 mg of *benzaldehyde R*
and 30.0 mg of *tribenoside impurity A CRS* to 100.0 ml
with *acetonitrile R*. Introduce 20.0 ml of this solution into a
50 ml volumetric flask, add 2.5 ml of *water R* and dilute to
50.0 ml with *acetonitrile R*.

Reference solution (b). Dissolve 50.0 mg of *tribenoside CRS*
in a mixture of 5 volumes of *water R* and 95 volumes of
acetonitrile R and dilute to 50.0 ml with the same mixture
of solvents.

Reference solution (c). Dissolve 12.0 mg of *benzyl ether R*
in a mixture of 5 volumes of *water R* and 95 volumes of
acetonitrile R and dilute to 100.0 ml with the same mixture
of solvents.

Column:

− *size*: l = 0.15 m, Ø = 4.6 mm,

− *stationary phase*: octadecylsilyl silica gel for
chromatography R (3 μm).

Mobile phase:

− *mobile phase A*: 0.1 per cent V/V solution of *phosphoric
acid R*,

− *mobile phase B*: acetonitrile R,

Time (min)	Mobile phase A (per cent V/V)	Mobile phase B (per cent V/V)
0 - 40	55 → 10	45 → 90
40 - 55	10	90
55 - 56	10 → 55	90 → 45
56 - 60	55	45

Flow rate: 1.3 ml/min.

Detection: spectrophotometer at 254 nm.

Injection: 20 μl; inject test solution (a) and reference
solutions (a), (b) and (c).

Relative retentions with reference to the β-anomer
of tribenoside (retention time = about 18 min):
α-anomer = about 1.1; impurity C = about 0.2;
impurity B = about 0.6; impurity D = about 0.8;
impurity A = about 1.4.

System suitability: reference solution (b):

− *resolution*: minimum 3.0 between the peaks due to the
α-anomer and to the β-anomer of tribenoside.

Limits:

− *impurity A*: not more than 1.7 times the area of the
corresponding peak in the chromatogram obtained with
reference solution (a) (0.5 per cent),

- *impurity C*: not more than twice the area of the corresponding peak in the chromatogram obtained with reference solution (a) (0.5 per cent); if the area of the peak due to impurity C in the chromatogram obtained with the test solution is greater than the area of the corresponding peak in the chromatogram obtained with reference solution (a) (0.25 per cent), dilute the test solution to obtain an area equal to or smaller than the area of the peak in the chromatogram obtained with reference solution (a); calculate the content of impurity C taking into account the dilution factor;

- *impurity D*: not more than the area of the principal peak in the chromatogram obtained with reference solution (c) (0.3 per cent),

- *any other impurity*: not more than the area of the peak due to impurity A in the chromatogram obtained with reference solution (a) (0.3 per cent),

- *total*: not more than 6.7 times the area of the peak due to impurity A in the chromatogram obtained with reference solution (a) (2.0 per cent),

- *disregard limit*: 0.17 times the area of the peak due to impurity A in the chromatogram obtained with reference solution (a) (0.05 per cent).

Heavy metals (*2.4.8*): maximum 20 ppm.

Dilute 5.0 ml of solution S to 20.0 ml with *methanol R*. 12 ml of the solution complies with limit test B. Prepare the standard using lead standard solution (1 ppm Pb) obtained by diluting *lead standard solution (100 ppm Pb) R* with *methanol R*.

ASSAY

Liquid chromatography (*2.2.29*) as described in the test for related substances with the following modification.

Injection: test solution (b) and reference solution (b).

Calculate the sum of the percentage contents of the α-anomer and the β-anomer of tribenoside.

STORAGE

Under nitrogen, in an airtight container.

IMPURITIES

A. R = CH$_2$-C$_6$H$_5$: 3,5,6-tri-*O*-benzyl-1,2-*O*-(1-methylethylidene)-α-D-glucofuranose,

B. R = H: 3,5-di-*O*-benzyl-1,2-*O*-(1-methylethylidene)-α-D-glucofuranose,

C. C$_6$H$_5$-CHO: benzaldehyde,

D. C$_6$H$_5$-CH$_2$-O-CH$_2$-C$_6$H$_5$: dibenzyl ether.

TRIMETHOPRIM

Trimethoprimum

C$_{14}$H$_{18}$N$_4$O$_3$ M_r 290.3

DEFINITION
5-(3,4,5-Trimethoxybenzyl)pyrimidine-2,4-diamine.
Content: 98.5 per cent to 101.0 per cent (dried substance).

CHARACTERS
Appearance: white or yellowish-white powder.
Solubility: very slightly soluble in water, slightly soluble in alcohol.

IDENTIFICATION
First identification: C.
Second identification: A, B, D.

A. Melting point (*2.2.14*): 199 °C to 203 °C.

B. Dissolve about 20 mg in *0.1 M sodium hydroxide* and dilute to 100.0 ml with the same solvent. Dilute 1.0 ml of this solution to 10.0 ml with *0.1 M sodium hydroxide*. Examined between 230 nm and 350 nm (*2.2.25*), the solution shows an absorption maximum at 287 nm. The specific absorbance at the maximum is 240 to 250.

C. Infrared absorption spectrophotometry (*2.2.24*).
   Preparation: discs.
   Comparison: trimethoprim CRS.

D. Dissolve about 25 mg, heating if necessary, in 5 ml of *0.005 M sulphuric acid* and add 2 ml of a 16 g/l solution of *potassium permanganate R* in *0.1 M sodium hydroxide*. Heat to boiling and add to the hot solution 0.4 ml of *formaldehyde R*. Mix, add 1 ml of *0.5 M sulphuric acid*, mix and heat again to boiling. Cool and filter. To the filtrate add 2 ml of *methylene chloride R* and shake vigorously. The organic layer, examined in ultraviolet light at 365 nm, shows green fluorescence.

TESTS

Appearance of solution. The solution is not more intensely coloured than reference solution BY$_7$ (*2.2.2, Method II*).

Dissolve 0.5 g in 10 ml of a mixture of 1 volume of *water R*, 4.5 volumes of *methanol R* and 5 volumes of *methylene chloride R*.

Related substances

A. Liquid chromatography (*2.2.29*).
   Test solution. Dissolve 25.0 mg of the substance to be examined in the mobile phase and dilute to 25.0 ml with the mobile phase.
   Reference solution (a). Dilute 1.0 ml of the test solution to 200.0 ml with the mobile phase.
   Reference solution (b). Dissolve 5.0 mg of trimethoprim CRS and 2.5 mg of *trimethoprim impurity E CRS* in the mobile phase and dilute to 100.0 ml with the mobile phase. Dilute 1.0 ml of the solution to 10.0 ml with the mobile phase.

Column:
- *size*: l = 0.250 m, Ø = 4.0 mm,
- *stationary phase*: *base-deactivated octadecylsilyl silica gel for chromatography R* (5 µm).

Mobile phase: mix 30 volumes of *methanol R* and 70 volumes of a 1.4 g/l solution of *sodium perchlorate R* adjusted to pH 3.6 with *phosphoric acid R*.

Flow rate: 1.3 ml/min.

Detection: spectrophotometer at 280 nm.

Injection: 20 µl loop injector.

Run time: 11 times the retention time of trimethoprim.

Relative retentions with reference to trimethoprim (retention time = about 5 min): impurity C = about 0.8; impurity E = about 0.9; impurity A = about 1.5; impurity D = about 2.0; impurity G = about 2.1; impurity B = about 2.3; impurity J = about 2.7; impurity F = about 4.0.

System suitability: reference solution (b):
- *resolution*: minimum of 2.5 between the peaks.

Limits:
- *correction factors*: for the calculation of contents, multiply the peak areas of the following impurities by the corresponding correction factor: impurity B = 0.43; impurity E = 0.53; impurity J = 0.66,
- *any impurity*: not more than 0.2 times the area of the principal peak in the chromatogram obtained with reference solution (a) (0.1 per cent),
- *total*: not more than 0.4 times the area of the principal peak in the chromatogram obtained with reference solution (a) (0.2 per cent),
- *disregard limit*: 0.04 times the area of the principal peak in the chromatogram obtained with reference solution (a) (0.02 per cent); disregard any peak corresponding to impurity H (relative retentions = about 10.3).

B. Liquid chromatography (*2.2.29*).

Test solution. Dissolve 25.0 mg of the substance to be examined in the mobile phase and dilute to 25.0 ml with the mobile phase.

Reference solution (a). Dilute 1.0 ml of the test solution to 200.0 ml with the mobile phase.

Reference solution (b). Dissolve 5.0 mg of *trimethoprim CRS* and 5.0 mg of *trimethoprim impurity B CRS* in the mobile phase and dilute to 100.0 ml with the mobile phase.

Column:
- *size*: l = 0.250 m, Ø = 4.6 mm,
- *stationary phase*: *nitrile silica gel for chromatography R* (5 µm) with a specific surface area of 350 m^2/g and a pore diameter of 10 nm.

Mobile phase: dissolve 1.14 g of *sodium hexane sulphonate R* in 600 ml of a 13.6 g/l solution of *potassium dihydrogen phosphate R*; adjust to pH 3.1 using *phosphoric acid R* and mix with 400 volumes of *methanol R*.

Flow rate: 0.8 ml/min.

Detection: spectrophotometer at 280 nm.

Injection: 20 µl loop injector.

Run time: 6 times the retention time of trimethoprim.

Relative retentions with reference to trimethoprim (retention time = about 4 min): impurity H = about 1.8; impurity I = about 4.9.

System suitability: reference solution (b):

- *resolution*: minimum of 2.0 between the peaks.

Limits:
- *correction factors*: for the calculation of contents, multiply the peak areas of the following impurities by the corresponding correction factor: impurity H = 0.50; impurity I = 0.28,
- *any impurity*: not more than 0.2 times the area of the principal peak in the chromatogram obtained with reference solution (a) (0.1 per cent),
- *total*: not more than 0.4 times the area of the principal peak in the chromatogram obtained with reference solution (a) (0.2 per cent),
- *disregard limit*: 0.04 times the area of the principal peak in the chromatogram obtained with reference solution (a) (0.02 per cent); disregard any peak corresponding to impurity B (relative retention = about 1.3).

Impurity K. Gas chromatography (*2.2.28*).

Test solution. Dissolve 0.500 g of the substance to be examined in 35.0 ml of *citrate buffer solution pH 5.0 R*, add 10.0 ml of *1,1-dimethylethyl methyl ether R*, shake thoroughly and centrifuge for 10 min. Use the upper layer.

Reference solution. Dilute 5.0 ml of *concentrated hydrochloric acid R* to 50.0 ml with *water R*. Add 12.5 mg of *aniline R* and shake thoroughly (solution A). To 35.0 ml of *citrate buffer solution pH 5.0 R* add 10.0 µl of solution A and 10.0 ml of *1,1-dimethylethyl methyl ether R*, shake thoroughly and centrifuge for 10 min. Use the upper layer.

Column:
- *material*: fused silica,
- *size*: l = 30 m, Ø = 0.53 mm,
- *stationary phase*: *poly(dimethyl)siloxane R* (film thickness 3 µm).

Carrier gas: *helium for chromatography R*.

Flow rate: 12 ml/min.

Temperature:
- *column*: 80 °C,
- *injection port*: 230 °C,
- *detector*: 270 °C.

Detection: nitrogen-phosphorus detector.

Injection: 3 µl.

Run time: 15 min.

System suitability: reference solution:
- *repeatability*: maximum relative standard deviation of 5.0 per cent after 6 injections.

Limits:
- *impurity K*: not more than the area of the corresponding peak in the chromatogram obtained with the reference solution (5 ppm).

Heavy metals (*2.4.8*): maximum 20 ppm.

1.0 g complies with limit test C. Prepare the standard using 2 ml of *lead standard solution (10 ppm Pb) R*

Loss on drying (*2.2.32*): maximum 1.0 per cent, determined on 1.000 g by drying in an oven at 100-105 °C.

Sulphated ash (*2.4.14*): maximum 0.1 per cent, determined on 1.0 g.

ASSAY

Dissolve 0.250 g in 50 ml of *anhydrous acetic acid R*. Titrate with *0.1 M perchloric acid*, determining the end-point potentiometrically (*2.2.20*).

1 ml of *0.1 M perchloric acid* is equivalent to 29.03 mg of $C_{14}H_{18}N_4O_3$.

IMPURITIES

By liquid chromatography A: A, B, C, D, E, F, G, H, J.

By liquid chromatography B: B, H, I.

By gas chromatography: K.

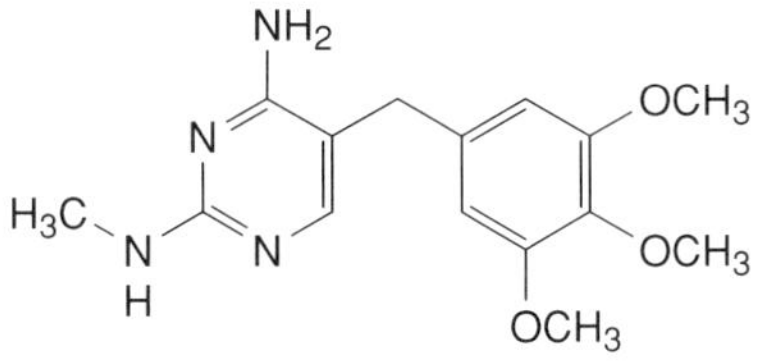

A. N^2-methyl-5-(3,4,5-trimethoxybenzyl)pyrimidine-2,4-diamine,

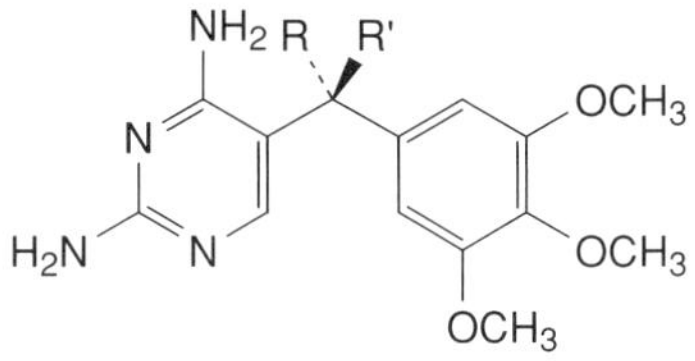

and enantiomer

B. R + R' = O: (2,4-diaminopyrimidin-5-yl)(3,4,5-trimethoxyphenyl)methanone,

C. R = OH, R' = H: (RS)-(2,4-diaminopyrimidin-5-yl)(3,4,5-trimethoxyphenyl)methanol,

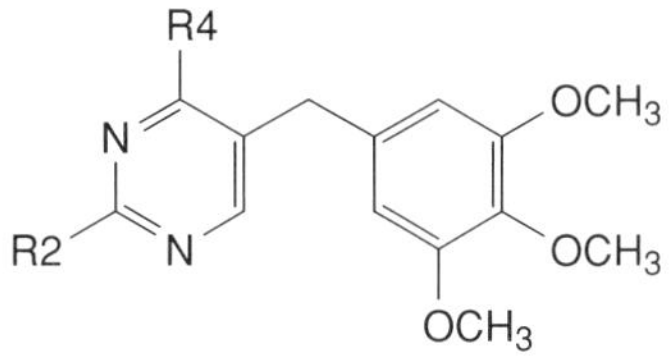

D. R2 = NH$_2$, R4 = OH: 2-amino-5-(3,4,5-trimethoxybenzyl)pyrimidin-4-ol,

E. R2 = OH, R4 = NH$_2$: 4-amino-5-(3,4,5-trimethoxybenzyl)pyrimidin-2-ol,

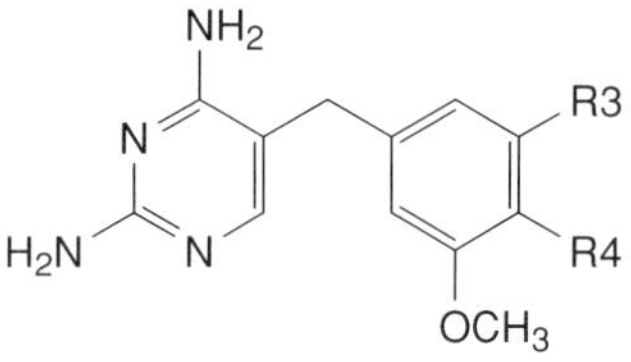

F. R3 = Br, R4 = OCH$_3$: 5-(3-bromo-4,5-dimethoxybenzyl)pyrimidine-2,4-diamine,

G. R3 = OCH$_3$, R4 = OC$_2$H$_5$: 5-(4-ethoxy-3,5-dimethoxybenzyl)pyrimidine-2,4-diamine,

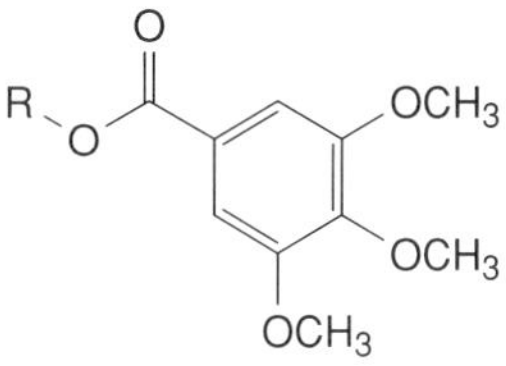

H. R = CH$_3$: methyl 3,4,5-trimethoxybenzoate,

J. R = H: 3,4,5-trimethoxybenzoic acid,

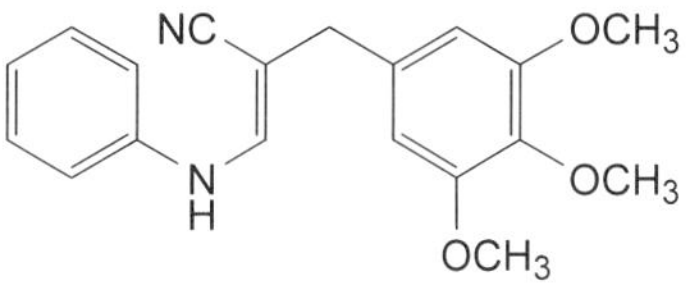

I. 3-(phenylamino)-2-(3,4,5-trimethoxybenzyl)prop-2-enenitrile,

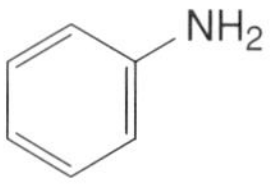

K. aniline.

V

04/2003:0749

VINCRISTINE SULPHATE

Vincristini sulfas

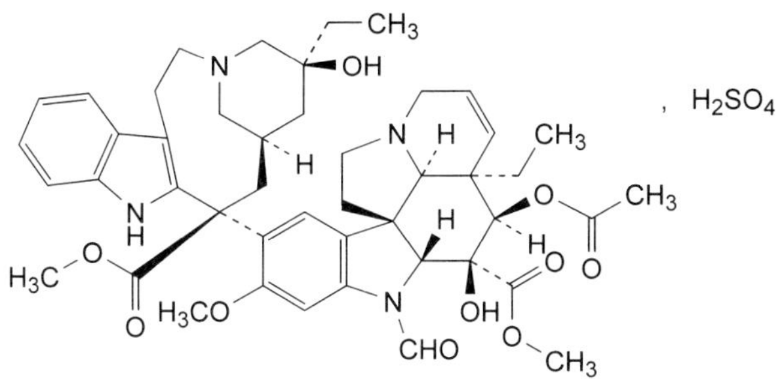

$C_{46}H_{58}N_4O_{14}S$ M_r 923

DEFINITION

Methyl (3aR,4R,5S,5aR,10bR,13aR)-4-(acetyloxy)-3a-ethyl-9-[(5S,7R,9S)-5-ethyl-5-hydroxy-9-(methoxycarbonyl)-1,4,5,6,7,8,9,10-octahydro-2H-3,7-methanoazacycloundecino[5,4-b]indol-9-yl]-6-formyl-5-hydroxy-8-methoxy-3a,4,5,5a,6,11,12,13a-octahydro-1H-indolizino[8,1-cd]carbazole-5-carboxylate sulphate.

Content: 95.0 per cent to 104.0 per cent (dried substance).

CHARACTERS

Appearance: white or slightly yellowish, crystalline powder, very hygroscopic.

Solubility: freely soluble in water, slightly soluble in alcohol.

IDENTIFICATION

Infrared absorption spectrophotometry (2.2.24).

Comparison: Ph. Eur. reference spectrum of vincristine sulphate.

TESTS

Solution S. Dissolve 50.0 mg in carbon dioxide-free water R and dilute to 10.0 ml with the same solvent. Keep the solution in iced water to carry out the test for related substances.

Appearance of solution. Solution S is clear (2.2.1) and not more intensely coloured than reference solution Y_7 (2.2.2, Method I).

pH (2.2.3): 3.5 to 4.5.

Dilute 2 ml of solution S to 10 ml with carbon dioxide-free water R.

Related substances. Liquid chromatography (2.2.29). Keep the solutions in iced water before use.

Test solution. Dilute 1.0 ml of solution S to 5.0 ml with water R.

Reference solution (a). Dissolve the contents of a vial of vincristine sulphate CRS in water R and dilute to 5.0 ml with the same solvent.

Reference solution (b). Dissolve 1.0 mg of vinblastine sulphate CRS in 1.0 ml of reference solution (a).

Reference solution (c). Dilute 1.0 ml of the test solution to 50.0 ml with water R.

Reference solution (d). Dilute 1.0 ml of reference solution (c) to 20.0 ml with water R.

Precolumn:

— stationary phase: octylsilyl silica gel for chromatography R.

Column:

— size: l = 0.25 m, Ø = 4.6 mm,

— stationary phase: octylsilyl silica gel for chromatography R (5 μm).

Mobile phase:

— mobile phase A: 1.5 per cent V/V solution of diethylamine R adjusted to pH 7.5 with phosphoric acid R,

— mobile phase B: methanol R,

Time (min)	Mobile phase A (per cent V/V)	Mobile phase B (per cent V/V)
0 - 12	38	62
12 - 27	38 → 8	62 → 92
27 - 29	8 → 38	92 → 62
29 - 34	38	62

Flow rate: 2 ml/min.

Detection: spectrophotometer at 297 nm.

Injection: 20 μl.

System suitability: reference solution (b):

— resolution: minimum 4 between the peaks due to vincristine and vinblastine.

Limits:

— any impurity: not more than the area of the principal peak in the chromatogram obtained with reference solution (c) (2.0 per cent),

— total: not more than 2.5 times the area of the principal peak in the chromatogram obtained with reference solution (c) (5.0 per cent),

— disregard limit: area of the peak in the chromatogram obtained with reference solution (d) (0.1 per cent).

The following chromatogram is published for information.

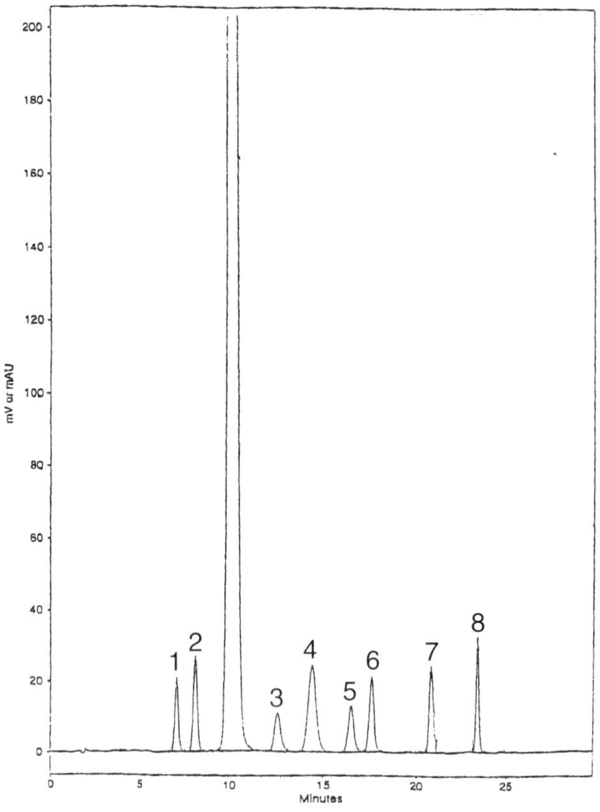

1. impurity A   5. impurity H
2. impurity D   6. impurity G
3. impurity E   7. impurity F
4. impurity C   8. impurity B

Figure 0749.-1. – *Chromatogram of vincristine sulphate spiked with the impurities*

Loss on drying: maximum 12.0 per cent, determined on 3 mg by thermogravimetry (*2.2.34*). Heat the substance to be examined to 200 °C increasing the temperature by 5 °C/min, under a current of *nitrogen for chromatography R*, at a flow rate of 40 ml/min.

Sterility (*2.6.1*). If intended for use in the manufacture of parenteral dosage forms without a further appropriate sterilisation procedure, it complies with the test for sterility.

ASSAY

Liquid chromatography (*2.2.29*) as described in the test for related substances, with the following modifications.

Mobile phase: mix 30 volumes of a 1.5 per cent *V/V* solution of *diethylamine R* adjusted to pH 7.5 with *phosphoric acid R* and 70 volumes of *methanol R*.

Flow rate: 1.0 ml/min.

Calculate the percentage content of $C_{46}H_{58}N_4O_{14}S$ using the chromatogram obtained with reference solution (a) and the declared content of *vincristine sulphate CRS*.

STORAGE

In an airtight, glass container, protected from light, at a temperature not exceeding − 20 °C. If the substance is sterile, store in a sterile, airtight, tamper-proof glass container.

LABELLING

The label states, where applicable, that the substance is sterile.

IMPURITIES

Qualified impurities: A, B, C, D, H.

Other detectable impurities: E, F, G.

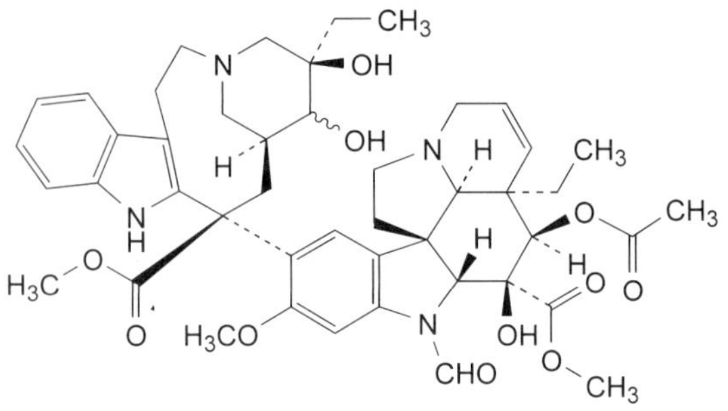

A. methyl (3aR,4R,5S,5aR,10bR,13aR)-4-(acetyloxy)-3a-ethyl-9-[(5R,7S,9S)-5-ethyl-5,6-dihydroxy-9-(methoxycarbonyl)-1,4,5,6,7,8,9,10-octahydro-2H-3,7-methanoazacycloundecino[5,4-b]indol-9-yl]-6-formyl-5-hydroxy-8-methoxy-3a,4,5,5a,6,11,12,13a-octahydro-1H-indolizino[8,1-*cd*]carbazole-5-carboxylate (3'-hydroxy-VCR),

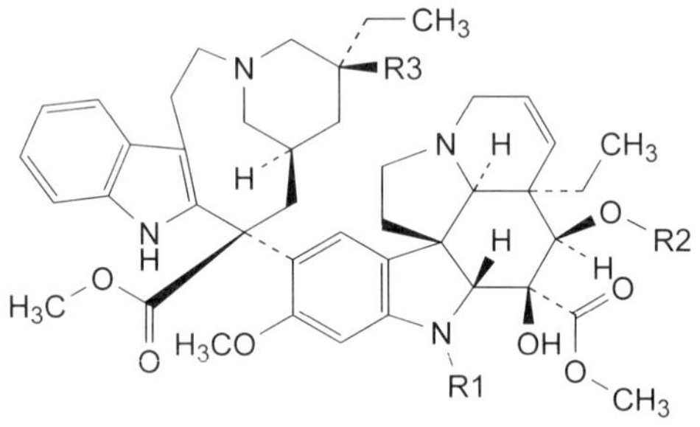

B. R1 = CHO, R2 = CO-CH$_3$, R3 = H: methyl (3aR,4R,5S,5aR,10bR,13aR)-4-(acetyloxy)-3a-ethyl-9-[(5R,7S,9S)-5-ethyl-9-(methoxycarbonyl)-1,4,5,6,7,8,9,10-octahydro-2H-3,7-methanoazacycloundecino[5,4-b]indol-9-yl]-6-formyl-5-hydroxy-8-methoxy-3a,4,5,5a,6,11,12,13a-octahydro-1H-indolizino[8,1-*cd*]carbazole-5-carboxylate (4'-deoxyvincristine),

C. R1 = H, R2 = CO-CH$_3$, R3 = OH: methyl (3aR,4R,5S,5aR,10bS,13aR)-4-(acetyloxy)-3a-ethyl-9-[(5S,7R,9S)-5-ethyl-5-hydroxy-9-(methoxycarbonyl)-1,4,5,6,7,8,9,10-octahydro-2H-3,7-methanoazacycloundecino[5,4-b]indol-9-yl]-5-hydroxy-8-methoxy-3a,4,5,5a,6,11,12,13a-octahydro-1H-indolizino[8,1-*cd*]carbazole-5-carboxylate (*N*-desmethylvinblastine),

D. R1 = CHO, R2 = H, R3 = OH: methyl (3aR,4R,5S,5aR,10bR,13aR)-3a-ethyl-9-[(5S,7R,9S)-5-ethyl-5-hydroxy-9-(methoxycarbonyl)-1,4,5,6,7,8,9,10-octahydro-2H-3,7-methanoazacycloundecino[5,4-b]indol-9-yl]-6-formyl-4,5-dihydroxy-8-methoxy-3a,4,5,5a,6,11,12,13a-octahydro-1H-indolizino[8,1-*cd*]carbazole-5-carboxylate (deacetylvincristine),

E. R1 = CH$_3$, R2 = H, R3 = OH: methyl (3aR,4R,5S,5aR,10bR,13aR)-3a-ethyl-9-[(5S,7R,9S)-5-ethyl-5-hydroxy-9-(methoxycarbonyl)-1,4,5,6,7,8,9,10-octahydro-2H-3,7-methanoazacycloundecino[5,4-b]indol-9-yl]-4,5-dihydroxy-8-methoxy-6-methyl-3a,4,5,5a,6,11,12,13a-octahydro-1H-indolizino[8,1-*cd*]carbazole-5-carboxylate (deacetylvinblastine),

H. R1 = CH$_3$, R2 = CO-CH$_3$, R3 = OH: vinblastine,

F. R = CH₃: methyl (3a*R*,4*R*,5*S*,5a*R*,10b*R*,13a*R*)-4-
(acetyloxy)-3a-ethyl-9-[(1a*S*,11*S*,13*S*,13a*R*)-1a-ethyl-11-
(methoxycarbonyl)-1a,4,5,10,11,12,13,13a-octahydro-2*H*-
3,13-methano-oxireno[9,10]azacycloundecino[5,4-*b*]indol-
11-yl]-5-hydroxy-8-methoxy-6-methyl-3a,4,5,5a,6,11,12,13a-
octahydro-1*H*-indolizino[8,1-*cd*]carbazole-5-carboxylate
(leurosine),

G. R = CHO: methyl (3a*R*,4*R*,5*S*,5a*R*,10b*R*,13a*R*)-4-
(acetyloxy)-3a-ethyl-9-[(1a*S*,11*S*,13*S*,13a*R*)-1a-ethyl-11-
(methoxycarbonyl)-1a,4,5,10,11,12,13,13a-octahydro-2*H*-
3,13-methano-oxireno[9,10]azacycloundecino[5,4-*b*]indol-
11-yl]-6-formyl-5-hydroxy-8-methoxy-3a,4,5,5a,6,11,12,13a-
octahydro-1*H*-indolizino[8,1-*cd*]carbazole-5-carboxylate
(formylleurosine).

W

04/2003:0698

WARFARIN SODIUM

Warfarinum natricum

and enantiomer

$C_{19}H_{15}NaO_4$ M_r 330.3

DEFINITION

Warfarin sodium contains not less than 98.0 per cent and not more than the equivalent of 102.0 per cent of sodium 2-oxo-3-[(1RS)-3-oxo-1-phenylbutyl]-2H-1-benzopyran-4-olate, calculated with reference to the anhydrous substance.

CHARACTERS

A white powder, hygroscopic, very soluble in water and in alcohol, soluble in acetone, very slightly soluble in methylene chloride.

IDENTIFICATION

First identification: B, D, E.

Second identification: A, C, D, E.

A. Dissolve 1 g in 25 ml of *water R*, add 2 ml of *dilute hydrochloric acid R* and filter. Reserve the filtrate for identification test E. The precipitate, washed with *water R* and dried at 100 °C to 105 °C, melts (*2.2.14*) at 159 °C to 163 °C.

B. Dissolve 1 g in 25 ml of *water R*, add 2 ml of *dilute hydrochloric acid R* and filter. Reserve the filtrate for identification test E. Examine the precipitate by infrared absorption spectrophotometry (*2.2.24*) comparing with the spectrum obtained with the precipitate prepared in the same manner from *warfarin sodium CRS*.

C. Examine the chromatograms obtained in the test for related substances. The principal spot in the chromatogram obtained with test solution (b) is similar in position and size to the principal spot in the chromatogram obtained with reference solution (b).

D. Dissolve 1 g in 10 ml of *water R*, add 5 ml of *nitric acid R* and filter. To the filtrate add 2 ml of *potassium dichromate solution R1* and shake for 5 min. Allow to stand for 20 min. The solution is not greenish-blue when compared with a blank.

E. The filtrate obtained in identification test A or B gives reaction (b) of sodium (*2.3.1*).

TESTS

Appearance of solution. Dissolve 1.0 g in *water R* and dilute to 20 ml with the same solvent. The solution is clear (*2.2.1*) and colourless (*2.2.2, Method II*).

pH (*2.2.3*). Dissolve 1.0 g in *carbon dioxide-free water R* and dilute to 100 ml with the same solvent. The pH of the solution is 7.6 to 8.6.

Related substances. Examine by thin-layer chromatography (*2.2.27*), using *silica gel GF₂₅₄ R* as the coating substance.

Test solution (a). Dissolve 0.20 g of the substance to be examined in *acetone R* and dilute to 10 ml with the same solvent.

Test solution (b). Dilute 2 ml of test solution (a) to 10 ml with *acetone R*.

Reference solution (a). Dilute 1 ml of test solution (b) to 200 ml with *acetone R*.

Reference solution (b). Dissolve 40 mg of *warfarin sodium CRS* in *acetone R* and dilute to 10 ml with the same solvent.

Reference solution (c). Dissolve 10 mg of *acenocoumarol CRS* in *acetone R*, add 1 ml of test solution (a) and dilute to 10 ml with *acetone R*.

Apply separately to the plate 20 μl of each solution. Develop over a path of 15 cm using a mixture of 20 volumes of *glacial acetic acid R*, 50 volumes of *methylene chloride R* and 50 volumes of *cyclohexane R*. Allow the plate to dry in air and examine in ultraviolet light at 254 nm. Any spot in the chromatogram obtained with test solution (a), apart from the principal spot, is not more intense than the spot in the chromatogram obtained with reference solution (a) (0.1 per cent). The test is not valid unless the chromatogram obtained with reference solution (c) shows two clearly separated spots and the chromatogram obtained with reference solution (a) shows a clearly visible spot.

Phenolic ketones. Dissolve 1.25 g in a 20 g/l solution of *sodium hydroxide R* and dilute to 10.0 ml with the same solvent. The absorbance (*2.2.25*), measured at 385 nm within 15 min of preparing the solution, is not greater than 0.20.

Water (*2.5.12*). Not more than 4.0 per cent, determined on 0.750 g by the semi-micro determination of water.

ASSAY

Dissolve 0.1000 g in *0.01 M sodium hydroxide* and dilute to 100.0 ml with the same solvent. Dilute 10.0 ml of this solution to 100.0 ml with *0.01 M sodium hydroxide*. Dilute 10.0 ml of the latter solution to 100.0 ml with *0.01 M sodium hydroxide*. Measure the absorbance (*2.2.25*) at the maximum at 308 nm.

Calculate the content of $C_{19}H_{15}NaO_4$ taking the specific absorbance to be 431.

STORAGE

Store in an airtight container, protected from light.

04/2003:0699

WARFARIN SODIUM CLATHRATE

Warfarinum natricum clathratum

and enantiomer

DEFINITION

Warfarin sodium clathrate contains not less than 98.0 per cent and not more than the equivalent of 102.0 per cent of sodium 2-oxo-3-[(1RS)-3-oxo-1-phenylbutyl]-2H-1-benzopyran-4-olate, calculated with reference to the anhydrous, propan-2-ol-free substance. Warfarin sodium clathrate contains approximately 92 per cent of warfarin sodium. It consists of warfarin sodium and propan-2-ol (molecular proportions 2:1) in the form of a clathrate. It contains not less than 8.0 per cent and not more than 8.5 per cent of propan-2-ol.

Monographs Q - Z

CHARACTERS

A white powder, very soluble in water, freely soluble in alcohol, soluble in acetone, very slightly soluble in methylene chloride.

IDENTIFICATION

First identification: B, D, E.

Second identification: A, C, D, E.

A. Dissolve 1 g in 25 ml of *water R*, add 2 ml of *dilute hydrochloric acid R* and filter. Reserve the filtrate for identification test E. The precipitate, washed with *water R* and dried at 100 °C to 105 °C, melts (*2.2.14*) at 159 °C to 163 °C.

B. Dissolve 1 g in 25 ml of *water R*, add 2 ml of *dilute hydrochloric acid R* and filter. Reserve the filtrate for identification test E. Examine the precipitate by infrared absorption spectrophotometry (*2.2.24*) comparing with the spectrum obtained with the precipitate prepared in the same manner from *warfarin sodium CRS*.

C. Examine the chromatograms obtained in the test for related substances. The principal spot in the chromatogram obtained with test solution (b) is similar in position and size to the principal spot in the chromatogram obtained with reference solution (b).

D. Dissolve 1 g in 10 ml of *water R*, add 5 ml of *nitric acid R* and filter. To the filtrate add 2 ml of *potassium dichromate solution R1* and shake for 5 min. Allow to stand for 20 min. The solution is greenish-blue when compared with a blank.

E. The filtrate obtained in identification test A or B gives reaction (b) of sodium (*2.3.1*).

TESTS

Appearance of solution. Dissolve 1.0 g in *water R* and dilute to 20 ml with the same solvent. The solution is clear (*2.2.1*) and colourless (*2.2.2, Method II*).

pH (*2.2.3*). Dissolve 1.0 g in *carbon dioxide-free water R* and dilute to 100 ml with the same solvent. The pH of the solution is 7.6 to 8.6.

Related substances. Examine by thin-layer chromatography (*2.2.27*), using *silica gel GF$_{254}$ R* as the coating substance.

Test solution (a). Dissolve 0.20 g of the substance to be examined in *acetone R* and dilute to 10 ml with the same solvent.

Test solution (b). Dilute 2 ml of test solution (a) to 10 ml with *acetone R*.

Reference solution (a). Dilute 1 ml of test solution (b) to 200 ml with *acetone R*.

Reference solution (b). Dissolve 40 mg of *warfarin sodium CRS* in *acetone R* and dilute to 10 ml with the same solvent.

Reference solution (c). Dissolve 10 mg of *acenocoumarol CRS* in *acetone R*, add 1 ml of test solution (a) and dilute to 10 ml with *acetone R*.

Apply separately to the plate 20 μl of each solution. Develop over a path of 15 cm using a mixture of 20 volumes of *glacial acetic acid R*, 50 volumes of *methylene chloride R* and 50 volumes of *cyclohexane R*. Allow the plate to dry in air and examine in ultraviolet light at 254 nm. Any spot in the chromatogram obtained with test solution (a), apart from the principal spot, is not more intense than the spot in the chromatogram obtained with reference solution (a) (0.1 per cent). The test is not valid unless the chromatogram obtained

with reference solution (c) shows two clearly separated spots and the chromatogram obtained with reference solution (a) shows a clearly visible spot.

Phenolic ketones. Dissolve 1.25 g in a 20 g/l solution of *sodium hydroxide R* and dilute to 10.0 ml with the same solvent. The absorbance (*2.2.25*), measured at 385 nm within 15 min of preparing the solution, is not greater than 0.20.

Propan-2-ol: 8.0 per cent *m/m* to 8.5 per cent *m/m*, determined by gas chromatography (*2.2.28*) using *propanol R* as internal standard.

Internal standard solution. Dilute 1.0 ml of *propanol R* to 200.0 ml with *water R*.

Test solution (a). Dissolve 0.250 g of the substance to be examined in *water R* and dilute to 5.0 ml with the same solvent.

Test solution (b). Dissolve 0.50 g of the substance to be examined in the internal standard solution and dilute to 10.0 ml with the internal standard solution.

Reference solution. Dilute 0.50 ml of *propan-2-ol R* to 100.0 ml with the internal standard solution.

The chromatographic procedure may be carried out using:

— a column 1.5 m long and 4 mm in internal diameter packed with *ethylvinylbenzene-divinylbenzene copolymer R* (125 μm to 150 μm),

— *nitrogen for chromatography R* as the carrier gas at a flow rate of 40 ml/min,

— a flame-ionisation detector,

maintaining the temperature of the column at 150 °C, that of the injection port at 180 °C and that of the detector at 200 °C. Inject the selected volumes of the test solutions and the reference solution. Calculate the content of propan-2-ol taking its density at 20 °C to be 0.785 g/ml.

Water (*2.5.12*). Not more than 0.1 per cent, determined on 2.500 g by the semi-micro determination of water.

ASSAY

Dissolve 0.1000 g in *0.01 M sodium hydroxide* and dilute to 100.0 ml with the same solvent. Dilute 10.0 ml of this solution to 100.0 ml with *0.01 M sodium hydroxide*. Dilute 10.0 ml of the latter solution to 100.0 ml with *0.01 M sodium hydroxide*. Measure the absorbance (*2.2.25*) at the maximum at 308 nm.

Calculate the content of $C_{19}H_{15}NaO_4$ taking the specific absorbance to be 431.

STORAGE

Store in an airtight container, protected from light.

07/2002:0169
corrected

WATER FOR INJECTIONS

Aqua ad iniectabilia

H_2O M_r 18.02

DEFINITION

Water for injections is water for the preparation of medicines for parenteral administration when water is used as vehicle (water for injections in bulk) and for dissolving or diluting substances or preparations for parenteral administration (sterilised water for injections).

Water for injections in bulk

PRODUCTION

Water for injections in bulk is obtained from water that complies with the regulations on water intended for human consumption laid down by the competent authority or from purified water by distillation in an apparatus of which the parts in contact with the water are of neutral glass, quartz or suitable metal and which is fitted with an effective device to prevent the entrainment of droplets. The correct maintenance of the apparatus is essential. The first portion of the distillate obtained when the apparatus begins to function is discarded and the distillate is collected.

During production and subsequent storage, appropriate measures are taken to ensure that the total viable aerobic count is adequately controlled and monitored. Appropriate alert and action limits are set so as to detect adverse trends. Under normal conditions, an appropriate action limit is a total viable aerobic count (2.6.12) of 10 micro-organisms per 100 ml when determined by membrane filtration, using agar medium S using at least 200 ml of water for injections in bulk and incubating at 30-35 °C for 5 days. For aseptic processing, stricter alert limits may need to be applied. Conductivity (2.2.38) (maximum 1.1 μS·cm^{-1} at 20 °C) and total organic carbon (2.2.44) (maximum 0.5 mg/l) are also controlled.

In order to ensure the appropriate quality of the water, validated procedures and in-process-monitoring of the electrical conductivity and regular microbial monitoring are applied.

Water for injections in bulk is stored and distributed in conditions designed to prevent growth of micro-organisms and to avoid any other contamination.

CHARACTERS

Clear, colourless, odourless and tasteless liquid.

TESTS

It complies with the tests prescribed in the section on Purified water in bulk of the monograph on *Purified Water (0008)* and with the addition of the following test.

Bacterial endotoxins (2.6.14): less than 0.25 IU/ml.

Sterilised water for injections

Sterilised water for injections is water for injections in bulk that has been distributed into suitable containers, closed and sterilised by heat in conditions which ensure that the product still complies with the test for bacterial endotoxins. Sterilised water for injections is free from any added substances.

Examined in suitable conditions of visibility, it is clear and colourless.

Each container contains a sufficient quantity of water for injections to permit the nominal volume to be withdrawn.

TESTS

It complies with the tests prescribed in the section on Purified water in containers of the monograph on *Purified Water (0008)* with modification of the tests for acidity or alkalinity, for oxidisable substances, for chlorides (if the nominal volume of the container is 100 ml or less) and for residue on evaporation. It also complies with the tests for particulate contamination, sterility and bacterial endotoxins.

Acidity or alkalinity. To 20 ml add 0.05 ml of *phenol red solution R*. If the solution is yellow, it becomes red on the addition of 0.1 ml of *0.01 M sodium hydroxide*; if red, it becomes yellow on the addition of 0.15 ml of *0.01 M hydrochloric acid*.

Conductivity (2.2.38): maximum 25 μS·cm^{-1} for containers with a nominal volume of 10 ml or less; maximum 5 μS·cm^{-1} for containers with a nominal volume greater than 10 ml.

Oxidisable substances. Boil 100 ml with 10 ml of *dilute sulphuric acid R*. Add 0.2 ml of *0.02 M potassium permanganate* and boil for 5 min. The solution remains faintly pink.

Chlorides (2.4.4): maximum 0.5 ppm for containers with a nominal volume of 100 ml or less.

15 ml complies with the limit test for chlorides. Prepare the standard using a mixture of 1.5 ml of *chloride standard solution (5 ppm Cl) R* and 13.5 ml of *water R*. Examine the solutions down the vertical axes of the tubes.

Residue on evaporation: maximum 4 mg (0.004 per cent) for containers with a nominal volume of 10 ml or less; maximum 3 mg (0.003 per cent) for containers with a nominal volume greater than 10 ml.

Evaporate 100 ml to dryness on a water-bath and dry in an oven at 100-105 °C.

Particulate contamination: sub-visible particles (2.9.19). It complies with the test.

Sterility (2.6.1). It complies with the test for sterility.

Bacterial endotoxins (2.6.14): less than 0.25 IU/ml.

04/2003:1379

WHEAT-GERM OIL, REFINED

Tritici aestivi oleum raffinatum

DEFINITION

Fatty oil obtained from the germ of the grain of *Triticum aestivum* L. by cold expression or by other suitable mechanical means and/or by extraction. It is then refined. A suitable antioxidant may be added.

CHARACTERS

Appearance: clear, light yellow liquid.

Solubility: practically insoluble in water and in alcohol, miscible with light petroleum (40 °C to 60 °C).

Relative density: about 0.925.

Refractive index: about 1.475.

IDENTIFICATION

A. Identification of fatty oils by thin-layer chromatography (2.3.2). The chromatogram obtained is similar to the type chromatogram for wheat-germ oil.

B. It complies with the test for composition of fatty acids (see Tests).

TESTS

Acid value (2.5.1): maximum 0.9. If intended for use in the manufacture of parenteral dosage forms: maximum 0.3.

Peroxide value (2.5.5): maximum 10.0. If intended for use in the manufacture of parenteral dosage forms: maximum 5.0.

Unsaponifiable matter (2.5.7): maximum 5.0 per cent, determined on 5.0 g.

Alkaline impurities (2.4.19). It complies with the test for alkaline impurities in fatty oils.

Composition of fatty acids. Gas chromatography (2.4.22, Method C). Use the mixture of calibrating substances in Table 2.4.22.-3.

Composition of the fatty-acid fraction of the oil:

– *palmitic acid*: 14.0 per cent to 19.0 per cent,

– *stearic acid*: maximum 2.0 per cent,

– *oleic acid*: 12.0 per cent to 23.0 per cent,

– *linoleic acid*: 52.0 per cent to 59.0 per cent,

– *linolenic acid*: 3.0 per cent to 10.0 per cent,

– *eicosenoic acid*: maximum 2.0 per cent.

Brassicasterol (*2.4.23*): maximum 0.3 per cent of brassicasterol in the sterol fraction of the oil.

Water (*2.5.32*). If intended for use in the manufacture of parenteral dosage forms: maximum 0.1 per cent, determined on 5.00 g. Use a mixture of equal volumes of *methanol R* and *methylene chloride R* as solvent.

STORAGE

In an airtight, well-filled container, protected from light.

LABELLING

The label states:

– the name and concentration of any added antioxidant,

– where applicable, that the substance is suitable for use in the manufacture of parenteral dosage forms,

– whether the oil is obtained by mechanical means, by extraction or by a combination of the two.

VACCINES FOR VETERINARY USE

Vaccines

04/2003:0963

PORCINE INFLUENZA VACCINE (INACTIVATED)

Vaccinum influenzae inactivatum ad suem

DEFINITION

Porcine influenza vaccine (inactivated) is an aqueous suspension, an oily emulsion or a freeze-dried preparation of one or more inactivated strains of swine or human influenza virus. Suitable strains contain both haemagglutinin and neuraminidase.

PRODUCTION

The virus is propagated in the allantoic cavity of fertilised hen eggs from a healthy flock or in suitable cell cultures (5.2.4). Each virus strain is cultivated separately. After cultivation, the viral suspensions are collected separately and inactivated by a method that avoids destruction of the immunogenicity. If necessary, they may be purified.

An amplification test for residual infectious influenza virus is carried out on each batch of antigen immediately after inactivation by passage in the same type of substrate as that used for production (eggs or cell cultures) or a substrate shown to be at least as sensitive. The quantity of inactivated virus used in the test is equivalent to not less than 10 doses of the vaccine. No live virus is detected.

The vaccine may contain one or more suitable adjuvants; it may be freeze-dried.

CHOICE OF VACCINE COMPOSITION

The choice of strains is based on the antigenic types and sub-types observed in Europe. The vaccine is shown to be satisfactory with respect to safety and immunogenicity for pigs. The following tests may be used during demonstration of safety (5.2.6) and efficacy (5.2.7).

Safety

A. A test is carried out in each category of animal for which the vaccine is intended (sows, fattening pigs). The animals used do not have antibodies against swine influenza virus. 2 doses of vaccine are injected by the intended route into each of not fewer than 10 animals. After 14 days, 1 dose of vaccine is injected into each of the animals. The animals are observed for a further 14 days. During the 28 days of the test, no abnormal local or systemic reaction is produced.

B. The animals used in the test for immunogenicity are also used to evaluate safety. The rectal temperature of each vaccinated animal is measured at the time of vaccination and 24 h and 48 h later. No abnormal effect on rectal temperature is noted nor other systemic reactions (for example, anorexia). The injection site is examined for local reactions at slaughter. No abnormal local reaction occurs.

C. The animals used for field trials are also used to evaluate safety. A test is carried out in each category of animals for which the vaccine is intended (sows, fattening pigs). Not fewer than 3 groups each of not fewer than 20 animals in at least 2 locations are used with corresponding groups of not fewer than 10 controls. The rectal temperature of each animal is measured at the time of vaccination and 24 h and 48 h later. No abnormal effect on rectal temperature is noted. The injection site is examined for local reactions at slaughter. No abnormal local reaction occurs.

Immunogenicity. The test described under Potency carried out using an epidemiologically relevant challenge strain or strains is suitable to demonstrate the immunogenicity of the vaccine.

IN-PROCESS TESTS

For vaccines produced in eggs, the content of bacterial endotoxins is determined on the virus harvest to monitor production.

BATCH POTENCY TEST

The test described below under Potency is not carried out for routine testing of batches of vaccine. It is carried out, for a given vaccine, on one or more occasions, as decided by or with the agreement of the competent authority; where the test is not carried out, a suitable validated test is carried out, the criteria for acceptance being set with reference to a batch of vaccine that has given satisfactory results in the test described under Potency. The following test may be used after a satisfactory correlation with the test described under Potency has been established by a statistical evaluation.

Inject subcutaneously into each of 5 seronegative guinea-pigs, 5 to 7 weeks old, a quarter of the dose stated on the label. Collect blood samples before the vaccination and 21 days after vaccination. Determine for each sample the level of specific antibodies against each virus subtype in the vaccine by haemagglutination-inhibition or another suitable test. The vaccine complies with the test if the level of antibodies is not lower than that found for a batch of vaccine that gave satisfactory results in the potency test in pigs (see Potency).

IDENTIFICATION

When injected into healthy, susceptible animals, the vaccine stimulates the production of specific antibodies against the influenza virus subtypes included in the vaccine. The antibodies may be detected by a suitable immunochemical method (2.7.1).

TESTS

Safety. Use 2 pigs, free from antibodies against swine influenza virus and not older than the minimum age stated for vaccination. Inject into each pig a double dose of vaccine by the route stated on the label. Observe the animals for 14 days and then inject into each animal 1 dose of vaccine. Observe the animals for 14 days. No abnormal local or systemic reaction occurs during the 28 days of the test.

Inactivation. If the vaccine has been prepared in eggs, inoculate 0.2 ml into the allantoic cavity of each of 10 fertilised hen eggs, 9 to 11 days old. Incubate at a suitable temperature for 3 days. The death of any embryo within 24 h of inoculation is considered as non-specific mortality and the egg is discarded. The test is not valid unless at least 80 per cent of the eggs survive. Collect the allantoic fluid of each egg, pool equal quantities and carry out a second passage on fertilised eggs in the same manner. Incubate for 4 days; the allantoic fluid of these eggs shows no haemagglutinating activity.

If the vaccine has been prepared in cell cultures, carry out a suitable test for residual infectious influenza virus using 2 passages in the same type of cell culture as used in the production of vaccine. No live virus is detected. If the vaccine contains an oily adjuvant that interferes with this test, where possible separate the aqueous phase from the vaccine by means that do not diminish the capacity to detect residual infectious influenza virus.

Extraneous viruses. On the pigs used for the safety test, carry out tests for antibodies. The vaccine does not stimulate the formation of antibodies other than those against influenza virus. In particular, no antibodies against viruses pathogenic for pigs or against viruses which could interfere with the diagnosis of infectious diseases of pigs (including viruses of the pestivirus group) are detected.

Sterility. The vaccine complies with the test for sterility prescribed in the monograph on *Vaccines for veterinary use (0062)*.

POTENCY

Carry out a potency test for each subtype used in the preparation of the vaccine. Use not fewer than 20 pigs of the minimum age recommended for vaccination and that do not have antibodies against swine influenza virus. Vaccinate not fewer than 10 pigs as recommended on the label and keep not fewer than 10 pigs as unvaccinated controls. Take a blood sample from all control pigs immediately before challenge. 3 weeks after the last administration of vaccine, challenge all the pigs with a suitable quantity of a virulent influenza field virus by the intratracheal route. Kill half of the vaccinated and control pigs 24 h after challenge and the other half 72 h after challenge. For each pig, measure the quantity of influenza virus in 2 lung tissue homogenates, one from the left apical, cardiac and diaphragmatic lobes, and the other from the corresponding right lung lobes. Take equivalent samples from each animal. The test is invalid if antibodies against influenza virus are found in any control pig immediately before challenge. The vaccine complies with the test if, at both times of measurement, the mean virus titre in the pooled lung tissue samples of vaccinated pigs is significantly lower than that for control pigs, when analysed by a suitable statistical method such as the Wilcoxon Mann-Whitney test.

Vaccines

HOMOEOPATHIC PREPARATIONS

Homoeopathic
preparations

04/2003:1038

HOMOEOPATHIC PREPARATIONS

Praeparationes homoeopathicas

DEFINITION

Homoeopathic preparations are prepared from substances, products or preparations called stocks, in accordance with a homoeopathic manufacturing procedure. A homoeopathic preparation is usually designated by the Latin name of the stock, followed by an indication of the degree of dilution.

Raw materials

Raw materials for the production of homoeopathic preparations may be of natural or synthetic origin.

For raw materials of zoological or human origin, adequate measures are taken to minimise the risk of agents of infection in the homoeopathic preparations. For this purpose, it is demonstrated that:

— the method of production includes a step or steps that have been shown to remove or inactivate agents of infection,

— where applicable, raw materials of zoological origin comply with the monograph on *Products with risk of transmitting agents of animal spongiform encephalopathies (1483)*,

— where applicable, the animals and the tissues used to obtain the raw materials comply with the health requirements of the competent authorities for animals for human consumption,

— for materials of human origin, the donor follows the recommendations applicable to human blood donors and to donated blood (see *Human plasma for fractionation (0853)*), unless otherwise justified and authorised.

A raw material of botanical, zoological or human origin may be used either in the fresh state or in the dried state. Where appropriate, fresh material may be kept deep-frozen. Raw materials of botanical origin comply with the requirements of the monograph on *Herbal drugs for homoeopathic preparations (2045)*.

Where justified and authorised for transportation or storage purposes, fresh plant material may be kept in ethanol (96 per cent *V/V*) or in alcohol of a suitable concentration, provided the whole material including the storage medium is used for processing.

Raw materials comply with any requirements of the relevant monographs of the European Pharmacopoeia.

Vehicles

Vehicles are excipients used for the preparation of certain stocks or for the potentisation process. They may include for example: purified water, alcohol of a suitable concentration, glycerol and lactose.

Vehicles comply with any requirements of the relevant monographs of the European Pharmacopoeia.

Stocks

Stocks are substances, products or preparations used as starting materials for the production of homoeopathic preparations. A stock is usually one of the following: a

mother tincture or a glycerol macerate, for raw materials of botanical, zoological or human origin, or the substance itself, for raw materials of chemical or mineral origin.

Mother tinctures comply with the requirements of the monograph on *Mother tinctures for homoeopathic preparations (2029)*.

Glycerol macerates are liquid preparations obtained from raw materials of botanical, zoological or human origin by using glycerol or a mixture of glycerol and either alcohol of a suitable concentration or a solution of sodium chloride of a suitable concentration.

Potentisation

Dilutions and triturations are obtained from stocks by a process of potentisation in accordance with a homoeopathic manufacturing procedure: this means successive dilutions and succussions, or successive appropriate triturations, or a combination of the 2 processes.

The potentisation steps are usually one of the following:

— 1 part of the stock plus 9 parts of the vehicle; they may be designated as "D", "DH" or "X" (decimal),

— 1 part of the stock plus 99 parts of the vehicle; they may be designated as "C" or "CH" (centesimal).

The number of potentisation steps defines the degree of dilution; for example, "D3", "3 DH" or "3X" means 3 decimal potentisation steps, and "C3", "3 CH" or "3C" means 3 centesimal potentisation steps.

"LM-" (or "Q-") potencies are manufactured according to a specific procedure.

Dosage forms

A dosage form of a homoeopathic preparation complies with any relevant dosage form monograph in the European Pharmacopoeia and with the following:

— for the purpose of dosage forms for homoeopathic use "active substances" are considered to be "dilutions or triturations of homoeopathic stocks",

— these dosage forms are prepared using appropriate excipients,

— the test for uniformity of content is normally not appropriate. However, in certain circumstances, it is required.

Homoeopathic dosage form "pillule"

Pillules for homoeopathic use are solid preparations obtained from sucrose, lactose or other suitable excipients. They may be prepared by impregnation of preformed pillules with a dilution or dilutions of homoeopathic stocks or by progressive addition of these excipients and the addition of a dilution or dilutions of homoeopathic stocks. They are intended for oral or sublingual use.

Homoeopathic dosage form "tablet"

Tablets for homoeopathic use are solid preparations obtained from sucrose, lactose or other suitable excipients according to the monograph on *Tablets (0478)*. They may either be prepared by compressing one or more solid active substances with the excipients or by impregnating preformed tablets with a dilution or dilutions of homoeopathic stocks. The preformed tablets for impregnation are obtained from sucrose, lactose or other suitable excipients according to the monograph on *Tablets (0478)*. They are intended for oral or sublingual use.

INDEX

To aid users the index includes a reference to the supplement where the latest version of a text can be found.

For example: Alfacalcidol...**4.2**-2656

means the monograph Alfacalcidol can be found on page 2656 of Supplement 4.2.

Note that where no reference for a supplement is made, the text can be found in the principal volume.

Monographs deleted from the Fourth Edition are not included in the index; a cumulative list of deleted texts is found in the Contents of this supplement, page xxviii.

Index

Index

Index

General Notices (1) apply to all monographs and other texts

See the information section on general monographs (cover pages)

Index

Index

Index

Notes

Notes